A Manual of

LABORATORY & DIAGNOSTIC TESTS

A Manual of LABORATORY & DIAGNOSTIC TESTS

Fifth Edition

FRANCES TALASKA FISCHBACH, *RN, BSN, MSN*
Associate Clinical Professor of Nursing
Department of Health Restoration
School of Nursing
University of Wisconsin–Milwaukee
Milwaukee, Wisconsin
Associate Professor of Nursing, Retired
School of Nursing
University of Wisconsin–Milwaukee
Milwaukee, Wisconsin

Lippincott
Philadelphia • New York

Sponsoring Editor: Lisa Stead
Coordinating Editorial Assistant: Sarah Andrus
Project Editor: Susan Deitch
Production Manager: Helen Ewan
Production Coordinator: Nannette Winski
Design Coordinator: Melissa Olson
Indexer: Betty Herr Hallinger

Fifth Edition

Library of Congress Cataloging in Publication Data
Fischbach, Frances Talaska.
A manual of laboratory & diagnostic tests / Frances Talaska Fischbach, — 5th ed.
p. cm.
Includes bibliographical references and index.
ISBN 0–397–55186–X
1. Diagnosis, Laboratory—Handbooks, manuals, etc. I. Title.
[DNLM: 1. Diagnosis, Laboratory. QY 25 F528m 1996]
RB38.2.F57 1996
616.07'5--dc20
DNLM/DLC
for Library of Congress *95-9601*
CIP

The material contained in this volume was submitted as previously unpublished material, except in the instances in which credit has been given to the source from which some of the illustrative material was derived.

Any procedure or practice described in this book should be applied by the health-care practitioner under appropriate supervision in accordance with professional standards of care used with regard to the unique circumstances that apply in each practice situation. Care has been taken to confirm the accuracy of information presented and to describe generally accepted practices. However, the author, editors, and publisher cannot accept any responsibility for errors or omissions or for any consequences from application of the information in this book and make no warranty, express or implied, with respect to the contents of the book.

The author and publisher have exerted every effort to ensure that drug selection and dosage set forth in this text are in accordance with current recommendations and practice at the time of publication. However, in view of ongoing research, changes in government regulations, and the constant flow of information relating to drug therapy and drug reactions, the reader is urged to check the package insert for each drug for any change in indications and dosage and for added warnings and precautions. This is particularly important when the recommended agent is a new or infrequently employed drug.

9 8 7 6 5 4 3

To Michael, Mary, Paul, and Margaret

● CONTRIBUTORS

Dave Arnold, BS, MS
Department of Pulmonary Medicine
St. Luke's Medical Center
Milwaukee, Wisconsin

Barbara Barron, MT (ASCP)
Supervisor of Diagnostic Immunology, Department of Pathology
Clement Zablocki VA Medical Center
Milwaukee, Wisconsin

Carol Colasacco, CT (ASCP), CMIAC
Cytotechnologist, Department of Pathology
Howard Young Medical Center
Woodruff, Wisconsin

Bernice Gestout DeBoer, RN, BSN, CPAN
Communication Specialist, Postanesthesia Recovery Nurse
St. Joseph's Hospital
Milwaukee, Wisconsin

Marshall B. Dunning, BS, MS, PhD
Associate Professor of Physiology, Department of Critical Care Pulmonary Medicine
Medical College of Wisconsin
Milwaukee, Wisconsin

Emma Felder, RN, BSN, MSN, PhD
Professor of Nursing, Department of Foundations
University of Wisconsin–Milwaukee
Milwaukee, Wisconsin

Michael Kenneth Kaplon, MD
Chief of Hematology, Oncology
Clement Zablocki VA Medical Center
Milwaukee, Wisconsin
Assistant Professor
Medical College of Wisconsin
Milwaukee, Wisconsin

Donna Soik Karweik, *MT (ASCP)*
Microbiologist, Department of Pathology
Clement Zablocki VA Medical Center
Milwaukee, Wisconsin

Mark S. Lubinsky, *MD*
Associate Professor, Department of Pediatrics
Medical College of Wisconsin
Director, Genetic Services
Children's Hospital of Wisconsin
Milwaukee, Wisconsin

Anne Witkowiak Nezworski, *RN, BSN*
Maternity and Newborn Specialist
Sacred Heart Hospital
Eau Claire, Wisconsin

Joseph Nezworski, *BS, RN, BSN*
Chief Deputy Medical Examiner
Eau Claire County
Eau Claire, Wisconsin

Richard Nuccio, *MAT, MBA, CNMT, (ASCP)*
Nuclear Clinical Educator
G.E. Medical Systems
Milwaukee, Wisconsin

Mary Ellen Paisley, *MT (ASCP)*
Blood Banking and Pre-transfusion Testing
Department of Pathology
Milwaukee County Medical Complex
Milwaukee, Wisconsin

Patricia Pomahac, *MT (ASCP)*
Supervisor, Diagnostic Immunology
Department of Pathology
United Regional Medical Services, Inc.
Milwaukee, Wisconsin

Mary Pat Haas Schmidt, *BS, MT*
Manager, Laboratory Services
Elm Grove Medical Associates
Instructor, Medical Technology
Milwaukee, Wisconsin

Jerry A. Schneider, *MD*
Professor of Pediatrics
Bernard L. Maas Chair in Inherited Metabolic Diseases
University of California–San Diego
La Jolla, California

Jean M. Schultz, *BS, RT, RDMS*
Director, Ultrasound Education
St. Luke's Medical Center
Milwaukee, Wisconsin

Eleanor C. Simms, *RN, BSN*
Community Health Nurse, Field Office
City of Baltimore Health Department
Baltimore, Maryland

Rosalie Wilson Steiner, *RN, BSN, MSN, PhD*
Community Health Specialist
Milwaukee, Wisconsin

Corrinne Strandell, *RN, BSN, MSN, PhD*
Research and Education Consultant
West Allis, Wisconsin

Keith Templin, *BS, DDS*
Assistant Professor of Dentistry
Marquette University
Milwaukee, Wisconsin

Teri Thode, *BS, EdM, RD, CHE*
Associate Professor of Dietetics, Program Coordinator
Mount Mary College
Milwaukee, Wisconsin

Beverly B. Wheeler, *RN, MSN, CS*
Cardiology/Cardiothoracic Nurse
Specialist
National Naval Medical Center
Bethesda, Maryland

● PREFACE

The fifth edition of *A Manual of Laboratory & Diagnostic Tests* has been completely revised and updated to reflect many new and important developments in the dynamic world of laboratory and diagnostic testing.

Technological Development and Changes in Population Needs

Within the past two decades, **technological development** has introduced total body and brain scanners, PET scanners, improved ultrasound and nuclear medicine procedures, genetic studies, tests for cancer, and a resurgence in testing after death. In addition, the government has drafted guidelines on mandatory drug testing, increasing the number of urine tests being conducted. The Agency for Health Care Policy and Research developed guidelines to help consumers regain control over healthcare, which have resulted in a greater emphasis on diagnostic and therapeutic management strategies for various diseases and illnesses.

Beyond these technological and governmental changes are **changes in population needs.** The "baby boom" generation is entering middle age; society is becoming more attuned to ethnic, cultural, and socioeconomic diversity; and the incidence of cancer, AIDS, and virulent infectious diseases is increasing. These trends, combined with a shift of diagnostic care from acute care hospital settings to outpatient community-based centers, challenge caregivers to provide standards-based, safe, effective, and informed care.

Consequently, a fifth edition of *A Manual of Laboratory & Diagnostic Tests* comes at a time when a comprehensive, up-to-date diagnostic reference manual that includes newer technologies, as well as time-honored classic tests, is demanded by healthcare professionals and students in the healthcare field.

Purpose

The purpose of the fifth edition of *A Manual of Laboratory & Diagnostic Tests* is to promote the delivery of safe, effective, and informed care for patients undergoing diagnostic tests and procedures. This is accomplished by providing necessary and required information for quality care planning, individualized patient assessment, analysis of patient needs, appropriate interventions, patient education, and timely evaluation of patient outcomes.

Potential risks and complications mandate that proper test protocols, factors that interfere with test results, need for possible follow-up testing, and necessity for collaboration among those involved in the testing process be a significant part of the information in this text.

New Elements

- Addition of more than **twenty** new tests, including soluble amylase beta protein precursor (sBPP) test for Alzheimer's disease, anti-cardiolipin antibody test for cardiac disease, maternal serum alphafetoprotein (MSAFP) test, parvovirus B-19 antibody test for use before organ transplantation, and tests after death
- Revision of all chapters to coincide with current laboratory and diagnostic practice standards
- Updated charts, tables, and figures
- Addition of two new appendices—Latex/Rubber Allergy Precautions and Intravenous Conscious Sedation Precautions
- Addition of patient preparation and patient aftercare information to all tests
- Updated bibliographies that represent a composite of selected references from medicine, nursing, physiology, psychology, medical technology, x-ray and ultrasound technology, nuclear medicine technology, forensic medicine, and other special methodologies such as magnetic resonance scanning and endoscopy.

Organization

The book is organized into sixteen chapters and nine appendices. Chapter 1 outlines the Caregivers' Responsibilities for Diagnostic Testing and includes descriptions of safe, effective, informed, pre- and posttest care. This chapter has been expanded to include cultural sensitivity, test limitations, specific influence, direct complications, test result availability, record keeping, and communication as key to desired outcomes. The reader is referred back to Chapter 1 throughout the text. Chapters 2 through 16 consist of the following groups of tests:

Blood Studies
Urine Studies
Stool Studies
Cerebrospinal Fluid Studies
Chemistry Studies
Microbiologic Studies
Immunodiagnostic Studies
Nuclear Medicine Studies
X-Ray Studies
Cytology and Genetic Studies
Endoscopic Studies
Ultrasound Studies
Pulmonary Function and Blood Gas Studies
Special System and Organ Function Studies
Prenatal Diagnosis and Tests of Fetal Well-Being

Tests include background material and explanation, interfering factors that contribute to false test results, procedure for specimen collection or test completion as it relates to patient involvement, clinical implications of abnormal findings and disease patterns, patient preparation, patient aftercare, and clinical alerts that signal special cautions. The outline format of the text permits easy information retrieval. In addition, age-related reference values are included with the normal values throughout the text, and numerous examples of test values and clinical considerations for newborn, infant, child, adolescent, and older adult groups have been added where appropriate.

Frances Talaska Fischbach

● ACKNOWLEDGMENTS

I want to give special praise and recognition to my husband, Jack Fischbach, for his competent research assistance; to my daughter, Margaret Fischbach, for her expert computer consultation and help in preparing the manuscript; and to my right-hand woman, Kathie Gordon, for carefully preparing and typing the manuscript and for her proficient assistance in all publishing matters.

I would also like to recognize the knowledgeable contributors to this fifth edition and all persons who provided information and ideas for manuscript revision. This work would not have been complete without the help and information provided by the librarians and staff of the Todd Wehr Library of the Medical College of Wisconsin, the Murphy Library of the Milwaukee County Medical Complex, and the Marquette University Library.

Appreciation is also due to those persons who encouraged and supported me and who helped with previous editions, especially my mother, Frances Nezworski Talaska; my daughters, Mary and Margaret; my daughter-in-law, Ann Shafranski Fischbach; Gloria Shutte Boge; Marshall B. Dunning; Timothy Philipp; Theresa Philipp; Barbara Niemczycki; Randle Pollard, M.D.; Julie Erickson; Rod Doering; Dolaine Genthe; Corrine Strandell; Mary Pat Schmidt; and Bernice DeBoer.

As always, many special thanks to the editorial and production staff at J.B. Lippincott, especially Sarah Andrus, who sustained me and helped so much from start to finish; to Tim Morgan, whose timely assistance got the project off to a good start; to Lisa Stead for revision administration; to Diana Intenzo for her watchful eye and direction; and to Susan Deitch for a great production!

Frances Talaska Fischbach, RN, BSN, MSN

CONTENTS

APPENDICES

A Manual of

LABORATORY & DIAGNOSTIC TESTS

1

Caregivers' Responsibilities for Diagnostic Testing

Frances Fischbach: A MANUAL OF LABORATORY & DIAGNOSTIC TESTS, Fifth Edition.

OVERVIEW OF RESPONSIBILITIES, STANDARDS, AND REQUISITE KNOWLEDGE

Basics of Informed Care

In this era of high technology, healthcare delivery involves many different disciplines and specialities. Consequently, the caregiver must have an understanding and working knowledge of modalities other than one's own area of expertise. This includes diagnostic evaluation. Basically, laboratory and diagnostic tests are tools to gain additional information about the patient. By and of themselves, they are not therapeutic. However, when joined with a thorough history and a physical examination, these tests may confirm a diagnosis or may provide valuable information about a patient's status and response to therapy that may not be apparent from the history and physical examination alone. Generally, a tiered approach to test selections is used. This approach includes

1. Basic screening (wellness groups and case finding)
2. Establishment of specific diagnoses
3. Differential diagnoses
4. Evaluation of current theories for management of follow-up care
5. Estimation of disease severity
6. Monitoring disease progress and course; response to treatment or progress toward recovery
7. Ordering certain tests in combination as part of a group or a panel of tests
8. Ordering regularly scheduled screening tests as part of routine on-going care (eg, monthly, yearly, every-other year)
9. Ordering tests related to specific events, signs and symptoms, or other situations (eg, for evidence in sexual assault, drug screens, GI bleeding, tests after death)

(See Chart 1-1, Examples of Selecting Tests.)

As an integral part of their practice, caregivers have long supported patients and their significant others in meeting the demands and challenges incumbent in the simplest to the most complex diagnostic testing. (See Chart 1-2, Basics of Informed Care.) These responsibilities extend to all phases of the testing process—the *pretest, intratest,* and *posttest* periods. Each phase requires that its own set of guidelines and standards be followed if the testing is to provide accurate and optimal results for the patient. Development of patient care standards and standards of professional practice are a key point in a collaborative approach to patient care during diagnostic evaluation. Standards of care set minimum requirements for professional practice and care of patients and protect the public against less-than-quality care. Many standards govern and guide caregiver responsibilities during diagnostic evaluation. (See Chart 1-3, Standards for Diagnostic Evaluation.)

The settings in which healthcare takes place, cultural diversity, and the physical, emotional, social, and spiritual state of the patient combine to re-

CHART 1-1
Examples of Selecting Tests

DIAGNOSTIC TEST	INDICATION
Stool occult blood	Yearly screening after age 45
Serum potassium	Yearly in patients taking diuretic agents or potassium supplements
Liver enzyme levels	Yearly if patient is taking hepatotoxic drugs; baseline for other patients
Serum amylase	In the presence of abdominal pain
T_4 index	Suspicion of hypo- or hyperthyroidism
Reticulocyte count	Undiagnosed anemia
Hematocrit and hemoglobin	Baseline study; abnormal bleeding
PAP cervical smear	Yearly
Urine culture	Pyuria
Syphilis serum fluorescent treponemal antibody (FTA) tests	Positive VDRL
Tuberculosis skin test	Easiest test to use for screening purposes for individuals younger than 35, or with a history of negative TB skin tests
Prothrombin time (PT)	During anticoagulant treatment
Prostate-specific antigen	Screening in men 50 and older for prostate cancer
Chest x-ray	Screening; follow-up of lung infiltrates; congestive heart failure; some cancers and anatomic deformities, post-trauma
Mammogram	Screen by age 40 in women, then every 12–18 months between ages 40 and 49, annually 50 and older; follow-up of breast cancer; also routine screening for family history of carcinoma
Colon x-rays and proctosigmoidoscopy	Hemoglobin-positive stools
Computed tomography (CT) scans	Before and after treatment for certain cancers, injuries, illness states such as suspected transient ischemic attack or cerebrovascular accident (CVA)
DNA testing of hair, blood, or semen samples	To gather evidence in certain criminal cases and to track parentage

Some tests are mandated by government agencies; others are deemed part of necessary care based on individual practitioner's judgment and expertise.

CHART 1-2
Basics of Informed Care

- Support patients
- Communicate effectively
- Use collaborative approach
- Follow standards
- Evaluate outcomes
- Intervene appropriately

flect how the patient will actually respond to the diagnostic procedure. It also must be emphasized that the care of the patient includes not only the patient, but also the significant others, who have a vested interest in the patient's health state. Diagnostic testing, both simple and sophisticated, takes place in many different settings. Certain tests (eg, cholesterol screening, blood glucose) can be done in the field, so to speak, where the service is brought to the patient's environment. Other tests (eg, electrocardiograms, complete blood count, and blood chemistry panels) are done in a physician's office, clinic, or hospital laboratory. Magnetic resonance imaging (MRI) and ultrasound procedures are commonly performed in free-standing diagnostic centers. The most complex tests such as endoscopic retrograde cholangiopancreatography (ERCP), cardiac catheterization, or bronchoscopy may require hospital admittance, at least as an outpatient or for an overnight stay. As testing equipment becomes more technologically sophisticated and risks associated with testing are reduced, the environment in which diagnostic procedures take place will also shift. No doubt, healthcare coverage and reimbursement will influence these trends, as will managed care and case management; collaboration among diverse healthcare disciplines and the patient will be key to providing optimal diagnostic services.

As society becomes more culturally blended, the need to appreciate and work within the realm of cultural diversity becomes imperative. Interacting and directing patients through diagnostic testing can present formidable challenges if one is not somewhat familiar and sensitive to the patient's healthcare belief system. Something as basic as communicating in the face of language differences may make it necessary to arrange for a relative or translator to be present during the preparation or procedure, or both.

The sensitivity of the caregivers to the foregoing issues will frequently influence the patients' and their significant others' response to the actual procedure, the ability of the patient to comply with specific test requirements, and the ability to tolerate the procedure to its expected and desired outcome. To be most effective, the care providers must be able to adopt a holistic perspective and attitude that translates itself into their caregiving and communication behaviors.

CHART 1–3
Standards

SOURCE OF STANDARDS FOR DIAGNOSTIC TESTING	STANDARDS FOR DIAGNOSTIC TESTING	EXAMPLES OF APPLIED STANDARDS FOR DIAGNOSTIC TESTING
Professional practice parameters of American Nurses Association (ANA), American Medical Association (AMA), American Society of Clinical Pathologists (ASCP), American College of Radiology, Centers for Disease Control and Prevention (CDC), JCAHO health care practice requirements	Use a decision-making model as a framework for choosing the proper test, the procedure, the interpretation of test results. Use laboratory and diagnostic procedures for screening, differential diagnoses, follow-up, and case management.	Test strategies include single tests or combinations or panels of tests. Panels can be performed in parallel or in a series or both.
	Order the correct test and properly perform the test in an accredited laboratory or diagnostic facility; accurately report test results; communicate and interpret test findings; treat or monitor the disease and the course of therapy; provide diagnosis as well as prognosis.	Patients receive information and care based on a documented assessment of need for diagnostic evaluation. Patients have the right to information necessary to enable them to make choices and decisions that reflect their need or wish for diagnostic care.

(continued)

CHART 1–3 *(continued)*

SOURCE OF STANDARDS FOR DIAGNOSTIC TESTING	STANDARDS FOR DIAGNOSTIC TESTING	EXAMPLES OF APPLIED STANDARDS FOR DIAGNOSTIC TESTING
Individual agency and institution policies and procedures and quality criteria	Latex allergy protocols, methodology of specimen collection. Standards statements for monitoring patients who receive intravenous conscious sedation for invasive diagnostic procedures. Statements on quality assurance or continuous quality improvement standards. Standards of professional practice. Standards of patient care.	The healthcare professional wears protective eyewear and gloves when handling all body fluids. Vital signs monitored and recorded for specific times before and after completion of procedure. Patients monitored for respiratory problems, bleeding, infection, or neurovascular changes. Recording data on care outcomes when defined care criteria are implemented and practiced.
State and federal government communicate disease reporting regulations	Medical laboratory personnel and other healthcare providers follow regulations to control the spread of communicable diseases by reporting disease conditions, outbreaks and unusual manifestations.	The healthcare professional reports instances with laboratory or clinical evidence of certain classes of diseases (eg, sexually transmitted disease, diphtheria, Lyme disease, and symptomatic HIV infection. (See Micro chapter for list of reportable diseases.) Persons diagnosed with hepatitis A may not handle food, care for patients, young children, or elderly for specific period of time.

Preparing patients for diagnostic or therapeutic procedures and providing follow-up care have long been requisite activities of professional practice. This care continues even after the patient's death. These activities may include not only death reporting so that proper postmortem investigations are done, but also talking to grieving families about autopsies and other after-death testing (see Chap. 15). Professionals need to have expertise in meeting diverse patient needs in helping patients and their families make decisions, in developing meaningful care plans, and in helping patients to adjust or modify their daily activities to meet the test requirements. These basic responsibilities can be divided into two main phases: the *pretest* phase and the *posttest* phase of diagnostic care. Occasionally, the professional may need to assist during the actual procedure. In these instances, institutional protocols would be followed.

PRETEST PHASE: PRINCIPLES OF SAFE, EFFECTIVE, INFORMED CARE

Requisite Knowledge, Vital Information and Basic Responsibilities

Basic Knowledge

1. Know test terminology, test purpose, actual test process and procedure, and normal test values or results.
   a. The clinical value of a test is related to its *sensitivity,* its *specificity,* and the *incidence of the disease* in the population tested. Sensitivity and specificity do not change when different populations of ill and well patients are tested.

Specificity refers to percentages of positive results in persons with a given disease. (When a positive result is obtained in all patients who have the disease, the specificity of the test is 100%.)

Sensitivity refers to percentage of negative results among people who do not have the disease. (When a negative result is obtained in all people who do not have the disease, the test has a sensitivity of 100%).

Incidence of disease refers to prevalence of disease in a population or community. The predictive value of the same test can be very different when applied to persons of differing age, sex, and geographic locations.

Predicted Values of a positive and negative test define the percentage of positive or negative results that are *true* positives or negatives. Predicted values may change markedly. Generally, the higher the prevalence of a specific disease (the percentage of persons who have this disease) within the population, the greater is the predictive value of a positive test result.

2. Review current as well as previous test results. The plan of care may need to be developed or changed because of these test results.
3. Sequentially gather diagnostic information from existing healthcare records. Review the most recent laboratory data first; then work sequentially backward to evaluate trends or changes in data.

History and Assessment

4. Obtain a relevant, current health history and perform an assessment if necessary.

- **a.** Identify conditions that could affect or be affected by the actual testing process as well as by the outcomes (eg, pregnancy, diabetes, cultural diversity, language barrier, physical impairment, or altered mental state).
  - **(1)** Identify contraindications to testing, such as allergies to iodine, latex, or certain medications or contrast media. Records of previous diagnostic procedures may provide clues to possible reactions.
  - **(2)** Assess for coping styles and teaching or knowledge needs.
- **b.** Address fears and phobias (eg, claustrophobia, "panic attacks," fear of blood). Ascertain what strategies the patient uses to deal with these reactions.
- **c.** Know that a patient may choose not to disclose drug or alcohol use or human immunodeficiency virus (HIV) and hepatitis risks.

5. Document appropriate data. Address patient concerns and questions. This information adds to the database for collaborative problem-solving activities between medical, laboratory, diagnostic, and nursing disciplines.

Correct Procedures

6. Follow procedures correctly. Verify that desired tests are appropriately ordered and that required information is complete, accurate, and legible. List all the patient's drugs, as these may affect test outcomes.

- **a.** Ensure that specimens are correctly obtained, preserved, handled, labeled, and delivered to the appropriate department. For example, it is not generally acceptable to draw blood samples from an extremity site that has an intravenous line infusing below the intended puncture site.
- **b.** Use infection control precautions for patients in isolation. Verify proper protocols when in doubt.

7. Coordinate patient activities with testing schedules to avoid conflicts with meal times, medications, treatments, or other diagnostic tests.

- **a.** Maintain NPO status when necessary.
- **b.** Administer proper medications in a timely manner. Schedule tests needing contrast substances in such a manner that they do not invalidate succeeding tests.

8. Alleviate stress, anxiety, or fear by encouraging verbalization and stress-reduction strategies. Administer pain medication or antiemetics PRN as ordered.

- **a.** Protect the patient's sense of modesty and provide for privacy and the least amount of embarrassment possible.
- **b.** If the patient is to receive IV conscious sedation, follow established

protocols to monitor and assist the patient until they return to a stable reactive state (see Appendix IV).

Minimizing Interference

9. Minimize test outcome deviations by correcting caregiver actions or activities that affect or interfere with accurate test results. These include the following:

a.

(1) Incorrect specimen collection, handling, or labeling process
(2) Wrong preservative or lack of designated preservative
(3) Delayed delivery of a collected specimen to the proper department
(4) Incorrect or incomplete patient preparation
(5) Hemolyzed blood samples
(6) Incomplete sample collection, especially of timed samples
(7) Old specimens that may contain deteriorated cells.

b. Patient factors that could affect or interfere with accurate test results include the following:

(1) Incorrect diet preparation
(2) Current drug therapy
(3) Time of day
(4) Pregnancy
(5) Age and sex
(6) Type of illness
(7) Plasma volume
(8) Position or activity at time specimen was obtained
(9) Postprandial status (time patient last ate)
(10) Level of patient knowledge and understanding
(11) Stress
(12) Nonadherence or noncompliance with instructions and pretest preparation
(13) Undisclosed drug or alcohol use

Avoiding Errors

10. To avoid errors, know how the test is performed and how the results are obtained and measured. Communication errors are more likely to cause incorrect results than technical errors. Properly label and identify every specimen. Determine what type of sample is needed and what the method of collection is. Other considerations relate to whether the test is invasive or noninvasive; if contrast substance media are injected or swallowed; if there is a need to fast; whether fluids are restricted or forced; if medications need to be administered; what the approximate length of the procedure is and whether a consent form and sedation are required. Test results should be reported as soon as possible. In some instances, the results must be communicated *Stat* (eg, a blood glucose report for a critically ill diabetic patient).

   a. Inform patients and their families or significant others of their responsibilities in the testing process.
   b. Accurately communicate, to both the patient and to healthcare staff, dietary restrictions or the collection process for single, multiple, or timed specimens.
   c. Forward appropriate information about changes to those people involved in the diagnostic process. Conscientious efforts toward clear, timely communication between departments can reduce errors and inconvenience, both to staff and to patients.

Proper Preparation

11. Prepare the patient correctly.
   a. Be aware of patients with special needs such as the physically disabled, ostomy patients, diabetic persons, children, the elderly, and the culturally diverse.
   b. Give accurate, precise instructions that are specific to each test for optimal results. For example, patients need to know when and what they can eat and drink, or how long they must fast before certain tests are performed.
   c. Recognize and encourage dialogue about the patient's fears or apprehensions. "Walking" a patient through imagery and relaxation techniques may help them cope with these emotions. Never underestimate the value of being a caring presence.
   d. Assess for ability to read and to understand instructions. Poor eyesight or hearing difficulties may impair ability to comply with testing. Help the patient with assistive devices such as eyeglasses and hearing aids if necessary.
   e. Assess for language and cultural barriers. Understand that each patient behaves according to a personal value and perceptual system, a personal set of beliefs and traditions, and cultural and ethnic influences.
   f. Document specific caregiving activities performed in all testing phases.

Patient Education

12. Educate patient and family about the testing process and what will be required of them. Record date, time, teaching done, and information given, and to whom it was given.
   a. Patients need both sensory and objective information so that they can create an image of what is going to occur. Clear, well thought out descriptions enable patients to "see" a realistic schema of what to expect. Avoid medical jargon. Adapt information to the patient's level of understanding. Sometimes "slang" terms may be necessary to "get a point across."
   b. Sensory information helps the patient interpret situations that are very different from usual experiences. Subjective features may in-

clude unusual physical sensations. Objective features characterize such things as equipment used or length and process of the procedure. Predictable sensations should be discussed so that patient and family know what to expect.

c. Encourage questions. Allow the patient to verbalize fears and concerns. Do not minimize or invalidate the patient's anxiety by making remarks such as "Don't worry." Develop "listening ears and eyes." Cue into nonverbal cues (body language). Above all, be nonjudgmental!

d. Tell patients that there is usually a waiting period ("turn-around time") before test results are relayed back to the physician, nursing unit, or patient. Recognize that this waiting period may be a time of great concern and anxiety for the patient and significant others.

13. Record information given and the patient's response to that information. Because something is "taught" does not necessarily mean that it is "learned" or accepted. The specific names of audiovisual and reading materials and handouts need to be documented correctly for audit, reimbursement, and accreditation purposes.

Testing Protocols

14. Develop protocols for consistent teaching and testing that encompass comprehensive *pretest* and *posttest* care.

a. Prepare patients for those aspects of the procedure that are experienced by the majority of patients. Caregivers can collaborate to collect data and to develop a list of more common patient experiences and responses and their reactions to these things.

Patient Independence

15. Allow the patient to maintain as much control of the diagnostic phase as possible to reduce stress.

a. Include the patient and significant others in decision-making. Because of things such as anxiety, language barriers, physical, or emotional impairments, the patient may not fully assimilate instructions and explanations. Therefore, validate the patient's understanding of what is presented. Request that the patient repeat taught instructions to evaluate retention and understanding of presented information.

b. Reinforce information about the diagnostic plan, procedures, time frames, and the patient's role in the diagnostic process.

Test Results

16. Knowledge of normal or reference values is vital.

a. Normal ranges can vary, to some degree, from laboratory to laboratory. Theoretically, "normal" can refer to the ideal health state, to average reference values, or to types of statistical distribution. Normal values are those that fall within 2 standard deviations (SD) from the mean value for the normal population.

b. The reported reference range for a test can vary according to the laboratory, the method used, the population tested, and the conditions of collection and preservation of specimens. Thus, each laboratory must specify its own normal ranges.

(1) Many factors may affect values and influence the determination (range). These may produce values that are normal under the prevailing conditions, but outside the limits determined under other circumstances. Age, sex, race, environment, posture, diurnal and other cyclic variations, foods, beverages, fasting or postprandial state, drugs, and exercise, may affect values derived.

(2) Interpretation of laboratory results must always be in the context of the actual condition of the patient. Hydration and nourishment, fasting state, mental status, or ability to comply with test protocols are but a few of the situations influencing test outcomes.

(3) The majority of normal values for blood tests are determined by measurement of "fasting" specimens.

Specific Influences

(4) Posture influence is important when plasma volume is measured because it is 12% to 15% greater in a person who has been supine for several hours. When the position changes from supine to standing, values change as follows: increase in Hb, RBC, HCT, calcium, K, P, AST, phosphatases, total protein, albumin, cholesterol, and triglycerides. When position changes from upright to supine, it results in a decrease in HCT, calcium, total protein, and cholesterol.

(5) A tourniquet applied for more than 1 minute produces an increase in protein (5%), iron (6.7%), AST (9.3%), cholesterol (5%); and a decrease in K^+ (6%) and creatinine (2.3%).

SI Values

c. Scientific publications and many professional organizations are changing the reporting of clinical laboratory data from conventional units to Système International (SI) units. Currently, much clinical laboratory data are reported in conventional units with SI units placed in parentheses.

d. The SI system uses seven dimensionally independent units of measurement to provide a logical and consistent measurement. For example, SI concentrations are written as amount per volume (moles or millimoles per liter), rather than as mass per volume (grams, milligrams, or milliequivalents per deciliter, 100 milliliters, or liter). Sometimes numerical values differ between systems. However, they may be the same. For example, chloride is the same—95 to 105 mEq/L (conventional) and 95 to 105 mmol/L (SI); (see Appendix I).

Margins of Error

17. Recognize margins of error. If a patient has a battery of chemistry tests, the possibility exists that some tests will be abnormal, purely owing to chance. This can occur because a significant margin of error arises from the arbitrary setting of limits. Moreover, if a laboratory test is considered normal up to the 95th percentile, then five times out of 100, the test will show an abnormality even though a patient is not ill. A second test performed on the same sample will probably yield the following: 0.95×0.95 or 90.25%. This means that 9.75 times out of 100 a test will show an abnormality even though the person has no underlying health disorder. Each successive testing will produce a higher percentage of abnormal results. The point here is that if the patient has a group of tests performed on one blood sample, the possibility that some of the tests will be abnormal, purely by chance, is not an uncommon occurrence.

Ethics and the Law

18. Consider legal and ethical implications. These include the patient's right to information, properly signed and witnessed consent forms, or explanations and instructions concerning risks, as well as benefits of tests.

- **a.** The patient must demonstrate appropriate use of cognitive and reasoning faculties to legally sign a valid consent. Conversely, a patient may not legally give consent while under the immediate influence of sedation, anesthetic agents, or certain classes of analgesics and tranquilizers. If the patient cannot validly and legally sign a consent form, an appropriately qualified individual may give consent for the patient.
- **b.** Guidelines and wishes set forth in advance directives or "living will"-type documents needs to be honored, especially in life-threatening situations. Such directives may preclude the more sophisticated invasive procedures form being performed.

19. A collaborative team approach is essential for responsible patient-centered care.

- **a.** The attending physician (or whoever orders the test) has a responsibility to inform the patient about test results and to discuss alternatives for follow-up care.
- **b.** Other caregivers provide additional information and clarification, and support the patient and family toward the best possible outcomes.
- **c.** The duty to maintain confidentiality of information, freedom of choice, reporting of infectious diseases, and respect for the dignity of the individual reflect basic ethical considerations.
- **d.** Patients and family have a right to consent, to question, or to refuse diagnostic tests.
- **e.** Caregivers have the right to know the diagnoses of the patients they care for so that they can minimize risks to their own well-being.

Cultural Sensitivity

20. Provide culturally sensitive care.

- **a.** Preserving the cultural well-being of any group of people helps them comply with testing and recover more easily from invasive or complex procedures.
- **b.** Sensitive questioning and observation may reveal that an individual has certain traditions, concerns, and practices related to health. Some cultures (Hmong) believe the soul resides in the head, and one should not touch an adult's head without permission. Patting a child on the head may violate this belief.
- **c.** Many cultures have diverse beliefs about diagnostic testing that involves blood sampling. For example, alarm about having blood specimens drawn or concerns related to the disposal of body fluids or tissue samples may require the healthcare worker to demonstrate the utmost sensitivity and tact when communicating and teaching information related to testing of blood. Learning about varied cultural beliefs, values, and practices supports one's healthcare practice when dealing with culturally diverse populations. If asked, many people will willingly share this information.

Infection Control

21. Follow accepted infection control protocols.

- **a.** The term *universal precautions* refers to a system of disease control that presupposes each direct contact with body fluids is potentially infectious, and that every employee exposed to these fluids needs to protect themselves. It is a method of preventing infections in certain classes of healthcare workers. Consequently, healthcare workers must be both informed and conscientious about adhering to strict infection control guidelines and behaviors. Moreover, they must be scrupulous about proper handwashing (see Appendix).
- **b.** Proper protective clothing and devices must be worn. Procurement and disposal of specimens according to OSHA standards must be adhered to.
- **c.** **Universal precautions must prevail!**

POSTTEST PHASE: PRINCIPLES OF SAFE, EFFECTIVE, INFORMED CARE

Requisite Knowledge, Vital Information and Basic Responsibilities

Abnormal Test Results

1. Interpret test outcomes correctly. Patterns or trends related to abnormal outcomes can sometimes provide more useful information than single-test outcome deviations. On the other hand, single tests can show normal results in persons with a proved disease.

a. Recognize abnormal test results and consider the implications for the patient's health state, both in the acute and the chronic stages of the disease as well as during screening.

b. The greater the degree of abnormality, the more likely the outcome is significant or representative of a more serious disorder.

c. Abnormal results may be caused by drugs. Consider this possibility when tests are abnormal. Be alert to use of over-the-counter drugs, vitamins, iron, and other minerals that may produce false-positive or false-negative results. Patients often do not disclose all medication used, either through forgetfulness or by intent. The classes of commonly prescribed drugs that most often affect laboratory test outcomes are anticoagulants, anticonvulsants, antihypertensives, anti-infectious agents, oral hypoglycemics, hormones, and psychotropic drugs. For more specific information, consult a detailed source or pharmacist about drugs the patient is taking (examples of sources: current literature, computer file-based data, pharmacist, and manufacturer's insert sheet).

d. Consider biocultural variations when interpreting test results. The table that follows provides examples of common variations. *Bio* (biological) refers to physics (body) *-evolved* structure and response and *cultural* refers to learned psychosocial responses. Biological processes and adjustments evolve from one's physical and emotional environments, in similar fashion, one's cultural framework is also influenced by this same environment.

Diagnostic Test	***Biocultural Variation***
Orthopedic x-rays	*Body proportions and tendencies: Blacks* exhibit longer arms and legs and shorter trunks than whites. *Black women* are wider shouldered and more narrow hipped, but with more abdominal adipose tissue than white women. *White* men exhibit more abdominal adipose tissue than black men. *American Indians* and *Asians* have larger trunks and shorter limbs than *blacks* and *whites*. *Asians* tend to be wider hipped and more narrow shouldered.
Bone density measurements	Black men have the densest bones followed by black women and white men with similar densities; white women have the least dense bones. Chinese, Japanese, and Eskimos' bone density is less than white Americans. Also, the density of bone decreases with age.
Dehydrogenase deficiency (G-6-PD) test for glucose-6-phosphate	

(continued)

	Blood Types			
Occurrence	*A*	*B*	*A−*	*B−*
Blacks	35%		65%	
Whites		100%		
Asians		2%–5%		2%–5%
Mediterranean		50%		50%

G6PD x-linked problems related to the deficiency occur mostly in males.

Individuals with B− deficiency experience hemolysis after eating fava beans. The A− and B− types are deficient in the G6PD enzyme and less likely to be parasitized. This lowers the parasite load, lessening the severity of the illness. See above for occurrence table.

Cholesterol levels	Blacks and whites have similar cholesterol levels at birth. During childhood, blacks develop higher levels than whites. However, black adults have lower levels than white adults.
Hemoglobin/ hematocrit levels	The normal hemoglobin level for blacks is 1 g lower than for other groups. Given similar social economic conditions, Asian–Americans and Mexican–Americans have hemoglobin/hematocrit levels higher than whites.
Sickle Cell Anemia	Sickle cell diseases affect more than 50,000 Americans. They are primarily of African heritage, but Mediterranean, Caribbean, South and Central American, Arabian, or East Indian ancestry can also exhibit this trait. Eight percent of the African–American population carries the sickle cell trait, and approximately 1 African–American child in every 375 is affected by sickle cell disease. It is among the most prevalent genetically transmitted diseases in the United States.

Clinical Alert

Correct test interpretation requires a knowledge of all drugs the patient is taking.

2. Help the patient and significant others to understand and cope with a positive or negative test outcome.
3. Recognize "panic values" that pose an immediate life-threatening situation. Report these findings to the attending physician or other designated person immediately. Document results and actions taken as soon as possible.
4. Almost all tests have limitations. Some tests cannot predict future outcomes or events. For example, an electrocardiogram (ECG) cannot pre-

dict a future myocardial infarction. It can merely tell what has already occurred. No test is perfect.

5. Devastating physical, psychological, and social consequences can result from being misdiagnosed with a serious disease because of false-positive or false-negative test results. Major alterations in lifestyles and relationships can be a consequence of these clinical aberrations (for example, misdiagnosis of acquired immunodeficiency syndrome [AIDS], syphilis, or cervical cancer).

Detect Complications

6. Observe for complications and take measures to prevent complications, promote patient safety, and foster well-being.

  a. *Posttest* assessments include evaluation of patient's behaviors, complaints, activities, and compliance within the emotional, physical, psychosocial, and spiritual dimensions. Alterations in any of these domains may signal a need for instituting safety and protective measures.

  b. Older patients and children may require closer and more lengthy monitoring and observation. Invasive sites should be observed and assessed for possible bleeding, circulatory problems, or infection.

  c. The patient who has received sedation, drugs, contrast medium (eg, iodine or barium), or radioactive medications needs to be evaluated and treated according to established protocols. (See Appendix concerning sedation protocols during diagnostic evaluations.)

  d. Infection control measures and aseptic techniques need to be a part of the routine care for all testing processes and procedures.

Test Result Availability

7. Collaborate with other disciplines to ensure that test results are made available to patient and staff as soon as possible. Time-critical diagnostic test information is of limited help to clinicians or the patient if the information is late, delayed, or never received. Even though computer networks and communication technology all contribute to faster information delivery, clinicians are often left waiting for crucial clinical data. Fax machines, computers, and wireless networks can be valuable access tools to vital patient data for the healthcare provider. Follow agency policy for transmission of diagnostic information by these modalities. Questions of confidentiality should be resolved and access to records and information should be on a need-to-know basis.

Follow-Up Care

8. Follow-up care should be consistent and should include clearly understood discharge instructions and infection control measures. If necessary, explain protocols for repeat testing. If designated, emphasize the importance of follow-up visits.

  a. Use discharge instructions to reinforce verbal information given at the patient's level of understanding.

b. If possible, allow time for listening, support, discussion, and problem solving according to the patient's needs.

Documentation

9. Record information about all phases of the diagnostic-testing process.

a. Accurately document the diagnostic activities and procedures performed in the *pretest, intratest,* and *posttest* phases because of legal, budgetary, reimbursement, and diagnostic-related grouping (DRG) implications and constraints.

b. Indicate that the purpose, side effects, risks, expected results and benefits, as well as alternative methods have been explained.

c. Medications, IV conscious sedation, beginning and end times, and patient responses need to be documented. Appropriately describe any adverse reactions, such as allergic reactions to contrast substances. (See conscious sedation standards in Appendix.)

d. Record data collected about specimens and their disposition, together with information about follow-up care and instructions.

e. Document reasons for a test refusal.

Record Keeping

10. Keep records of laboratory and diagnostic test data. Issues can revolve around compact record storage, such as on microfilm and computer-based records, and archival storage of certain laboratory test outcomes, such as blood donor records. Many blood bank records, such as donor history forms, must now be kept indefinitely owing to the need to review the records in cases of possible transfusion-transmitted diseases.

a. When an individual tests positive for human immunodeficiency virus (HIV; the virus implicated in the acquired immunodeficiency syndrome [AIDS]) or for human T-cell lymphotropic virus type I, it is necessary to review donor records at blood donor centers to determine whether the individual ever donated blood.

b. If blood was donated by the infected person, the recipients of those blood components must be contacted and informed. This process is called "look back." Because many years may pass between the time of donation and transfusion and the time the donor tests positive for the virus, blood donor medical history records must be stored indefinitely.

Disclosure Guidelines

11. Follow disclosure guidelines.

a. Ethical standards, with the professional nurse acting as patient advocate, may be a source of conflict and anxiety. Accepted guidelines for telling a patient about test results can alleviate some of this frustration. Under normal conditions, the patient has the right to be informed of test results.

(1) Although the physician is responsible for providing initial information, the nurse or other designated individuals need to facilitate and support the patient's right to know.

(2) Bringing the patient and the family together to inform them about test results can do much to open communication and prevent the so-called "conspiracy of silence."

Patient Response to Outcome

12. Be familiar with crisis intervention skills for patients who experience difficulty dealing with the posttest phase.

a. Encourage the patient to take as much control of the situation as possible.

b. Recognize that the different stages of behavioral responses may last several weeks (see the following).

Immediate Response	***Secondary Response***
Acute emotional turmoil, shock, disbelief about diagnosis, denial.	Insomnia, anorexia, difficulty concentrating, depression, difficulty in performing work-related responsibilities and tasks.
Anxiety will usually last several days until the person assimilates the information.	Depression may last several weeks as the person begins to incorporate the information and to participate realistically in a treatment plan and lifestyle adaptation.

Comfort Measures

13. Use the following strategies to lessen the impact of a threatening situation.

a. Offer appropriate comfort measures.

b. Help patients work through feelings of anxiety and depression and reassure them that these feelings and emotions are normal. Be a therapeutic listener.

c. Assist the patient and family to make necessary lifestyle and self-concept adjustments.

d. Teach that risk factors associated with certain diseases can be reduced through lifestyle changes.

Expected Outcomes

14. Evaluate outcomes

a. Be familiar with the normal values–expected outcomes. The patient should be able to describe the testing purpose, testing process and procedure, and should properly perform expected activities associated with testing. Sometimes assistance may be necessary. If test outcomes are abnormal, the patient should be encouraged to comply with repeat testing and to make appropriate lifestyle changes. Deal with anxiety or fears in a timely manner.

b. Know how to interpret abnormal test values and outcomes. Compare actual outcomes or abnormal test patterns with normal expected outcomes. Sometimes, anticipated outcomes cannot be achieved. Some collaborative diagnoses that could apply to these situations include the following:

(1) Inability to fully participate in teaching/learning process as evidenced by verbal and nonverbal cues. Inability to perform expected activities related to the testing process or follow-up care.

(2) Noncompliance with test preparation guidelines and *posttest* activities related to denial of health status.

(3) Refusal to submit to diagnostic tests related to fear of results.

(4) Other nursing diagnoses related to diagnostic testing include noncompliance with test protocols; inability to collect specimens without assistance; difficulty in obtaining valid specimens in a timely manner; inaccurately performing procedure steps; and inability to participate in procedure to test completion.

The reasons for these responses can be numerous and varied: lack of appropriate problem-solving behaviors; inappropriate behaviors; uncertainty or denial about test outcomes; signs and symptoms of complications (eg, allergic response, shock, bleeding, nausea, vomiting, retention of barium); inability to cope with test outcomes; extreme depression and abnormal emotional patterns of response; and refusal to take control of the situation.

COMMUNICATION IS KEY

At the heart or core of informed care is the ability to communicate effectively. Frequently, because of time constraints, communication must take place within a "compressed" time frame. Thus, the importance of communicating effectively cannot be emphasized enough. It is key to achieving desired outcomes and preventing misunderstanding and errors. One must always keep in mind that the human person is an integration of body, mind, and spirit, and that these three entities are intimately bound together to make each of us the unique individuals that we are. Skillful assessment of physical, emotional, psychosocial, and spiritual dimensions provides a sound database from which to plan communication and teaching–instruction strategies.

Individuals have different needs and changing capacities for learning as they progress from child to adult to older adult. Therefore, it is important for the caregiver to know the different developmental levels and stages and how clear communication can be achieved at any level.

For the pediatric patient, teaching tools might include tours of the diagnostic area, play therapy, films or videos, actual models of equipment that can be touched or manipulated, and written materials and pictures. Shorter attention spans and the unpredictable nature of children can make this a challenge. Mentally retarded or mentally ill patients might need significant others close by who can guide communication between caretaker and patient. Demonstrating gentle, simple, nurturing behavior usually works well with children.

Adolescents may be at the stage of developing their own unique identity toward adulthood. Teaching might be more effective without parents present. (However, at some point, include parents!) Drawings, illustrations, or videos are helpful. Because body image is so very important at this stage, honest, supportive behaviors are necessary, especially if some alteration in physical appearance will be necessary (eg, no make-up allowed).

The opportunity to actively participate and to ask questions is important for adults. They bring to the communication process their lifetime of perceptions. This can be a proverbial "two-edged sword." Listening well to verbal as well as nonverbal messages cannot be overemphasized. Interacting with patients who have Alzheimer's disease can present special challenges. The presence of a significant other who shows finesse in communicating with this type of patient may be key to performing a successful procedure.

An environment that is quiet, private, and free of distractions is ideal for clear communication. Determine by what name or title the patient wishes to be addressed. *Referring to a patient as a room number, procedure, or disease is demeaning and inexcusable!*

Nonverbal communication behaviors, such as proper eye contact, a firm handshake, sense of respect, and ***appropriate*** humor can reduce anxiety. Do not dismiss the power of touch, the sense of time devoted to the patient, and the use of a light and positive voice. These things make first impressions and *lasting* impressions.

Each person engaged in the entire process of performing a test or procedure is a link in an ongoing communication continuum. This continuum is as effective as the weakest link that joins all activities and all communication together.

CONCLUSION

As professionals, we need to maintain the perception that we are dealing with people not so unlike ourselves in many ways. These individuals come to us with their perceptions of what the diagnostic process and their illness means to them and their loved ones, what strategies they use to cope, what resources are available for their use, and what knowledge they have about themselves. As caregivers and patient advocates, then, we have to be willing to try to "take on the mind" of another—to identify with that patient's point of view. In other words, we must be willing to show empathy. Once we reach that point, we can then begin to understand each other and to communicate with one another beyond a merely superficial level.

BIBLIOGRAPHY

Banja J: Ethics, The incompetent chart. Case Management 4(1): 28–30, Jan/Feb/Mar 1993

Buffington J: How much do you know about laboratory studies? Nursing '91 21(12): 46–49, December 1991

Christopher M, Lajkowicz C: Patient teaching by the book. RN 48–50, July 1993

Ditmer WM et al: Pocket Guide to Diagnostic Tests. Norwalk, CT, Appleton & Lane, 1992

Donovan NM: Confidentiality versus duty to warn. Nursing and Health Care, 12(8): 432–436, October 1992

Eddy DM (ed): Common Screening Tests. Philadelphia, American College of Physicians, 1991

Editorial: Fostering patient empowerment. Cancer Practice 2(5): 327, September/October 1994

Escarie JJ et al: Racial differences in the elderly's use of medical practices and diagnostic tests. American Journal of Public Health 83(7): 948–954, 1993

Farrice L: Does a smile cost extra? Laboratory Medicine 21(7): 409–410, July 1990

Feste L: Guidelines for FAXing patient health information. Journal of AHMA 62 (6): 29–34, June 1991

Fischbach FT: Quick Reference to Common Laboratory and Diagnostic Tests. Philadelphia, JB Lippincott, 1995

Fischbach FT: Documenting Care—Communication; Nursing Process; Documentation Standards. Philadelphia, FA Davis, 1991

Gold J: Ask about latex. RN 57(6): 32–34, June 1994

Joel LA: Changing standards in consumer–provider relations. American Journal of Nursing 94(6): 7, June 1994

Kisabett RM: Mayo Medicine Laboratories 1994 test catalog. Rochester, MN

Long CO, Greenerd DS: Four strategies for keeping patients satisfied. American Journal of Nursing 94(6): 26–27, June 1994

McHugh NG, Christman NJ, Johnson JE: Preparatory information: What helps and why. American Journal of Nursing 82: 780–782, 1992

[OSHA] Occupational Safety and Health Administration: Blood banking, pathogens and acute care facilities. US Department of Labor 312(8), 1992

Riordan B, Zana RH: When your patient is a Hmong refugee. American Journal of Nursing 52–53, March 1992

Speicher CE: The Right Test. A Physician's Guide to Laboratory Medicine, 2nd ed. Philadelphia, WB Saunders, 1993

US Department of Health and Human Services: Healthy People 2000: National Health Promotion and Disease Prevention Objectives. 91–50, 212 Washington, DC, US Government Printing Office, 1991

Veatch RM: Medical Ethics. Boston, Jones and Bartlett, 1989

Wallach J: Interpretation of Diagnostic Tests, 5th ed. Boston, Little, Brown & Co, 1992

2

Blood Studies

OVERVIEW OF BASIC BLOOD TESTS ●

Composition of Blood

The average person circulates about 5 L of blood, (1/13 of body weight), of which 3 L is plasma and 2 L is cells. Plasma fluid derives from the intestines and organs and provides a vehicle for cell measurement. The cells are produced primarily by bone marrow and account for blood "solids." Blood cells are classified as white cells (leukocytes), red cells (erythrocytes), and platelets (thrombocytes). White cells are further categorized as granulocytes, lymphocytes, and monocytes.

The size of cells differs: white cells are the largest, red cells fall into the middle, and platelets are the smallest. To compare, for every 500 red cells, there are approximately 30 platelets and a single white cell.

Blood Disorders

Tests in this chapter address disorders of cell production (hematopoiesis), synthesis, and function. Blood and bone marrow examination constitutes the major means of determining certain blood disorders. Specimens are obtained through capillary skin punctures (finger, toe, heel) arterial and venous sampling, or bone marrow aspiration.

● BLOOD SPECIMEN COLLECTION PROCEDURES

Proper specimen collection presumes correct technique and accurate timing when necessary.

CAPILLARY PUNCTURE, SKIN PUNCTURE ●

Capillary blood is preferred for a peripheral blood smear.

1. Obtain capillary blood from fingertips or earlobes (adults); the great toe or the heel (infants).
2. Disinfect puncture site, dry the site, and puncture skin with sterile disposable lancet no deeper than 2 mm. If povidone-iodine is used, allow to dry thoroughly.
3. Wipe away the initial drop of blood. Collect subsequent drops in a microtube and prepare slides from this sample.
4. Observe universal precautions (Appendix IX). Check for latex allergy. If present, do not use latex-containing products (Appendix II).

Clinical Alert

1. Do not squeeze the site to obtain blood because this alters blood composition and invalidates test values.
2. Warming the extremity or placing it in a dependent position may facilitate specimen retrieval.

Patient Preparation

Instruct patient about purpose and procedure of test.

Patient Aftercare

Apply small dressing or adhesive strip to site. Evaluate puncture site for bleeding or oozing. Apply compression or pressure to the site if it continues to bleed. Evaluate patient's medication history for anticoagulant or acetylsalicylic acid (aspirin; ASA)–type drug ingestion.

VENIPUNCTURE ●

Venipuncture allows procurement of larger quantities of blood for testing. Usually, the antecubital veins are the veins of choice because of access ease. Blood values remain constant no matter what actual venipuncture site is selected.

1. Position and tighten a tourniquet on the upper arm to produce venous congestion.

NOTE: *A blood pressure cuff inflated to a point between systolic and diastolic pressure values can be used.*

2. Ask the patient to close and open the fist in the selected arm several times. Select an accessible vein.
3. Cleanse the puncture site and dry it properly with sterile gauze. Povidone-iodine must dry thoroughly.
4. Puncture the vein according to accepted technique. Usually, for an adult, anything smaller than a 21-gauge needle might make blood withdrawal somewhat more difficult.

NOTE: *The Vacutainer system consists of vacuum tubes (Vacutainer tubes), a tube holder, and a disposable multisample collecting needle.*

5. Once the vein is entered with the collecting needle, blood will fill the attached vacuum tubes automatically because of negative pressure within the collection tube.
6. Remove the tourniquet before removing the needle from the puncture site or bleeding will occur.
7. Remove needle. Apply pressure and sterile dressing strip to site.
8. The preservative or anticoagulant added to the collection tube depends on the test ordered. In general, most hematology tests use ethylenediaminetetraacetic acid (EDTA) anticoagulant. Even slightly clotted blood invalidates the test, and the sample must be redrawn.
9. Observe universal precautions (Appendix IX). If latex allergy is suspected, use latex-free supplies and equipment (Appendix II).

Patient Preparation

1. Instruct patient about sampling procedure. Assess for circulation or bleeding problems or allergy to latex.
2. Reassure patient that mild discomfort may be felt when the needle is inserted.
3. Place the arm in a fully extended position, with palmar surface facing upward (for antecubital access).

Clinical Alert

In patients with leukemia, agranulocytosis, or lowered resistance, the finger-stick and ear lobe puncture are more likely to cause infection and bleeding than venipuncture. Should a capillary sample be necessary, the cleansing agent should remain in contact with the skin for at least 5 to 10 minutes. Povidone-iodine is the cleansing agent of choice and should be allowed to dry. It may then be wiped off with alcohol and the site dried with sterile gauze before puncture.

4. If withdrawal of the sample is difficult, warm the extremity with warm towels or blankets. Allow the extremity to remain in a dependent position for several minutes before venipuncture.

Patient Aftercare

1. If oozing or bleeding from the puncture site continues for an unusually long time, elevate the area and apply a pressure dressing. Observe the patient closely. Check for anticoagulant and ASA-type ingestion.
2. If the patient feels dizzy or faint, put the head down between the knees or have patient lie flat and breathe deeply. A cool towel may be applied to head or back of neck. Should the patient remain unconscious, notify the physician immediately.
3. Hematomas can be prevented by use of proper technique (not sticking needle through the vein), release of the tourniquet before the needle is withdrawn, application of sufficient pressure over the puncture site, and maintenance of an extended extremity until bleeding stops.

Clinical Alert

1. Never draw blood from the same extremity being used for intravenous medications, fluids, or transfusions. If no other site is available, then make sure the venipuncture site is below the IV site. Avoid areas that are edematous, paralyzed, on the same side as a mastectomy, or have infections or skin conditions present. Venipuncture may cause infection, circulatory impairment, or retarded healing.
2. Prolonged tourniquet application causes statis and hemoconcentration.

BONE MARROW ASPIRATION

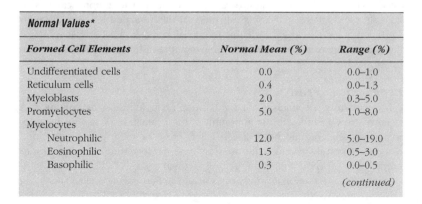

Normal Values*

Formed Cell Elements	*Normal Mean (%)*	*Range (%)*
Undifferentiated cells	0.0	0.0–1.0
Reticulum cells	0.4	0.0–1.3
Myeloblasts	2.0	0.3–5.0
Promyelocytes	5.0	1.0–8.0
Myelocytes		
Neutrophilic	12.0	5.0–19.0
Eosinophilic	1.5	0.5–3.0
Basophilic	0.3	0.0–0.5

(continued)

Normal Values* *(continued)*

Formed Cell Elements	*Normal Mean (%)*	*Range (%)*
Metamyelocytes		
Neutrophilic	25.6	17.5–33.7
Eosinophilic	1.5	0.5–3.0
Basophilic	0.3	0.0–0.5
Metamyelocytes		
Neutrophilic	25.6	17.5–33.7
Eosinophilic	0.4	0.0–1.0
Basophilic	0.0	0.0–0.2
Segmented granulocytes		
Neutrophilic	20.0	11.6–30.0
Eosinophilic	2.0	0.5–4.0
Basophilic	0.2	0.0–3.7
Monocytes	2.0	1.6–4.3
Lymphocytes	10.0	3.0–2.4
Megakaryocytes	0.4	0.0–3.0
Plasma cells	0.9	0.0–2.0
Erythroid series		
Pronormoblasts	0.5	0.2–4.2
Basophilic normoblasts	1.6	0.25–4.8
Polychromatic normoblasts	10.4	3.5–20.5
Orthochromatic normoblasts	6.4	3.0–25
Promegaloblasts	0	0
Basophilic megaloblasts	0	0
Polychromatic megaloblasts	0	0
Orthochromatic megaloblasts	0	0
Myeloid/erythroid ratio (M/E) ratio of WBC to nucleated RBC	2:1–4:1	

*These values are only for adults.

Background

Bone marrow is located within cancellous bone and long-bone cavities. It consists of a pattern of vessels and nerves, differentiated and undifferentiated hemotopoietic cells, reticuloendothelial cells, and fatty tissue. All of these are increased by endosteum, the membrane lining the bone marrow cavity.

Explanation of Test

A bone marrow specimen is obtained through needle biopsy or aspiration. A bone marrow examination is important in the evaluation of several hematologic disorders and infectious diseases. The presence or suspicion of a blood disorder is not always an indication for bone marrow studies. A decision to employ this procedure is made on an individual basis.

Sometimes, the aspirate does not contain hematopoietic cells. This is referred to as a "dry tap" and occurs when hematopoietic activity is so sparse that there are no cells to be withdrawn, or when the marrow contains so many tightly packed cells that they cannot be suctioned out of the marrow. In such cases, a bone marrow biopsy would be advantageous.

Procedure

1. Follow universal precautions. Check for latex allergy. If allergy is present, do not use latex-containing products. Position the patient on the back or side according to site selected. The posterior iliac crest is the preferred site in all patients older than 12 to 18 months of age. Alternative sites include the anterior iliac crest, sternum, spinous vertebral processes T-10 through L-4, the ribs, and the tibia in children.

The sternum is not generally used in children because the bone cavity is too shallow, the risk of mediastinal and cardiac perforation is too great, and the child may be uncooperative.

2. Shave, cleanse, and drape the site as for any minor surgical procedure.

3. The physician injects local anesthetic (procaine or lidocaine). This may cause a burning sensation.

4. The physician introduces a short, rigid, sharp-pointed needle with stylet through the periosteum into the marrow cavity. The stylet is removed, and 0.2 to 0.5 ml of marrow fluid is aspirated. When the stylet needle enters the marrow, the patient may experience a feeling of pressure. Moderate discomfort *may* also be felt as aspiration is done, especially in the iliac crest. The Jameshedi needle is commonly used for biopsy, although the Westermani–Jensen modification of the Vim–Silverman needle may also be used. A skin incision (3 mm) is often made.

6. The needle–stylet combination is passed through the incision, subcutaneous tissue, and bone cortex.

7. Once the stylet is removed, the biopsy needle is advanced with a twisting motion toward the anterior superior iliac spine.

8. After adequate penetration of the base (3 cm), the needle is rotated or "rocked" in several directions several times. This "frees up" the specimen. Once this is done, the needle is then slowly withdrawn.

9. The biopsy specimen is pushed out "backwards" from the needle and may be used to make touch preparations or may be immediately placed in fixative. Slide smears are made at the bedside.

10. Pressure is applied to the puncture site until bleeding ceases. The site is then dressed.

11. Specimens are properly labeled and routed to the appropriate department.

Clinical Implications

1. A specific and diagnostic bone marrow picture provides clues to many diseases. The presence, absence, and ratio of cells are characteristic of the suspected disease.

2. Bone marrow examination may reveal the following abnormal cell patterns.
   a. Multiple myeloma
   b. Chronic or acute leukemias
   c. Anemia, including vitamin B_{12}, folic acid, iron and pyridoxine (vitamin B_6) deficiencies
   d. Toxic states that produce marrow depression or destruction
   e. Neoplastic diseases in which the marrow is invaded by tumor cells (metastatic carcinoma, myeloproliferative, and lymphoproliferative diseases)
   f. Agranulocytosis (a decrease in the production of certain types of white cells). This occurs when bone marrow activity is severely depressed, usually as a result of radiation therapy or chemotherapeutic drugs. Implications for the patient focus on risk for death due to overwhelming infection.
   g. Platelet-clotting dysfunction
   h. Some types of infectious diseases, especially histoplasmosis and tuberculosis
   i. Deficiency of body iron stores
   j. Lipid or glycogen storage disease

Patient Preparation

1. Instruct the patient about the test procedure, purpose, benefits, and risks of the test.
2. A legal consent form must be properly signed and witnessed. Bone marrow aspiration is usually contraindicated in the presence of hemophilia and other bleeding dyscrasias. However, risk versus benefit may dictate choice made.
3. Reassure the patient that analgesics will be available if needed.
4. Iliac crest biopsies or aspirations may be uncomfortable. Squeezing a pillow may be helpful as a distraction technique.
5. Observe universal precautions.

Clinical Alert

1. Complications can include bleeding and sternal fractures. Osteomyelitis or injury to heart or great vessels is rare but can occur if the sternal site is used.
2. Manual and pressure dressings over the puncture site usually control excessive bleeding. Remove dressing in 24 hours. Redress site if necessary.
3. Fever, headache, unusual pain, redness, or pus at biopsy site may indicate infection (later event). Instruct patient to report unusual symptoms to physician immediately.

Patient Aftercare

1. Monitor vital signs until stable and assess site for excess drainage or bleeding.
2. Recommend bed rest for 30 minutes; then resume normal activities.
3. Administer analgesics or sedatives, as necessary. Soreness over the puncture site for 3 to 4 days after procedure is normal. Continued pain may indicate fracture.
4. Interpret test outcomes and monitor appropriately.
5. Follow Chapter 1 guidelines for safe, effective, informed *posttest* care.

● BASIC BLOOD TESTS

HEMOGRAM ●

A hemogram includes platelet count, white blood count (WBC), red blood count (RBC), hematocrit (HCT), and indices. Complete blood count (CBC) is a hemogram plus differential count.

COMPLETE BLOOD COUNT (CBC) ●

The complete blood count (CBC) is a basic screening test and is one of the most frequently ordered laboratory procedures. The findings in the CBC give valuable diagnostic information about the hematologic and other body systems, prognosis, response to treatment, and recovery. The CBC consists of a series of tests that determine number, variety, percentage, concentrations, and quality of blood cells:

White blood count (WBC)
Differential white cell count (Diff)
Red blood count (RBC)
Hematocrit (HCT)
Hemoglobin (Hb)
Red blood cell indices
Mean corpuscular volume (MCV)
Mean corpuscular hemoglobin (MCH)
Mean corpuscular hemoglobin concentration (MCHC)
Stained red cell examination (film or peripheral blood smear)
Platelet count (often included in CBC)

These tests are described in detail in the following pages.

Normal Values for Hemogram

Age	*WBC* × 10^3	*RBC* × 10^6	*Hb g/dl*	*HCT (%)*	*MCV fl*
Birth–2 wk	9.0–30.0	4.1–6.1	14.5–24.5	44–64	
2–8 wk	2.0–21.0	4.0–6.0	12.5–20.5	39–59	98–112
2–6 mo	5.0–19.0	3.8–5.6	10.7–17.3	35–49	83–97

(continued)

Normal Values for Hemogram *(continued)*

Age	*WBC × 10^3*	*RBC× 10^6*	*Hb g/dl*	*HCT (%)*	*MCV fl*
6 mo–1 yr	5.0–19.0	3.8–5.2	9.9–14.5	29–43	73–87
1–6 yr	5.0–19.0	3.9–5.3	9.5–14.1	30–40	70–84
6–16 yr	4.8–10.8	4.0–5.2	10.3–14.9	32–42	73–87
16–18 yr	4.8–10.8	4.2–5.4	11.1–15.7	34–44	75–89
>18 yr males	5.0–10.0	4.5–5.5	14.0–17.4	42–52	84–96
>18 yr females	5.0–10.0	4.0–5.0	12.0–16.0	36–48	

Age	*MCH pg*	*MCHC g/dl*	*PLTS × 10^3*	*RDW (%)*	*MPV fl*
Birth–2 wk	34–40	33–37	150–450		
2–8 wk	30–36	32–36			
2–6 mo	27–33	31–35			
6 mo–1 yr	24–30	32–36			
1–6 yr	23–29	31–35			
6–16 yr	24–30	32–36			
16–18 yr	25–31	32–36			
>18 yr	28–34	32–36	140–400	11.5–14.5	7.4–10.4

Standard Patient Preparation for Hemogram, CBC, and Differential (All Components)

1. Explain test procedure. Explain that slight discomfort may be felt when skin is punctured. Refer to venipuncture procedure for additional information.
2. Avoid stress if possible because altered physiological states influence and change normal hemogram values.
3. Select hemogram components ordered at regular intervals (eg, daily, every other day), should be consistently drawn at the same time of day for accurate comparison; natural body rhythms cause fluctuations in lab values at certain times of the day.
4. Dehydration or overhydration can dramatically alter values (eg, large volumes of IV fluid can "dilute" the blood and values will present as lower counts). Both of these states should be communicated to the lab.
5. Fasting is not necessary. However, fat-laden meals may alter some test results.

Standard Patient Aftercare for Hemogram, CBC, and Differential (All Components)

1. Apply manual pressure and dressings to the puncture site after removing the needle.
2. Monitor puncture site for oozing or hematoma formation. Maintain pressure dressing on the site if necessary. Notify physician of unusual problems with the bleeding.

Clinical Alert

NEVER apply a total circumferential dressing and wrap *because* this may compromise circulation and nerve function if constriction, for whatever cause, occurs.

3. Resume normal activities and diet.
4. Bruising at the puncture site is not uncommon. Signs of inflammation are unusual and should be reported if inflamed area appears larger, if "red streaks" develop, or if drainage occurs.

TESTS OF WHITE BLOOD CELLS

WHITE BLOOD CELL COUNT (WBC) (LEUKOCYTE COUNT)

Normal Values

Adults:	$5–10^3/\mu l$ or $5–10^9/L$	
Children:	0–2 wk	9.0–30.0
	2–8 wk	5.0–21.0
	2 mo–6 yr	5.0–19.0
	6–18 yr	4.8–10.8

Background

White blood cells or leukocytes are divided into two main groups: granulocytes and agranulocytes. The granulocytes receive their name from the granules that are present in the cytoplasm of neutrophils, basophils, and eosinophils. However, each of these cells also contains a multilobed nucleus, which accounts for their also being called *polymorphonuclear leukocytes.* In laboratory terminology, they are often called "polys" (PMNs). The nongranulocytes, which consist of the lymphocytes and monocytes, do not contain granules and have nonlobular nuclei. They are not necessarily spherical; thus, the term *mononuclear leukocytes* is applied to these cells.

The endocrine system is an important regulator of the number of leukocytes in the blood. Hormones affect production of the leukocytes in the blood-forming organs, their storage and release from the tissue, and their disintegration. A local inflammatory process exerts a definite chemical effect on the mobilization of the leukocytes. The lifespan of leukocytes varies from 13 to 20 days, after which the cells are destroyed in the lymphatic system; many are excreted from the body in fecal matter.

Leukocytes fight infection and defend the body by a process called *phagocytosis* in which the leukocytes actually encapsulate foreign organisms.

White blood cells (WBCs) also produce, transport, and distribute antibodies as part of the immune response.

Explanation of Test

The leukocyte count serves as a useful guide to the severity of the disease process. Specific patterns of leukocyte response can be expected in different types of diseases. The differential count (of the numbers of different types of leukocytes) identifies persons with increased susceptibility to infection. A leukocyte function test may be done to determine the white blood cells' ability to phagocytose and destroy bacteria. Leukocyte and differential counts, by themselves, are of little value as aids to diagnosis unless the results are related to the clinical condition of the patient; only then is a correct and useful interpretation possible.

Procedure

1. Obtain a venous, anticoagulated, EDTA blood sample of 5 ml, or a finger-stick sample.
2. Record the time when specimen was obtained (eg, 7:00 AM).
3. Blood is processed either manually or automatically using the Coulter counter.

Clinical Implications

1. *Leukocytosis* (white blood cell count above 10,000/μl or $10^3/mm^3/\mu l$ is usually due to an increase of only *one* type of white cell and is given the name of the type of cell that shows the main increase:
   a. Neutrophilic leukocytosis or neutrophilia
   b. Lymphocytic leukocytosis or lymphocytosis
   c. Eosinophilic leukocytosis or eosinophilia
   d. Monocytic leukocytosis or monocytosis
   e. Basophilic leukocytosis or basophilia
2. An increase in circulating leukocytes is rarely due to a proportional increase in leukocytes of all types. When it occurs, it is usually due to hemoconcentration.
3. In certain diseases (such as measles, pertussis, and sepsis), the increase of leukocytes is so great that the blood picture suggests leukemia. *Leukocytosis of a temporary nature* (leukemoid reaction) must be distinguished from leukemia. In leukemia, the leukocytosis is permanent and progressive.
4. Leukocytosis occurs in acute infections in which the degree of increase of white cells depends on the severity of the infection, the patient's resistance, the patient's age, and the marrow efficiency and reserve.
5. Other causes of leukocytosis include
   a. Leukemia
   b. Trauma or tissue injury as occurs in surgery
   c. Malignant neoplasms, especially bronchogenic carcinoma

d. Toxins, uremia, coma, eclampsia, thyroid storm, and bacterial
e. Drugs, especially ether, chloroform, quinine, epinephrine (Adrenalin), colony-stimulating factors
f. Acute hemolysis
g. Hemorrhage (acute)
h. After splenectomy
i. Polycythemia vera
j. Tissue necrosis

6. Occasionally leukocytosis is found when there is no evidence of clinical disease. Such findings suggest the presence of:
a. Sunlight, ultraviolet irradiation
b. Physiologic leukocytosis due to excitement, stress exercise, pain, cold or heat, anesthesia
c. Nausea, vomiting, seizures

7. Steroid therapy modifies the leukocyte response.
a. When ACTH is given to a healthy person, leukocytosis occurs.
b. When ACTH is given to a patient with severe infection, the infection can spread rapidly without producing the expected leukocytosis; thus, what would normally be an important sign is obscured.

8. Hematologic disorders; recovery from marrow suppression, hemolysis, asplenia, myeloproliferative disorders

9. *Leukopenia* (a decrease of white blood cells below 4000, or 4.0×10^3 mm^3, occurs during the following
a. Viral infections, some bacterial infections, overwhelming bacterial infections
b. Hypersplenism
c. Bone-marrow depression caused by drugs
(1) Antimetabolites
(2) Barbiturates
(3) Benzine
(4) Antibiotics
(5) Antihistamines
(6) Anticonvulsants
(7) Antithyroid drugs
(8) Arsenicals
(9) Cancer chemotherapy causes a decrease in leukocytes; leukocyte count is used as a link to disease
(10) Cardiovascular drugs
(11) Diuretics
(12) Analgesics and anti-inflammatory drugs
Also, by heavy-metal intoxication and radiation (ionizing)
d. Primary bone marrow disorders
(1) Leukemia (aleukemic)
(2) Pernicious anemia
(3) Aplastic anemia
(4) Myelodysplastic syndromes
(5) Congenital disorders
(6) Kostmann's syndrome
(7) Reticular agenesis
(8) Cartilage–hair/hypoplasia
(9) Shwachman–Diamond syndrome
(10) Chédiak–Higashi syndrome
e. Immune-associated neutropenia
f. Marrow-occupying diseases: fungal infection, metastatic tumor

g. Hypersplenism
h. Iron-deficiency anemia

Clinical Alert

1. White blood cell count below 500 or 0.5×10^3 WBC represents a panic value.
2. White blood cell count above 30,000 or 30.0×10^3 is a panic value.

Interfering Factors

1. Hourly rhythm: There is an early-morning low level and late-afternoon high peak.
2. Age: In newborns and infants, the count is high (10,000–20,000) and gradually decreases in children until the adult values are reached at about age 21.

Patient Preparation

1. Explain test purpose and procedure.
2. Refer to standard *pretest* care for hemogram, CBC, and differential on page 32. Also, see Chapter 1 guidelines for safe, effective, informed *pretest* care.

Patient Aftercare

1. Interpret test outcome and monitor appropriately. Refer to standard *posttest* care for hemogram, CBC, and differential on page 32. Also, follow Chapter 1 guidelines for safe, effective, informed *posttest* care.
2. In prolonged severe granulocytopenia or pancytopenia, give no fresh fruits or vegetables because the kitchen, especially in a hospital, may be a source of food contamination. When leukocytes are low, a person can develop pseudomonal or fungal infection from fresh fruits and vegetables. Use minimal-bacteria diet or commercially sterile diet. All food must be served from a single serving or a new package. Consider leukemia diet. See dietary department for restrictions, such as cooked food only and careful food preparation. Do not give intramuscular injections. Do not take rectal temperature or give suppositories or enemas. Do not use razor blades. Do not give aspirin or nonsteroidal anti-inflammatory drugs (produce abnormal platelet dysfunction). Watch carefully for any signs or symptoms of infection. Without white cells to produce inflammation, serious infections can present very subtle findings. Often patients will have only a fever.

DIFFERENTIAL WHITE BLOOD CELL COUNT
(DIFF; DIFFERENTIAL LEUKOCYTE COUNT)

Normal Values

Age	*Bands % STAB*	*Segs % VENT*	*Eos %*	*Basos %*	*Lymphs %*	*Monos %*	*Metas %*
Birth–1 wk	10–18	32–62	0–2	0–1	26–36	0–6	
1–2 wk	8–16	19–49	0–4	0–0	38–46	0–9	
2–4 wk	7–15	14–34	0–3	0–0	43–53	0–9	
4–8 wk	7–13	15–35	0–3	0–1	41–71	0–7	
2–6 mo	5–11	15–35	0–3	0–1	42–72	0–6	
6 mo–1 yr	6–12	13–33	0–3	0–0	46–76	0–5	
1–6 yr	5–11	13–33	0–3	0–0	46–76	0–5	
6–16 yr	5–11	32–54	0–3	0–1	27–57	0–5	
16–18 yr	5–11	34–64	0–3	0–1	25–45	0–5	
>18 yr	3–6	50–62	0–3	0–1	25–40	3–7	0–1

Background
The total leukocyte count of the circulating white blood cells is differentiated according to the five types of leukocyte cells, each of which performs a specific function.

Cell	*These Cells Function to Combat*
Neutrophils	Pyogenic infections
Eosinophils	Allergic disorders and parasitic infestations
Basophils	Parasitic infections
Lymphocytes	Viral infections (measles, rubella, chickenpox, infectious mononucleosis)
Monocytes	Severe infections, by phagocytosis

Explanation of Test
The differential count is expressed as a percentage of the total number of white cells. The distribution of the number and type of cells and the degree of increase or decrease are diagnostically significant. The percentage is the *relative* number of each type of leukocyte in the blood. The absolute count is obtained mathematically by multiplying the percentile value of one type of leukocyte by the total leukocyte count. Formula:

$$\begin{matrix}\text{Absolute value} \\ \text{WBC/mm}^3\end{matrix} = \begin{matrix}\text{Relative value} \\ (\%)\end{matrix} \times \begin{matrix}\text{Total WBC count} \\ (\text{cells/mm}^3)\end{matrix}$$

The differential count alone has limited value; it must always be interpreted in relation to the total leukocyte count. If the percentage of one type of cell is increased, it can be inferred that cells of that type are relatively more numerous than normal, but it is not known if this reflects an absolute decrease in cells of another type or an actual increase in the number of cells that are relatively increased. On the other hand, if the relative percentile values of the differential are known and if the total leukocyte count is known, it is possible to calculate absolute values that are not subject to misinterpretation.

SEGMENTED NEUTROPHILS (POLYMORPHONUCLEAR NEUTROPHILS, PMNS, "SEGS," OR "POLYS") ●

Normal Values

50%–60% of total white cell count
3000–7000/mm^3 absolute count
0%–3% of the total count of stabs or band cells

Background

Neutrophils, the most numerous and important type of white cells in the body's reaction to inflammation, constitute a primary defense against microbial invasion through the process of phagocytosis. These cells can also cause some body tissue damage by their release of enzymes and endogenous pyrogenes. In their immature stage of development, neutrophils are referred to as "stab" or "band" cells. The term *band* stems from the appearance of the nucleus that has not assumed the lobed shape of the mature cell.

Explanation of Test

This test determines the presence of neutrophilia or neutropenia. Neutrophilia is the increase of the absolute number of neutrophils in response to invading organisms and tumor cells. Neutropenia occurs when too few neutrophils are produced in the marrow, too many stored in the blood vessel margin, or too many have been called into action and have been used up.

Procedure

Obtain a 7-ml blood sample in EDTA coagulant. Count as part of the differential.

Clinical Implications

1. *Neutrophilia* (increased absolute number and percentage of neutrophils; > 8000/mm^3 > 0% neutrophils) occurs in
   - **a.** Acute, localized and general bacterial infections
   - **b.** Inflammation (eg, rheumatic fever [RA], acute gout)
   - **c.** Intoxications: metabolic (eg, gout and uremia) and poisoning by chemicals and drugs
   - **d.** Acute hemorrhage

   - **e.** Acute hemolysis of RBCs
   - **f.** Myeloproliferative diseases (eg, myelogenous leukemia)
   - **g.** Tissue necrosis due to myocardiainfarction, tumors, burns, gangrene, carcinoma, or sarcoma
   - **h.** Some viral and rickettsial diseases

2. Segmented neutrophils/band neutrophils ratio: normally 1% to 3% of neutrophils are *band* forms (immature neutrophils).
   - **a.** Degenerative shift to left: in some overwhelming infections, there is an increase in band (immature) forms with no leukocytosis (poor prognosis).
   - **b.** Regenerative shift to left: increased band (immature) forms with leukocytes (good prognosis) in bacterial infections.
   - **c.** Shift to the right: few band (immature) cells with increased segmented neutrophils can occur in liver disease, megaloblastic anemia, hemolysis, drugs, cancer, and allergies.
   - **d.** Hypersegmentation of neutrophils with no band (immature) cells are found in megaloblastic anemias (eg, pernicious anemia [PA] and chronic morphine addiction).

3. Neutropenia (decreased absolute number of neutrophils) occurs in
   - **a.** Acute, overwhelming bacterial infections (poor prognosis)
   - **b.** Viral infections (eg, influenza, infectious hepatitis, mononucleosis)
   - **c.** Rickettsial diseases, some parasitic diseases (malaria)
   - **d.** Drugs, chemicals, toxic agents, and radiation
   - **e.** Blood diseases (eg, aplastic and pernicious anemia, acute lymphoblastic leukemia)
   - **f.** Hormonal disorders (eg, Addison's disease, thyrotoxicosis, acromegaly)
   - **g.** Anaphylactic shock
   - **h.** Hypersplenism
   - **i.** Liver disease

4. See the table entitled Leukocyte Abnormalities and Diseases.

Interfering Factors

1. Physiologic conditions such as stress, excitement, and exercise temporarily cause increased neutrophils.

2. Obstetric labor and delivery: neutrophilia.

3. Steroid administration: neutrophilia peaks in 4 to 6 hours and returns to normal in 24 hours (in severe infection, expected neutrophilia does not occur).

4. Exposure to extreme heat or cold.

5. Age
   - **a.** Children respond to infection with a greater degree of neutrophilic leukocytosis than adults.
   - **b.** Some elderly patients respond weakly or not at all, even when the infection is severe.

Leukocyte Abnormalities and Diseases

Abnormality	*Description*	*Associated Diseases*
Toxic granulation	Coarse black or purple cytoplasmic granules	Infections or inflammatory diseases
Döhle bodies	Small (1–2 μm) blue cytoplasmic inclusions in neutrophils	Infections or inflammatory diseases, burns, myelocytic leukemia, myeloproliferative syndromes, cyclophosphamide therapy
Pelger–Huet anomalies	Neutrophil with bilobed nucleus or no segmentation of nucleus. Chromatin is coarse and cytoplasm is pink with normal granulation.	Hereditary, myelocytic leukemias, myeloproliferative syndromes
May–Hegglin anomaly	Basophilic, cytoplasmic inclusions of leukocytes; similar to Döhle bodies	May–Hegglin syndrome (hereditary), includes thrombocytopenia and giant platelets.
Alder's anomaly	Prominent azurophilic granulation in leukocytes; similar to toxic granulation; granulation is seen better with Giemsa stain.	Hereditary, gargoylism
Chédiak–Higashi anomaly	Gray-green, large cytoplasmic inclusions resembling Döhle bodies	Chédiak–Higashi syndrome
LE (lupus erythematosus) cells	Neutrophilic leukocyte with a *homogenous* red-purple inclusion that distends the cell's cytoplasm.	Lupus erythematosus and other collagen diseases, chronic hepatitis, drug reactions, serum sickness

Tart cell	Neutrophilic leukocyte with a phagocytosed nucleus of a granulocyte that retains some nuclear structure	Drug reactions (eg, penicillin, procainamide)
Myeloid "shift to left"	Presence of bands, myelocytes, metamyelocytes, or promyelocytes	Infections, intoxications, tissue necrosis, myeloproliferative syndrome, leukemia (chronic myelocytic), leukemoid reaction, pernicious anemia, hyposplenism
Hypersegmented neutrophil	Mature neutrophil with more than 5 distinct lobes	Megaloblastic anemia, hereditary constitutional hypersegmentation of neutrophils; rarely, iron-deficiency anemia; malignancy, or infection
Leukemic cells (lymphoblasts, myeloblasts, etc.)	Presence of lymphoblasts, myeloblasts, monoblasts, myelomonoblasts, promyelocytes (none normally present in peripheral blood)	Leukemia (acute or chronic), leukemoid reaction, severe infectious or inflammatory diseases, myeloproliferative syndrome, intoxications, malignancies, recovery from bone marrow suppression; infectious mononucleosis, myelophthisis
Auer bodies	Rodlike, 1–4 to 6-μm long, red-purple, refractile inclusions in neutrophils	Acute myelocytic leukemia
Smudge cell	Disintegrating nucleus of a ruptured white cell	Increased numbers in leukemic blood, particularly in CML or CLL when WBC count is greater than 100,000/mm^3

6. Resistance
   a. People of any age who are weak and debilitated may fail to respond with a significant neutrophilia.
   b. When an infection becomes overwhelming, the patient's resistance is exhausted and, as death approaches, the number of neutrophils decreases greatly.
7. Myelosuppressive chemotherapy

Patient Preparation

1. Explain test purpose and procedure.
2. Refer to standard *pretest* care for hemogram, CBC, and differential on page 32. Also, see Chapter 1 guidelines for safe, effective, informed *pretest* care

Patient Aftercare

1. Interpret test outcomes and monitor appropriately for neutrophilia or neutropenia.

> **Clinical Alert**
>
> Agranulocytosis (marked neutropenia and leukopenia) is extremely dangerous and is often fatal because the body is unprotected against invading agents. Patients with agranulocytosis must be protected from infection by means of reverse isolation techniques with strictest emphasis on handwashing technique.

2. Refer to standard *posttest* care for hemogram, CBC, and differential on page 32. Also, follow Chapter 1 guidelines for safe, effective, informed *posttest* care.

EOSINOPHILS

Normal Values

1%–4% of total leukocyte count (relative value), or
50–250/mm^3 (absolute value) or 50–250 × 10^6/L

Background

Eosinophils, capable of phagocytosis, ingest antigen–antibody complexes and become active in the later stages of inflammation. Eosinophils are not bactericidal but do respond to allergic and parasitic diseases.

Explanation of Test

This test is used to diagnose allergic infections, severity of infestations with worms and other large parasites, and monitor the response to treatment.

Procedure

1. Obtain a 7-ml blood sample in EDTA anticoagulant.
2. Note the time the blood sample is obtained (eg, 3:00 PM).
3. A manual WBC is performed, 100 cells counted, and the percentage of eosinophils is reported.
4. An absolute eosinophile count is also available, done with a special eosinophile stain.

Clinical Implications

1. *Eosinophilia:* an increase of circulating eosinophils greater than 5% or more than 500/mm^3 occurs in
   a. Allergies, hay fever, asthma, drug reactions
   b. Parasitic disease and trichinosis tapeworm, especially with tissue invasion
   c. Addison's disease
   d. Hodgkin's disease and lymphoma, myeloproliferative disorders
   e. Chronic skin diseases (eg, psoriasis, pemphigus, scabies)
   f. systemic eosinophilia associated with pulmonary infiltration
   g. Some infections (scarlet fever, chlamydia)
   h. Familial eosinophilia (rare), hypereosinic syndrome
   i. Polyarteritis nodosa, SLE, collagen diseases, connective tissue disorders
   j. Gastrointestinal diseases (eg, ulcerative colitis, Crohn's disease)
   k. Immunodeficiency disorders (Wiskott–Aldrich syndrome)
   l. Malignant tumors, Hodgkin's disease, T-cell leukemia
   m. Many drug reactions
2. *Eosinopenia* (a decrease in the amount of circulating eosinophils) is usually due to an increased adrenal steroid production that accompanies most conditions of bodily stress and is associated with:
   a. Cushing's syndrome
   b. Use of certain drugs such as ACTH, epinephrine, thyroxine, prostaglandins
   c. Infections with neutrophilia
3. Eosinophils disappear early in pyogenic infections where there is a leukocytosis with a marked shift to the left (increase in immature white cells).
4. *Eosinophilic myelocytes* are counted separately because they have a greater significance, being found only in leukemia or leukemoid blood pictures.

Interfering Factors

1. Hourly rhythm: The normal eosinophil count is lowest in the morning, then rises from noon until after midnight. For this reason, serial eosinophil counts should be repeated at the same time each day.
2. Stressful situations, such as in burns, postoperative states, lupus erythematosus, electroshock, eclampsia, and labor will cause a decreased count.

Patient Preparation

1. Explain test purpose and procedure.
2. Refer to standard patient care for hemogram, CBC, and differential on page 32. Also, see Chapter 1 guidelines for safe, effective, informed *pretest* care.

Patient Aftercare

1. Interpret test outcomes and monitor appropriately.
2. Use special precautions if patient is receiving steroid therapy, epinephrine, thyroxine, or prostaglandins. Eosinophilia can be masked by steroid use; infections can be fatal. (It is not clear why eosinophils disappear promptly from the blood following injection of ACTH.)
3. Refer to standard *posttest* care for hemogram, CBC, and differential on page 32. Also, see Chapter 1 guidelines for safe, effective, informed *posttest* care.

BASOPHILS ●

Normal Values

0.5%–1.0% of the total leukocyte count, or 25–100/mm^3

Background

Basophils constitute a small percentage of the total leukocyte count, are considered phagocytic, and contain heparin, histamines, and serotonin. Tissue basophils are also called *mast* cells; similar to blood basophils, they store and produce heparin, histamine, and serotonin. Normally, mast cells are not found in peripheral blood and are rarely seen in healthy bone marrow.

Explanation of Test

Basophil counts are used to study allergic reactions. There is a positive correlation between high basophil counts and high concentrations of blood histamines, although this correlation does not imply cause and effect.

Procedure

Obtain a 7-ml blood sample in EDTA and count as part of the differential.

Clinical Implications

1. *Increased count* (basophilia) is associated most commonly with granulocytic and basophilic leukemia, myeloid metaplasia, and Hodgkin's disease
2. It is less commonly associated with
   - **a.** Inflammation, allergy, or sinusitis
   - **b.** Polycythemia vera
   - **c.** Chronic hemolytic anemia
   - **d.** Following splenectomy
   - **e.** Following radiation
   - **f.** Endocrine problems (eg, myxedema, diabetes)
   - **g.** Infections, including tuberculosis, smallpox, chickenpox, influenza
   - **h.** Foreign protein ingestion

3. *Decreased count* (basopenia) associated with
   a. Acute phase of infection
   b. Hyperthyroidism
   c. Stress reactions (eg, myocardial infarction and bleeding, peptic ulcer, stress situations)
   d. Following prolonged steroid therapy
   e. Hereditary absence of basophils
4. *Presence of numbers of tissue mast cells* (tissue basophils) is associated with
   a. Rheumatoid arthritis
   b. Urticaria, asthma
   c. Anaphylactic shock
   d. Hypoadrenalism
   e. Lymphoma
   f. Macroglobulinemia
   g. Mast cell leukemia
   h. Lymphoma invading bone marrow
   i. Urticaria pigmentosa
   j. Asthma
   k. Chronic liver and renal disease
   l. Osteoporosis
   m. Systemic mastocytosis
5. Refer to standard hemogram, CBC, and differential *pre-* and *posttest* on page 32.

MONOCYTES (MONOMORPHONUCLEAR MONOCYTES)

Normal Values
2%–6% of total leukocyte count, or 100–600/mm^3

Background
These agranulocytes, the largest cells of normal blood, are the body's second line of defense against infection. Histiocytes, which are large macrophagic phagocytes, are classified as *monocytes* in a differential leukocyte count. Histiocytes and monocytes are capable of reversible transformation from one to the other.

These phagocytic cells, of varying size and mobility, remove injured and dead cells, microorganisms, and insoluble particles from the circulating blood. Monocytes escaping from the upper and lower respiratory tracts and the gastrointestinal and genitourinary organs perform a scavenger function, clearing the body of debris. These phagocytic cells produce the antiviral agent *interferon.*

Explanation of Test
This test counts monocytes that circulate in certain specific conditions, such as tuberculosis, leprosy, lipid storage disease, and subacute bacterial endocarditis (infectious leukocytosis).

Procedure
Obtain a 7-ml blood sample in EDTA and count as part of differential.

Clinical Implications
1. *Monocytosis:* a monocyte increase in > 800/mm^3 occurs in

a. Monocytic leukemia, other leukemias
b. Myeloproliferative disorders, such as multiple myeloma
c. Hodgkin's disease and other lymphomas
d. Recovery state of acute infections (favorable sign)
e. Lipid storage diseases
f. Some parasitic and rickettsia diseases
g. Certain bacterial diseases, as tuberculosis and subacute endocarditis
h. Chronic ulcerative colitis, enteritis, and sprue
i. Collagen diseases and sarcoidosis

2. Phagocytic monocytes (macrophages) may be found in small numbers in the blood in many conditions:
   a. Severe infections
   b. Lupus erythematosus
   c. Hemolytic anemias
   d. Agranulocytosis
   e. Thrombocytopenic purpura
3. *Decreased monocyte count* (not usually identified with specific diseases)
   a. Prednisone treatment
   b. Hairy cell leukemia
   c. Rheumatoid arthritis
   d. HIV infection

Patient Preparation

1. Explain test purpose and procedure.
2. Refer to standard hemogram, CBC, and differential *pretest* care on page 32. Also, see Chapter 1 guidelines for safe, effective, informed *pretest* care.

Patient Aftercare

1. Interpret test outcomes and monitor appropriately for leukemia and infection.
2. Refer to standard hemogram, CBC, and differential *posttest* care on page 32. Also, follow Chapter 1 guidelines for safe, effective, informed *posttest* care.

LYMPHOCYTES (MONOMORPHONUCLEAR LYMPHOCYTES) ●

Normal Values

20%–40% of total leukocyte count (relative value), or 1000–4000/mm^3

Background

These agranulocytes are small, motile cells that migrate to areas of inflammation in both the early and late stages of the process. They are the source of serum immunoglobulins and of cellular immune response, and they play an important role in immunologic reactions. All lymphocytes are manufactured in the bone marrow. (The B-cell lymphocyte matures there; other lymphocytes—T cells—mature in the thymus gland.) The B cells control the antigen–antibody response that is specific to the offending antigen and is said to have "memory." The T cells, the master immune cells, include the T_4 helper cells, killer cells, cytotic cells and suppressor T8 cells (see Chap. 8 for further tests of T cells).

Explanation of Test

This test measures the number of lymphocytes in the peripheral blood. Relative lymphocytosis is present in various diseases and is especially prominent in disorders with neutropenia.

Procedure

1. Obtain 7 ml of EDTA anticoagulated blood.
2. Lymphocytes are counted as part of the differential count.

Clinical Implications

1. *Lymphocytosis:* >4000 mm^3 in adults, >7200 mm^3 in children, and >9000 mm^3 in infants occurs in
   a. Lymphatic leukemia: acute and chronic lymphoma
   b. Infectious lymphocytosis (occurs mainly in children)
   c. Infectious mononucleosis
      (1) Caused by Epstein–Barr virus
      (2) Most common in adolescents and young adults
      (3) Characterized by atypical lymphocytes—Downey cells—large, deeply indented, with deep blue (basophilic) cytoplasm
      (4) Differential diagnosis: positive heterophil test
   d. Other viral diseases
      (1) Upper respiratory
      (2) Cytomegalovirus
      (3) Measles
      (4) Mumps
      (5) Chickenpox
      (6) Infectious hepatitis
      (7) Toxoplasmosis
   e. Some bacterial diseases, such as tuberculosis, brucellosis, and pertussis
   f. Crohn's disease, ulcerative colitis
   g. Serum sickness, drug hypersensitivity
   h. Hypoadrenalism
   i. Hypothyroidism (Graves' disease)
2. *Lymphopenia*—$<1000/\text{mm}^3$, adults; $<2500/\text{mm}^3$, children—occurs in
   a. Chemotherapy, radiation treatment (immunosuppressive medications
   b. After administration of ACTH and cortisone (steroids) and ACTH-producing pituitary tumors
   c. Increased loss through GI tract owing to obstruction of lymphatic drainage (eg, tumor, Whipple's disease, intestinal lymphectasia)
   d. Aplastic anemia
   e. Hodgkin's disease and other malignancies
   f. Inherited immune disorders, acquired immunodeficiency syndrome (AIDS), and AIDS—immune dysfunction
   g. Far advanced tuberculosis
   h. Severe debilitating illness of any kind
   i. Congestive heart failure
   j. Renal failure

Abnormal Lymphocytes

Abnormality	*Description*	*Associated Diseases*
Atypical lymphocytes Reactive lymphocytes "Downey" cells	Lymphocytes, some with vacuolated cytoplasm, irregularly shaped nucleus, increased numbers of cytoplasmic azurophilic granules, peripheral basophilia, or some with more abundant basophilic cytoplasm	Infectious mononucleosis, viral hepatitis, and other viral infections, tuberculosis, drug (eg, penicillin) sensitivity, posttransfusion syndrome

Patient Preparation

1. Explain test purpose and procedure.
2. Refer to standard hemogram, CBC, and differential *pretest* care on page 32. Also, see Chapter 1 guidelines for safe, effective, informed *pretest* care.

Patient Aftercare

Clinical Alert

A decreased lymphocyte count of fewer than 500/mm^3 means that a patient is dangerously susceptible to infection, especially viral infections. *Institute measures to protect patient from infection.*

1. Interpret test outcomes and monitor appropriately for lymphocytosis or lymphopenia.
2. Refer to standard hemogram, CBC, and differential *posttest* care on page 32. Also, follow Chapter 1 guidelines for safe, effective, informed *posttest* care.

● STAINS FOR LEUKEMIA

Several special WBC-staining methods are used to diagnose leukemia, amyloid disease, lymphoma, erythroleukemia, differentiate erythema myelosis from sideroblastic anemia, monitor progress, response to therapy, and detect early relapse. Amyloid refers to starchlike substances deposited in certain diseases (eg, tuberculosis, osteomyelitis, leprosy, Hodgkin's disease, and carcinoma).

SUDAN BLACK B (SBB) STAIN

Normal Values
Lymophocytes do not stain; granulocytes and monocytes do stain.

Clinical Implications
Positive staining of primitive (blast) cells indicates myelogenous origin of cells. SBB is positive in acute granulocytic leukemia. SBB is negative in acute lymphocytic leukemia and plasma cell leukemia. SBB is weakly positive for monocytes and platelets.

Procedure
Obtain bone marrow aspirate. Prepare slide, stain with SBB, and scan microscopically. Use normal smear as contrast.

PERIODIC ACID–SCHIFF (PAS) STAIN

Normal Values
Negative in presence of lymphoblasts and megaloblasts.

Clinical Implications
PAS is positive in acute lymphocytic leukemia (Large blocks of PAS-positive material), erythroleukemia, severe iron-deficiency anemia, thalassemia, amyloidosis, strongly positive lymphocytes in the circulatory blood suggest malignant lymphomas, in Hodgkin's and non-Hodgkin's lymphoma and infectious mononucleosis, megakaryocytic leukemia, acute monocytic leukemia—discrete, small granules are positive in hairy cell leukemia.

Procedure
Obtain bone marrow aspirate. Prepare slide, stain with PAS and scan microscopically.

TERMINAL DEOXYNUCLEOTIDYL TRANSFERASE (TDT) STAIN

Normal Values
0%–2% in bone marrow; negative in peripheral blood or lymph nodes.

Clinical Implications
TDT is positive in acute lymphocytic leukemia, lymphoblastic lymphoma, chronic myelogenous leukemia—"blast crisis," acute undifferentiated leukemia.

Procedure
Heparinized blood (10 ml) or EDTA anticoagulated bone marrow aspirate (2 ml). Glass slides are dried, stored at room temperature for up to 5 days, processed, and stained.

LEUKOCYTE ALKALINE PHOSPHATASE (LAP) STAIN ●

Normal Values

30–130 LAP units.

Clinical Implications

Decreased LPA values range from 0 to 13, meaning that none or little alkaline phosphatase activity is demonstrable. Chronic granulocytic anemia, paroxysmal nocturnal hemoglobinuria, aplastic anemia, cirrhosis of the liver, hereditary hypophosphatasia, diabetes mellitus, idopathic thrombocytopenic purpura, and sideroblastic anemia. LAP values are above normal in neutrophilic leukemoid reactions. (A leukemoid reaction is a higher white count that looks like leukemia, but is not.) Polycythemia vera, thrombocytopenia, infection, myelofibrosis, pregnancy, steroid therapy, Down syndrome, "hairy" cell leukemia, Hodgkin's disease, multiple myeloma, and infections with elevated white count.

Procedure

Obtain specimen by capillary puncture: venous blood, EDTA, or bone marrow aspirate. Prepare smear and air-dry, stain with LAP.

TARTRATE-RESISTANT ACID PHOSPHATASE (TRAP) STAIN ●

Normal Values

No TRAP activity.

Clinical Implications

TRAP present in the leukemic cells of most patients with hairy cell leukemia (a disease primarily of older men), 5% of patients with otherwise typical hairy cell leukemia lack the enzyme. TRAP occasionally occurs in malignant cells of patients with lymphoproliferative disorders other than hairy cell leukemia. Histiocytes have weakly positive reactions.

Procedure

Obtain venous blood sample (5 ml) or capillary puncture. Blood smear is incubated with TRAP, counterstained and examined microscopically.

BUFFY COAT SMEAR ●

Normal Values

In health, the buffy coat of the blood contains normal white cell components, mononuclear cells, platelets, and metamyelocytes.

Clinical Implications

Abnormal cells may indicate: leukemia and infiltration of bone marrow by solid tumors or fibrosis.

Procedure

Obtain venous blood sample with EDTA coagulant. Finger stick may be done. White cells concentrate between red cell layer and plasma, known as "buffy" layer. Slide is stained and examined microscopically. Differential may be done.

Patient Preparation

1. Explain test purposes and procedures. If bone marrow aspiration is done, see pages 27 for special care.
2. See Chapter 1 guidelines for safe, effective, informed, *pretest* care.

Patient Aftercare

1. Interpret test outcomes, counsel and monitor appropriately for leukemia, amyloid disease, anemia, and infection.
2. Follow Chapter 1 guidelines for safe, effective, informed *posttest* care.

● RED BLOOD CELL TESTS

Many tests look at the red blood cells: their number, size, amount of hemoglobin, rate of production, percentage composition of the blood. The red blood cell count (RBC), hematocrit (HCT), and hemoglobin (Hb) are closely related but are different ways to look at the adequacy of red blood cell production. The same conditions cause respective rise and fall in each of these indicators.

RED BLOOD CELL COUNT (RBC; ERYTHROCYTE COUNT) ●

Normal Values

Men: 4.2–5.4 × 10^6/µl (average 4.8) or 4.2–5.4 × 10^{12}/L
Women: 3.6–5.0 × 10^6/µl (average 4.3) or 3.6–5.0 × 10^{12}/L

Age	*RBC × 10^6*
Birth–2 wk	4.1–6.1
2–8 wk	4.0–6.0
2–6 mo	3.8–5.6
6 mo–1 yr	3.8–5.2
1–6 yr	3.9–5.3
6–16 yr	4.0–5.2
16–18 yr	4.2–5.4
>18 yr (males)	4.5–5.5
>18 yr (females)	4.0–5.0

Background

The main function of the red blood cell (erythrocyte) is to carry oxygen from the lungs to the body tissue and to transfer carbon dioxide from the tissues to the lungs. This process is achieved by means of the *hemoglobin* (Hb) in the red cells that combines easily with oxygen and carbon dioxide and gives arterial blood a bright red appearance. Because venous blood has a low oxygen content, it appears dark red. To enable the maximum amount of hemoglobin to be used, the red cell is shaped like a biconcave disk, which affords more surface area for the hemoglobin to combine with oxygen. The cell is also able to change its shape when necessary to permit its passage through the smaller capillaries.

Explanation of Test

The RBC count, an important measurement in the determination of anemia or polycythemia, determines the total number of red blood cells or erythrocytes found in a cubic millimeter (mm^3) of blood.

Procedure

1. Obtain 7 ml of EDTA venous blood.
2. Automated electronic devices are generally used to determine the number of red blood cells.
3. Note patient age and time of day on laboratory slip.

Clinical Implications

1. *Decreased RBC Values* occur in
  a. Anemia, a condition in which there is a reduction in the number of circulating RBCs, in the amount of hemoglobin, or in the volume of packed cells (hematocrit), or a combination thereof.
    (1) Is associated with cell production and destruction, blood loss, dietary insufficiency of iron and certain vitamins that are essential in the production of RBCs. See pages 62, 63, and 64 for classification of anemias based on the underlying mechanisms of anemia and for the discussion of the purpose and the clinical implications of the reticulocyte count (pp 67–72).
    (2) Disorders such as
      (a) Hodgkin's disease and other lymphomas
      (b) Multiple myeloma, myeloproliferative disorders
      (c) Leukemia, especially occult
      (d) Lupus erythematosus
      (e) Addison's disease
      (f) Rheumatic fever
      (g) Subacute endocarditis
      (h) List is not meant to be all-inclusive.

Clinical Alert

Refer to pages 60 and 61 for a discussion of the composite of the clinical implications of decreased RBC count, hematocrit, and hemoglobin values (closely related, but different, ways to look at the adequacy of RBC production). The same underlying conditions will cause a *decrease* in each of these three tests of red blood cell production.

2. *Increased RBC values* or erythrocytosis in
   a. Primary erythrocytosis
      (1) Polycythemia vera (myeloproliferative disorder)
      (2) Erythrocytosis–erythremia (increased RBC production in bone marrow)
   b. Secondary erythrocytosis in
      (1) Renal disease
      (2) Extrarenal tumors
      (3) High altitude
      (4) Pulmonary disease
      (5) Cardiovascular disease
      (6) Alveolar hypoventilation
      (7) Hemoglobinopathy
      (8) Tobacco/carboxyhemoglobin
   c. Relative erythrocytosis (decrease in plasma volume)
      (1) Dehydration (vomiting, diarrhea)
      (2) Gaisbock's syndrome
      (3) Stress
      (4) Tobacco use
      (5) Overuse of diuretics

Clinical Alert

Please refer to page 60 for discussion of the combined clinical implications of *increased* RBC count, hematocrit, and hemoglobin values (as stated earlier, closely related, but different, ways to look at the adequacy of RBC production). The same underlying conditions will cause an *increase* in each of these three tests of red blood cell production.

Interfering Factors

1. Posture: When blood sample is obtained from a healthy person in a recumbent position, the count is lower than normal. (If the patient is anemic, the count will be even lower.)

2. Dehydration: Hemoconcentration in dehydrated adults, caused by severe burns, untreated intestinal obstruction, and severe, persistent vomiting, may obscure significant anemia.

3. Age: the normal RBC of a newborn is higher than that of an adult, with a rapid drop to the lowest point in life at 2 to 4 months. The normal adult level is reached at age 14 and is maintained until old age, when there is a gradual drop (see page 51).

4. Altitude: The higher the altitude, the greater the increase in RBC. Decreased oxygen content of the air stimulates the RBC to increase (erythrocytosis).
5. Pregnancy: There is a relative decrease in RBC when the body fluid increases in pregnancy, with the normal number of erythrocytes becoming more diluted.
6. There are *many* factors that may cause *reduced* RBCs. The drugs that may cause *increased* RBCs are gentamicin and methyldopa.
7. The blood sample tube EDTA must be three-fourths filled (at least, or values will be invalid).
8. The blood sample may not be clotted (even slightly) or the values will be invalid.

Patient Preparation

1. Explain test purpose and procedure.
2. Refer to standard hemogram, CBC, differential *pretest* care on page 32.
3. Have patient avoid extensive exercise, stress, or excitement preceding the test. This causes elevated counts of doubtful clinical value.
4. Avoid overhydration or dehydration if possible, which causes invalid results. If patient is receiving IV fluids, note on requisition.
5. Note any medications patient is taking.
6. See Chapter 1 guidelines for safe, effective, informed *pretest* care.

Patient Aftercare

1. Interpret test outcomes and monitor appropriately for anemia and erythrocytosis.
2. Refer to standard hemogram, CBC, differential *posttest* care on page 32. See Chapter 1 guidelines for safe, effective, informed *posttest* care.
3. Resume normal activities and diet.

HEMATOCRIT(HCT); **PACKED CELL VOLUME** (PCV) ●

Normal Values

	Percentage
ADULT	
Female	36–48
Male	42–52
CHILDREN	
0–2 wk	44–64
2–8 wk	39–59
2–6 mo	35–49
6 mo–1 yr	29–43
1–6 yr	30–40
6–16 yr	32–42
16–18 yr	34–44

NOTE: *If blood is drawn from a capillary puncture and a microhematocrit done, values are slightly lower.*

Background
The word *hematocrit* means "to separate blood," which underscores the mechanism of the test, because the plasma and blood cells are separated by centrifugation.

Explanation of Test
Hematocrit is part of the complete blood count. This test determines red blood cell mass. The results are expressed as the percentage of packed red cells in a volume of whole blood. It is an important measurement in the determination of anemia or polycythemia.

Procedure
1. When doing a capillary puncture (finger puncture), the microcapillary tube is three-fourths filled with blood, directly from puncture site. These tubes are coated with an anticoagulant.
2. The tubes are centrifuged in a microcentrifuge and the height of packed cells is measured.
3. The measurement is recorded as a percentage of the total amount of blood in the capillary tube.
4. A hematocrit can be done on the automated hematology instruments, in which case a 7-ml anticoagulated venous blood sample is obtained.

Clinical Implications
1. *Decreased hematocrit values* are an indicator of anemia, a condition in which there is a reduction in the hematocrit (volume of packed cells), amount of hemoglobin, and the number of circulating RBCs. A hematocrit of 30 or less means the patient is moderately to severely anemic. This also occurs in
   - **a.** Leukemia
   - **b.** Hyperthyroidism
   - **c.** Cirrhosis
   - **d.** Acute, massive blood loss
   - **e.** Hemolytic reaction—this condition may be found in transfusion of incompatible blood, or as a reaction to chemicals or drugs, infectious agents, or physical agents (eg, severe burn or prosthetic heart valves)
2. The hematocrit may or may not be reliable immediately after even a moderate loss of blood and immediately after transfusions. However, HCT is a good indicator of how much blood has been lost up to the time the blood sample is obtained.
3. Hematocrit may be normal following acute hemorrhage. During the recovery phase, the HCT and RBC will drop markedly.
4. Usually, the HCT parallels the RBC when the cells are of a normal size. As the number of normal-sized erythrocytes increases, so does the HCT.

a. However, for the patient with microcytic or macrocytic anemia, this relationship does not hold true.
b. If a patient has an iron-deficiency anemia with small red cells, the HCT decreases because the microcytic cells pack to a smaller volume. The RBC, however, may be normal.

> **Clinical Alert**
>
> Please refer to pages 60–61 for a discussion of the combined clinical implications of *decreased* hematocrit, hemoglobin, and RBC count (closely related, but different ways to look at the adequacy of RBC production. The same underlying conditions will cause a *decrease* in each of these three tests' values).

5. *Increased hematocrit* occurs in polycythemia, an increase in the number of RBCs that is based upon the HCT and hemoglobin values, and also in
a. Erythrocytosis
b. Severe dehydration
c. Shock, when hemoconcentrates rise considerably

Interfering Factors

1. People living in high altitudes will have high HCT values, the same as in Hb and RBC.
2. Normally, the value slightly decreases in the physiologic hydremia of pregnancy.
3. The normal values for the HCT vary with the age and sex of the individual. The normal value for infants is higher because the newborn has many macrocytic red cells. Hematocrits in females are usually slightly lower than in males.
4. There is also a tendency toward lower values in men and women after age 60, corresponding to lower values for erythrocyte counts in this age group.

Patient Preparation

1. Explain test purpose and procedure.
2. Refer to standard *pretest* care for hemogram, CBC and differential. Also, see Chapter 1 guidelines for safe, effective, informed *pretest* care.

> **Clinical Alert**
>
> Hematocrit of < 20.0% can lead to cardiac failure and death.
> Hematocrit of > 60% is associated with spontaneous clotting of blood.

Patient Aftercare

1. Interpret test results and monitor for anemia or polycythemia.
2. Refer to RBC/hemogram standard *posttest* care for hemogram, CBC, and RBC. Also, follow Chapter 1 guidelines for safe, effective, informed *posttest* care.

HEMOGLOBIN (Hb) ●

Normal Values

Adult	
Female	12.0–16.0 g/dl, or 1.86–2.48 nmol/L
Male	14.0–17.4 g/dl
Children	
0–2 wk	14.5–24.5 g/dl
2–8 wk	12.5–20.5 g/dl
2–6 mo	10.7–17.3 g/dl
6 mo–1 yr	9.9–14.5 g/dl
1–6 yr	9.5–14.1 g/dl
6–16 yr	10.3–14.9 g/dl
16–18 yr	11.1–15.7 g/dl

Background

Hemoglobin, the main component of erythrocytes, serves as the vehicle for the transportation of oxygen and carbon dioxide. It is composed of amino acids that form a single protein called *globin,* and a compound called *heme,* which contains iron atoms and the red pigment porphyrin. The iron pigment is that portion of the hemoglobin that combines readily with oxygen and gives blood its characteristic red color. Each gram of hemoglobin can carry 1.34 ml of oxygen. The oxygen-combining capacity of the blood is directly proportional to the hemoglobin concentration, rather than to the number of RBC, because some red cells contain more hemoglobin than others. This is why hemoglobin determinations are important in the evaluation of anemia.

Hemoglobin also serves as an important buffer in the extracellular fluid. In tissue, the oxygen concentration is lower, and the carbon dioxide level and hydrogen ion concentration are higher. At a lower pH, more oxygen dissociates from hemoglobin. The unoxygenated hemoglobin binds to hydrogen ions, thus raising the pH. As carbon dioxide diffuses into the red cell, carbonic anhydrase converts carbon dioxide to bicarbonate and protons. As the protons are bound to hemoglobin, the bicarbonate ions leave the cell. For every bicarbonate ion leaving the cell, a chloride ion enters. The efficiency of this buffer system depends on the ability of carbon dioxide or bicarbonate to be eliminated in the lungs and kidneys, respectively.

Explanation of Test

Hemoglobin determination is part of a complete blood count. It screens for disease associated with anemia, determines the severity of anemia, follows the response to treatment for anemia, and evaluates polycythemia.

Procedure

1. A venous blood EDTA sample of 7 ml is obtained. The Vacutainer tube must be filled at least three-fourths full. Automated electronic devices are generally used to determine the Hb value; however, a manual colorimetric procedure is also widely used.
2. The blood sample must not be clotted or results are invalid.

Clinical Implications

1. *Decreased levels of hemoglobin* are found in anemia states (a condition in which there is a reduction of hemoglobin, hematocrit, and/or RBC numbers). It is difficult to say explicitly which hemoglobin level represents the presence of anemia *per se* because of the variable adaptability and efficiency of the body in response to blood hemoglobin concentrations. This level must be evaluated along with the erythrocyte count and the hematocrit.
   - **a.** Hyperthyroidism
   - **b.** Cirrhosis of the liver
   - **c.** Severe hemorrhage
   - **d.** Hemolytic reactions caused by
     - **(1)** Transfusions of incompatible blood
     - **(2)** Reactions to chemicals and drugs
     - **(3)** Reactions to infectious agents
     - **(4)** Reactions to physical agents (severe burns and artificial heart valves)
     - **(5)** Various systemic diseases:
       - **(a)** Hodgkin's disease
       - **(b)** Leukemia
       - **(c)** Lymphoma
       - **(d)** Systemic lupus erythematosus
       - **(e)** Carcinomatosis
       - **(f)** Sarcoidosis
       - **(g)** Renal cortical necrosis
       - **(h)** List is not meant to be all-inclusive

Clinical Alert

Please refer to pages 60–61 for a discussion of the combined clinical implications of *decreased* hemoglobin, hematocrit, and RBC count (closely related, but different, ways to look at the adequacy of RBC production. The same underlying conditions will cause a *decrease* in each of these test values).

2. *Increased levels of hemoglobin* are found in hemoconcentration of the

blood (any condition such as polycythemia and severe burns in which the number of circulating erythrocytes rises above normal)
   - **a.** Chronic obstructive pulmonary disease
   - **b.** Congestive heart failure
   - **c.** Polycythemia vera
3. *Variance in levels of hemoglobin*
   - **a.** Occurs after transfusions, hemorrhages, burns (Hb and HCT are both high during and immediately after hemorrhage).
   - **b.** Hemoglobin and HCT give valuable information in an emergency situation if interpreted not in an isolated fashion, but in conjunction with other pertinent laboratory data. Keep in mind that there are very few tests in laboratory medicine that can be considered diagnostic all on their own.

> **Clinical Alert**
>
> Please refer to page 60 for a discussion of the combined clinical implications of an *increased* hemoglobin, *increased* hematocrit, and *increased* RBC numbers (closely related tests done to determine the RBC mass).

Interfering Factors

1. People living at high altitudes will have increased values, just as in hematocrit values.
2. Excessive fluid intake will cause a decreased value.
3. Normally, the value is higher in infants before active erythropoiesis begins.
4. Hemoglobin levels are normally decreased in pregnancy.
5. Drugs that may cause *increased* levels of hemoglobin include gentamicin and methyldopa.
6. There are many drugs that may cause *decreased* levels of hemoglobin.

Patient Preparation

1. Explain test purpose and procedure. Assess medication history.
2. Refer to standard *pretest* care for hemogram, CBC, and differential. Also, see Chapter 1 guidelines for safe, effective, informed *pretest* care.

Patient Aftercare

1. Interpret test results and monitor appropriately.

> **Clinical Alert**
>
> The panic hemoglobin value is <5.0 g/dl, which leads to heart failure and death. A value higher than 20 g/dl leads to clogging of capillaries owing to hemoconcentration.

2. Refer to standard *posttest* care for hemogram, CBC, and differential. Also, follow Chapter 1 guidelines for safe, effective, informed *posttest* care.

Clinical Implications of Polycythemia, Increased RBC Count, Hematocrit, or Hemoglobin Values

A. *Polycythemia* is the term used to describe an abnormal increase in the number of red blood cells. Although there are several tests to determine the red blood cell mass, these tests are expensive and somewhat cumbersome. For screening purposes, we rely on the hematocrit and hemoglobin to evaluate polycythemia.

B. *Classification of polycythemias*

- **1.** Relative: an increase in hemoglobin, hematocrit or RBCs caused by a decrease in the plasma volume (eg, dehydration and spurious [stress or smoker] erythrocytosis)
- **2.** Absolute or true polycythemia
  - **a.** Primary (eg, polycythemia vera, erythremia or erythrocytosis)
  - **b.** Secondary
    - **(1)** Appropriate: an appropriate bone marrow response to physiological conditions
      - **(a)** Altitude
      - **(b)** Cardiopulmonary disorder
      - **(c)** Increased affinity for oxygen
    - **(2)** Inappropriate: an overproduction of red cells not necessary to deliver oxygen to the tissues
      - **(a)** Renal tumor or cyst
      - **(b)** Hepatoma
      - **(c)** Cerebellar hemangioblastoma

Clinical Implications of Anemia, Decreased RBC Count, Hematocrit, and Hemoglobin Values

A. *Anemia* is the term used to describe a condition in which there is a reduction in the number of circulating RBCs, the amount of hemoglobin, or the volume of packed cells (hematocrit), or any combination thereof. A pathophysiologic classification of anemia based on the underlying mechanisms of anemias follows. Anemias are further explained on pages 62–64.

B. *Classification of anemias*

- **1.** Hypoproliferative anemias occur with inadequate production of red blood cells
  - **a.** Marrow aplasias
  - **b.** Myelophthisic anemia
  - **c.** Anemia with blood dyscrasias
  - **d.** Anemia of chronic disease
  - **e.** Anemia with organ failure
- **2.** Maturation defect anemias
  - **a.** Cytoplasmic: hypochromic anemias
  - **b.** Nuclear: megaloblastic anemias
  - **c.** Combined: myelodysplastic syndromes

3. Hyperproliferative anemias occur with decrease in the hemoglobin or hematocrit, in spite of an increased production of RBCs.
   a. Hemorrhagic: acute blood loss
   b. Hemolytic: a premature accelerated destruction of the RBCs
      (1) Immune hemolysis
      (2) Primary membrane
      (3) Hemoglobinopathies
      (4) Hypersplenism
      (5) Enzymopathies
      (6) Toxic hemolysis: physical–chemical
      (7) Traumatic or microangiopathic hemolysis
      (8) Parasitic infections
4. Dilutional anemias
   a. Pregnancy
   b. Splenomegaly

RED BLOOD CELL INDICES

Background
These indices define the size and hemoglobin content of the red blood cell and consist of the mean corpuscular volume (MCV), mean corpuscular hemoglobin (MCH), and mean corpuscular hemoglobin concentration (MCHC).

Explanation of Tests
The red blood cell indices are used in differentiating anemias. When these are used together with an examination of the red cells on the stained smear, a clear picture of red cell morphology may be ascertained. On the basis of the red blood cell indices, the erythrocytes can be characterized as normal in every respect, or as abnormal in volume or hemoglobin content. In deficient states, the anemias can be classified by cell size as macrocytic, normocytic, simple microcytic, or by cell size and color as microcytic hypochromic. An explanation of each individual measurement follows.

Patient Preparation for MCV, MCH, MCHC
1. Explain purpose and procedure for testing. Assess for possible causes of anemia. No fasting is required.
2. See Chapter 1 guidelines for safe, effective, informed *pretest* care.

Patient Aftercare for MCV, MCH, MCHC
1. Interpret test results and monitor appropriately for anemia. Counsel appropriately for proper diet, medication, related hormone and enzyme problems, and genetically linked disorders.
2. Follow Chapter 1 guidelines for safe, effective, informed *posttest* care.

MEAN CORPUSCULAR VOLUME (MCV)

Normal Values
82–98 femto liters (fl) or μm^3 (higher values in infants and newborns)

Explanation of Test

Individual cell size is the best index for classifying anemias. This index expresses the volume occupied by a single red cell and is a measure in cubic microns (μm^3) of the mean volume. The MCV indicates whether the red blood cell size appears normal (normocytic), smaller (microcytic), or larger (macrocytic) if the MCV is less than 87 μm^3, the red cells are microcytic; if the MCV is greater than 103 μm^3, the red cells are macrocytic; if the MCV is within the normal range, the red blood cells are normocytic.

Procedure

The volume of the red blood cells is calculated from the red blood cell counts (the number of cells per cubic millimeter of blood) and from the hematocrit (the proportion of the blood occupied by the red blood cells) and is expressed as percentage. Formula:

$$\text{MCV} = \frac{\text{HCT }\% \times 10}{\text{RBC } (10^{12}/\text{L})}$$

Clinical Implications

The MCV results are the basis of classification used in the evaluation of an anemia. The following categorizations aid in the orderly investigation:

Anemias Characterized by Deficient Hemoglobin Synthesis
Hypochromic Erythrocytes (RBCs) (MCV 50–82 fl)
DISORDERS OF IRON METABOLISM Iron-deficiency anemia: the most prevalent worldwide cause of anemia. The major causes of iron deficiency are dietary inadequacy, malabsorption, increased iron loss, and increased iron requirements. Anemia of chronic disease, hereditary atransferrinemia Congenital hypochromic–microcytic anemia with iron overload (Shahidi–Nathan–Diamond syndrome)
DISORDERS OF PORPHYRIN AND HEME SYNTHESIS Acquired sideroblastic anemias Idiopathic refractory sideroblastic anemia, complicating other diseases associated with drugs or toxin (ethanol, INH, lead) Hereditary sideroblastic anemias X chromosome-linked, autosomal
DISORDERS OF GLOBIN SYNTHESIS The thalassemias, hemoglobinopathies, characterized by unstable hemoglobins

(continued)

Anemias Characterized by Deficient Hemoglobin Synthesis *(continued)*

Normocytic Normochromic Anemias (MCV 82–98 µm³) or fl

ANEMIA WITH APPROPRIATE BONE MARROW RESPONSE

Acute posthemmorhagic anemia

Hemolytic anemia (may be macrocytic when there is pronounced reticulocytosis)

ANEMIA WITH IMPAIRED MARROW RESPONSE

Marrow Hypoplasia

Aplastic anemia, pure red cell aplasia

Marrow Infiltration

Infiltration by malignant cells, myelofibrosis, inherited storage diseases

Decreased Erythropoietin Production

Kidney and liver disease, endocrine deficiencies, malnutrition, anemia of chronic disease

Macrocytic Anemias (MCV 100–160 µm³ or fl)

COBALAMIN DEFICIENCY

Decreased Ingestion

lack of animal products, strict vegetarianism

Impaired Absorption

intrinsic factor deficiency, pernicious anemia, gastrectomy (total and partial), destruction of gastric mucosa by caustics, anti-IF antibody in gastric juice, abnormal intrinsic factor molecule, intrinsic intestinal disease, familial selective malabsorption (Imerslund's syndrome) Ileal resection, ileitis, sprue, celiac disease, infiltrative intestinal disease (eg, lymphoma, scleroderma) drug-induced malabsorption

Competitive Parasites

Fish tapeworm infestations (*Diphyllobothrium latum*); bacteria in diverticulum of bowel, blind loops

Increased Requirements

Chronic pancreatic disease, pregnancy, neoplastic disease, hyperthyroidism

Impaired Utilization

Enzyme deficiencies, abnormal serum cobalamin binding protein, lack of transcobalamin II, nitrous oxide administration

FOLATE DEFICIENCY

Decreased Ingestion

Lack of vegetables, alcoholism, infancy

Impaired Absorption

Intestinal short circuits, steatorrhea, sprue, celiac disease, intrinsic intestinal disease, anticonvulsants, oral contraceptives, other drugs

(continued)

Anemias Characterized by Deficient Hemoglobin Synthesis *(continued)*
Increased Requirement Pregnancy, infancy, hyperthyroidism, hyperactive hematopoiesis, neoplastic disease, exfoliative skin disease
Impaired Utilization folic acid antagonists: methotrexate, triamterene, trimethoprim, enzyme deficiencies.
Increased Loss Hemodialysis
UNRESPONSIVE TO COBALAMIN OR FOLATE *Metabolic Inhibitors* Purine synthesis: 6-mercaptopurine, 6-thioguanine, azathioprine; pyrimidine synthesis: 6-azauridine; thymidylate synthesis: methotrexate, 5-fluorouracil; deoxybonucleotide synthesis: hydroxyurea, cytarabine, severe iron deficiency
Inborn Errors Lesch-Nyhan syndrome, hereditary orotic aciduria, deficiency of formimino transferase, methyltransferase, etc.

Interfering Factors

1. Demographic population of macrocytes and microcytes can give a normal MCV. Examination of blood film will confirm this.
2. Increased reticulocytes can increase MCV.

MEAN CORPUSCULAR HEMOGLOBIN CONCENTRATION (MCHC) ●

Normal Values

31–37 g/dl or 41.81–57.4 mmol Hb per liter.

Explanation of Test

This test measures the average concentration of hemoglobin in the red blood cells. The MCHC is most valuable in monitoring therapy for anemia because the two most accurate hematologic determinations (hemoglobin and hematocrit) are used in calculation of this test.

Procedure

The MCHC is a calculated value. It is an expression of the average concentration of hemoglobin in the red blood cells and, as such, it gives the ratio of the weight of hemoglobin to the volume of the red blood cell. Formula:

$$\frac{\text{Hb (g/dl)} \times 100}{\text{HCT (\%)}} = \text{g/dl}$$

Clinical Implications

1. *Decreased MCHC values* signify that a unit volume of packed RBCs contains less hemoglobin than normal:
   - **a.** Iron deficiency
   - **b.** Macrocytic anemias, chronic blood loss anemia
   - **c.** Pyridoxine-responsive anemia
   - **d.** Thalassemia
2. Hypochromic anemia is characterized by an MCHC of 30 or less.
3. *Increased MCHC values* usually indicate spherocytosis; RBCs cannot accommodate more than 37 g/dl hemoglobin, also newborns and infants.

Interfering Factors

1. The MCHC may be falsely high in the presence of lipemia, cold agglutinins, or rouleaux, and with high heparin concentrations.
2. Regarding calculations, no MCHC occurs over 37 g/dl because higher values are impossible.

MEAN CORPUSCULAR HEMOGLOBIN (MCH) ●

Normal Values

26–34 picograms (pg)/cell or 0.40–0.53 fmol/cell (Normally higher in newborns and infants)

Explanation of Test

The MCH is a measure of the average weight of hemoglobin per red blood cell. This index is of value in diagnosing severely anemic patients.

Procedure

1. The MCH is a calculated value. It is an expression of the average weight of hemoglobin in the red blood cell. The MCH is expressed as picograms of hemoglobin per red blood cell.
2. Formula:

$$\frac{\text{Hemoglobin/dl} \times 10}{\text{RBC } (10^{12}/\text{L}) = \text{pg } (10^{12}/\text{L})}$$

Clinical Implications

1. An increase of the MCH is associated with macrocytic anemia.
2. A decrease of the MCH is associated with microcytic anemia.

Interfering Factors

1. Hyperlipidemia will falsely elevate the MCH.

2. WBC counts greater than 50,000/mm^3 will falsely raise the hemoglobin value, and this falsely elevates the MCH.
3. High heparin concentrations falsely elevate MCH.

RED CELL SIZE DISTRIBUTION WIDTH (RDW) ●

Normal Values
11.5–14.5 CV%

Explanation of Test
This automated method of measurement is helpful in the investigation of some hematologic disorders and in monitoring response to therapy. The RDW is essentially an indication of the degree of anisocytosis (abnormal variation in size of RBC). Normal RBCs have a slight degree of variation.

Procedure
1. The RDW is determined and calculated by the analyzer.
2. RDW should be used with caution and should not replace other diagnostic tests.

Clinical Implications
1. Changes in coefficients of variation (CV) occur in
   a. Pernicious anemia (CV = 12.9%)
   b. Posthemorrhagic anemia (CV = 9.9%)
   c. Can be helpful in distinguishing uncomplicated heterozygous thalassemia (low MCV, normal RDW) from iron-deficiency (low MCV, high RDW).
   d. Can be helpful in distinguishing anemia of chronic disease, with a low normal MCV (normal RDW), from early iron-deficiency anemia (low normal MCV, elevated RDW).
2. Increased RDW occurs in
   a. Iron deficiency
   b. Vitamin B_{12} or folate deficiency
   c. Abnormal hemoglobin
   d. Thalassemia
   e. Immune hemolytic anemia

Interfering Factors
1. Not helpful for persons who do not have anemia.
2. **Patient Preparation** and **Patient Aftercare** are the same as that observed for the Red Cell Indices on page 61.

STAINED RED CELL EXAMINATION (FILM; STAINED ERYTHROCYTE EXAMINATION) ●

Normal Values
Size: Normocytic (normal size: 7–8 μm

Color: Normochromic (normal)

Shape: Normocyte (biconcave disk)

Structure: Normocytes or erythrocytes (anucleated cells)

Explanation of Test

The stained film examination determines variations and abnormalities in erythrocyte size, shape, structure, hemoglobin content, and staining properties. It is useful in diagnosing blood disorders such as anemia, thalassemia, and other hemoglobinopathies. This examination also serves as a guide to therapy and as an indicator of harmful effects of chemotherapy and radiation. The leukocytes are also examined at this time.

Procedure

1. A 7-ml blood sample in EDTA is collected. A stained blood smear is studied under a microscope to determine size, shape, and other characteristics of the RBC.
2. A capillary smear may also be used and may be preferred for detection of some abnormalities.

Clinical Implications

1. *Variations in staining, color, shape, and red cell inclusion* are indicative of red blood cell abnormalities (see table entitled Peripheral Red Blood Cell Abnormalities).

> **Clinical Alert**
>
> Marked abnormalities in size and shape of RBCs without a known cause are an indication for more complete blood studies.

2. **Patient Preparation** and **Patient Aftercare** are the same as described for Red Cell Indices on page 61.

RETICULOCYTE COUNT

Normal Values

Men: 0.5%–1.5% of total erythrocytes
Women: 0.5%–2.5% of total erythrocytes
Children: 0.5%–4% of total erythrocytes
Infants: 2%–5% of total erythrocytes
Reticulocyte index = 1.0
Absolute reticulocyte count = % reticulocytes × erythrocyte count 25–85 × 10^3 cells/μl or 25–85 × 10^9 cells/L

Background

A *reticulocyte,* a young, immature, nonnucleated red blood cell, contains reticular material (RNA) that stains a gray-blue when tested in the laboratory. Reticulum is present in newly released blood cells for 1 to 2 days before the cell reaches its full mature state. Normally a small number of these cells are found in circulating blood. For the reticulocyte count to be meaningful, it must be viewed in relation to the total number of erythrocytes.

Peripheral Red Blood Cell Abnormalities

Abnormality	*Description*	*Associated Diseases*
Anisocytosis diameter	Abnormal variation in size (normal diameter = 6–8 μm)	Any severe anemia (eg, iron-deficiency, megalobastic)
Microcytosis	Small cells, less than 6 μm (MCV < 80 fl)	Iron-deficiency and iron-loading (sideroblastic) anemia, thalassemia, lead poisoning
Macrocytosis	Large cells, greater than 8 μm (MCV > 100 fl) MCV/M > 94 fl MCV/F > 97 fl	Megaloblastic anemia, liver disease, hypothyroidism, hemolytic anemia (reticulocytes), multiple myeloma, physiologic macrocytosis of newborn, myelophthisis
Macroovalocytosis	Large (> 8 μm) oval cells	Megaloblastic anemia
Hypochromia	Pale cells with decreased concentration of hemoglobin (MCHC < 31 g/dl)	Iron-deficiency and iron-loading (sideroblastic) anemia, thalassemia, lead poisoning, transferrin deficiency, anemia of chronic disease (inflammatory diseases, eg, rheumatoid arthritis, collagen diseases, malignancies)
Poikilocytosis	Abnormal variation in shape	Any severe anemia (eg, megaloblastic iron-deficiency, myeloproliferative syndrome, hemolytic); certain shapes are diagnostically helpful (see following, Spherocytosis through teardrop cells)

Spherocytosis	Spherical cells without pale centers; often small (ie, microspherocytosis)	Hereditary spherocytosis, Coombs-positive hemolytic anemia; small numbers are seen in any hemolytic anemia and after transfusion of stored blood
Ovalocytosis	Oval cells	Hereditary elliptocytosis, iron deficiency
Stomatocytosis	Red cells with slitlike, instead of circular, areas of central pallor	Congenital hemolytic anemia, thalassemia, burns, lupus erythematosus, lead poisoning, liver disease, artifact
Sickle cells	Crescent-shaped cells	Sickle cell hemoglobinopathies
Target cells	Cells with a dark center and periphery and a clear ring in between	Liver disease, thalassemia, hemoglobinopathies (S, C, SC, S-thalassemia)
Schistocytes	Irregularly contracted cells (severe poikilocytosis), fragmented cells	Uremia, carcinoma, hemolytic–uremic syndrome, disseminated intravascular coagulation, microangiopathic hemolytic anemia, toxins (lead, phenylhydrazine), burns, thrombotic thrombocytopenic purpura
"Burr" cells	Cells irregularly spaced, spinous processes	Hemolytic anemias, liver disease ("spur cell" anemia), normal infants, uremia, microangiopathic hemolytic anemia, disseminated intravascular coagulation, thrombotic thrombocytopenic purpura, pyruvate kinase deficiency, carcinoma

(continued)

Peripheral Red Blood Cell Abnormalities *(continued)*

Abnormality	*Description*	*Associated Diseases*
Acanthocytosis	Small cells with thorny projections	Abetalipoproteinemia (hereditary acanthocytosis or Bassen–Kornzweig disease)
Teardrop cells	Cells shaped like teardrops	Myeloproliferative syndrome, myelophthisic anemia (neoplastic, granulomatous, or fibrotic marrow infiltration), anemia with extramedullary hematopoiesis or ineffective erythropoiesis
Nucleated red cells	Erythrocytes with nuclei still present; may be normoblastic or megaloblastic	Hemolytic anemias, leukemias, myeloproliferative syndrome, polycythemia vera, myelophthisic anemia (neoplastic, granulomatous, or fibrotic marrow infiltration), multiple myeloma, extramedullary hematopoiesis, megaloblastic anemias, any severe anemia
Howell–Jolly bodies	Spherical purple bodies (Wright stain) within or on erythrocytes; nuclear debris	Hyposplenism, pernicious anemia

Heinz inclusion bodies	Small round inclusions seen under phase microscopy or with supravital staining	Congenital hemolytic anemias (eg, glucose-6-phosphate dehydrogenase deficiency), hemolytic anemia secondary to drugs (dapsone, phenacetin), thalassemia (HbH), hemoglobinopathies (Hb Zurich, Koln, Ube, I, etc.)
Pappenheimer bodies (siderocytes)	Siderotic granules, staining blue with Wright or Prussian blue stains	Iron-loading anemias, hyposplenism, hemolytic anemias
Cabot's rings	Purple, fine, ringlike, intraerythrocytic structure	Pernicious anemia, lead poisoning
Basophilic stippling	Punctate stippling when Wright-stained	Hemolytic anemia, punctate stippling seen in lead poisoning (mitochondrial RNA and iron), thalassemia
Rouleaux	Aggregated erythrocytes regularly stacked on one another	Multiple myeloma, Waldenstrom's macroglobulinemia, cord blood, pregnancy, hypergammaglobulinemia, hyperfibrinogenemia
Polychromasia	RBCs containing RNA, staining a pinkish blue; stains supravitally as reticular network with new methylene blue	Hemolytic anemia, blood loss, uremia, following treatment of iron-deficiency or megaloblastic anemias

Explanation of Test

A reticulocyte count is used to differentiate anemias caused by bone marrow failure from those caused by hemorrhage or hemolysis (red cell destruction); to check the effectiveness of treatment in pernicious anemia or the recovery of bone marrow function in aplastic anemia; and to determine the effects of radioactive substances on exposed workers.

Procedure

1. Obtain an anticoagulated (EDTA) venous blood sample.
2. The blood sample is mixed with a supravital stain, such as brilliant cresyl blue. After the stain is allowed to react with the blood, a smear is prepared with this mixture and scanned under a microscope. The reticulocytes are counted and calculated.

Clinical Implications

1. *Increased reticulocyte counts* (reticulocytosis) indicate that increased RBC production is occurring as the bone marrow replaces cells lost or prematurely destroyed. Identifying reticulocytosis may lead to the recognition of an otherwise occult disease, such as hidden chronic hemorrhage or unrecognized hemolysis (sickle cell anemia and thalassemia). Increased levels are obtained in
   - **a.** Hemolytic anemia
     - **(1)** Immune
     - **(2)** Primary RBC membrane problems
     - **(3)** Hemoglobinopathic and sickle cell disease
     - **(4)** RBC enzyme deficits
     - **(5)** Toxin exposure
     - **(6)** Traumatic or microorganiopathic
     - **(7)** Hypersplenism
     - **(8)** Parasitic infections disease
   - **b.** Three to four days following hemorrhage
   - **c.** Following treatment of anemias
     - **(1)** Increase may be used as an index of the effectiveness of treatment.
     - **(2)** After adequate doses of iron in iron-deficiency anemia, the rise in reticulocytes may exceed 20%.
     - **(3)** There is a proportional increase when pernicious anemia is treated by transfusion or with vitamin B_{12} therapy.
2. *Decreased counts* means that bone marrow is not producing enough erythrocytes and occurs in
   - **a.** Iron-deficiency anemia
   - **b.** Aplastic anemia (a persistent deficiency of reticulocytes suggests a poor prognosis)
   - **c.** Untreated pernicious anemia
   - **d.** Chronic infection
   - **e.** Radiation therapy
   - **f.** Endocrine problems
   - **g.** Tumor in marrow (bone marrow failure
   - **h.** Myelodysplastic syndromes

Interfering Factors

1. Reticulocytes normally increase in infants and pregnancy.
2. Recently transfused patients have a lower count owing to delutional effect.
3. The presence of Howell–Jolly bodies falsely elevates the count when using automated methods.

Patient Preparation

1. Explain test purpose and procedure. Refer to hemogram for similar *pre-* and *posttest* care. Also, see Chapter 1 guidelines for safe, effective, informed *pretest* care.
2. Note medications. Some drugs cause aplastic anemia.

Patient Aftercare

1. Interpret test outcome and monitor appropriately for anemias.
2. Follow Chapter 1 guidelines for safe, effective, informed *posttest* care.

SEDIMENTATION RATE; SED RATE; ERYTHROCYTE SEDIMENTATION RATE (ESR) ●

Normal Values

Method	*Values*	
Westergren	Men	0–15 mm/hr
	Women	0–20 mm/hr
	Children	0–10 mm/hr

Background

Sedimentation occurs when the erythrocytes clump or aggregate together in a columnlike manner (rouleaux formation). These changes are related to alterations in the plasma proteins.

Explanation of Test

Erythrocyte sedimentation rate (ESR) is the rate at which erythrocytes settle out of anticoagulated blood in 1 hour. This test is based on the fact that inflammatory and necrotic processes cause an alteration in blood proteins, resulting in an aggregation of red cells, which make them heavier and more likely to fall rapidly when placed in a special vertical test tube. The faster the sedimentation rate, or settling of cells, the higher the ESR. The ESR should not be used to screen asymptomatic patients for disease. It is most useful for the diagnosis and monitoring of temporal arteritis and polymyalgia rheumatica. The sedimentation rate is not diagnostic of any particular disease, but rather is an indication that a disease process is ongoing and must be investigated.

Procedure

Obtain an anticoagulated EDTA venous sample of 7 ml. The specimen is suctioned into a graduated sedimentation tube and allowed to settle for exactly 1 hour. The amount of settling is the patient's sedimentation rate.

Clinical Implications

1. *Increased sedimentation* rates are found in
- **a.** All collagen diseases, SLE
- **b.** Infections, pneumonia, syphilis
- **c.** Inflammatory diseases
- **d.** Carcinoma, lymphoma, neoplasms
- **e.** Acute heavy metallic poisoning
- **f.** Cell or tissue destruction
- **g.** Toxemia
- **h.** Waldenstrom's macroglobulinemia
- **i.** Nephritis, nephrosis
- **j.** Subacute bacterial endocarditis
- **k.** Anemia
- **l.** Rheumatoid arthritis, gout, arthritis

2. *Normal (no increase)* sedimentation rate is found in
- **a.** Polycythemia vera, erythrocytosis
- **b.** Sickle cell anemia, hemoglobin C disease
- **c.** Congestive heart failure
- **d.** Hypofibrinogenemia (from any cause)
- **e.** Pyruvate kinase deficiency
- **f.** Hereditary spherocytosis

3. *Normal or varied values* are found in
- **a.** Acute disease: The change in rate may lag behind the temperature elevation and leukocytosis for 6 to 24 hours, reaching a peak after several days.
- **b.** Convalescence: The increased rate tends to persist longer than the temperature or the leukocytosis.
- **c.** Unruptured acute appendicitis (early): Even when suppurative or gangrenous, the rate is normal, but if abscess or peritonitis develops, the rate increases rapidly.
- **d.** Musculoseletal conditions
  - **(1)** In rheumatic, gonorrheal, and acute gouty arthritis, the rate is significantly increased.
  - **(2)** In osteoarthritis, the rate is slightly increased.
  - **(3)** In neuritis, myositis, and lumbago, the rate is within normal range.
- **e.** Cardiovascular conditions
  - **(1)** In myocardial infarction, the ESR is increased.
  - **(2)** In angina pectoris, the rate is not increased.
- **f.** Malignant diseases
  - **(1)** In multiple myeloma, lymphoma, and metastic cancer, the rate is very high.
  - **(2)** However, there is little correlation between the degree of elevation of the ESR and the prognosis in any one case.

g. Uncomplicated viral disease and infectious mononucleosis
h. Active renal failure with heart failure
i. Active allergy
j. Peptic ulcer

Clinical Alert

Extreme elevation of sedimentation rate is found with malignant lymphocarcinoma of the colon and breast, myeloma, and rheumatoid arthritis.

Interfering Factors

1. Do not allow the blood sample to stand more than 24 hours before the test is started; causes the rate to decrease.
2. In refrigerated blood the sedimentation is increased. Refrigerated blood should be allowed to return to room temperature before the test is performed.
3. Factors leading to increased rate include
   - **a.** The presence of fibrinogen, globulins, and cholesterol
   - **b.** Pregnancy after 12 weeks until about the fourth week postpartum
   - **c.** Young children
   - **d.** Menstruation
   - **e.** Certain drugs (eg, heparin and oral contraceptives)
   - **f.** High hemoglobin values
4. The sedimentation rate may be very high (up to 69 mm/hr—Westergren) in apparently healthy women aged 70 to 89.
5. Factors leading to reduced rates include
   - **a.** High blood sugar, high albumin level, and high phospholipid levels
   - **b.** Decreased fibrinogen level in the blood of newborns
   - **c.** Certain drugs (eg, steroids, high-dose aspirin)

Patient Preparation

1. Explain test purpose and procedure. Obtain appropriate medication history. Fasting is not necessary, but a fatty meal may cause plasma alterations.
2. See Chapter 1 guidelines for safe, effective, informed *pretest* care.

Patient Aftercare

1. Resume normal activities and diet.
2. Interpret test outcome, counsel and monitor appropriately for rheumatic disorders and inflammatory conditions.
3. See Chapter 1 guidelines for safe, effective, informed *posttest* care.

● TESTS FOR PORPHYRIA

Tests of blood, urine, and stool are done to diagnose porphyria, an abnormal accumulation of porphyrins in body fluids. Prophyrias are a group of diseases caused by a deficit in the enzymes involved in porphyrin metabolism and abnormalities in the production of the metalloporphyrin heme. These tests are indicated in persons who have unexplained neurologic manifestations, unexplained abdominal pain, cutaneous blisters, or the presence of a relevant family history. Test results may identify clinical conditions associated with abnormal heme production. These clinical states include anemia and the genetic (hereditary) or acquired (lead poisoning, alcohol) enzyme disorders associated with abnormal accumulation of the porphyrins (porphyria). Accumulation of porphyrins occurs in the blood plasma, serum, erythrocytes, urine, and feces. A discussion of erythrocyte totals and fractionation of erythrocytes and plasma follows. For details of urine, serum, and stool testing for porphyrias, see pages 227 *(Urine),* 273 *(Feces),* and 76–77 *(Serum).* Also, see Uroporphyrinogen in Chapter 6 for other blood testing.

ERYTHROPOIETIC PORPHYRINS; ERYTHROCYTE TOTAL ●

Normal Values

< 35 μg/dl whole blood
17–77 μg/dl packed red cells (normal values reflect heme precursors)

Background

Normally there is a small amount of excess porphyrin at the completion of heme synthesis. This excess is cell-free erythrocyte protoporphyrin (FEP). The amount of FEP in the erythrocyte is elevated when the iron supply is diminished.

Explanation of Test

This test is useful in diagnosing metabolic RBC disorders such as erythropoietic protoporphyria. It is also used to support the diagnosis of lead poisoning, especially in children 6 months to 5 years of age.

Procedure

1. Obtain a 5-ml sample of anticoagulated venous blood, EDTA, heparin, or oxalate anticoagulant may be used.
2. Protect blood sample from light.
3. The blood cells are washed and then tested for porphyrins.
4. Hematocrit value must be known for test interpretation.

Clinical Implications

1. Increased erythrocyte protoporphyrins are associated with

   - **a.** Protoporphyria
   - **b.** Lead poisoning
   - **c.** Halogenated solvents and many drugs
   - **d.** Iron-deficiency anemias
   - **e.** Acquired iodopathic sideroblastic anemia
2. Slight increase in
   - **a.** Exposure to environmental pollutants
   - **b.** Hodgkin's disease
   - **c.** Leukemia
   - **d.** Azotemia
   - **e.** Hemolytic anemia
3. Normal in thalassemia minor and, therefore, can be used to differentiate this from iron-deficiency anemia.

Patient Preparation

1. Explain test purpose and sampling procedure.
2. Note on lab slip or computer any medications patient is taking that cause intermittent porphyria. Discontinue before testing after checking with physician.
3. See Chapter 1 guidelines for safe, effective, informed *pretest* care.

Patient Aftercare

1. Interpret test outcome and monitor appropriately for porphyria or lead poisoning.

Clinical Alert

Critical value greater than 300 µg/dl

2. See Chapter 1 guidelines for safe, effective, informed *posttest* care.

PORPHYRINS; FRACTIONATION OF ERYTHROCYTES AND OF PLASMA

Normal Values

A report is provided in micrograms per deciliter (µg/dl; see your laboratory reference values).

Background

The primary prophyrins of erythrocytes (RBCs) are protoporphyrin, uroporphyrin, and coproporphyrin.

Explanation of Test

Fractionation of *erythrocytes* is used to differentiate congenital erythropoietic coproporphyria from erythropoietic protoporphyria and confirm a diagnosis of protoporphyria. This test establishes a specific type of porphyria by naming the specific porphyrin in *plasma.* In persons with renal failure, plasma fractionation can help determine whether the porphyria is due to a deficiency of uroporphyrinogenic decarboxylase or is due to failure of the renal system to excrete porphyrinogens.

Procedure

1. Five ml of anticoagulated blood is drawn: EDTA heparin or oxalate can be used as an anticoagulant.
2. Protect specimen from light.

Clinical Implications

1. Increased erythrocyte porphyrins are associated with
   a. Congenital erythropoietic protoporphyria
   b. Protoporphyria—autosomal dominant deficiency of heme synthetase
   c. Intoxication porphyria (lead)
   d. Iron-deficiency anemias
2. Increased plasma porphyrins are associated with
   a. Congenital erythropoietic protoporphyria
   b. Coproporphyria
   c. Porphyria cutanea tarda

Patient Preparation

1. Advise patient of test procedure.
2. Note on requisition any drugs the patient is taking.
3. Before testing, drugs that are known to cause intermittent porphyria should be discontinued after checking with physician.
4. See Chapter 1 guidelines for safe, effective, informed *pretest* care.

Patient Aftercare

1. Resume medications.
2. Interpret test outcome and monitor appropriately for porphyria or lead poisoning.
3. Caution persons diagnosed with porphyria (with cutaneous manifestations) to avoid sun exposure.
4. Advise persons diagnosed with porphyria (with neurologic symptoms) that attacks can be precipitated by infections, various phases of the menstrual cycle, fasting states, and by certain drugs. A listing of drugs that may precipitate acute attacks follows: Apronalide, barbiturates, chlordiazepoxide, chloroquine, chlorpropamide, dichloralphenazone, ergot preparations, estrogens, ethanol, glutethimide, griseofulvin, hydantoins, imipramine, meprobamate, methsuximide, methyldopa, methyprylon, novonal, sulfonamides.
5. Follow Chapter 1 guidelines for safe, effective, informed *posttest* care.

Clincial Alert

1. A test for uroporphyrinogen-1-synthase (UIS) can be done to identify persons at risk for acute intermittent porphyria; it also detects latent stage intermittent porphyria as well as confirms diagnosis during an acute episode.
2. Normal value is 8–16.8 nmol/L or 1.27–200 ml/g of hemoglobin in females; 79–14.7 nmol/L in males. A value of less than 6 nmol/L is diagnostic of acute intermittent porphyria.

ADDITIONAL TESTS FOR HEMOLYTIC ANEMIA

Several RBC enzyme and fragility tests can be done to screen, detect, and confirm the cause of chronic hemolytic anemia. Many persons with hemolytic anemia will have no clinical signs or symptoms. Abnormal test outcomes are associated with inherited deficiencies, abnormal hemoglobins, and exposure to chemicals and drugs. Definitive test results indicate some type of injury to the RBC, or oxidated activity that interferes with normal hemoglobin function, and/or increased RBC fragility.

PYRUVATE KINASE (PK)

Normal Values

13–17 units (U)/g hemoglobin if deficiency in congenital hemolytic anemia (with low ATP in RBC which causes a membrane defect).

Background

Acquired deficiency caused by ingestion of oral contraceptives. Metabolic liver diseases, acute leukemias, aphasias.

Procedure

Obtain venous blood sample of at least 2 ml to which EDTA is added.

GLUTATHIONE REDUCTASE (GR)

Normal Values

5–9 μg of hemoglobin.

Clinical Implications

Decreased is rare hereditary deficiency, after ingestion of fava beans. *Increased* in diabetes, G6PD deficiency, drug-induced (nicotinic acid, primaquine). GR activity reflects riboflavin nutrition.

Procedure
Obtain venous blood sample of at least 3 ml. EDTA or heparin used as anticoagulant.

ERYTHROCYTE FRAGILITY (OSMOTIC FRAGILITY AND AUTOHEMOLYSIS) ●

Normal Values and Background
Spherocytes are more susceptible to hemolysis and show the increased osmotic fragility (> 0.5%) that occurs in hemolytic anemia, hereditary spherocytosis, hemolytic disease of newborn; severely thinner cells (hypochromic pyruvate kinase deficiency and target cells) have decreased osmotic fragility (< 0.30%) in hypochromic cells, iron deficiency anemia, hemoglobin C and S disease, thalassemia, liver disease, owing to macrocyte or target cells and postsplenectomy. Test is not diagnostic of hereditary spherocytosis.

Procedure
Obtain 7-ml venous blood sample using heparin as anticoagulant. Erythrocytes are exposed to varying dilutions of sodium chloride. Hemolysis is read on spectrophotometer (optical density measurement).

GLUCOSE-6-PHOSPHATE DEHYDROGENASE (G6PD) ●

Normal Values
Adults: 2.4–5.1 U/ml/RBC; Infants: 1.5–2.2 U/ml/RBCs. If screening test, G6PD activity is within normal limits.

Background
G6PD is a sex-linked disorder. There are more than 500 variants of this sex-linked (X chromosome) condition. Type A, found in blacks; Mediterranean type, found in both white (Greek, Sardinian, Sephardic Jew) and Orientals.

Clinical Implications
Decreased levels also in rare congenital nonspherocytic anemia and nonimmunologic hemolytic disease of newborn. *Increased* in pernicious anemia, idiopathic hemocytopenic purpura, hepatic coma, hyperthyroidism, myocardial infarction, chronic blood loss, and other megaloblastic anemias.

Procedure
Obtain a blood sample of at least 5 ml. EDTA or heparin is anticoagulant used.

Interfering Factors
Marked reticulocytosis may give a falsely high G6PD.

HEINZ BODIES/EHRLICH STAIN

Normal Values

Present in G6PD deficiency (40% of cells have five or more Heinz bodies), in African, Mediterranean, and Oriental ancestry, congenital Heinz body hemolytic anemia, splenectomized patients, acute hemolytic crises, and unstated hemolytic disorders; in hemolytic anemias caused by drug poisoning, 50% to 75% of RBCs contain Heinz bodies.

Procedure

Obtain a venous blood sample, anticoagulated with heparin. Cells are mixed with a supravital stain and examined microscopically.

2,3-DIPHOSPHOGLYCERATE (2,3-DPG)

Normal Values

Male: 4.2–5.4 μmol/ml of packed cells; 9.2–17.4 μmol/g of hemoglobin
Female: 4.5–6.1 μmol/ml of packed cells; 8.4–18.8 μmol/g of hemoglobin

Clinical Implications

Increases in hypoxia, emphysema, pulmonary disease, cyanotic heart disease, acute leukemia, pyruvate kinase deficiency, sickle cell anemia, hyperthyroidism, uremia, and chronic renal failure; differentiates anemia. *Decreases* in polycythemia, respiratory distress syndrome, 2,3-DPG cermutase deficiency, acidosis, stored blood.

Interfering Factors

High altitudes increase 2,3-DPG.

Procedure

Obtain venous blood sample of at least 3 ml, anticoagulated with heparin. Place on ice immediately. 2,3-DPG is stable for only 2 hours.

Clinical Alert

If blood with decreased 2,3-DPG is used for transfusion, the hemoglobin may not release 0_2 when needed.

Patient Preparation

1. Explain test purposes and procedure. No exercising before tests.
2. Withhold transfusion until after blood samples are drawn (especially osmotic fragility).
3. See Chapter 1 guidelines for safe, effective, informed *pretest* care.

Patient Aftercare

1. Interpret test results and monitor appropriately for hemolytic anemia, hypoxia, or polycythemia.
2. Follow Chapter 1 guidelines for safe, effective, informed *posttest* care.

Clinical Alert

Many prescribed drugs interfere with the normal functioning of hemoglobin in susceptible persons, especially sulfonamides, antipyretics, analgesics, large doses of vitamin K, and nitrofurans.

IRON TESTS

IRON, TOTAL IRON-BINDING CAPACITY (TIBC), AND TRANSFERRIN TESTS

Normal Values

Iron
Males: 75–175 μg/dl
Females: 65–165 μg/dl
Newborn: 100–250 μg/dl
Child: 50–120 μg/dl

Transferrin
Adult: 200–400 mg/dl
Newborn: 130–275 mg/dl
Child: 203–360 mg/dl

Total Iron-Binding Capacity
Iron Binding Capacity (TIBC)
240–450 μg/dl
FeF: 100–400 μg/dl

Transferring (Iron) % Saturation
Males: 0%–5%
Females: 15%–50%

Background

Iron is necessary for the production of hemoglobin. Iron is contained in several components. Transferrin (also called *siderophilin*), a transport protein and beta-globulin, regulates iron absorption. High levels of transferrin relate to the ability of the body to deal with infections. Total iron-binding capacity (TIBC) correlates with serum transferrin, but the relationship is not linear. A serum iron test without a TIBC and transferrin has very limited value except for cases of iron poisoning. Transferrin saturation is a better index of iron saturation evaluated as:

$$\% \text{ Saturation} = \frac{\text{Serum iron} \times 100}{\text{TIBC}}$$

Explanation of Test

The test combinations of transferrin, iron, and TIBC are helpful in the differential diagnosis of anemia, assessment of iron-deficiency anemia, evaluation of thalassemia, sideroblastic anemia, and hemochromatosis.

Procedure

Obtain a venous blood sample of 10 ml.

Clinical Implications

1. *Transferrin increases* in
   - **a.** Iron deficiency anemia
   - **b.** Pregnancy
   - **c.** Estrogen therapy
   - **d.** Oral contraceptives
2. *Transferrin decreases* in
   - **a.** Microcytic anemia of chronic disease
   - **b.** Protein deficiency or loss from burns
   - **c.** Chronic infection
   - **d.** Malnutrition
   - **e.** Renal disease (nephrosis)
   - **f.** Genetic deficiency
3. *Iron decreases* in
   - **a.** Iron deficiency
   - **b.** Chronic blood loss
   - **c.** Chronic diseases (eg, lupus, rheumatoid arthritis, chronic infections)
   - **d.** Third trimester of pregnancy
   - **e.** Remission of pernicious anemia
   - **f.** Hypothyroidism
4. *Iron increases* in
   - **a.** Hemolytic anemias, especially thalassemia
   - **b.** Acute iron poisoning (children)
   - **c.** Iron-overload syndromes
   - **d.** Hemochromatosis
   - **e.** Transfusions (multiple)
   - **f.** Acute hepatitis
   - **g.** Recent intramuscular iron
   - **h.** Acute hepatic necroses
   - **i.** Lead poisoning
   - **j.** Acute leukemia
   - **k.** Nephrosis
5. Total serum iron binding capacity (TIBC) *increases* in
   - **a.** Iron deficiency
   - **b.** Use of contraceptives
   - **c.** Pregnancy
   - **d.** Acute and chronic blood loss
   - **e.** Acute hepatitis
6. TIBC *decreases* in
   - **a.** Hypoproteinemia (malnutrition and burns)
   - **b.** Hemochromatosis
   - **c.** Anemia (infection and chronic disease)
   - **d.** Cirrhosis of liver
   - **e.** Nephroses and other renal diseases
   - **f.** Non–iron-defined anemias
7. Iron saturated (transferrin saturation) index *increases* in
   - **a.** Hemochromatosis
   - **b.** Increased iron intake
   - **c.** Thalassemia
   - **d.** Vitamin B_6 deficiency
   - **e.** Aplastic anemia
   - **f.** Hemosiderosis

8. Iron saturation (transferrin saturation) index *decreased* in
   a. Iron-deficiency anemias
   b. Malignancy (standard and small intestine)
   c. Anemia of infection and chronic disease
   d. Iron neoplasms

Interfering Factors

1. Iron-chelating drugs affect outcome.
2. Drugs that may cause increased iron-binding capacity include chloramphenicol, fluorides, estrogens, and oral contraceptives.
3. Hemolysis of blood sample.

Patient Preparation

1. Explain test purpose and procedure.
2. Draw fasting blood in the morning when levels are higher.
3. Draw iron sample before iron therapy is initiated or blood transfusion.
4. If patient has received a transfusion, delay iron testing for 4 days.
5. Any iron-chelating drug such as deferoxamine (Desferal) must be avoided.
6. Avoid sleep deprivation or extreme stress, which will cause lower iron levels.
7. Note on lab slip or computer screen if patient is taking oral contraceptives or receiving estrogen therapy.
8. See Chapter 1 guidelines for safe, effective, informed *pretest* care.

Patient Aftercare

1. Resume normal activities.
2. Interpret test outcome and monitor appropriately. The combination of low serum iron, high TIBC, and high transferrin levels indicates iron deficiency. Diagnosis of iron deficiency may lead further to detection of adenocarcinoma of GI tract, a point that cannot be overemphasized. A significant minority of patients with megaloblastic anemias (20%–40%) have coexisting iron deficiency. Megaloblastic anemia can interfere with the interpretation of iron studies; repeat iron studies 1 to 3 months after folate or B_{12} replacement.
3. Use Chapter 1 guidelines for safe, effective informed *posttest* care.

Clinical Alert

1. Critical iron values: intoxicated child, 280–2550 μg/dl; falsely poisoned child, > 1800 μg/dl.
2. Symptoms of iron poisoning include abdominal pain, vomiting, bloody diarrhea, cyanosis, and convulsions.

FERRITIN

Normal Values

Men: 18–270 ng/ml or μg/L
Women: 18–160 ng/ml or μg/L
Children: 7–140 ng/ml or μg/L
Newborns: 25–200 ng/ml or μg/L
1 mo: 50–200 ng/ml or μg/L
2–5 mo: 50–200 ng/ml or μg/L

Background

Ferritin, a complex of ferric (Fs^{2F}) hydroxide and a protein, apoferritin originates in the reticuloendothelial system. Ferritin reflects the body iron stores and is a good indication of iron storage status.

Explanation of Test

The ferritin test is more sensitive than the iron or TIBC for diagnosing iron deficiency or overload.

Ferritin, Iron, and Iron Saturation Changes in Anemias*

	Ferritin	Iron	Iron Saturation
Hemorrhage, acute	N	D	D
Hemorrhage, chronic	D	D	D
Iron deficiency	D	D	D
Aplastic anemia	D	I	I
Megaloblastic anemia	I	D	D
Hemolytic anemia	I	I	I
Sideroblastic anemia	I	I	I
Thalassemia major	I	I	I
Thalassemia minor	I	N/I	N/I
Bone marrow neoplasia	N/I	I	I
Uremia, nephrosis, or nephrotic syndrome	N/I	D/I	D
Liver disease	N/I	N/I	N/I
Chronic disorders	I	D	D

*N = no change; D = decrease; I = increase

Procedure

Obtain a venous sample of 6 ml.

Clinical Implications

1. *Decreased ferritin values* usually indicate iron-deficiency anemia (< 10 ng/ml).
2. *Increased ferritin values* occur in iron excess (7400 ng/ml or μg/L) and
   a. Iron overload from hemochromatosis
   b. Oral or parenteral iron administration

c. Inflammatory diseases
d. Acute and chronic liver disease
e. Acute myoblastic and lymphoblastic leukemia
f. Other malignancies (Hodgkin's disease, breast carcinoma, malignant lymphoma)
g. Megaloblastic anemia
h. Hemolytic anemia
i. Thalassemia (normal or sometimes higher)

Interfering Factors
1. Recently administered radioactive medications cause spurious results.
2. Oral contraceptives interfere with testing.

Clinical Alert

The best and most reliable evaluation of total body iron stores is by bone marrow aspiration and biopsy.

Patient Preparation
1. Explain test purpose and procedure. Fasting is not necessary.
2. Radioactive medications may not be given for 3 to 4 days before testing.
3. Refrain from alcohol (higher levels of ferritin in alcoholism).
4. See Chapter 1 guidelines for safe, effective, informed *pretest* care.

Patient Aftercare
1. Resume normal activities.
2. Interpret test results and monitor appropriately for iron-deficiency anemia or ferritin increases. When iron and TIBC tests are used together with ferritin, they can better distinguish between iron-deficiency anemia and the anemia of chronic disease.
3. See Chapter 1 guidelines for safe, effective, informed *posttest* care.

● TESTS FOR HEMOGLOBIN DISORDERS

HEMOGLOBIN ELECTROPHORESIS ●

Normal Values
Hemoglobin A_1: > 9.5–9.8% **No** abnormal hemoglobin variants.
Hemoglobin A_2: 1.5–3.5%
Hemoglobin F: 0–2%

Background

Normal and abnormal hemoglobins can be detected by electrophoresis, which matches hemolyzed red cell material against standard bands for the various hemoglobins known. The most common forms of normal adult hemoglobins are hemoglobin A_1, A_2, and F (fetal hemoglobin). Of the various types of abnormal hemoglobin (hemoglobinopathies), the best known are hemoglobin S (responsible for sickle cell anemia) and hemoglobin C (results in a mild hemolytic anemia). The most common abnormality is a significant increase in hemoglobin A_2, diagnostic of α-thalassemia minor. The α-thalassemia trait is in and of itself a harmless condition. More than 350 variants of hemoglobin have been recognized and identified by capital letters such as HbA or G-Philadelphia.

Clinical Alert

The results may be questionable if a blood transfusion has been given in the preceding months before testing.

FETAL HEMOGLOBIN (HEMOGLOBIN F; HBF) (ALKALI-RESISTANT HEMOGLOBIN) ●

Normal Values

Adults: 0%–2%
Newborns: 60%–90%; by 6 months: 2%

Background

Fetal hemoglobin (hemoglobin F), is a normal hemoglobin manufactured in the red blood cells of the fetus and infant and composes 50% to 90% of the hemoglobin in the newborn. The remaining portion of the hemoglobin in the newborn is made up of hemoglobin A_1 and A_2, the adult types.

Explanation of Test

Determination of hemoglobin F is used to diagnose thalassemia, an inherited abnormality in the manufacture of hemoglobin, characterized by microcytic, hypochromic anemia. Under normal conditions, the manufacture of fetal hemoglobin is replaced by the manufacture of adult hemoglobin during the first year of life. But if hemoglobin F persists and constitutes more than 5% of the hemoglobin after 6 months of age, an abnormality should be expected, especially thalassemia.

Procedure

A 7-ml venous blood EDTA sample is used for hemoglobin electrophoresis.

Clinical Implications

1. *Increased values of HbF* are found in
   - **a.** Thalassemias (major and minor)
   - **b.** Hereditary familial fetal hemoglobinemia
   - **c.** Spherocytic anemia
   - **d.** Sickle cell anemia
   - **e.** Hemoglobin H disease
   - **f.** Anemia, as a compensatory mechanism
   - **g.** Leakage of fetal blood into the maternal blood stream
   - **h.** Aplastic anemia
   - **i.** Acute and chronic leukemia
   - **j.** Myeloproliferative disorders
   - **k.** Untreated pernicious anemia
   - **l.** Metastatic carcinoma to the bone marrow
   - **m.** Multiple myeloma and lymphoma

Clinical Alert

In *thalassemia minor,* continued production of fetal hemoglobin may occur on a minor scale with values of 5% to 10%, and the patient usually lives. In *thalassemia major,* the values may reach 40% to 90%. This continued production of hemoglobin F leads to a severe anemia, and death usually occurs.

Interfering Factors

1. If analysis of specimen is delayed for more than 2 to 3 hours, the specimen may falsely appear to have higher quantities of hemoglobin F.
2. Infants small for gestational age or with chronic intrauterine anoxia will have persistent, elevated levels of HbF.
3. Increased during anticonvulsant drug therapy.
4. Increased in non–hemoglobin-related diseases, such as diabetes, hyper- and hypothyroidism, and macroglobulinemia.

Patient Preparation

1. Explain test purpose and procedure.
2. Test should be done before transfusion.
3. See Chapter 1 guidelines for safe, effective, informed *pretest* care.

Patient Aftercare

1. Interpret test outcome, counsel, and monitor appropriately for thalassemia and anemia.
2. Follow Chapter 1 guidelines for safe, effective, informed *posttest* care.

HEMOGLOBIN S (SICKLE CELL TEST; SICKLEDEX)

Normal Values

Adult: None present

Background

Sickle cell anemia is caused by an abnormal form of hemoglobin, known as *hemoglobin S*. In this condition, hemoglobin becomes more viscous and precipitates or bonds in a way such that it causes the red cells to assume a sickle shape. The abnormally shaped cells are unable to pass freely through the capillary system, resulting in increased viscosity of the blood and sluggish circulation. This can cause a backup of cells in the capillary system, resulting in a stoppage of blood supply to certain organs.

Explanation of Test

This blood measurement is routinely done as a screening test for sickle cell anemia or trait and to confirm these disorders. This test detects hemoglobin S, the product of an inherited, recessive gene. An examination is made of the erythrocytes for the sickle-shaped forms characteristic of sickle cell anemia or trait. This is done by removing oxygen from the erythrocyte. In erythrocytes with normal hemoglobin the shape is retained, but erythrocytes containing hemoglobin S will assume a sickle shape. However, the distinction between sickle cell trait and sickle cell disease is done by electrophoresis, which identifies a hemoglobin pattern.

Procedure

A 5-ml venous blood sample with EDTA is obtained. The Sickledex test or hemoglobin electrophoresis is done. Electrophoresis is more accurate and should be done in all positive Sickledex screens.

Clinical Implications

1. *Positive test* (hemoglobin S present) means that great numbers of erythrocytes have assumed the typical sickle cell (crescent) shape. Positive tests are 99% accurate.

   a. *Sickle cell trait*

      (1) Definite confirmation of sickle cell trait in a given person by hemoglobin electrophoresis reveals the following A/S heterozygous pattern: Hemoglobin S 20%–40%, hemoglobin A_1 60%–80%, hemoglobin F small amount. This means that the patient has inherited a normal hemoglobin gene from one parent and a hemoglobin S gene from the other (heterozygous pattern). This patient does not have any clinical manifestations of the disease, but some of the children of this patient may inherit the disease if the person's mate has the recessive gene pattern.

      (2) The diagnosis of sickle cell trait does not affect longevity and is not accompanied by signs and symptoms of sickle cell anemia.

      (3) Sickle cell trait can lead to renal papillary necrosis, hematuria, and to an increased risk of pulmonary embolus.

   b. *Sickle cell anemia*

      (1) Definite confirmation of sickle cell anemia by hemoglobin electrophoresis reveals the following S/S homozygous pattern:

Hemoglobin S 80%–100%, hemoglobin F makes up the rest; hemoglobin A_1 0% or small amount. This means that an abnormal S gene has been inherited from both parents (homozygous pattern). Such a patient has all the clinical manifestations of the disease.

Interfering Factors

1. False-negative results occur in:
   a. Infants younger than 3 months
   b. Polycythemia
   c. Protein abnormalities
2. False-positive results occur up to 4 months after transfusions with RBCs having sickle cell trait.
3. HgbD migrates to same place as HgbF in electrophoresis.

Clinical Alert

A positive Sickledex test must be confirmed by electrophoresis.

Patient Preparation

1. Explain purpose and procedure.
2. Provide genetic counseling.
3. Follow Chapter 1 guidelines for safe, effective, informed *pretest* care.

Patient Aftercare

1. Interpret test outcome, counsel, and monitor appropriately.
2. A positive diagnosis of sickle cell disorder has genetic implications, including the need for genetic counseling.
3. A person with sickle cell disease should avoid situations in which hypoxia may occur, such as traveling to high-altitude regions and in an unpressurized aircraft; also, very strenuous exercise.
4. Because of general anesthetics and the state of shock creating hypoxia, surgical or maternity patients with sickle cell disease need very close observation.
5. See Chapter 1 guidelines for safe, effective, informed *posttest* care.

METHEMOGLOBIN, HEMOGLOBIN M

Normal Values

0.4–1.5% of total hemoglobin > 10% critical value
0.06–0.24 g/dl or 9.3–37.2 μmol/L

Background

Methemoglobin is formed when the iron in the heme portion of deoxygenated hemoglobin is oxidized to a ferric form, rather than a ferrous form. In the ferric form, oxygen and iron cannot combine. The formation of methemoglobin is a normal process and is kept within bounds by the reduction of methemoglobin to hemoglobin. Methemoglobin causes a shift to the left of the oxyhemoglobin dissociation curve. When a high concentration of methemoglobin is produced in the erythrocytes, it reduces the capacity of the red blood cells to combine with oxygen. Thus, anoxia and cyanosis result.

Explanation of Test

This test is used to diagnose hereditary or acquired methemoglobinemia in patients with symptoms of anoxia or cyanosis and no evidence of cardiovascular or pulmonary disease. *Hemoglobin M* is an inherited disorder of the hemoglobin that produces cyanosis.

Procedure

1. A venous or arterial blood sample, anticoagulated with heparin, is obtained.
2. Place on ice immediately and transport to lab.

Clinical Implications

1. *Hereditary methemoglobinemia* (uncommon) is associated with a hemoglobin M content as high as 40% of the total hemoglobin (hemoglobin structure variant).
2. *Acquired methemoglobinemia* is associated with
   - **a.** Black water fever
   - **b.** Paroxysmal hemoglobinuria
   - **c.** Clostridial infection
   - **d.** Ingestion of colored wax crayons or chalk
   - **e.** Exposure to excessive radiation
3. The most common cause is toxic effect of drugs or chemicals:
   - **a.** Aniline dyes and derivatives
   - **b.** Sulfonamides, sulfones
   - **c.** Nitrates and nitrites; nitroglycerin
   - **d.** Ionizing radiation
   - **e.** Phenacetin (acetophenatin)
   - **f.** Chlorates
   - **g.** Quinones
   - **h.** Ferrous sulfate
   - **i.** Benzocaine, lidocaine

Interfering Factors

1. Eating Polish sausage and spinach, foods rich in nitrite and nitrate.
2. Absorption of silver nitrate used to treat extensive burns.
3. Excessive intake of Bromo-Seltzer is a common cause of methemoglobinemia. (The patient appears cyanotic, but otherwise feels well.)
4. Smoking.
5. Bismuth preparations for diarrhea.

Patient Preparation

1. Advise patient of purpose of test. Assess for history of Bromo-Seltzer, toxic drugs, or chemical ingestion.
2. See Chapter 1 guidelines for safe, effective, informed *pretest* care.

Patient Aftercare

1. Interpret test outcome, counsel for cause of cyanosis, and monitor appropriately for anoxia.
2. Treatment includes intravenous methylene blue and oral ascorbic acid.
3. Follow Chapter 1 guidelines for safe, effective, informed *posttest* care.

> **Clinical Alert**
>
> Because fetal hemoglobin is more easily converted to methemoglobin than is adult hemoglobin, infants are more susceptible than adults to methemoglobinemia, which may be caused by drinking well water containing nitrites. Bismuth preparations for diarrhea may also be reduced to nitrites by bowel action.

SULFHEMOGLOBIN

Normal Values

None present: 0–1.0% of total hemoglobin

Background

Sulfhemoglobin is an abnormal hemoglobin pigment produced by the combination of inorganic sulfides with hemoglobin. Sulfhemoglobinemia presents as a cyanosis.

Explanation of Test

This test is indicated in persons with cyanosis. Sulfhemoglobinemia may occur in associated with the administration of various drugs and toxins. The symptoms are few, but cyanosis is intense, even though the concentration seldom exceeds 10%.

Procedure

A 5-ml venous sample of blood is drawn and is anticoagulated with EDTA.

Clinical Implications

1. Sulfhemoglobin is observed in patients who take oxidant drugs, such as phenacetin (excessive intake of Bromo-Seltzer), sulfonamides, and acetanilid.
2. Sulfhemoglobin is formed rarely without exposure to drugs or toxins, as in chronic constipation and purging.

Patient Preparation

1. Explain test purpose and procedure. Assess for exposure to drugs and toxins.
2. See Chapter 1 guidelines for safe, effective, informed *pretest* care.

Patient Aftercare

1. Interpret test outcome, counsel for cause of cyanosis and use of certain medications.
2. See Chapter 1 guidelines for safe, effective informed *posttest* care.

CARBOXYHEMOGLOBIN; CARBON MONOXIDE (CO) ●

Normal Values

0%–2.0% of total hemoglobin or 0–0.020
In heavy smokers: 6%–8.0% or 0.06–0.08
In light smokers: 4%–5% or 0.04–0.05

Background

Carboxyhemoglobin is formed when hemoglobin is exposed to carbon monoxide. The affinity of hemoglobin for carbon monoxide is 218 times greater than for oxygen. Carbon monoxide poisoning causes anoxia because the carboxyhemoglobin formed does not permit hemoglobin to combine with oxygen, and that which does bind is not readily released to the tissues.

Explanation of Test

This test is done to detect carbon monoxide poisoning. Because carboxyhemoglobin is incapable of transporting oxygen, hypoxia results, causing headache, nausea, vomiting, vertigo, collapse, or convulsions. Death may result from anoxia and irreversible tissue changes. Carboxyhemoglobin produces a cherry red or violet color of the blood and skin, but may not be present in chronic exposure. The most common cause of carbon monoxide toxicity is automobile exhaust fumes, coal gas, water gas, and smoke inhalation from fires, although smoking is a minor cause.

Procedure

A heparinized venous blood sample of 5 ml is drawn and put on ice. Keep sample tightly capped and transport to lab immediately.

Clinical Implications

1. Carboxyhemoglobin is increased in CO poisoning from many sources, including smoking; it is also found in
   - **a.** Hemolytic disease
   - **b.** Blood in intestines
   - **c.** A direct correlation has been found between CO and symptoms of heart disease, angina, and myocardial infarction.

Patient Preparation

1. Advise patient of purpose of test.
2. Draw blood sample before oxygen therapy has started.
3. See Chapter 1 guidelines for safe, effective, informed *pretest* care.

Patient Aftercare

1. Interpret test outcome and monitor appropriately.
2. Treatment consists of removal of patient from source of carbon monoxide.
3. Oxygen therapy is initiated either by supplemental oxygen at atmospheric pressure or by hyperbaric oxygen.
4. See Chapter 1 guidelines for safe, effective, informed *posttest* care.

Clinical Alert

1. With values of 10%–20%, the person may be asymptomatic.
2. 20%–30%: headache, nausea, vomiting, loss of judgment
3. 30%–40%: tachycardia, hyperpnea, hypotension, confusion
4. 50%–60%: loss of consciousness
5. 60%: convulsion, respiratory arrest, death

MYOGLOBIN (Mb)

Normal Values

Male: 19–92 μg/L
Female: 12–76 μg/L

Background

Myoglobin is the oxygen-binding protein of striated muscle. It resembles hemoglobin, but is unable to release oxygen except at extremely low tension. Injury to skeletal muscle will result in release of myoglobin.

Explanation of Test

Myoglobin tests are used as an index of muscle damage in myocardial infarction and to detect polymyositis and muscle injuries.

Procedure

Obtain a venous blood sample of at least 5 ml.

Clinical Implications

1. *Increased myoglobin values* are associated with
   a. Myocardial infarction (elevates earlier than CK)
   b. Other muscle injury (trauma, exercise, open-heart surgery)
   c. Polymyositis and progressive muscular dystrophy
   d. Various muscle enzyme deficiencies

   e. Metabolic stress (eg, carbon dioxide poisoning, hypoglycemia, hypokalemia, or water intoxication)
   f. Inflammatory myopathy (eg, systemic lupus erythematosus)
   g. Toxin exposure: narcotics, Malayan sea snake toxin
   h. Malignant hyperthelia
   i. Severe renal failure
2. *Decreased myoglobin values* are found in circulating antibodies to myoglobin (many patients with polymyositis); also in
   a. Rheumatoid arthritis
   b. Myasthenia gravis

Patient Preparation

1. Advise patient of test purpose.
2. Radioisotopes must be avoided until after blood is drawn.
3. Avoid vigorous exercise before test, which may elevate myoglobin.
4. See Chapter 1 guidelines for safe, effective, informed *pretest* care.

Patient Aftercare

1. Resume normal activities.
2. Interpret test outcomes, counsel, and monitor appropriately for myocardial infarction, muscle inflammation, and metabolic stress.
3. See Chapter 1 guidelines for safe, effective, informed *posttest* care.

Clinical Alert

Myoglobin has less clinical usefulness than CK-MB for the diagnosis of myocardial muscle damage. The diagnostic value of the test for detecting MI is strongly debated.

HAPTOGLOBIN (Hp)

Normal Values

Newborns: absent in 90%
Infants: 0–30 mg/dl
Children: 40–180 mg/dl
Adults: 40–270 mg/dl

Background

Haptoglobin, a transport glycoprotein synthesized solely in the liver, is structurally similar to hemoglobin. It is the first line of defense for the preservation of iron (located in the heme portion of hemoglobin) in the human body.

Explanation of Test

Haptoglobin measurement is primarily used as a confirmatory test for the presence of increased intravascular hemolysis. Haptoglobin will increase in any condition that causes tissue damage, such as infections and cancer. A decrease in haptoglobin in most persons with normal liver function is most likely due to an increased consumption of Hp. Any disease state that can cause an increase in intravascular hemolysis usually causes a decrease in haptoglobin. The concentration of haptoglobin is inversely related to the degree of hemolysis, as well as to the length of time of the hemolytic episode.

Procedure

A venous blood sample of at least 2 ml is obtained. The serum is measured for haptoglobin by a radial immunodiffusion method. A single determination is of limited value.

Clinical Implications

1. *Haptoglobin levels are decreased in acquired disorders,* such as
   - **a.** Transfusion reactions
   - **b.** Erythroblastosis fetalis
   - **c.** Systemic lupus erythematosus
   - **d.** Autoimmune hemolytic anemia
   - **e.** Other hemoglobinemias caused by intravascular hemorrhages, especially artificial heart valves
   - **f.** Malarial infestation
   - **g.** Paroxysmal nocturnal hemoglobinuria
   - **h.** Liver disease, especially cirrhosis
   - **i.** Thrombotic thrombocytopenic purpura
   - **j.** Drug-induced hemolytic anemia (methyldopa)
   - **k.** Uremia
   - **l.** Hypertension
   - **m.** Oral contraceptive use
2. *Hepatoglobin levels are also decreased in some inherited disorders,* such as
   - **a.** Sickle cell disease
   - **b.** G6PD and PK deficiency
   - **c.** Hereditary spherocytosis
   - **d.** Thalassemia and megaloblastic anemias
   - **e.** Generally observed in 1% of black and Oriental populations
3. *Hepatoglobin levels are increased* in
   - **a.** Infection and inflammation (acute and chronic)
   - **b.** Neoplasias, lymphomas
   - **c.** Biliary obstruction (33%)
   - **d.** Nephritis
   - **e.** Granulomatous disease
   - **f.** Steroid or androgen use
   - **g.** Ulcerative colitis
   - **h.** Peptic ulcer
   - **i.** Arterial disease
   - **j.** Acute rheumatic disease and other collagen diseases
   - **k.** Myocardial infarction (after) and other tissue destruction

Patient Preparation

1. Advise patient of test purpose.
2. Avoid use of oral contraceptives and androgens before blood is drawn. Check with physician.
3. Follow Chapter 1 guidelines for safe, effective, informed *pretest* care.

Patient Aftercare

1. Resume normal activities and medications.
2. Interpret test results. Repeat testing may be necessary. Monitor appropriately for abnormal bleeding.
3. See Chapter 1 guidelines for safe, effective, informed *posttest* care.

HEMOGLOBIN BART'S ●

Normal Values

None in children and adults; newborns < 0.5%

Background

Bart's is an unstable hemoglobin with high oxygen affinity. When there is complete absence of production of the chain of hemoglobin and deletion of all four globin genes, the disorder is known as Bart's hydrops fetalis. Both parents of the affected infant have heterozygous thalassemia and are almost exclusively Southeast Asians. Affected infants are either stillborn or die shortly after birth.

Explanation of Test

This test determines the percentage of Bart's abnormal hemoglobin in cord blood and identifies α-thalassemia hemoglobinopathies.

Procedure

A sample of cord blood is obtained, and a hemoglobin electrophoresis is performed.

Clinical Implications

Increased levels are associated with stillborn infants with homozygous α-thalassemia.

Patient Preparation

1. Explain test purpose and procedure to parents.
2. Obstetric complications may lead to significant morbidity and mortality for the mother of these infants.
3. Provide genetic counseling in a sensitive manner.
4. See Chapter 1 guidelines for safe, effective, informed *pretest* care.

Patient Aftercare

1. Interpret test outcome and counsel parents.
2. See Chapter 1 guidelines for safe, effective, informed *posttest* care.

PAROXYSMAL NOCTURNAL HEMOGLOBINURIA (PNH) TEST ●

Normal Values

Negative

Background

Paroxysmal nocturnal hemoglobinuria, was first described by a patient who noted hemoglobinuria after sleep. In many patients, the hemolysis is quite irregular or occult. Paroxysmal nocturnal hemoglobinuria (PNH) is a hemolytic anemia, in which there is also the production of defective platelets and granulocytes. The diagnostic feature of PNH is the increased sensitivity of the erythrocytes to complement-mediated lysis. Although patients with PNH can present with hemoglobinuria or a hemolytic anemia, they may also present with iron deficiency (because of urinary loss), bleeding secondary to thrombocytopenia, thrombosis, renal abnormalities, or neurologic abnormalities.

Explanation of Test

These tests are carried out to make a definitive diagnosis of PNH. The basis of these tests is that the cells peculiar to PNH have membrane defects, making them extrasensitive to complement in the plasma. Cells from patients with PNH will undergo marked hemolysis after 15 minutes in the laboratory test.

Procedure

Obtain a venous blood sample of 2 ml that is anticoagulated with 4 ml of EDTA blood. The patient's red cells are mixed with normal serum and also with the patient's own serum, acidified, incubated at 37°C, and examined for hemolysis. Normally, there should be no lysis of the red cells in this test.

Clinical Implications

1. These tests are almost never positive in any disease other than PNH and are seldom negative in patients with PNH.
2. The tests are performed on patients who have hemoglobinuria, bone marrow aplasia (hypoplasia), or undiagnosed hemolytic anemias. These tests may be useful in the evaluation of patients with unexplained thrombosis or acute leukemia.

Interfering Factors

False-positive results may be obtained when blood contains large numbers of spherocytes, or in patients with hereditary erythroblastic multinuclearity associated with a positive acidified serum test.

Patient Preparation

1. Explain test purpose.
2. See Chapter 1 guidelines for safe, effective, informed *pretest* care.

Patient Aftercare

1. Interpret test results, counsel, and monitor appropriately for anemia.
2. See Chapter 1 guidelines for safe, effective, informed *posttest* care.

● OTHER BLOOD TESTS FOR ANEMIA

VITAMIN B_{12} (VB_{12}) ●

Normal Values

Vitamin B_{12}: 100–700 pg/ml or 74–517 pmol/L
Newborn: 160–1300 pg/ml
Vitamin B_{12} (unsaturated binding capacity): 743–1632 pg/ml

Background

Vitamin B_{12}, also known as the antipernicious anemia factor, is necessary for the production of red blood cells. It is obtained only from ingesting animal protein and requires an intrinsic factor for absorption. Both vitamin B_{12} and folic acid depend on a normally functioning intestinal mucosa for their absorption and are important for the production of red blood cells. Levels of vitamin B_{12} and folate are usually tested in conjunction with one another because the diagnosis of macrocytic anemia requires measurement of both B_{12} and folate.

Explanation of Test

This determination is used in the differential diagnosis of anemia and conditions marked by high turnover of myeloid cells, as in the leukemias. When binding capacity is measured, it is the unsaturated fraction that is determined. The measurement of unsaturated vitamin B_{12}-binding capacity (UBBC) is valuable in distinguishing between untreated polycythemia vera and other conditions in which there is an elevated hematocrit.

Procedure

1. A fasting venous blood sample of at least 5 ml is obtained.
2. The specimen must be obtained before an injection of vitamin B_{12} is administered.

Clinical Implications

1. *Decreased vitamin B_{12} levels* of less than 100 pg/ml are associated with
   - **a.** Pernicious anemia (megaloblastic anemia)
   - **b.** Malabsorption syndromes and inflammatory bowel disease
   - **c.** Fish tapeworm infestation
   - **d.** Primary hypothyroidism
   - **e.** Loss of gastric mucosa, as in gastrectomy and resection

f. Zollinger–Ellison syndrome
g. Blind loop syndromes (bacterial overgrowth)
h. Vegetarian diets
i. Folic acid deficiency
j. Iron deficiency

2. *Increased vitamin B_{12} levels* of greater than 700 pg/ml are associated with
   a. Chronic granulocytic leukemia
   b. Myelomonocytic leukemia
   c. Liver disease (hepatitis, cirrhosis)
   d. Some cases of cancer, especially with liver metastasis
   e. Polycythemia vera
   f. Congestive heart failure
3. Increased unsaturated vitamin B_{12} binding found in more than 66% of cases of polycythemia vera. This test is normal in secondary relative polycythemia, aiding in the differential diagnosis of these two states; also in
   a. Reactive leukocytosis (leukemoid reaction).
   b. Chronic myelogenous leukemia.

Interfering Factors

Increases are seen with

1. Pregnancy
2. Oral contraceptive use
3. Aged persons
4. High vitamin C and A doses
5. Smoking
6. Drugs capable of interfering with B_{12} absorption

Patient Preparation

1. Explain test purpose and procedure.
2. Overnight fasting from food is necessary. Water is permitted.
3. Withhold vitamin B_{12} injection before the blood is drawn.
4. Follow Chapter 1 guidelines for safe, effective, informed *pretest* care.

Patient Aftercare

1. Resume normal activities and diet.
2. Interpret test results, counsel, and monitor appropriately for anemia, leukemia, or polycythemia.
3. See Chapter 1 guidelines for safe, effective, informed *posttest* care.

> **Clinical Alert**
>
> Persons who have recently received therapeutic or diagnostic doses of radionuclides will have unreliable results.

FOLIC ACID (FOLATE)

Normal Values

2–20 ng/ml

Background

Folic acid is needed for normal red and white blood cell function and the production of cellular genes. Folic acid is a more potent growth promoter than vitamin B_{12}, although both depend on the normal functioning of intestinal mucosa for their absorption. Folic acid, like B_{12}, is required for DNA production. Folic acid is formed by bacteria in the intestines, stored in the liver, and present in eggs, milk, leafy vegetables, yeast, liver, fruits, and other elements of a well-balanced diet.

Explanation of Test

This test is indicated in the differential diagnosis of megaloblastic anemia, and in the investigation of folic acid deficiency, iron deficiency, and hypersegmental granulocytes. The folic acid level must remain at a decreased level for 20 weeks or more before anemia develops. The test is usually done in conjunction with determination of vitamin B_{12} levels.

Procedure

Obtain a fasting venous sample of 10 ml. Protect sample from light.

Clinical Implications

1. *Decreased* folic acid levels are associated with
- **a.** Inadequate intake owing to alcoholism, chronic disease, malnutrition, diet devoid of fresh vegetables, and anorexia
- **b.** Malabsorption of folic acid as in small-bowel disease
- **c.** Excessive utilization of folic acid by the body in pregnancy and hypothyroidism
- **d.** Megaloblastic (macrocytic) anemia
- **e.** Hemolytic anemia—sickle cell, phenocytosis, PNH
- **f.** Liver disease associated with cirrhosis, alcoholism, hepatoma
- **g.** Adult celiac disease, sprue
- **h.** Exfoliative dermatitis
- **i.** Carcinomas (mainly metastatic), acute leukemia
- **j.** Crohn's disease, ulcerative colitis
- **k.** Infantile hyperthyroidism
- **l.** Myelofibrosis
- **m.** Drugs that are folic antagonists (interfere with nucleic acid synthesis), such as
  - **(1)** Anticonvulsants (phenytoin)
  - **(2)** Aminopterin and methotrexate used in leukemia treatment
  - **(3)** Antimalarials
  - **(4)** Alcohol (ethanol)
  - **(5)** Oral contraceptives

2. *Increased* folic acid levels are associated with
- **a.** Blind loop syndrome
- **b.** Vegetarian diet
- **c.** Pernicious anemia
- **d.** Blood transfusion

Interfering Factors

1. Drugs that are folic acid antagonists
2. False elevation in hemolyzed specimens
3. False increase in iron-deficiency anemia

> **Clinical Alert**
>
> Elderly persons or those having inadequate diets develop folate-deficient megaloblastic anemia.

Patient Preparation

1. Explain test purpose and procedure. Obtain pertinent medication history.
2. Fasting from food for 8 hours before testing; water is permitted.
3. Blood must be drawn before B_{12} injection.
4. No radioisotopes can be administered for 24 hours before specimen is drawn.
5. See Chapter 1 guidelines for safe, effective, informed *pretest* care.

Patient Aftercare

1. Resume normal activities and medications.
2. Interpret test results, counsel and monitor appropriately for anemia.
3. See Chapter 1 guidelines for safe, effective, informed *posttest* care.

● TESTS OF HEMOSTASIS AND COAGULATION

OVERVIEW OF TESTING FOR ABNORMAL BLEEDING AND CLOTTING

Hemostasis and coagulation tests are generally done in the presence of bleeding disorders, vascular injury or trauma, and coagulopathies. Reflex vasoconstriction is the normal response to vascular insult once the first-line defenses (skin and tissue) are breached. In larger vessels, vasoconstriction may be the primary mechanism for hemostasis. With smaller vessels, vasoconstriction reduces the size of the area that must be occluded by the hemostatic plug. Part of this cascade of sequential clotting events relates to the fact that platelets adhere to the injured and exposed subendothelial tissues. This phenomenon initiates the sequence of the complex clotting mechanism whereby thrombin and fibrin are formed and deposited to aid in intravascular clotting.

The entire mechanism of coagulation and fibrinolysis (removal of fibrin clot) is one of balance. It may be best understood by referring to diagrams in this section. Abnormal bleeding does not always indicate coagulopathy in much the same way that lack of bleeding does not necessarily indicate absence of a bleeding disorder.

The most common cause of hemorrhage is thrombocytopenia (platelet deficiency). Liver disease, uremia, disseminated intravascular coagulation disorder (DIC), and anticoagulant administration account for most other routine hemorrhagic problems. Hemophilia and other inherited factor deficiencies are seen less frequently. Bleeding tendencies are associated with delays in clot formation or in premature clot lysis. Thrombosis is associated with inappropriate clot activation or localization of the blood coagulation process. Finally, clotting disorders are divided into two classes: those caused by impaired coagulation, and those caused by hypercoagulability. See table entitled The Complex Chain of Coagulation Reactions.

HYPERCOAGULABILITY STATES ●

Two general forms of hypercoagulability exist: (1) hyperreactivity of the platelet system (results in arterial thrombosis), and (2) accelerated activity of the clotting system (results in venous thrombosis). Hypercoagulability refers to an unnatural tendency toward thrombosis. The thrombus is the actual insoluble mass (fibrin or platelets) present in the bloodstream or chambers of the heart.

Conditions and classifications associated with hypercoagulability include the following:

PLATELET ABNORMALITIES. These conditions are associated with arteriosclerosis, diabetes mellitus, elevated blood lipids or cholesterol levels, elevated platelet levels, and smoking. Arterial thrombosis may be related to blood flow disturbances, vessel wall changes, and increased platelet sensitivity to factors causing platelet adherence and aggregation.

CLOTTING SYSTEM ABNORMALITIES. These are associated with congestive heart failure, immobility, artificial surfaces (eg, artificial heart valves), damaged vasculature, oral contraceptive or estrogen use, pregnancy and the postpartum state, and the postsurgical state. Other influences include malignancy, myeloproliferative (bone marrow) disorders, obesity, lupus disorders, and genetic predisposition.

VENOUS THROMBOSIS. This can be related to status of blood flow, coagulation alterations, or increases in procoagulation factors or decreases in anticoagulation factors (see Proteins Involved in Blood Coagulation, Table 2-1).

DISORDERS OF HEMOSTASIS ●

CONGENITAL VASCULAR ABNORMALITIES—VESSEL WALL STRUCTURE DEFECTS. Defects of the actual blood vessel are poorly defined and difficult to test for.

1. Hereditary telangiectasia is the most commonly recognized vascular ab-

The Complex Chain of Coagulation Reactions

A balance normally exists between the factors that stimulate formation of thrombin and forces acting to delay thrombin formation. This balance maintains circulating blood as a fluid. When injury occurs or blood is removed from a vessel, this balance is upset and coagulation occurs. Blood clotting involves four progressive stages. The roman numerals assigned to the coagulation factors identify their order of discovery, rather than their involvement in the stages of clot formation.

Stage	Components of Stages	Clotting Factors*	
STAGE I (3–5 MIN)		*INTERNATIONAL NOMENCLATURE*	
Phase I—Platelet activity. Platelets serve as a source of thromboplastin.	90% of all coagulation disorders are due to defects in phase I. Platelet counts <1 million/mm^3 indicate moderate interference with phase I activity.	Factor I:	fibrinogen
		Factor II:	prothrombin (vitamin K functions in the production of prothrombin)
Phase II—Thromboplastin (factor III, an enzyme thought to be liberated by damaged cells, is formed by six different factors plus calcium.)	Calcium, Factor V, Factor VIII, Factor IX, Factor X, Factor XI, Factor XII } are involved in the formation of tissue thromboplastin (intrinsic prothrombin activation)	Factor III:	tissue thromboplastin
		Factor IV:	calcium ions
		Factor V:	platelet phospholipids and calcium ions
		Factor VI:	This factor is no longer considered to be a distinct part of coagulation.

STAGE II (8–15 SEC) Prothrombin factor II, is converted to thrombin in the presence of calcium	Factor II, Factor X, Factor VII, Factor V } are involved in the conversion of fibrinogen to fibrin	Factor VII:	a coenzyme (stable factor)
		Factor VIII:	antihemophilic globulin
		Factor IX:	Christmas factor (hemophilia)
		Factor X:	Stuart–Power factor. Factor X must be activated to convert prothrombin to thrombin
STAGE III (1 SEC) Thrombin interacts with fibrinogen (factor I) to form the framework of the clot.	At the end of stage III, factor XIII functions in the stabilization of the clot.	Factor XI:	plasma thromboplastin antecedent (PTA)
		Factor XII:	Hageman factor
		Factor XIII:	fibrin-stabilizing factor (FSF)
STAGE IV Fibrinolytic system (antagonistic system to the clotting mechanism; check-and-balance system is activated)	Removal of fibrin clot through fibrinolysis Plasminogen is converted to plasmin, which breaks clot into fibrin split products.		

*Note:** The 13 clotting factors of the blood are proteins. They are present in the blood plasma in an inactive form.

TABLE 2-1
Proteins Involved in Blood Coagulation

Proteins	*Synonym*	*Plasma Concentrations [mg/dl (μm)]*	*Function*
Fibrinogen	Factor I	300 (9)	Gels to form clot
Factor II	Prothrombin	15 (2)	Activates I, V, VIII, XIII, protein C, and platelets
Factor V	Proaccelerin	2 (0.05)	Supports X_a activation of II
Factor VII	Stable factor	0.1 (0.02)	Activates IX and X
Factor VIII	Antihemophilic factor	0.1 (0.003)	Supports IX_a activation of X
Factor IX	Christmas factor	1 (0.2)	Activates X
Factor X	Stuart–Prower factor	1 (0.2)	Activates II
Factor XI	Plasma thromboplastin antecedent	0.5 (0.03)	Activates XII and prekallikrein
Factor XII	Hageman factor	2 (0.2)	Activates XI and prekallikrein
Factor XIII	Fibrin-stabilizing factor	3 (0.08)	Crosslinks fibrin and other proteins
von Willebrand's factor	Factor VIII-related antigen	2 (0.05)	Binds VIII, mediates platelet adhesion

Prekallikrein	—	2 (0.3)	Activates XII and prekallikrein, cleaves HMWK
High molecular weight, kininogen (HMWK)	—	2 (0.2)	Supports reciprocal activation of XII, XI, and prekallikrein
Fibronectin	—	40 (1)	Mediates cell adhesion
Major antithrombin	Antithrombin III	20 (2.5)	Inhibits II_a, X_b, and other proteases; cofactor for heparin
Minor antithrombin	Heparin cofactor II	5 (0.6)	Inhibits II_a, cofactor for heparin and dermatan sulfate
Protein C	—	0.4 (0.06)	Inactivates V and VIII
Protein S	—	3 (0.4)	Cofactor for protein Ca, binds C4b-binding protein
Plasminogen	—	10 (1.2)	Lyses fibrin and other proteins
α_2-Antiplasmin	—	3 (0.5)	Inhibits plasmin
Prourokinase	—	—	Activates plasminogen
Tissue plasminogen activator (TPA)	—	—	Activates plasminogen
Plasminogen activator inhibitor I	—	—	Inactivates TPA
Plasminogen activator inhibitor II	—	—	Inactivates urokinase

normality. Laboratory studies are normal, so diagnosis must be made from clinical signs and symptoms. Patients frequently report epistaxis and symptoms of anemia.

2. Congenital hemangiomata; Kasabach–Merritt syndrome.

ACQUIRED VASCULAR ABNORMALITIES—VESSEL WALL STRUCTURE. Causes include Schönlein–Henoch purpura as an allergic response to infection or drugs, diabetes mellitus, rickettsial diseases, septicemia, and amyloidosis present with some degree of vascular abnormalities. Purpura also can be associated with steroid therapy and easy bruising in females (infectious purpura) or can be a result of drug use.

HEREDITARY CONNECTIVE TISSUE DISORDERS. These include Ehlers–Danlos syndrome (hyperplastic skin and hyperflexible joints) and pseudoxanthoma elasticum (rare connective tissue disorder).

ACQUIRED CONNECTIVE TISSUE DEFECTS. These can be caused by scurvy (vitamin C deficiency) or senile purpura.

QUALITATIVE PLATELET ABNORMALITIES. These can be divided into subclasses:

1. Thrombocytopenia (decreased < 150,000/mm^3 platelet count), caused by decreased production, increased platelet use or destruction, or hypersplenism. Contributing factors include bone marrow disease, autoimmune diseases, DIC, bacterial and viral infection, chemotherapy, radiation, multiple transfusions, and certain drugs (eg, NSAIDs, thiazides, estrogens).
2. Thrombocytosis (elevated platelet counts caused by hemorrhage, iron-deficiency anemia, inflammation, and splenectomy).

Clinical Alert

Elevated platelets predispose toward thrombosis.

3. Thrombocythemia (platelet counts > 1 million/mm^3) caused by granulocytic leukemia, polycythemia vera, or myeloid metaplasia.

Clinical Alert

When platelets are substantially elevated, hemorrhage can occur.

QUANTITATIVE PLATELET ABNORMALITIES. These are associated with Glanzmann's thrombasthenia, a hereditary autosomal recessive disorder that can produce severe bleeding, especially with trauma and surgical procedures; platelet factor 3 differences associated with aggregation, adhesion, or release defects can be manifested in storage-pool disease, May–Hegglin anomaly, Bernard–Soulier syndrome, and Wiskott–Aldrich syndrome. Dialysis and drugs, such as aspirin, other anti-inflammatory agents, dipyridamole, and prostaglandin E can also be tied to platelet abnormalities.

CONGENITAL COAGULATION ABNORMALITIES. These include hemophilia A and B (deficiencies of factors VIII and IX), rare autosomal recessive traits (hemophilia C), and autosomal dominant traits (eg, von Willebrand's disease).

ACQUIRED COAGULATION ABNORMALITIES. These are associated with several disease states.

1. Circulatory anticoagulant activity may be evident in the presence of antifactor VIII, rheumatoid arthritis, immediate postpartum period, systemic lupus erythematosus, or multiple myeloma.
2. Vitamin D deficiency may be caused by oral anticoagulants, biliary obstruction and malabsorption syndrome, or intestinal sterilization by antibiotic therapy. Newborns are prone to vitamin D deficiency.
3. Disseminated intravascular coagulation causes continuous production of thrombin, which, in turn, consumes the other clotting factors and results in uncontrolled bleeding (DIC).
4. Primary fibrinolysis is the situation whereby isolated activation of the fibrinolytic mechanism occurs without prior coagulation activity, such as in streptokinase therapy, severe liver disease, prostate cancer, and more rarely, in electroshock.
5. Most coagulation factors are manufactured in the liver. Consequently, in liver disease the extent of coagulation abnormalities is directly proportional to the severity of the liver disease.

TESTS FOR DISSEMINATED INTRAVASCULAR COAGULATION (DIC)

Disseminated intravascular coagulation (DIC) is an acquired hemorrhagic syndrome characterized by uncontrolled formation and deposition of fibrin thrombi. There is continuous generation of thrombin that causes depletion ("consumption") of the coagulation factors and results in uncontrolled bleeding. Also, fibrinolysis is activated in DIC. This further adds to the hemostasis defect caused by the consumption of clotting factors. Multiple coagulation test abnormalities found in DIC include

1. Prothrombin time (PT): prolonged
2. Partial thromboplastin time (PTT) or activated PTT: prolonged
3. Bleeding time: prolonged
4. Fibrinogen: decreased
5. Platelet count: decreased
6. Fibrinolysin test: increased
7. Fibrin split products: positive

8. Thrombin time (TT or TCT): prolonged
9. Clotting factors II, V, VIII, X: decreased
10. Fibrinopeptide: increased

Disseminated intravascular coagulation is a secondary condition caused by another disease. To treat DIC, the underlying disease must always be treated.

Causes of DIC include septicemia, malignancies and cancer, obstetric emergencies, cirrhosis of liver, sickle cell disease, trauma or crushing injuries, malaria, incompatible blood transfusions, cold hemoglobinuria or paroxysmal nocturnal hemoglobinuria, and abnormal protein or collagen diseases.

Paradoxically, the treatment for uncontrolled bleeding in DIC is heparin administration. The heparin blocks thrombin formation, which then blocks consumption of the other clotting factors and results in hemostasis.

Laboratory Investigation of Hemostasis

Usually, at least a 20-ml blood sample is obtained by the two-syringe technique. In the first syringe a 5-ml blood sample is obtained and discarded. Then 15 to 20 ml of blood is drawn into the second syringe and saved for examination. Sodium citrate additive acts as an anticoagulant. A butterfly needle may be used to prevent backflow or to make sampling easier in the case of a "difficult draw." Coagulation studies (*coagulation profiles, coag panels, coagulograms*), are used for screening or as diagnostic tools for evaluation of symptoms, such as easy or spontaneous bruising, petechiae, prolonged bleeding (eg, from cuts), abnormal nosebleeds, heavy menstrual flow, family history of coagulopathies, or gastrointestinal bleeding (Table 2-2).

1. These five primary screening tests are initially performed to diagnose suspected coagulation disorders:
   a. Platelet count, size, and shape
   b. Bleeding time—reflects data about the ability of platelets to function normally and of the capillaries to constrict their walls
   c. Partial thromboplastin time—determines the overall ability of the blood to clot (PTT)
   d. Prothrombin time—measures the function of second-stage clotting factors (PT)
   e. fibrinogen level
2. Factor assays are definitive coagulation studies of a specific clotting factor (eg, factor VIII for hemophilia). These would be done if the screening test indicated a problem with a specific factor(s).
3. Fibrinolysis is used to address problems of the fibrinolytic system. This includes studies of

a. Euglobulin clot lysis: identifies increased plasminogen activator activity. (Plasmin is *not* usually present in the blood plasma.)
b. Factor XIII: fibrin stabilizing factor
c. Fibrin split products (eg, protamine sulfate test)

4. The investigation of hypercoagulable status (thrombotic tendency or thromboembolic disorders) covers both primary (deficiencies of antithrombin III, proteins C and S, factor XII, and fibrinolytic mechanisms) and secondary (acquired platelet disorders and acquired diseases of coagulation and fibrinolytic impairment) causes. These include
   a. PT
   b. PTT
   c. Fibrinogen test
   d. Antiplatelet factors (eg, prostacyclin)
   e. Anticoagulant factors (eg, antithrombin III, proteins C and S, lupus anticoagulant)
   f. Fibrinolysis tests (eg, FDP, euglobulin lysis time, fibrin monomers)
   g. Thrombin time (TCT)

NOTE: *The lupus inhibitor (LI) /lupus anticoagulant (LA) is an antibody (against the phospholipid used in the PT/PTT test) responsible for inhibition of the prothrombin time, partial thromboplastin time, or both. To demonstrate the lupus anticoagulant, one must show that an inhibitor is present: 1 ml of patient's plasma is mixed with 1 ml of normal plasma and a PTT test of the mixture is then done. When an inhibitor of any sort is present, the PTT will not return to normal range. An inhibitor of the lupus type can be shown by correcting the PTT through using platelets as a phospholipid source or by demonstrating a characteristic pattern in the PTT that results from sequential dilution of the phospholipid reagent. Lupus anticoagulants may be associated with false-positive VDRL reports and another antiphospholipid—the anticardiolipid antibody lipin.*

Clinical Alert

Conditions associated with the presence of the lupus anticoagulant include

1. Systemic lupus erythematosus (one-third of patients).
2. Other autoimmune diseases (rheumatoid arthritis, Raynaud's syndrome).
3. Spontaneous abortions (associated with presence of anticardiolipid autoantibody).
4. Lupus anticoagulant is more often associated with thromboembolism, rather than with bleeding problems.

TABLE 2-2
Laboratory Tests to Measure Hemostasis

Name of Test	*Vascular Function*	*Platelet Function*	*Stage 1*	*Stage 2*	*Stage 3*	*Stage 4*
Tourniquet test	X	X				
Bleeding time	X	X				
Platelet count		X				
Platelet adhesiveness		X				
Platelet aggregation		X				
Aspirin tolerance		X				
Platelet factor 3 assay		X				
Clot retraction		X				
Prothrombin consumption		X	X			
Lee–White clotting time		X	X			
Siliconized clotting time		X	X			
Activated clotting time		X	X			
Recalcification time		X	X			
Activated recalcification time		X	X			
Partial thromboplastin time			X			
Activated partial thromboplastin			X			
Thromboplastin generation test			X			
Hicks–Pitney test			X			
Prothrombin time—quick						

Thrombotest*		X		
Stypven time*		X		
Circulating anticoagulant factor I.D. substitution	X	X	X	
Factor assay	X	X	X	
Thrombin time				X
Reptilase time			X	X
Fibrinogen assay			X	
Factor XIII assay			X	
Whole blood clot lysis				X
Dilute blood clot lysis				X
Euglobulin lysis time				X
Fibrin plate lysis				X
Serial thrombin time			X	X
Plasminogen assay				X
Protamine sulfate			X	X
Ethanol gelatin			X	X
TRCH II†				X
Staph clumping				X
Latex agglutination for FSP				X

*Monitors oral and coagulant therapy

†Tanned red cell hemagglutination inhibition immunoassay

These tests measure all facets of hemostasis: vascular function, platelets, and clotting factors.

(Based on table in Kennedy J: Laboratory Investigation of Hemostasis. Dade Monograph. Miami, American Hospital Supply, 1973)

Clinical Alert

1. All patients with hemorrhagic or thrombotic tendencies, or undergoing coagulation studies, should be observed closely for possible bleeding emergencies. A comprehensive history and physical exam should be done.
2. Blood samples for coagulation studies should be drawn last if other blood studies are indicated.
3. Procedure alert: When a blood sample is obtained for PT, PTT, and TT, sodium citrate is used as the anticoagulant in the sampling tubes.

Patient Assessment for Bleeding Tendency

1. Examine all skin for bruising.
2. Record petechiae associated with use of blood pressure cuffs or tourniquets.
3. Note bleeding from the nose or gums for no apparent cause.
4. Estimate blood quantity in vomitus, expectorated mucus, urine, stools, and menstrual flow.
5. Note prolonged bleeding from injection sites.
6. Watch for symptoms, especially changes in levels of consciousness or neurologic checks that may signal an "intracranial bleed."
7. Determine whether the patient is taking anticoagulants or aspirin.

BLEEDING TIME (IVY METHOD; TEMPLATE BLEEDING TIME) ●

Normal Values

3–10 minutes in most laboratories
Ivy method 2–9.5 minutes—forearm with template

Background

Bleeding time measures the primary phase of hemostasis: the interaction of the platelet with the blood vessel wall and the formation of the hemostatic plug. Bleeding time is the best single-screening test for platelet function disorders and is one of the primary screening tests for coagulation disorders. A small stab wound is made in either the earlobe or forearm; the bleeding time is recorded, and a measurement is made of the rate at which a platelet clot is formed. The duration of bleeding from a punctured capillary depends on the quantity and quality of platelets and the ability of the blood vessel wall to constrict.

Explanation of Test

The bleeding time test is of significant value in detecting vascular abnormalities and of moderate value in detecting platelet abnormalities or deficiencies.

Its principal use today is in the diagnosis of von Willebrand's disease, an inherited defective molecule of factor VIII, and a type of pseudohemophilia. It has been established that aspirin may cause abnormal bleeding in some normal persons, but the bleeding time has not proved to be consistently valuable in identifying such persons. Although the bleeding time is classically recognized as prolonged in thrombocytopenia, the test is an indirect method of identifying the condition.

Procedure

In the Ivy method, the area three finger-widths below the antecubital space is cleansed with alcohol and allowed to dry.

1. A blood pressure cuff is placed on the arm above the elbow and inflated to 40 mm Hg.
2. A cleansed area of the forearm, without superficial veins, is selected. The skin is stretched laterally and tautly between the thumb and forefinger.
3. The skin is punctured with a sterile disposable template to a uniform depth of 3 mm and width of 5 mm.
4. A stopwatch is started. The edge of a 4″ × 4″ filter paper is used to blot the blood through capillary action by gently touching the drop every 30 seconds. The wound itself is not disturbed. The blood pressure gauge is removed when bleeding stops spontaneously. A sterile dressing is applied when the test is completed.
5. The results of both procedures are reported in this way: The endpoint is reached when blood is no longer blotted from the ear or forearm puncture. It is reported in minutes and half minutes (eg, 5 min to 30 sec).

Clinical Implications

1. Bleeding time is prolonged when the level of platelets is decreased or when platelets are qualitatively abnormal, as in
   - **a.** Thrombocytopenia (less than 50,000)
   - **b.** Platelet dysfunction syndromes
   - **c.** Decrease or abnormality in plasma factors, such as von Willebrand's factor and fibrinogen
   - **d.** Abnormalities in walls of the small blood vessels, vascular disease
   - **e.** Advanced renal failure
   - **f.** Severe liver disease
   - **g.** Leukemia, lymphoproliferative disease
   - **h.** Aplastic anemia
   - **i.** DIC disease
2. In von Willebrand's disease, bleeding time can be normal or will be prolonged if aspirin is taken before testing (aspirin tolerance test).
3. A single prolonged bleeding time does not prove the existence of hemorrhagic disease. Since a larger vessel can be punctured, the puncture

should be repeated on an alternative body site, and the two values obtained should be averaged.
4. Bleeding time is normal in the presence of coagulation disorders, with the exception of platelet dysfunction or vascular disease.

Interfering Factors

1. Normal values for bleeding time vary when the puncture site is not of uniform depth and width.
2. Touching the test site during this test will break off fibrin particles and prolong the bleeding time.
3. Excessive alcohol consumption (as in alcoholics) may cause increased bleeding time.
4. Prolonged bleeding time can reflect ingestion of 10 g of aspirin (acetylsalicylic acid) up to 5 days before the test.
5. Other drugs that may cause increased bleeding times include dextran, streptokinase–streptodornase (fibrinolytic agents), mithramycin, pantothenyl alcohol.
6. Extreme hot or cold conditions can alter the results.

Patient Preparation

1. Explain test purpose and procedure. See **Patient Assessment** on page 114.
2. Instruct patient to abstain from aspirin and aspirinlike drugs for at least 7 days before the test.
3. Advise the patient to abstain from alcohol before the test.
4. Inform the patient that scar tissue may form at puncture site.
5. If the patient has an infectious skin disease, the test should be postponed.
6. See Chapter 1 guidelines for safe, effective, informed *pretest* care.

Patient Aftercare

1. Interpret test outcome and monitor appropriately for prolonged bleeding. See **Patient Assessment** for bleeding tendencies on page 114.
2. See Chapter 1 guidelines for safe, effective, informed *posttest* care.

Clinical Alert

1. Critical value is > 15 min
2. If the puncture site is still bleeding after 15 minutes, discontinue the test and apply pressure to the site. Document and report to physician.

TOURNIQUET TEST (RUMPEL-LEEDE POSITIVE-PRESSURE TEST; CAPILLARY FRAGILITY TEST; NEGATIVE-PRESSURE TEST) ●

Normal Values

Normal = no petechiae or negative = one to two petechiae

Positive = occasional (five to ten) petechiae

1+ = a few petechiae anterior forearm; 2+ = many petechiae anterior forearm; 3+ multiple petechiae whole arm and top of hand; 4+ = confluent petechiae all areas of arm and top of hand.

Normal in presence of coagulation and vascular disorders.

Background

This test measures capillary integrity. Thrombocytopenia, toxic vascular reactions, and hereditary vascular disorders produce positive results. Generally, large petechiae are a result of thrombocytopenia and pinpoint petechiae are more often associated with vascular permeability.

Explanation of Test

This test demonstrates capillary fragility. Positive or negative pressure is applied to various areas of the body by a blood pressure cuff or a suction cup. The degree of capillary fragility is reflected in the number of petechiae (nonraised, round red spots) that appear in a designated area. The forearm, wrists, hands, and fingers are examined for petechiae. Petechial distribution is usually irregular. The test is graded 1+ to 4+, depending on whether few or many petechial areas are visible.

Procedure

In the positive-pressure tourniquet test, a blood pressure cuff located on the upper arm is inflated to 70 to 90 mm Hg pressure or midway between systolic and diastolic pressures. The inflated cuff is removed after 5 minutes. The arm, wrist, and hand are then inspected for petechiae. In the negative-pressure test, a lubricated suction cup, 2 cm in diameter, is applied to the upper arm skin. Negative pressure is applied for 1 minute. Then the suction cup is released. Five minutes later the skin is inspected for petechiae.

Clinical Implications

1. Increased petechiae formation occurs in the presence of
   - **a.** Thrombocytopenia
   - **b.** Thrombasthenia
   - **c.** Vascular purpura
   - **d.** Senile purpura
   - **e.** Scurvy
   - **f.** Aplastic anemia
   - **g.** Hemophilia
   - **h.** Allergic purpura

2. The number and size of petechiae are roughly proportional to the bleeding tendency and, possibly, to the degree of thrombocytopenia. However, the test can also be positive because of capillary fragility in the presence of a normal platelet count (see **Normal Values**).

Interfering Factors

1. Menstruation: capillary fragility is normally increased before menstruation.
2. Capillary fragility is increased in measles and influenza.
3. Age: Women older than 40, with decreasing estrogen levels, may show a positive test (not indicative of a coagulation disorder).
4. Prolonged use of steroids increases capillary fragility.
5. Variation: owing to differences in texture, thickness, and temperature of the skin.

Patient Preparation

1. Explain test purpose and procedure. See special **Patient Assessment** for bleeding tendencies on page 114.
2. Examine patient's arm for any preexisting petechiae, ecchymoses, or skin infection that would influence results.
3. See Chapter 1 guidelines for safe, effective, informed *pretest* care.

> **Clinical Alert**
>
> Do not repeat this test on the same arm for at least 1 week.

Patient Aftercare

1. Interpret test outcome and monitor appropriately for bleeding tendency. Repeat testing may be necessary. Use opposite arm for repeat test.
2. See Chapter 1 guidelines for safe, effective, informed *posttest* care.

PLATELET COUNT

Normal Values

Adults: 140–400 × $10^3/mm^3$

Children: 150–450 × $10^3/mm^3$

Phase platelets—the normal value—can be slightly higher, or the same as the standard method.

Background

Platelets (or thrombocytes) are the smallest of the formed elements in the blood. These cells are nonnucleated, round or oval, flattened, disk-shaped structures. Platelet activity is necessary for blood clotting, vascular integrity and vasoconstriction, and the adhesion and aggregation activity in the formation of a platelet plug that occludes (plugs) breaks in small vessels. Platelet (thrombocyte) development takes place primarily in the bone marrow. The life span of a platelet is about 7.5 days. Normally, two-thirds of all the body platelets are found in the circulating blood, and one-third are in the spleen.

Explanation of Test

This test is indicated when the platelet count is below normal. It is helpful for evaluating bleeding disorders that occur with liver disease, thrombocytopenia, uremia, anticoagulant therapy, and following the course of diseases associated with bone marrow failure.

Other tests of platelet function include bleeding time (measures activity of platelets, adhesiveness, and platelet factor 3 content or release) and special function tests, such as platelet aggregation.

Procedure

A 7-ml venous blood sample is mixed with an anticoagulant EDTA tube.

Clinical Implications

1. *Abnormally increased numbers* of platelets (thrombocythemia/thrombocytosis 100,000 count) occur in
    - **a.** Malignancies
    - **b.** Chronic myelogenous and granulocytic leukemia
    - **c.** Polycythemia vera and primary thrombocytosis
    - **d.** Splenectomy, postoperative
    - **e.** Trauma, exercise
    - **f.** Asphyxiation
    - **g.** Rheumatoid arthritis and other collagen diseases
    - **h.** Iron-deficiency and posthemor rhagic anemias
    - **i.** Acute infections, inflammatory diseases
    - **j.** Hodgkin's disease, lymphomas
    - **k.** Chronic pancreatitis
    - **l.** Tuberculosis
    - **m.** Recovery from bone marrow suppression (thrombocytopenia)

Clinical Alert

1. In 50% of patients who exhibit unexpected platelet increases, a malignancy will be found.
2. In patients with an extremely elevated platelet count (1 million/mm^3), from a myeloproliferative disorder, assess for bleeding because of abnormal platelet function.

2. *Abnormally decreased numbers* of platelets (thrombocytopenia) occur in
    - **a.** Idiopathic thrombocytopenic purpura (ITP)
    - **b.** Pernicious, aplastic, and hemolytic anemias
    - **c.** After massive blood transfusion (dilution effect)
    - **d.** Viral, bacterial, and rickettsial infections
    - **e.** Congestive heart failure
    - **f.** Exposure to DDT and other chemicals
    - **g.** During cancer chemotherapy and radiation
    - **h.** HIV infection
    - **i.** Lesions involving the bone marrow

- **j.** Toxic effects of many drugs; dosages do not have to be high to be toxic. Toxic thrombocytopenia depends on the ability of the body to metabolize and secrete the toxic substance.
- **k.** DIC and thrombotic thrombocytopenic purpura (TTC)
- **l.** Inherited syndromes as Bernard–Soulier syndrome, May–Hegglin anomaly, Wiskott–Aldrich syndrome
- **m.** Fanconi's syndrome
- **n.** Liver disease
- **o.** Hyperthyroidism, hypothyroidism
- **p.** Renal vein thrombosis

Clinical Alert

1. Panic values: A *decrease in platelets* of < 20,000 mm^3 is associated with a tendency to spontaneous bleeding, prolonged bleeding time, petechiae, and ecchymosis.
2. Platelet counts of greater than 50,000 mm^3 are not generally associated with spontaneous bleeding.

Interfering Factors

1. Counts normally increase at high altitudes, after strenuous exercise, excitement and in winter.
2. They normally decrease before menstruation.

Patient Preparation

1. Explain test purpose and procedure.
2. Avoid strenuous exercise before blood is drawn.
3. Note what medications patient is taking.
4. See Chapter 1 guidelines for safe, effective, informed *pretest* care.

Patient Aftercare

1. Interpret test outcomes and monitor appropriately. Observe for signs and symptoms of GI bleeding, hemolysis, hematuria, petechiae, vaginal bleeding, epistasis, and bleeding from gums. When hemorrhage is apparent, use emergency measures to control bleeding and notify attending physician.
2. See Chapter 1 guidelines for safe, effective, informed *posttest* care.

MEAN PLATELET VOLUME

Normal Values

7.4–10.4 fl
25 μm in diameter

Explanation of Test

This test provides information about platelet size. This test is done to study various hematologic disorders, such as thrombocytopenic purpura, leukemia, and evaluation of alcoholics under treatment.

Procedure

The mean platelet volume is determined and calculated by an analyzer.

Clinical Implications

1. *Increases* in proportion of platelets exceeding 10.4 fl in volume occur in
   - **a.** Idiopathic thrombocytopenic purpura (autoimmune) in apparent remission
   - **b.** Thrombocytopenia caused by sepsis
   - **c.** DIC
   - **d.** Massive hemorrhage
   - **e.** Myeloproliferative disorders
   - **f.** Acute and chronic myelogenous leukemia
   - **g.** Splenectomy
   - **h.** Vasculitis
   - **i.** Megaloblastic anemia
2. *Decreases* occur in Wiskott-Aldrich syndrome.

PLATELET AGGREGATION ●

Normal Values

A normal pattern of platelet aggregation. Interpretation in the context of the patient's history, including medications and acute medical problems.

Explanation of Test

This platelet function test aids in the diagnosis of von Willebrand's disease, Glanzmann's disease, and other platelet disorders. Platelet aggregation or release are absent in a variety of deficiency conditions, termed *thrombocytopathy*.

Procedure

Obtain a 5-ml venous blood sample (anticoagulated in a tube containing sodium citrate). The sample is kept at room temperature (*never refrigerate*) and must be run within 30 minutes of drawing blood. When platelets aggregate, the transmission of light through a sample of platelet-rich plasma (PRP) is increased. This increase in light transmission can be used as an index of the aggregation in response to various agonists.

Clinical Implications

1. Abnormal platelet aggregation occurs in *congenital diseases* (decreased aggregation)
   - **a.** Bernard–Soulier syndrome
   - **b.** Glanzmann's thrombasthenia
   - **c.** Storage pool diseases
   - **d.** Thrombocytopenia with absent radius
   - **e.** Wiskott–Aldrich syndrome

   f. Albinism
   g. Chédiak–Higashi syndrome
   h. May–Hegglin anomaly
   i. Various connective tissue disorders
   j. von Willebrand's disorder
   k. β-Thalassemia minor

2. Abnormal platelet aggregation also occurs in *acquired disorders* (decreased aggregation)
   a. Uremia
   b. Antiplatelet antibodies
   c. Cardiopulmonary bypass
   d. Myeloproliferative disorders
   e. Dysproteinemias
   f. Idiopathic thrombocytopenic purpura
   g. Gray platelet syndrome
   h. Use of drugs and aspirin, some antibiotics, anti-inflammatory, pyrotropic and others
   i. Thrombothenia

3. Increased aggregation occurs in primary and secondary Raynaud's syndrome.

Patient Preparation

1. Explain test purpose and procedure.
2. For 10 days before the test, drugs that inhibit platelet aggregation are contraindicated. These include aspirin, antihistamines, steroids, cocaine, anti-inflammatories, and theophylline.
3. On the day of the test, avoid caffeine.
4. Avoid warfarin (Coumadin) for 2 weeks and heparin therapy for 1 week before testing.
5. See Chapter 1 guidelines for safe, effective, informed *pretest* care.

Patient Aftercare

1. Interpret test outcome and monitor appropriately.
2. Resume medications and normal diet.
3. See Chapter 1 guidelines for safe, effective, informed *posttest* care.

THROMBIN TIME (TT); THROMBIN CLOTTING TIME (TCT) ●

Normal Values

7.0–12.0 seconds. However, "normals" can vary widely according to different laboratories' interpretations.

Explanation of Test

Stage III fibrinogen defects can be detected by thrombin time. It can detect DIC and hypofibrinogenemia and may also be used for monitoring streptokinase therapy. The test actually measures time needed for plasma to clot when thrombin is added. Normally, a clot will form rapidly; if it does not, a fibrinogen deficiency is present (Fig. 2-1).

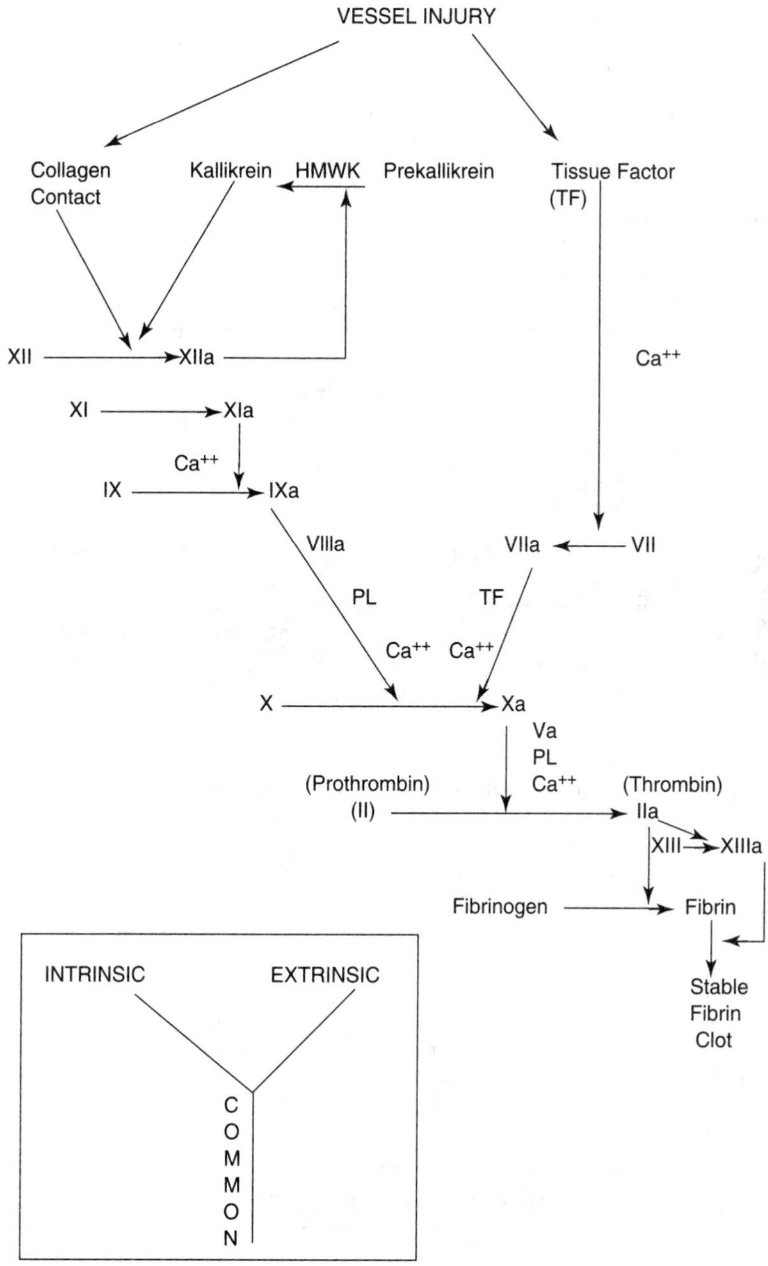

FIGURE 2-1

Intrinsic, extrinsic, and common pathways of coagulation. Vessel injury initiates intrinsic pathway through contact activation by exposed collagen. Extrinsic pathway is initiated by endothelial release of tissue factor (ie, tissue thromboplastin). Extrinsic and intrinsic pathway each initiate common pathway to create stable fibrin clot. (Lotspeich-Steininger, C.A., et al. (1992). *Clinical Hematology*. Philadelphia, J. B. Lippincott Co.)

Procedure

With the procedure for two-tube specimen collection, a 7-ml venous blood sample is anticoagulated with sodium citrate and put on ice.

Clinical Implications

1. Prolonged TT time occurs in
   - **a.** Hypofibrinogenemia
   - **b.** Therapy with heparin or heparinlike anticoagulants
   - **c.** Disseminated intravascular coagulopathy (DIC)
   - **d.** Fibrinolysis
   - **e.** Multiple myeloma
   - **f.** The presence of large amounts of fibrin or fibrinogen breakdown products (FBPs)
   - **g.** Uremia
   - **h.** Severe liver diseases
2. Shortened thrombin time occurs in
   - **a.** Hyperfibrinogenemia
   - **b.** Elevated hematocrit (> 755%)

> **Clinical Alert**
>
> Thrombin time is *severely* prolonged in the presence of afibrinogenemia (< 80 mg/dl of fibrinogen).

Interfering Factors

Heparin prolongs thrombin time. Interpret test results within this context.

Patient Preparation

1. Explain test purpose and procedure.
2. If possible, no heparin should be administered for 2 days before testing.
3. See Chapter 1 guidelines for safe, effective, informed *pretest* care.

Patient Aftercare

1. Resume normal activities and medications as ordered.
2. Interpret test outcomes and monitor appropriately. Check for excess bleeding.
3. See Chapter 1 guidelines for safe, effective, informed *posttest* care.

PARTIAL THROMBOPLASTIN TIME (PTT); **ACTIVATED PARTIAL THROMBOPLASTIN TIME** (APTT) ●

Normal Values

PTT: 30–45 sec
APTT: 21–35 sec
Check with your laboratory concerning therapeutic range values for heparin therapy.

Background

The PTT, a one-stage clotting test, screens for coagulation disorders. Specifically, it can detect deficiencies of the intrinsic thromboplastin system and will also reveal defects in the extrinsic coagulation mechanism pathway.

> **NOTE:** *The PTT and APTT test for the same functions. APTT is a more sensitive version of PTT that is used to monitor heparin therapy.*

Explanation of Test

The APTT is the preferred test to monitor heparin therapy. It can also detect circulating anticoagulants.

Procedure

1. A 7-ml venous blood sample is anticoagulated with sodium citrate and put on ice until the test can be run. Use the two-tube method.
2. Do not draw blood samples from a heparin lock or heparinized catheter.

Clinical Implications

1. The *APTT is prolonged* in
   - **a.** All congenital deficiencies of intrinsic system coagulation factors, including hemophilia A and hemophilia B
   - **b.** Congenital deficiency of Fitzgerald factor and Fletcher factor (prekallikrein)
   - **c.** Heparin therapy
   - **d.** Warfarin (Coumadin)-like therapy
   - **e.** Vitamin K deficiency
   - **f.** Hypofibrinogenemia
   - **g.** Liver disease
   - **h.** Disseminated intravascular coagulopathy (DIC)—chronic or acute
   - **i.** Fibrin breakdown products (FBPs)
2. The APTT and PT will detect approximately 95% of coagulation abnormalities. When APTT is performed in conjunction with a PT, a further clarification of coagulation defects is possible. For example, a normal PT and an abnormal PTT means that the defect lies within the first stage of the clotting cascade (factors VIII, IX, X, XI, and/or XII). A normal PTT and abnormal PT suggests a possible factor VII deficiency. The pattern of a prolonged PT and PTT suggests a deficiency of factors I, II, V, or X.
3. *Shortened APTT* occurs in:
   - **a.** Extensive cancer, except when the liver is involved
   - **b.** Immediately after acute hemorrhage
   - **c.** Very early stages of disseminated intravascular coagulopathy (DIC)
4. *Circulating anticoagulants* (inhibitors) usually occur as inhibitors of a specific factor (eg, factor VIII). These are most commonly seen in the development of antifactor VIII or antifactor IX in 5% to 10% of hemophiliac patients. Anticoagulants that develop in the treated hemophiliac are detected through prolonged APTT. Circulating anticoagulants are also associated with other conditions such as

a. Following many plasma transfusions
b. Drug reactions
c. Tuberculosis
d. Chronic glomerulonephritis
e. Systemic lupus erythematosus
f. Rheumatoid arthritis

Clinical Alert

APTT > 100 sec signifies spontaneous bleeding.

5. *Heparin therapy:* Heparin is a *direct* anticoagulant.
  a. In the blood, heparin combines with an alpha-globulin (heparin cofactor) to form a potent antithrombin.
  b. Intravenous heparin injection produces an immediate anticoagulant effect; it is chosen when rapid anticoagulant effects are desired.
  c. Because the half-life of heparin is 3 hours, APTT is measured 3 hours after heparin administration.
  d. Therapeutic APTT levels are ordinarily maintained at 2 to 2 1/2 times normal values.
  e. To evaluate heparin effects blood is tested
    (1) For baseline values before initiating therapy
    (2) One hour before next dose is due (when a 4-hour administration cycle is ordered)
    (3) According to the patient's status (ie, bleeding)

Patient Preparation

1. Explain test purpose and procedure.
2. Draw blood sample 1 hour before next dose of heparin. The heparin dose given relates to the APTT result.
3. See Chapter 1 guidelines for safe, effective, informed, *pretest* care.

Patient Aftercare

1. Interpret test outcome and monitor appropriately. Protamine sulfate is the antidote for heparin overdose or for reversal of heparin anticoagulation therapy.
2. Follow Chapter 1 guidelines for safe, effective, informed *posttest* care.
3. Watch for signs of spontaneous bleeding, notify physician, and treat accordingly.
4. In case of spontaneous bleeding, notify physician immediately.
5. Alert the patient to watch for bleeding gums, hematuria, oozing from wounds, excessive bruising.
6. Instruct the patient to use electric shaver instead of blade and to exercise caution in all activities.

7. Avoid use of aspirin or ASA-like drugs as these contribute to bleeding tendencies (unless specifically prescribed).

AUTOMATED COAGULATION TIME (ACT)

Therapeutic Range

ACT: 150–180

This test evaluates intrinsic coagulation status more accurately than the PTT or APTT. The patient's own platelet factor 3 is actively used and calcium variations are minimized. The clotting time responds both linearly to heparin level changes and to wider ranges of heparin concentrations than does the APTT.

The ACT can be a bedside procedure and requires only 0.4 ml of blood. Heparin infusion or reversal with protamine then can be titrated almost immediately according to ACT results. Additionally, ACT is routinely used during dialysis, coronary artery bypass procedure, arteriograms, and percutaneous transluminal coronary arteriography (PTCA).

PROTHROMBIN TIME (PRO TIME; PT)

Normal Values

11.0–13.0 sec (can be variable according to laboratory methodology)

Therapeutic Levels

1. Therapeutic levels are at a prothrombin time (PC) ratio of 2.0–2.5.
2. Recommended therapeutic ranges in International Normal Ratio (INRs) are as follows:

	INR	*Target*
PREOPERATIVE ORAL ANTICOAGULANT STARTED 2 WEEKS BEFORE SURGERY		
Nonhip surgery	1.5–2.5	2.0
Hip surgery	2.0–3.0	2.5
Primary and secondary prevention of deep vein thrombosis	2.0–3.0	2.5
Prevention of systemic embolism in patients with atrial fibrillation	2.0–3.0	2.5
Recurrent systemic embolism	3.0–4.5	3.5
Prevention of recurrent deep vein thrombosis (two or more episodes)	2.5–4.0	3.0
Cardiac stents	3.0–4.5	3.5
Prevention of arterial thrombosis including patients with mechanical heart valves	3.0–4.5	3.5

DEFINITIONS

P/C ratio = Prothrombin time ratio: The observed patient PT divided by the laboratory PT mean normal value.

INR = International Normalized Ratio: A comparative rating of PT ratios (INR represents the observed PT ratio adjusted by the International Reference Thromboplastin).

ISI = International Sensitivity Index: A comparative rating of thromboplastin (supplied by the manufacturer of the reagent).

Background

Prothrombin is a protein, produced by the liver, that acts in the clotting of blood. Prothrombin production depends on adequate vitamin K intake and absorption. During the clotting process, prothrombin is converted to thrombin. The prothrombin content of the blood will be reduced in patients with liver disease.

Explanation of Test

Prothrombin time is one of the four most important screening tests used in diagnostic coagulation studies. It directly measures a potential defect in stage II of the clotting mechanism through analysis of the clotting ability of five plasma coagulation factors (prothrombin, fibrinogen, factor V, factor VII, and factor X). This is known as the "prothrombin time" and is commonly ordered during management of oral anticoagulant (warfarin; Coumadin) therapy.

Procedure

1. A 5-ml venous blood sample is drawn (by the two-tube technique) into a tube containing a calcium-binding anticoagulant (sodium citrate). The ratio of sodium citrate to blood is critical.
2. Blue top vacuum tubes will keep prothrombin levels stable at room temperature if left capped.

Oral Anticoagulant Therapy

Oral anticoagulant drugs (eg, warfarin [Coumadin] and dicumarol) are commonly prescribed to treat blood clots. These are *indirect* anticoagulants (as compared with heparin, which is a *direct* anticoagulant). However, if necessary, heparin is the initial choice for initiating treatment because it acts rapidly and also partially lyses the clot.

1. These drugs act through the liver to delay coagulation by interfering with the action of vitamin K–related factors (II, VII, IX, and X) that promote clotting.
2. Oral anticoagulants delay vitamin K formation and cause prothrombin time to increase owing to *decreased* factors II, VII, IX, and X.
3. The usual procedure is to run a PT test every day. Once the PT is deter-

mined, the anticoagulant dose is adjusted until the therapeutic range is reached. Then, weekly to monthly, PT testing continues for the duration of therapy.

4. Warfarin (Coumadin) takes 48 to 72 hours to cause a measurable change in the PT.

Drug Therapy and PT Protocols

1. Patients with cardiac problems are usually maintained at a PT level 2 to 2.5 times normal (baseline) values.

2. Using the INR values allows more sensitive control.

3. For treatment of blood clots, the PT is maintained within 2 to 2.5 times normal. If the PT drops below this range, treatment may be ineffective and old clots may expand, or new clots may form. Conversely, if the PT rises above 30 seconds, bleeding or hemorrhage may occur.

Clinical Implications

1. Conditions showing *increased PT levels* include
- **a.** Prothrombin deficiency (factor II) also factors V, VII, X
- **b.** Vitamin K deficiency
- **c.** Hemorrhagic disease of the newborn
- **d.** Liver disease (eg, alcoholic hepatitis)
- **e.** Current anticoagulant therapy outside the therapeutic range
- **f.** Biliary obstruction
- **g.** Salicylate intoxication
- **h.** Hypervitaminosis A
- **i.** Disseminated intravascular coagulation (DIC)
- **j.** Zollinger–Ellison syndrome
- **k.** Hypofibrinogenemia (factor I deficiency)
- **l.** Systemic lupus erythematosus (SLE)

2. Conditions *that decrease the PT* include
- **a.** Ovarian hyperfunction
- **b.** Regional enteritis/ileitis

3. Conditions that *do not affect* the PT include
- **a.** Polycythemia vera
- **b.** Tannin disease
- **c.** Christmas disease (factor IX deficiency)
- **d.** Hemophilia A (factor VIII)
- **e.** von Willebrand's deficiency
- **f.** Platelet disorders—idiopathic thrombocytopenic purpura (ITP)

Interfering Factors

1. Diet: ingestion of excessive green, leafy vegetables (increases the body's absorption of vitamin K, which promotes blood clotting).

2. Alcoholism and excessive alcohol ingestion raise PT levels.

3. Diarrhea and vomiting decrease PT because of dehydration.

4. Quality of venipuncture: PT can be shortened if technique is relatively traumatic.

5. Influence of prescribed medications (eg, isoniazid [INH], phenothiazides, cephalosporins, cholestyramines, phenylbutazone, metronidazole, oral hypoglycemics, phenytoin).

Patient Preparation

1. Explain the purpose, procedure, and need for frequent testing. Emphasize the need for regular monitoring through frequent blood testing if on long-term therapy. *Do not refer to anticoagulants as "blood thinners."* One explanation might be: "Your blood will be tested periodically to determine the pro time, which is an indication of how quickly the blood clots." The anticoagulant dose will be adjusted according to PT results.
2. Caution against self-medication. Ascertain what drugs the patient has been taking. Many drugs, including over-the-counter medications, alter the effects of the anticoagulants and the PT values. Aspirin, acetaminophen, and laxative products should be avoided unless specifically ordered by the physician.
3. Instruct the patient never to start or to discontinue any drug without the doctor's permission. This will affect PT values and may also interfere with the healing process.
4. Counsel about diet. Excessive amounts of green, leafy vegetables (eg, spinach, broccoli) will increase vitamin K levels and could interfere with anticoagulant metabolism. Caution against using razor blades for shaving, trimming, and such. Electric shavers should be used.
5. These guidelines also apply to aftercare.

Patient Aftercare

1. Interpret test outcomes and monitor appropriately.
2. Avoid intramuscular injections during anticoagulant therapy because hematomas may form at the injection site. As the PT increases to upper limits (> 30 minutes), carefully assess for bleeding from different areas. It may be necessary to perform neurologic assessments (if cranial bleeding is suspected), lung assessments and auscultation, GI and GU assessments, or other assessments as appropriate. Instruct the patient to observe for bleeding from gums, in the urine, or other unusual bleeding. Advise that care should be exercised in all activities lest accidental injury occur.
3. Patients who are being monitored by PT for long-term anticoagulant therapy should not take any other drugs unless specifically prescribed.
4. When unexpected adjustments in anticoagulant dosages are required to maintain a stable PT, or when there are erratic changes in PT levels, a drug interaction should be suspected and further investigation should take place.
5. Changes in exercise intensity should be done gradually or even avoided. Active sports and contact sports should be avoided because of potential for injury.
6. See Chapter 1 guidelines for safe, effective, informed *posttest* care.

Clinical Alert

Critical Value

1. If P/C ratio is greater than 2.5 or longer than 30.0 seconds, notify physician.
2. If PT is excessively prolonged (> 40 sec), vitamin K may be ordered.
3. Baseline PT levels should be drawn before anticoagulant administration.

COAGULANT FACTORS (FACTOR ASSAY)

Normal Values

Factor II: 80%–120% of normal
Factor V: 50%–150% of normal
Factor VII: 65%–140% of normal or 65–135 AU
Factor VIII: 55%–145% of normal or 55–145 AU
Factor IX: 60%–140% of normal or 60–140 AU
Factor X: 45%–155% of normal or 45–155 AU
Factor XI: 65%–135% of normal or 65–135 AU
Factor XII: 50%–150% of normal or 50–150 AU
Ristocetin–von Willebrand factor: 45%–140% of normal or 45–140 AU
Factor VIII antigen: 50–150 mg/dl
Factor VIII-related antigen: 45%–185% of normal or 45–185 AU
Fletcher factor (prekallikrein): 80%–120% of normal

Explanation of Test

This test of specific factors of coagulation is done in the investigation of inherited and acquired bleeding disorders. For example, tests of factor VIII-related antigen are used in the differential diagnosis of classic hemophilia and von Willebrand's disease in patients in whom there is no family history of bleeding and when bleeding times may be borderline or abnormal. A test for ristocetin cofactor is done to help diagnose von Willebrand's disease by determining the degree or rate of platelet aggregation that is taking place.

Procedure

1. A 5-ml venous blood sample is drawn by the two-tube method and is added to a collection tube containing sodium citrate as the anticoagulant. Blood is drawn from a nonrelated person at the same time to serve as a control.
2. Samples are capped and iced.

Clinical Implications

1. *Inherited deficiencies*
   a. All of the specific factors—VII, VIII, IX, X, XI, and XII—may be defi-

cient on a familial basis, eg, factor VII is decreased in hypoproconvertinemia (autosomal recessive); factor VIII is decreased in classic hemophilia A and von Willebrand's disease (inherited autosomally); factor IX is decreased in Christmas disease or hemophilia B (sex-linked recessive); and factor XI is decreased in hemophilia C, occurring preponderantly in persons of Jewish decent (autosomal dominant).

2. *Acquired disorders*

a. Factor VII is also decreased in acquired disorders such as

(1) Liver disease
(2) Treatment with coumarin-type drugs
(3) Hemorrhagic disease of the newborn
(4) Kwashiorkor

b. Factor VIII increases are associated with

(1) Late normal pregnancy
(2) Thromboembolic conditions
(3) Coronary artery disease
(4) Postoperative period
(5) Rebound activity after sudden cessation of a coumarin-type drug
(6) Hyperthyroidism
(7) Myeloma
(8) Macroglobulinemia
(9) Hypoglycemia
(10) Cushing's syndrome
(11) DIC

c. Factor IX levels are decreased in:

(1) Uncompensated cirrhosis (40% of cases)
(2) Nephrotic syndrome
(3) Development of circulating anticoagulants against factor IX
(4) Normal newborn
(5) Dicumarol and related anticoagulant drugs cause a decrease after 48 to 72 hours of treatment
(6) DIC

d. Factor XI decreased levels are associated with

(1) Liver disease
(2) Intestinal malabsorption of vitamin K
(3) Occasional development of circulatory anticoagulants against factor IX
(4) Congenital heart disease
(5) Paroxysmal nocturnal hemoglobinuria
(6) DIC

e. Factor XII level is decreased in the nephrotic syndrome.

f. Factor VIII inhibitors (anticoagulants capable of specifically neutralizing a coagulation factor and, thereby, disrupting hemostasis) are associated with

(1) Hemophilia A
(2) Immunologic reactions

g. Factor VIII-related antigen is low in von Willebrand's disease and normal in hemophilia.

h. Ristocetin cofactor is decreased in von Willebrand's disease and Bernard–Soulier disease, an intrinsic platelet defect.

i. Factor X is increased during normal pregnancy.

j. Factor XI is decreased in newborns and with use of anticoagulant therapy.

k. Factor XIII is decreased in newborns and in normal pregnancy and increased after exercise.

l. Factor XIII levels are decreased in
- **(1)** Postoperative patients
- **(2)** Liver disease
- **(3)** Persistent increased fibrinogen levels
- **(4)** Myeloma
- **(5)** Lead poisoning
- **(6)** Pernicious anemia
- **(7)** Agammaglobulinemia

PLASMINOGEN/PLASMIN

Normal Values

Plasminogen activity:

Males: 76%–124%
Females: 65%–153%
Infants: 27%–59% of normal

Background

Plasminogen is a glycoprotein present in plasma as the inactive protein zymogen at a concentration of about 200 μg/ml. Decreased plasminogen activity may be an acquired or familial condition.

Explanation of Test

These measurements of fibrinolysis determine the level of plasminogen, the inactive precursor of plasmin, and of the active enzyme plasmin, which has the ability to dissolve formed fibrin clots. Also, the test is useful for monitoring streptokinase therapy in arterial thrombosis.

Procedure

1. A 5-ml venous blood sample is added to a collection tube containing sodium citrate. The two-tube method is used.
2. The sample is iced and immediately transported to the laboratory.
3. The test must be started within 30 minutes of the draw.

Clinical Implications

1. Decreases in plasminogen activity occur in
   - **a.** Some familial or isolated cases of idiopathic deep vein thrombosis
   - **b.** DIC and systemic fibrinolysis
   - **c.** Liver disease and cirrhosis
   - **d.** Neonatal hygiene membrane disease
   - **e.** Diabetes with thrombosis
2. Decreased levels of plasminogen or abnormally functioning plasminogen can lead to venous and arterial clotting (thrombosis).

Patient Preparation

1. Explain test purpose and procedure.
2. See Chapter 1 guidelines for safe, effective, informed *pretest* care.

Patient Aftercare

1. Interpret test outcomes and monitor appropriately for thrombotic tendency.
2. See Chapter 1 guidelines for safe, effective, informed *posttest* care.

FIBRINOLYSIS/EUGLOBULIN LYSIS TIME

Normal Values

Euglobulin lysis—no lysis of plasma clot at 37°C in 60 to 120 minutes. The clot is observed for 24 hours.

Background

Primary fibrinolysis, without any sign of intravascular coagulation, is extremely rare. Secondary fibrinolysis is usually seen and follows or occurs simultaneously with intravascular coagulation. This secondary fibrinolysis is thought to be a protective mechanism against generalized clotting.

Explanation of Test

This test is done to evaluate a fibrinolytic crisis. (No single test has been universally accepted for the complete diagnosis and management of fibrinolytic states.)

Procedure

1. A 5-ml venous blood sample is collected in a tube containing sodium citrate.
2. The sample is iced and immediately transported to the laboratory.
3. The test must be started within 30 minutes of the draw.

> **Clinical Alert**
>
> A lysis time of less than 1 hour signifies that abnormal fibrinolysis is occurring.

Clinical Implications

1. *Increased fibrinolysis* occurs (with)
   a. Within 48 hours after surgery (The fibrinolytic activity continues to increase for the next 6 days.)
   b. Incompatible blood transfusions
   c. Cancer of prostate or pancreas
   d. Cirrhosis (some cases)
   e. During lung and cardiac surgery
   f. Obstetric complications (eg, antepartum hemorrhage, amniotic embolism, septic abortion, death of fetus, hydatidiform mole)
   g. Long-term DIC
   h. Hypofibrinogenemia
   i. Administration of plasminogen activators (eg, TPA, streptokinase, or urokinase [can be used to monitor])

2. *Decreased fibrinolysis* occurs in diabetes and first 48 hours after surgery.

Interfering Factors

1. Increased fibrinolysis occurs with moderate exercise and increasing age.
2. Decreased fibrinolysis occurs in
   a. Arterial blood, when compared with venous blood. This difference is greater in arteriosclerosis (especially in young persons)
   b. Postmenopausal women
   c. Normal newborns
3. Fibrin degradation products interfere with fibrinolysis.
   a. False-negative results can occur if fibrinolysis is far advanced.
   b. False-positive results can be caused by very low fibrinogen levels.

Patient Preparation

1. Advise patient of test purpose and procedure.
2. See Chapter 1 guidelines for safe, effective, informed *pretest* care.

Patient Aftercare

1. Interpret test results and monitor appropriately.
2. See Chapter 1 guidelines for safe, effective, informed *posttest* care.

FIBRIN SPLIT PRODUCTS (FSP); **FIBRIN DEGRADATION PRODUCTS** (FDP) ●

Normal Values

Negative at 1:4 dilution or < 10 μg/ml

Background

When fibrin is split by plasmin, positive tests for fibrin degradation or split products, identified by letters X, Y, D, and E, are produced. These products have an anticoagulant action and inhibit clotting when there is an excess in the circulation. Increased levels of fibrin degradation products may occur with a variety of pathologic processes in which clot formation and lysis occur.

Explanation of Test

This test is done to establish the diagnosis of disseminated intravascular coagulation (DIC) and other thromboembolic disorders.

Procedure

1. A venous blood sample of at least 4.5 ml is placed in a tube containing thrombin and an inhibitor of fibrinolysis (reptilase, aprotinin, and calcium).
2. Blood must be completely clotted for test to be valid.

Clinical Implications

1. Increased FSP/FDP are associated with any condition associated with DIC. See page 110 for examples. They are also found in
   a. Venous thrombosis
   b. Primary fibrinolysis
   c. Following thoracic and cardiac surgery and renal transplantation
   d. Acute myocardial infarction
   e. Pulmonary embolism
   f. Carcinoma

Interfering Factors

1. Because all of the laboratory methods are sensitive to fibrinogen as well as FDP, it is essential that no unclotted fibrinogen be left in the serum preparation. False-positive reactions could result if any fibrinogen is present.
2. False-positive results occur with heparin therapy.
3. The presence of rheumatoid factor (RA) may give falsely high values.

Patient Preparation

1. Explain test purpose and procedure.
2. See Chapter 1 guidelines for safe, effective, informed *pretest* care.

Patient Aftercare

1. Interpret test results and monitor appropriately for DIC and thrombosis.
2. See Chapter 1 guidelines for safe, effective, informed *posttest* care.

> **Clinical Alert**
>
> Patients with very high levels of FSP/FDP have blood that does not clot or clots poorly.
> **Critical Value: >160 μg/ml**

D-DIMER

Normal Values

< 250 mg/ml
Qualitative: no D-dimer fragments present.

Background

The D-dimers are produced by the action of plasmin on crosslinked fibrin. They are not produced by the action of plasmin on unclotted fibrinogen.

Explanation of Test

This test is used in the diagnosis of DIC disease. The D-dimer test is more specific for DIC than are tests for fibrin split products (FSPs). It verifies in vivo fibrinolysis because it is specific for only fibrin degradation products and not fibrinogen degradation productions.

Procedure

A venous blood sample of 4.5 ml is collected into a tube containing sodium citrate (same tube as for PT/PTT).

Clinical Implications

1. Increased D-dimer values are associated with
   a. DIC
   b. Arterial or venous thrombosis
   c. Secondary fibrinolysis
   d. Pulmonary embolism
   e. Late in pregnancy, postpartum
   f. Blood taken within 2 days of surgery
   g. Malignancy
2. D-dimer is negative in primary fibrinolysis.

Interfering Factors

1. False-positive test results are obtained with high titers of rheumatoid factors.
2. False-positive D-dimer levels increase as the tumor marker CA-125 for ovarian cancer increases.

Patient Preparation

1. Explain test purpose and procedure. See information about tests for DIC on page 110.
2. See Chapter 1 guidelines for safe, effective, informed *pretest* care.

Patient Aftercare

1. Interpret test outcome and monitor appropriately for DIC or thrombin.
2. See Chapter 1 guidelines for safe, effective, informed *posttest* care.

FIBRINOPEPTIDE-A (FPA) ●

Normal Values

None present

Explanation of Test

This measurement is the most sensitive assay done to determine thrombin action. Fibrinopeptide A reflects the amount of active intravascular blood clotting, as in a subclinical DIC, which is common in patients with leukemia of various types and may be associated with tumor progression. The FPA elevations can occur without intravascular thrombosis, decreasing the value of a positive test.

Procedure

A venous blood sample of 4.5 ml is collected in a tube containing aprotinin to prevent activation.

Clinical Implications

1. FPA levels are *increased* in
   a. DIC
   b. Leukemia of various types
   c. Venous thrombosis and pulmonary embolus
   d. Infections
   e. Postoperative patients
   f. Patients with widespread solid tumors
2. FPA levels are *decreased* when clinical remission of leukemia is achieved with chemotherapy.

Interfering Factors

1. A traumatic venous puncture may result in falsely elevated levels.
2. The biologic half-life imposes limitations on the interpretation of a negative FPA test (stable for 2 hours or more).

> **Clinical Alert**
>
> Disseminated intravascular coagulation occurs commonly in association with death of tumor cells in acute promyelocytic leukemia. For this reason, heparin is used prophylactically and in association with the initiation of chemotherapy for promyelocytic leukemia. In contrast, DIC occurs less commonly during the treatment of acute myelomonocytic leukemia and acute lymphocyte leukemia. Evidence for DIC should be sought in every patient with leukemia, before initiation of treatment.

Patient Preparation

1. Explain test purpose and procedure.
2. Avoid prolonged use of tourniquet.
3. See Chapter 1 guidelines for safe, effective, informed *pretest* care.

Patient Aftercare

1. Interpret test outcome and monitor appropriately for DIC and thrombosis.
2. See Chapter 1 guidelines for safe, effective, informed *posttest* care.
3. Resume normal activities.

FIBRINOGEN

Normal Values

Fibrinogen: 200–400 mg/dl or 2.0–4.0 g/L

Background

Fibrinogen is a complex protein (polypeptide) that, with enzyme action, is converted to fibrin. The fibrin, along with platelets, forms the network for the common blood clot. Although of primary importance as a coagulation protein, fibrinogen is also an acute-phase protein reactant. It is increased in diseases involving tissue damage or inflammation.

Explanation of Test

This test is done to investigate abnormal PT, APTT, and TT (thrombin time) as well as to screen for DIC and fibrin–fibrinogenolysis.

Procedure

1. A venous blood sample is added to a collection tube containing sodium citrate.
2. The two-tube method is used.

Clinical Implications

1. *Increased fibrinogen values* occur in
   a. Inflammation (RA, pneumonia, TB, streptomycin)
   b. Acute myocardial infarction
   c. Nephrotic syndrome
   d. Cancer, multiple myeloma, Hodgkin's disease
   e. Compensated DIC
   f. Pregnancy, eclampsia
   g. Various cerebral accidents and diseases
2. *Decreased values of fibrinogen* occur in
   a. Liver disease
   b. DIC
   c. Cancer
   d. Fibrinolysis, primary and secondary
   e. Hereditary and congenital hypofibrinogenemia
   f. Dysfibrinogenemia

Interfering Factors

1. High levels of heparin interfere with test results.
2. High levels of FDP/FSP cause low values.
3. Use of oral contraceptives.
4. Elevated antithrombin III may cause decreased fibrinogen levels.

Clinical Alert

Values < 50 mg/dl can cause hemorrhage after traumatic surgery.

Patient Preparation

1. Explain test purpose and procedure.
2. Aggressive muscular exercise should be avoided before test.
3. See Chapter 1 guidelines for safe, effective, informed *pretest* care.

Patient Aftercare

1. Interpret test outcome and monitor appropriately for DIC and response to treatment. If fibrinogen is low, cryoprecipitate is the preferred product for therapeutic replacement.
2. See Chapter 1 guidelines for safe, effective, informed *posttest* care.

PROTEIN C (PC ANTIGEN) ●

Normal Values

71%–142% of increased functional activity

Background

Protein C, a vitamin K–dependent protein that prevents thrombosis, is produced in the liver and circulated in the plasma. It functions as an anticoagulant by inactivating factors V and VIII. Protein C is also a profibrinolytic agent (enhances fibrinolysis). The protein C mechanism thus functions to prevent extension of intravascular thrombi.

Explanation of Test

This test evaluates patients with severe thrombosis and those for whom there is an increased risk and predisposition to thrombosis. Patients with partial protein C or with partial protein S deficiency (heterozygotes) may suffer venous thrombotic episodes, usually in early adult years. There may be deep vein thromboses, episodes of thrombophlebitis or pulmonary emboli, and manifestations of a hypercoagulable state. Heterozygous protein C–deficient patients are of type I, with decreased C antigen, or type II, with normal C antigen levels, but decreased functional activity.

Procedure

1. A venous blood sample is anticoagulated with sodium esterase.
2. The two-tube method is used.

Clinical Implications

1. Decreased values of protein C are associated with
   - **a.** Severe thrombotic complications in the neonatal period
   - **b.** Increased risk of activation thrombosis
   - **c.** Warfarin (Coumadin)-induced skin necroses (some instances)
   - **d.** DIC, especially when it occurs with cancer (presumably owing to consumption by cofactor thrombin–thrombomodulin–catalyst activities. Thrombomodulin is a potentiator of protein C)
   - **e.** Neonatal purpura fulminans
   - **f.** Pulmonary embolus occurring mainly in teenaged years
2. A deficiency of protein C may also be congenital (35%–58%) or caused by

a. Cirrhosis (13%–25%)
b. Use of warfarin (28%–60%)
c. Vitamin K deficiency
d. Certain medications

Clinical Alert

Homozygous protein C–deficient patients have absent or near absent levels of C antigen and usually succumb in infancy with the picture of purpura fulminans neonatalis, including lower extremity skin ecchymoses, anemia, fever, and shock.

Patient Preparation

1. Explain test purpose and procedure.
2. See Chapter 1 guidelines for safe, effective, informed *pretest* care.

Patient Aftercare

1. Interpret test outcome and monitor appropriately for thrombosis. In the case of a protein C deficiency, educate the patient concerning the symptoms and implications of the disease. The risk factors include obesity, oral contraceptive use, varicose veins, infection, trauma, surgery, pregnancy, immobility, and congestive heart failure.
2. See Chapter 1 guidelines for safe, effective, informed *posttest* care.

PROTEIN S

Normal Values

Male: 78%–130% of normal
Female: 70%–120% of normal

Background

Both protein S and protein C are dependent on vitamin K for their production and function. The deficiency of either one is associated with a tendency toward thrombosis. Protein S serves as a cofactor to enhance the anticoagulant effects of activated protein C. Slightly over half of protein S is complexed with C4b-binding protein and is inactive.

Explanation of Test

This measurement is indicated for the investigation of hypercoagulable states such as thrombosis. The test may be useful in patients with recurrent or familial thrombosis and may be helpful in genetic counseling for these diseases.

Procedure

1. A venous blood sample is anticoagulated with sodium citrate.
2. The two-tube method is used.

Clinical Implications

1. *Decreased values* are associated with protein S deficiency. Familial protein S deficiency is associated with recurrent thrombosis. Abnormal plasma distribution of protein S occurs in functional protein S deficiency. In type I, the free protein S is decreased, although the level of total protein may be normal. In type II, total protein is markedly reduced.
2. Hypercoagulable state acquired protein S deficiency is found in
   a. Diabetic nephropathy
   b. Chronic renal failure caused by hypertension
   c. Cerebral venous thrombosis
   d. Coumarin-induced skin necrosis

Patient Preparation

1. Explain test purpose and procedure.
2. See Chapter 1 guidelines for safe, effective, informed *pretest* care..

Patient Aftercare

1. Interpret test outcome and monitor appropriately for thrombotic tendency.
2. See Chapter 1 guidelines for safe, effective, informed *posttest* care.

ANTITHROMBIN III (AT-III) OR HEPARIN COFACTOR ACTIVITY ●

Normal Values

Immunologic method: 84%–120% of normal (30% lower in serum than in person) 22–39 mg/dl

Functional method

Infants: 1–30 days, 26%–61% (premature); 44%–76% (full-term)

Adults and infants over 6 months: 77%–122%

Background

Antithrombin III inhibits the activity of activated factors XII, XI, IX, and X, as well as II. Antithrombin III is the main physiologic inhibitor of activated factor X, on which it appears to exert its most critical effect. Antithrombin III is a "heparin cofactor." Heparin interacts with AT-III and thrombin, increasing the rate of thrombin neutralization (inhibition), but decreasing the total quantity (of thrombin) inhibited.

Explanation of Test

This test detects a decreased level of antithrombin that is indicative of thrombotic tendency. Only the test of functional activity gives a direct clue to thrombotic tendency. In some families, several members may have a combination of recurrent thromboembolism and reduced plasma antithrombin (30%–60%). A significant number of patients with mesenteric venous thrombosis may have AT-III deficiency. It has been recommended that patients with such thrombotic disease be screened for AT-III levels to identify those patients who may benefit from coumarin anticoagulant prophylaxis.

Procedure

1. A venous blood sample (4.5 ml) is anticoagulated with sodium citrate.
2. The two-tube method is used.
3. The sample is iced and immediately transported to the laboratory.

Clinical Implications

1. *Increased values* are associated with
   a. Acute hepatitis
   b. Renal transplant
   c. Inflammation
   d. Menstruation
   e. Use of warfarin (Coumadin) anticoagulant
   f. Hyperglobulinemia
2. *Decreased values* are associated with
   a. Congenital deficiency (hereditary)
   b. Liver transplant and partial liver removal
   c. DIC
   d. Nephrotic syndrome
   e. Active thrombotic disease (deep vein thrombosis)
   f. Cirrhosis, chronic liver failure
   g. Carcinoma
   h. Pulmonary embolism
   i. Last trimester of pregnancy and early postpartum
   j. Fibrinolytic disorders
   k. After surgery (major)
   l. Deep vein thrombosis, thrombophlebitis
   m. Gram-negative septicemia

Interfering Factors

1. With heparin therapy, antithrombin decreases after 3 days of therapy.
2. Oral contraceptives

Patient Preparation

1. Explain test purpose and procedure.
2. See Chapter 1 guidelines for safe, effective, informed *pretest* care.

Patient Aftercare

1. Interpret test outcome and monitor appropriately for thrombotic tendency.
2. If patient has decreased levels of antithrombin III, a coumarin-type anticoagulant would be used as a prophylaxis.
3. See Chapter 1 guidelines for safe, effective, informed *posttest* care.

PROSTACYCLIN (6-Keto-PGF$_{1\alpha}$) ●

Normal Values

72 pg/ml

Explanation of Test

This diagnostic aid detects the presence of prostacyclin (an inhibitor of platelet aggregation and a potent vasodilator). This method evaluates several thrombotic diseases, such as venous thrombosis, thrombotic thrombocytopenic purpura, angina with occlusion (as opposed to spasm), and acute myocardial infarction.

Procedure

A venous blood sample is obtained.

Clinical Implications

1. *Decreased prostacyclin levels* occur in
   a. Hypercoagulability states and thrombotic disease
   b. Hypertension
   c. Atherosclerosis
   d. Diabetes mellitus
2. *Increased levels* occur in
   a. Congestive heart failure
   b. Graves' disease (returns to normal during therapy)
   c. Some tumors of breast and possibly of the prostate

Patient Preparation

1. Explain test purpose and procedure.
2. See Chapter 1 guidelines for safe, effective, informed *pretest* care.

Patient Aftercare

1. Interpret test outcome and monitor appropriately for thrombotic tendencies.
2. See Chapter 1 guidelines for safe, effective, informed *posttest* care.

CLOT RETRACTION ●

Normal Values

After 1 hour the blood clot appreciably shrinks or retracts from the sides of the test tube, becomes more firm, and maintains its molded shape when it is removed from the container in which it has formed. Clot retraction is nearly complete in 4 hours, and definitely completed in 24 hours. If clot retraction is normal and complete, approximately half the total volume is clot and the other half is serum.

Explanation of Test

This test is a rough measurement used to confirm a platelet problem, such as thrombocytopenia. In this test, blood is allowed to clot in a test tube without an anticoagulant. This test is based on the fact that whole blood that clots normally will retract or recede from the sides of its container, resulting in the separation of transparent serum and the contracted blood clot. Because platelets play a major part in the mechanism of clot retraction, this reaction is impaired when platelets are decreased or function abnormally. This reaction is also influenced by the fibrinogen content of the plasma, the ratio of the plasma volume to red cell mass, and the activity of a retraction-promoting principle in the serum.

Procedure

1. About 5 ml of venous blood is collected in a tube without anticoagulant.
2. Clot begins separating from the tube walls in 30 minutes to 1 hour; the clot usually separates completely in 12 to 24 hours. For 72 hours the retracted clot does not change appreciably.

Clinical Implications

There is a distinct parallel between the quality of the clot and the number of platelets. A defective clot is soft and soggy, is readily torn and, after removal from its container, flattens out as a shapeless mass from which serum continues to ooze.

1. *Poor or decreased clot retraction* occurs in thrombocytopenia, von Willebrand's disease when platelets are deficient in quality, and disorders caused by increase in red cell mass.
2. *Clot retraction appears to be increased* in severe anemia and hypofibrinogenemia as a result of small clot formation occurring from an increase in plasma volume.

Interfering Factors

1. If the hematocrit is high because of polycythemia or hemocontraction, clot retraction will be decreased.
2. In increased fibrinolysis, the clot will lyse in 10 to 30 minutes, and it will appear that no retraction has taken place. Increased fibrinolysis occurs with DIC or α_2-antiplasmin deficiency.

Patient Preparation

1. Explain test purpose and procedure.
2. See Chapter 1 guidelines for safe, effective, informed *pretest* care.

Patient Aftercare

1. Interpret test outcome and monitor appropriately for thrombocytopenia and anemia.
2. See Chapter 1 guidelines for safe, effective, informed *posttest* care.

BIBLIOGRAPHY

Ansell JE: Imprecision of prothrombin time monitoring of oral anticoagulation. American Journal Clinical Pathology 98: 237–239, 1992

Brown S: Behind the numbers on the CBC. RN 53(2): 46–51, February 1990

Bick R: Disseminated intravascular coagulation, Laboratory Medicine 23(3): March 1992

Bick R: Hypercoagulability and thrombosis. Laboratory Medicine 23(4): April 1992

Gaedeke-Norris MK: Lab test tips—how to evaluate platelet values. Nursing 91 21(2):20, February 1991

Gawlikowski J: White cells at war. AJN, March 1992

Hirsch DR et al: Bleeding time and other laboratory tests to monitor the safety and efficacy of thrombolytic therapy. Chest 94(4):124S–131S, April 1990

Kjeldsberg C et al: Practical Diagnoses of Hematologic Disorders. Chicago, ASCP Press, American Society of Clinical Pathologists, 1991

Koepke JA: Prothrombin time controls (Tip on Technology). MLO, October 1992.

Linz L: Elevation of hemoglobin, MCH or MCTC by paraprotein. How to recognize and correct the interference. Clinical Laboratory Science 7(4): 211–212, July/August 1994

Lotspeich-Steininger CA et al (eds): Clinical Hematology, Principles, Procedures, Correlations. Philadelphia, JB Lippincott, 1992

Medical Science Laboratories: Laboratory Handbook. Lexicomp Inc., OH, 1992

Meier FA, Shifman RB: The INR and Monitoring Oral Anticoagulation—Data Analysis and Critique. A-Probe 91-10A. Northfield, IL, College of American Pathologists, 1992

Millam D: How to teach good venipuncture technique. AJN, July 1993

Moran R: Hemoglobin F and measurement of oxygen saturation and fractional oxyhemoglobin. Clinical Laboratory Practice 7(3): 162–164, May/June 1994

Rice L: Anemia: Using a rational approach to diagnosis. Consultant 30(7): 39–40, 43–44, 47–49, July 1990

Tietz NB (ed): Clinical Guide to Laboratory Tests, 3rd ed. Philadelphia, WB Saunders, 1995

Varah N, Smith J, Baugh R: Heparin monitoring in the coronary care unit after percutaneous transluminal coronary angioplasty. Heart & Lung 19(3): 265–270, 1990

Wallach J: Interpretation of Laboratory Tests, 5th ed. Little, Brown & Company, 1992

Williams WJ, Beutler B, Erslen AJ et al: Hematology, 4th ed. New York, McGraw-Hill, 1990

3

Urine Studies

OVERVIEW OF URINE STUDIES ●

Urine Formation

Urine, a very complex fluid, is composed of 95% water and 5% solids. It is the end product of metabolism carried out by billions of cells in the renal and urinary system and results in an average output of 1 to 1.5 L of urine per day, dependent on fluid intake. A wide variety of waste metabolic products are excreted through the urine.

Urine formation takes place in the kidneys, two small fist-sized organs located outside the peritoneal cavity on each side of the spine, at about the level of the last thoracic and first two lumbar vertebrae. The kidneys, together with the skin and the respiratory system, are the chief excretory organs of the body. Each kidney is a highly discriminatory organ that maintains the internal environment of the body by selectively excreting or retaining various substances according to specific body needs. The importance of urine formation and excretion as a regulatory function is profoundly emphasized when dealing with situations in which kidney function is suddenly lost. In these circumstances, death can occur within a few days.

The main functional unit of the kidney is the nephron. There are about 1 million nephrons per kidney, each composed of two main parts: a glomerulus, which is essentially a filtering system, and a tubule, through which the filtered liquid passes. Each glomerulus consists of a capillary network surrounded by a membrane called *Bowman's capsule,* which continues on to form the beginning of the renal tubule. The afferent arteriole carries blood from the renal artery into the glomerulus, where it divides to form a capillary network. These capillaries reunite to form the efferent arteriole through which blood leaves the glomerulus. The blood vessels then follow the course of the tubule to form the surrounding capillary network.

A large amount of circulating blood flows through the kidneys: 25% of blood from the left side of the heart passes through the kidneys. One liter of urine is the end product of more than 1000 L of circulating blood passing through the kidneys.

Urine formation begins in the glomerular capillaries, with dissolved substances passing into the proximal tubule as a result of the force of blood pressure in the large afferent arteriole and the pressure in Bowman's capsule. As the filtrate passes along the tubule, more solutes are added by excretion from the capillary blood and secretions from the tubular epithelial cells. Certain solutes and water pass back into the blood through the mechanism of tubular reabsorption. Finally, urine concentration and dilution occur in the renal medulla. The kidney has the remarkable ability to dilute or concentrate urine, according to the needs of the individual, and to regulate sodium excretion. Blood chemistry, blood pressure, fluid balance, nutrient intake, together with the general state of health, are key elements in this entire metabolic process.

Urine contains thousands of dissolved substances, although the three principal constituents are water, urea, and sodium chloride. More solids are excreted from the body through urine than by any other method. Urine composition depends greatly on the quality and the quantity of the excreted waste material. Some constituents of the blood, such as glucose, have a renal threshold; that is, a certain elevated level must be reached in the blood before this constituent will be excreted in the urine. Almost all substances found in the urine are also found in the blood, although in different concentrations. Urea, for example, is present in the blood, but at a much lower concentration than in the urine.

URINE TESTING

Urinalysis is an essential procedure for those individuals undergoing hospital admissions and physical examinations. It is one of the most useful indicators of a healthy or diseased state. The analysis of urine has two purposes. The first is to detect abnormalities in which the kidneys function normally but excrete abnormal amounts of metabolic end products specific to a particular disease. The second purpose is to detect conditions that may adversely affect the function of the kidneys or urinary tract. Diseased kidneys cannot function normally to regulate the volume and composition of body fluids or maintain homeostasis. Urinalysis is useful in the diagnoses of nephrosis (degeneration of kidney without inflammation); nephritis (inflammation of kidney), including pyelonephritis (bacterial infection), or glomerulonephritis (without infection); and cystitis (inflammation of bladder).

Laboratory Testing

First, the physical characteristics of the urine are analyzed and recorded. Second, a series of chemical tests are run. A chemically impregnated dipstick may be used for many of these. Standardized results can be obtained by processing the urine-touched dipstick through special automated instrumentation. Third, the urine sediment is examined under the microscope.

DIPSTICKS

Although laboratory facilities allow a wide range of urine tests, some types of tablets, tapes, and dipstick tests are available for urinalysis outside the lab setting. They can be used and read directly by patients and other healthcare providers.

Similar in appearance to pieces of blotter paper on a paper or plastic strip, dipsticks actually function as miniature laboratories. These chemically impregnated reagent strips provide quick determination of pH, protein, glucose, ketones, bilirubin, hemoglobin (blood), nitrite, leukocyte esterase, urobilinogen, and specific gravity. The tip of the dipstick is impregnated with chemicals that react with specific substances in the urine to produce color-coded visual results. In some tests, the shape or depth of color produced relates to the concentration of the substance in the urine. Color controls are provided against which the actual color produced by the urine sample can be compared. The reaction times of the impregnated chemicals are standardized for each category of dipstick; it is vital that color changes be matched to the control chart at the correct elapsed time after each stick is dipped into the urine specimen. Instructions that accompany each type of dipstick outline the procedure. When more than one type of test is incorporated on a single stick (eg, pH, protein, glucose), the chemical reagents for each test are separated by a water-impermeable barrier made of plastic so that results do not become altered.

In addition to dipsticks, other reagent strips, chemical tablets, and treated slides for special determinations, such as bacteria, phenylketonuria (PKU), mucopolysaccharides, salicylate, and cystinuria, are available for urine analysis.

Procedure

1. Use a fresh urine sample (within 1 hour of collection or a sample that has been refrigerated).
2. Read or review directions for use of the reagent. Periodically check for changes in procedure.
3. Dip a reagent strip into well-mixed urine, then remove and compare each reagent area on the dipstick with the corresponding color control chart within the established time frames. Correlate color comparisons as closely as possible.

Interfering Factors

1. If dipsticks are kept in the urine sample too long, the impregnated chemicals in the strip may be overly dissolved and could produce inaccurate readings and values.
2. If the reagent chemicals on the impregnated pad become mixed, the readings will be inaccurate. To avoid this, shake off excess urine after withdrawing dipstick from sample.

Clinical Alert

1. Precise timing is essential. If not timed correctly, color changes may produce invalid or false results.
2. When not in use, the container for the reagent materials should be kept tightly closed to keep the contents dry and should be stored in a dry environment. If the reagents absorb moisture from the air before they are used, they will not produce accurate results. If a desiccant comes with the reagents, it should be kept in the container.
3. Certain drugs may give false-positive reactions.
4. Use fresh urine (within 1 hour of collection or a refrigerated sample). Failure to follow this precaution can lead to invalid results such as the following:
   a. Glucose level may drop
   b. Ketones dissipate
   c. Color will deepen
   d. Urinary sediment will deteriorate
   e. Bacteria (if present) will multiply
   f. pH becomes more alkaline
   g. Bilirubin and urobilinogen may be oxidized (if exposed to light for long periods of time).

Types of Urine Specimens

During the course of 24 hours, the composition and concentration of urine changes continuously. Urine concentration varies according to water intake and *pretest* activities. For this reason, various types of urine specimens, such as the following, are collected:

First morning specimen
Single random specimen
Timed short-term specimen
Timed long-term specimen (12-hr or 24-hr)
Catheterized specimen or specimen from an indwelling catheter
Double-voided specimens (test for sugar and acetone)
Clean-catch (midstream) specimen (urine culture and cytologic analyses—see Chap. 7)

COLLECTION OF URINE: RANDOM, SECOND (DOUBLE-VOIDED), CATHETER, AND CLEAN-CATCH MIDSTREAM URINE TESTS

Standard urinalysis specimens can be collected any time, whereas first morning, fasting, or timed specimens require collection at specific times of day. Patient preparation and education will vary according to type of specimen required (Table 3-1) and patient's ability to cooperate with specimen collection. Clear instructions and assessment of patient's understanding of the

TABLE 3-1
24-Hour Urine Collection Data

Test	*Preservative*	*Protocols*
Acid mucopolysaccharides	20 ml toluene	Add at start of collection
Aldosterone	1 g boric acid/100 ml urine	
Amylase	None	Refrigerate during collection
Arsenic	None	Refrigerate during collection
Cadmium	None	Refrigerate during collection
Calcium	None	Refrigerate during collection
Catecholamines	20 ml 8 *N** acetic acid	Refrigerate during collection
Chloride	None	Refrigerate during collection
Copper	None	Refrigerate during collection
Cortisol (free)	None	Refrigerate during collection
Creatinine	None	Refrigerate during collection
Creatinine clearance	None	Refrigerate during collection
Cyclic AMP	None	Refrigerate during collection
Cystine	None	Refrigerate during collection
Δ-Aminolevulinic acid (ALA)	1 ml of 33% glacial acetic acid/10 ml urine	Refrigerate during collection
Electrolytes Na	None	Refrigerate during collection
Estrogens	None	Refrigerate during collection
5-HIAA (serotonin)	1 g boric acid	Refrigerate during collection
Histamine	None	Freeze portion after collection
Homogentisic acid	None	Freeze portion after collection
Hydroxyproline	None	
FSH/LH	1.0 g boric acid	
17-Hydroxycorticosteroids	1.0 g boric acid	Do not refrigerate
17-Ketogenic steroid (Porter–Silber)	1.0 g boric acid	Do not refrigerate
17-Ketosteroids (total)	1.0 g boric acid	Do not refrigerate
Magnesium	None	
Metanephrine (total)	2.0 ml acetic acid	
Oxalate	None	Refrigerate during collection
Phosphorus (inorganic)	None	Refrigerate during collection
Pregnanediol	None	Refrigerate during collection
Protein (total)	See Total Protein	Refrigerate during collection
Porphobilinogens	None	Refrigerate during collection; protect from light
Potassium (K), sodium (Na)	None	Refrigerate during collection
Porphyrins (uro/copro)	None (preservative added on receipt in lab)	Refrigerate during collection; protect from light
Thiocyanate	None	Refrigerate during collection
Total protein	None	Refrigerate during collection
Urea nitrogen	None	Refrigerate during collection
Uric acid	None	Refrigerate during collection
Vanillylmandelic acid (VMA)	20 ml SN acetic acid before collection	

**N* = normal

process are the key to a successful outcome. Assess the patient's usual urinating patterns and encourage fluid intake, unless contraindicated. Provide verbal and written directions for self-collection of specimens. Assess for presence of interfering factors: failure to follow collection instructions, inadequate fluid intake, certain medications, and patient's use of illegal drugs may affect test results. Certain foods, or any type of food consumption in certain instances, may also affect test results.

URINE, SINGLE, RANDOM SPECIMEN ●

More testing is done on a random sample of freshly voided urine. Because the composition of urine changes over the course of the day, the time of day when the specimen is collected may influence the findings. The first-voided morning specimen is particularly valuable, for it is usually more concentrated and, thus, more likely to reveal abnormalities, as well as the presence of formed substances. It is also relatively free of dietary influences and changes owing to physical activity because the specimen is collected after a period of fasting and rest. Because urinalysis measures the concentration of substances, the results will vary according to the time of day the specimen is collected. Significant cellular abnormalities that show up in a morning specimen may be missed in dilute urine collected later in the day.

Procedure

1. Observe universal precautions (Appendix IX) and agency protocols. The patient is instructed to void directly into a clean, dry container or bedpan. The specimen is then directly transferred into an appropriate container. Women should always have a clean, voided specimen if a microscopic examination is ordered (see Chap. 7).
2. Specimens from infants and young children can be collected into a disposable collection apparatus consisting of a plastic bag with an adhesive backing around the opening that can be fastened to the perineal area or around the penis to permit voiding directly into the bag. The specimen bag should be carefully removed and the urine transferred to an appropriate specimen container.
3. All specimens should be covered tightly, labeled properly, and immediately sent to the laboratory.
4. If a urine specimen is likely to be contaminated with drainage, vaginal discharge, or menstrual blood, a clean specimen must be obtained using the same procedure as for bacteriologic examination (see Collection of Specimens for Culture in Chap. 7).
5. If a urine specimen is obtained from an indwelling catheter, it may be necessary to clamp off the catheter for about 15 minutes before obtaining the sample. Clean the specimen port (in the tubing) with antiseptic before aspirating the urine sample with a needle and syringe.
6. Observe universal precautions when handling urine specimens.

Interfering Factors

1. Feces, discharges, vaginal secretions, and menstrual blood will contaminate the urine specimen. A clean-voided specimen must be obtained.
2. If the specimen is not refrigerated within 1 hour of collection, the following changes in composition may occur:
   a. Bacteria in the urine "split" the urea, convert it to ammonia, and produce an alkaline urine.
   b. Urine casts decompose after several hours.
   c. Red blood cells are lysed by hypotonic urine.
   d. Very low or very high pH may affect cellular components (see pH section).

Therefore, specimens should be immediately refrigerated if any delay before analysis is expected.

URINE TIMED (2-HR); **LONG-TERM SPECIMEN** (24-HR) ●

Explanation of Test

Some diseases or conditions require a timed or 24-hour urine specimen in order to evaluate kidney function accurately (see Table 3-1). Substances excreted by the kidney are not excreted at the same rate or in the same amounts during different periods of the day and night; therefore, a random urine specimen might not give an accurate picture of the processes taking place over a 24-hour period. For measurement of total urine protein, creatinine, electrolytes, and so forth, more accurate information is obtained from urine collected over a 24-hour period. The 24-hour collection involves collecting the urine specimen into a suitable receptacle and either adding a preservative to it or keeping it refrigerated, or both.

Procedure

1. At the beginning of a 24-hour–timed urine specimen collection (or any other timed specimen collection), the patient is asked to void. This first specimen is *discarded,* and the time noted.
2. The time the test begins and the time the collection should end are labeled on the container. As a reminder, it may be helpful to post a sign above the toilet: "24-hour collection in progress," with the beginning and end time noted.
3. All urine voided over the next 24 hours is collected into a large container (usually glass or polyethylene) and labeled with the patient's name, timeframe for collection, test ordered, and other pertinent information. It is not necessary to measure the volume of urine unless specifically required.
4. To conclude the collection, the patient must void 24 hours after the first voiding. Urine from this last voiding must be added to the specimen in the container.

   NOTE: *Because the patient may not always be able to void on request, the last specimen should be obtained as closely as possible to the stated end-time of the test.*

5. Storage
   a. Nonrefrigerated samples may be kept in a specified area or in the patient's bathroom.
   b. If refrigeration is necessary, the urine specimen must either be refrigerated immediately after the patient has voided or the collection bottle must be placed into an iced container.

Special Considerations

1. In a healthcare facility, responsibility for the collection of urine specimens should be specifically assigned.
2. When instructing a patient about 24-hour urine collections, make certain the patient understands they must empty the bladder at the time the 24-hour collection starts and that this specimen must be discarded.
3. Do not predate and pretime requisitions for serial collections. It is difficult for some patients to void at specific times. Instead, mark actual times of collection on containers.
4. Documenting exact times the specimens are obtained is crucial to many urine tests.
5. Instruct the patient to urinate as near the end of the collection time period as possible.
6. When a preservative is added to the collection container (eg, hydrochloric acid preservative in 24-hour urine collection of vanillylmandelic acid), the patient must take precautions against spilling the contents. Instructions concerning spillage need to be addressed before the test begins.
7. Preservatives used are determined by the urine substance for which the test is designed. The laboratory usually provides the container and proper preservative when the test is ordered. If in doubt, verify this with laboratory personnel.

Interfering Factors

1. Failure of the patient or attending personnel to follow the procedure is the most common source of error.
   a. The patient should be given both verbal and written instructions. If unable to comprehend these, a significant other should be instructed in the process.
   b. If required, the proper preservative must be used (see preservative chart on page 152).
2. Instruct the patient to use toilet paper *after* transferring the urine to the 24-hour collection container. Toilet paper placed in the specimen decreases the actual amount of urine available and contaminates the specimen.
3. Feces contaminates the specimen. Patients should void first and transfer the urine to the collection receptacle before defecating.
4. If other discharges, secretions, or heavy menstrual flow are present, the test may have to be postponed or an indwelling catheter may need to be in-

serted to keep the specimen free of contamination. In some cases, thorough cleansing of the perineal or urethral area before voiding may be sufficient. If in doubt, communicate with lab personnel and patient's physician.

Patient Preparation

Most 24-hour urine specimen collections start in the early morning around 7:00 AM (0700). Instruct the patient to do the following:

1. Empty the bladder completely on awakening and then discard this urine specimen. Record the time the voided specimen is discarded and the time the test is begun.
2. Save all urine voided during the next 24 hours, including the first specimen voided the next morning.
3. The urine voided the next morning (as close to the ending time as possible) is added to the collection container. The 24-hour test is then terminated and the time recorded.
4. A bedpan, urinal, wide-mouth container, special toilet device, or the collection container itself can be used to catch urine. It is probably easier for women to void into another wide-mouth receptacle first and then *carefully* transfer the entire specimen to the collection bottle. Men may find it simpler to void directly into the 24-hour collection container.
5. It is most important that *all* urine be saved in the 24-hour container. Ideally, the container should be refrigerated or placed in ice.
6. Test results are calculated on the basis of a 24-hour output. Unless ***all*** urine is saved, results will not be accurate. Moreover, these tests are usually expensive, more complicated, and are necessary for the evaluation and treatment of the patient's condition.

● ROUTINE URINALYSIS (UA) AND RELATED TESTS

Normal Values

General Characteristics and Measurements	***Chemical Determinations***	***Microscopic Examination of Sediment***
Color: pale yellow to amber	Glucose: negative	Casts negative: occasional hyaline casts
Appearance: clear to slightly hazy	Ketones: negative	Red blood cells: negative or rare
		(continued)

General Characteristics and Measurements	*Chemical Determinations*	*Microscopic Examination of Sediment*
Specific gravity: 1.015–1.025 with a normal fluid intake	Blood: negative	Crystals: negative
pH: 4.5–8.0—average person has a pH of about 5–6	Protein: negative	White blood cells: negative or rare
Volume: 1500/24 hr	Bilirubin: negative Urobilinogen: 0.1–1.0 Nitrate for bacteria: negative Leukocyte esterase: negative	Epithelial cells: few

Explanation of Test

The process of urinalysis determines the various following properties of urine: color, odor, turbidity, specific gravity, pH, glucose, ketones, blood, protein, bilirubin, urobilinogen, nitrate, and leukocyte esterase, as well as other abnormal constituents revealed by microscopic examination of the urine sediment. A 10-ml urine specimen is usually sufficient for conducting these tests.

URINE VOLUME ●

Normal Values

Volume: 750–2500 ml/24 hr; 25–30 ml/hr

Background

Urine volume measurements are part of assessment for fluid balance and kidney function. The normal volume of urine voided by the average adult in a 24-hour time period ranges from 600 ml to 2000 ml; the normal amount is about 1500 ml. The amount voided over any period is directly related to the individual's fluid intake, temperature and climate, and amount of perspiration that occurs. Children void smaller quantities than adults, but the total volume voided is greater in proportion to their body size.

The night urine produced is about 400 ml, making the day/night ratio approximately 2:1 to 4:1.

Explanation of Test

Urine volume measurements are indicated in the assessment of fluid balance and kidney function. *Polyuria* is an increase in the volume of excreted urine. It is a physiologic response to increased fluid intake, ingested diuretic medications and drinks, chilling of the body, nervousness, large-volume intravenous fluid infusion, or certain disease processes, such as diabetes or certain renal diseases.

Oliguria is decreased urinary output. The extreme form of this process is *anuria*, a total lack of urine production.

Procedure

1. Collect a 24-hour urine specimen and keep refrigerated or on ice.
2. Record the exact collection starting time and collection end time on the specimen container and in the patient's healthcare record.
3. When the collection is completed, transfer the specimen container to the laboratory refrigerator. Make out the proper forms and document accordingly.
4. Volume is ascertained by measuring the entire urine amount in a graduated and appropriately calibrated pitcher or other receptacle. The total volume is recorded as urine volume in milliliters, or cubic centimeters, per 24 hours.

Clinical Implications

1. Polyuria: increased urine output with elevated blood urea nitrogen (BUN)/creatinine levels is found in
   - **a.** Diabetic ketoacidosis
   - **b.** Partial obstruction of urinary tract
   - **c.** Some types of tubular necrosis (aminoglycosides)
2. Polyuria with normal BUN/creatinine
   - **a.** Diabetes mellitus and diabetes insipidus
   - **b.** Neurotic states
   - **c.** Certain tumors of brain and spinal cord
   - **d.** Acromegaly
   - **e.** Myxedema
3. Oliguria: < 200 ml/24 hr; < 15–20 ml/kg/24 hr in children may result from
   - **a.** Various renal causes
     - **(1)** Renal ischemia
     - **(2)** Renal disease caused by toxic agents (certain drugs are toxic to the renal system)
     - **(3)** Glomerulonephritis, nephritis
   - **b.** Dehydration caused by prolonged vomiting, diarrhea, or excessive diaphoresis.
   - **c.** Obstruction of some area of the urinary tract/system (mechanical)
   - **d.** Cardiac insufficiency
4. Anuria: < 100 ml/24 hr, may result from
   - **a.** Complete urinary tract obstruction
   - **b.** Acute cortical necrosis (cortex of the kidney)
   - **c.** Glomerulonephritis (acute)
   - **d.** Acute tubular necrosis
   - **e.** Hemolytic transfusion reaction

Interfering Factors

1. Polyuria
   a. Intravenous glucose or saline
   b. Pharmacologic agents, such as thiazides and other diuretics
   c. Coffee, alcohol, tea, caffeine
2. Oliguria
   a. Water deprivation, dehydration
   b. Excessive salt intake

Patient Preparation

1. Explain purpose and procedure of test.
2. Withhold diuretics for 3 days before test.
3. Avoid excessive water (liquid) and excessive salt intake. Advise patients to avoid salty foods and added salt to diet. Eliminate caffeine and alcohol. Determine patient's usual liquid intake and request that intake not be increased beyond this daily amount during testing.
4. Follow guidelines in Chapter 1 for safe, effective, *pretest* care.

Patient Aftercare

1. Patient can resume normal fluid and dietary intake and medications, unless specifically ordered otherwise.
2. Interpret test outcomes and counsel appropriately.
3. Follow guidelines in Chapter 1 for safe, effective, *posttest* care.

URINE SPECIFIC GRAVITY (SG) ●

Normal Values

SG: 1.003–1.035 (usually between 1.010 and 1.025) with normal hydration and volume
SG: 1.025–1.030+ (concentrated urine)
SG: 1.001–1.010 (dilute urine)
SG: 1.001–1.018 in infants of < 2 years

Explanation of Test

Specific gravity is a measurement of the kidneys' ability to concentrate urine. The test compares the weight of urine against the weight of distilled water, which has a specific gravity of 1.000. Because urine is a solution of minerals, salts, and compounds dissolved in water, the specific gravity is obviously greater than 1.000. The relative difference between the specific gravity of distilled water and the specific gravity of urine reflects the degree of concentration of the urine specimen; specific gravity correlates roughly with osmolality.

The range of urine's specific gravity depends on the state of hydration and varies with urine volume and the load of solids to be excreted under standardized conditions; when fluid intake is restricted or increased, specific gravity measures the concentrating and diluting functions of the kidney. Loss of these functions is an indication of renal dysfunction.

Procedure

1. Specific gravity can be tested using a multiple test dipstick that has a separate reagent area for specific gravity (most common method).
2. Refractometer: Specific gravity can be determined with a refractometer or total solids meter. The refractive index is the ratio of light velocity in air to the velocity of light in solution. A drop of urine is placed on a clear glass plate of the urinometer and another "plate" is pressed on top of the urine sample. The degree of velocity difference is "read" through a telescopelike lens on the refractometer. Specific gravity values within the instrument are calibrated, and the line of demarkation registers the specific gravity value.
3. The urinometer is the most widely known, but least accurate, method. It has been used for many years and consists of a bulb-shaped instrument that contains a scale calibrated in specific gravity readings. Urine is transferred into a small test tube–like cylinder about 1/2 full. The urinometer is floated in the urine. Specific gravity is read off the urinometer at the meniscus level of the urine.
4. Specimen collection
   a. For regular urinalysis testing, about 2 ml of a random sample is needed for urinometer testing.
   b. When special evaluation of specific gravity is ordered separately from the urinalysis, the patient should fast for 12 hours before specimen collection.

Clinical Implications

1. *Normal*

   Specific gravity values usually vary inversely with amounts of urine excreted (decrease in urine volume = increase in specific gravity). However, the following are examples of conditions in which this relationship is not valid:
   a. Diabetes: increased urine volume; increased specific gravity
   b. Hypertension: normal volume; decreased specific gravity
   c. Early chronic renal disease: increased volume; decreased specific gravity
2. *Low specific gravity* (1.001–1.010)
   a. Diabetes insipidus
      (1) Low specific gravity and large urine volume.
      (2) Caused by absence or decrease of antidiuretic hormone (ADH). Antidiuretic hormone triggers kidney absorption of water; without it, kidneys produce an excessive amount of urine that is not reabsorbed (sometimes 15–20 L a day).

b. Glomerulonephritis (kidney inflammation without infection) and pyelonephritis (kidney inflammation with bacterial infection, but not in the acute type of this disease). Specific gravity can be low in glomerulonephritis.

(1) Decreased urine volume; low specific gravity

(2) Tubular damage affects the kidneys' ability to concentrate urine.

c. Severe renal damage

Fixed low specific gravity (1.010) that varies little from specimen to specimen

3. *Increased specific gravity* (1.025–1.030)

a. Diabetes mellitus or nephrosis in which abnormally large amounts of glucose or protein (100–750 mg/dl) increase the specific gravity up to 1.050.

b. Excessive water loss (dehydration, fever, vomiting, diarrhea).

c. Increased secretion of antidiuretic hormone (ADH) and diuretic effects related to the stress of a surgical procedure.

4. *Fixed specific gravity* (isosthenuric; SG = 1.010). Urine with a fixed low specific gravity that does not vary from specimen to specimen is indicative of severe renal damage, with disturbance of both the concentrating and diluting abilities of the kidney.

5. Hepatic disease

6. Congestive cardiac failure

Interfering Factors

1. Radiopaque x-ray contrast media, minerals, and dextrin may cause false high specific gravity readings when specific gravity is read through a refractometer.
2. Temperature of urine specimens affects specific gravity; cold specimens will produce false high values.
3. Highly buffered alkaline urine also may cause low readings (with dipsticks only).
4. Elevated readings may occur in the presence of moderate (100–750 mg/dl) amounts of protein.
5. Detergent residue (on specimen containers) can produce elevated specific gravity results.

Patient Preparation

1. Explain the purpose and procedure for urine collection.
2. Follow guidelines in Chapter 1 for safe, effective, informed *pretest* care.

Patient Aftercare

1. Interpret test outcomes, counsel, and monitor appropriately for conditions associated with altered specific gravity.
2. Follow Chapter 1 guidelines for safe, effective, informed *posttest* care.

URINE OSMOLALITY

Normal Values

300–900 mOsm/kg/ 24 hr
50–1200 mOsm/kg in a random sample

Background

Osmolality, a more exact measurement of urine concentration than specific gravity, depends on the number of particles of solute in a unit of solution. More information concerning renal function can be obtained if the serum osmolality is run at the same time as the urine osmolality. The normal ratio between urine and serum is 1:3. A high urinary/serum ratio is seen with concentrated urine. With poor concentrating ability, the ratio is low.

Explanation of Test

Whenever a more precise measurement than specific gravity is indicated to evaluate the concentrating and diluting ability of the kidney, this test is done. Urine osmolality during water restriction is an accurate test of decreased kidney function. It is also used to diagnose diabetes insipidus and to rule out compulsive water drinking.

Procedure:

This is a 24-hour urine collection test.

1. At approximately 7:00 AM, the patient voids. This urine is not saved.
2. The first urine test specimen is collected and used at 8:00 AM. All the urine voided until 7:00 AM the next day is saved in a special 24-hour collection container kept on ice or refrigerated.
3. At end of test, label specimen and send to laboratory.

Clinical Implications

1. *Osmolality is increased* in
   - **a.** Renal disease
   - **b.** Congestive heart failure
   - **c.** Addison's disease
   - **d.** Inappropriate ADH secretion (SIADH)
   - **e.** Dehydration
   - **f.** Amyloidosis
2. *Osmolality is decreased* in
   - **a.** Aldosteronism
   - **b.** Diabetes insipidus
   - **c.** Hypokalemia
   - **d.** Hypercalcemia
   - **e.** Compulsive water drinking

Interfering Factors

1. Intravenous sodium administration affects results.
2. Intravenous dextrose and water administration affects results.

Patient Preparation

1. Explain purpose and procedure of the test to the patient.
2. A high-protein diet is prescribed for 3 days before testing.
3. No liquids are to be taken with the evening meal **before** the test. No food or liquids should be taken after the evening meal until collection. Check with your laboratory if patient has diabetes.
4. Follow guidelines in Chapter 1 for safe, effective, informed *pretest* care.

Patient Aftercare

1. Provide the patient with foods and fluids as soon as the 8:00 AM urine sample is obtained.
2. Interpret test outcomes and monitor appropriately.
3. Follow guidelines in Chapter 1 for safe, effective, *posttest* care.

URINE APPEARANCE ●

Normal Values

Fresh urine is clear to slightly hazy.

Background

The first observation made about a urine specimen is usually its appearance to the eye.

Explanation of Test

Cloudy urine signals a possible abnormality, such as pus, red blood cells, or bacteria. Conversely, excretion of cloudy urine may not be abnormal because a change in urine pH may cause precipitation of normal urinary components within the bladder. Alkaline urine may appear cloudy because of phosphates; acid urine may appear cloudy because of urates.

Procedure

Observe the clarity of a fresh urine sample. Document findings.

Clinical Implications

1. Pathologic urines are often turbid or cloudy; however, many normal urines can also appear cloudy.
2. Urine turbidity may result from urinary tract infections.
3. Urine may be cloudy because of red blood cells, white blood cells, or bacteria.

Interfering Factors

1. Following ingestion of food, urates or phosphates may produce cloudiness in normal urine.
2. Semen or vaginal discharges mixed with urine are common causes of turbidity.

3. "Greasy" cloudiness may be caused by large amounts of fat.
4. Often normal urine will develop a haze or turbidity after refrigeration or standing at room temperature because of crystal precipitates.

URINE COLOR

Normal Values

The normal color of urine is pale yellow to amber; specific gravity ranges from 1.011 to 1.019; the urine output averages 1 to 1.5 L/day.

Straw-colored urine is normal and indicates a low specific gravity, usually under 1.010. (The exception may be a patient with an elevated blood glucose level whose urine is very pale yellow, but has a high specific gravity.)

Amber-colored urine is normal and indicates a high specific gravity and a small output of urine. Specific gravity may be greater than 1.020 and output may be less than 1 L/day.

Explanation of Test

Urine specimens may vary in color from pale yellow to dark amber. The darker amber color may be directly related to the urine concentration or specific gravity. Urine color is primarily a result of urochrome (pigments present in the diet or formed from bile metabolism). Sometimes the color of urine may change because of abnormal pigment by-products from certain disease states.

Procedure

Observe and record the color of freshly voided urine.

Clinical Implications

1. A nearly *colorless* urine may be due to
   - **a.** Large fluid intake
   - **b.** Reduction in perspiration
   - **c.** Chronic interstitial nephritis
   - **d.** Untreated diabetes mellitus
   - **e.** Diabetes insipidus
   - **f.** Alcohol ingestion
   - **g.** Diuretic therapy
   - **h.** Nervousness
2. An *orange-colored* urine may be due to
   - **a.** Dehydration
   - **b.** Concentrated urine
   - **c.** Restricted fluid intake
   - **d.** Excess sweating
   - **e.** Fever
   - **f.** Small quantities of bile pigment
   - **g.** Certain urinary tract medications (eg, phenazopyridine)
3. A *brownish yellow* or *greenish yellow* color may indicate bilirubin in the urine.
   - **a.** However, not all dark urines contain bilirubin.
   - **b.** Stale urine containing bilirubin may be green because of an oxidation of the bilirubin to biliverdin.

   c. Bilirubin crystals in urine sediment may produce an opalescent appearance.
   d. *Yellow foam* or *green foam* after voiding may be due to biliverdin bile pigment.
   e. Green color may be caused by pseudomonal infection.
4. A *red* or *reddish to dark brown* color may indicate hemoglobinuria and may be due to blood, porphyrins, hemoglobin, or myoglobin in the urine.
5. A *port wine* color may be the result of porphyrins or a mixture of methemoglobin and oxyhemoglobin in the urine.
6. *Dark brown* urine may contain porphyrins, melanin, or blood.
7. *Brown-black* urine may be due to great amounts of hemoglobin, Lysol poisoning, or melanin.
8. *Black* urine results from alkaptonuria, a disease of tyrosine metabolism.
9. *Smoky* color may be caused by red blood cells.
10. *Milky* urine is associated with fat, cystinuria, pus, and many WBCs, or phosphates (not pathologic).

Interfering Factors

1. Normal urine color darkens on standing because of the oxidation of urobilinogen to urobilin. This decomposition process starts about 30 minutes after voiding.
2. Some foods cause changes in urine color:
   a. Beets will turn the urine *red.*
   b. Rhubarb can cause *brown* urine.
3. Many drugs alter the color of urine:
   a. Cascara and senna laxatives in the presence of acid urine will turn the urine *reddish brown;* in the presence of alkaline urine, they will turn the urine *red.*
   b. Phenazopyridine (Pyridium), aminopyrine, or oral anticoagulants may cause an *orange* color.
   c. *Orange* to *orange-red* may be due to phenazopyridine or ethoxazene.
   d. *Orange* to *purple-red* may be due to chlorzoxazone.
   e. *Orange-yellow* in the presence of alkaline urine may be caused by sulfasalazine, anisindione, or phenindione.
   f. *Rust-yellow* to *brownish* may be a result of sulfonamides or nitrofurantoins.
   g. *Pink* to *red* or *red-brown* may be due to phenytoin (diphenylhydantoin; Dilantin), dioocytl calcium sulfosuccinate (Doxidan), phenolphthalein (Ex-Lax), or thiodiphenylamine (phenothiazine).
   h. *Magenta* may be due to phenolphthalein.
   i. *Red* may be due to aminopyrine, phenazopyridine, Neotropin, Prontosil, aniline dyes, without PSP and without BSP dyes in alkaline urine, phenolphthalein or phenazopyridine in acid urine, or deferoxamine (Desferal).

- **j.** *Purple-red* may be due to phenolphthalein in alkaline urine.
- **k.** *Dark brown* may be due to phenolic drugs or phenylhydrazine.
- **l.** *Brown-black* may be due to iron sobitex (Jecotofer) or cascara.
- **m.** *Bright yellow* may be due to riboflavin or phenazopyridine in alkaline urine.
- **n.** *Blue* or *green* may be due to methylene blue, vitamin B complex, or amitriptyline.
- **o.** Urine that *darkens* on standing may be due to antiparkinsonian agents, such as levodopa or Sinemet.
- **p.** *Dark-colored* urine may be due to iron salts.
- **q.** *Pink* to *brown* may be due to phenothiazine tranquilizer.
- **r.** *Pale blue* may be due to triamterene (Dyrenium).

Clinical Alert

1. If the urine is red, do not assume drug causation. Check the urine for hemoglobin. Question the patient about hematuria and activity or recent injury or infection. Sometimes vigorous exercise can bring on hematuria.
2. Red urine that has a negative outcome for occult blood testing is an indication that porphyria may be present. Report at once and document test results.
3. Other grossly abnormal colors such as black or brown should be documented and reported.

Patient Preparation

Assess color of urine; instruct patient to monitor and to report abnormal urine colors.

Patient Aftercare

1. Interpret abnormal colors and counsel appropriately.
2. Explain that follow-up testing may be needed.

URINE ODOR

Normal, freshly voided urine has a characteristic odor owing to the presence of volatile acids. It is not generally offensive.

Normal Values

Fresh urine from most healthy persons has a characteristic aromatic odor.

Procedure

Smell the urine and record perceptions.

Clinical Implications

1. The urine of patients with diabetes mellitus may have a fruity (acetone) odor because of ketosis.
2. Urinary tract infections produce a foul-smelling urine owing to presence of bacteria.
3. The urine of infants with an inherited disorder of amino acid metabolism smells like maple or burnt sugar; hence, the name "maple sugar urine disease."
4. Cystinuria and homocystinuria evoke a sulfurous odor.
5. Oasthouse urine disease has a smell associated with the smell of a brewery (yeasts, hops).
6. In phenylketonuria, a musty, mousy smell may be evident.
7. Tyrosenemia is characterized by a cabbagelike or "fishy" urine odor.
8. Butyric/hexanoic acidemia produces a urine odor resembling sweaty feet.

Interfering Factors

1. Some foods, such as asparagus, produce characteristic urine odors.
2. After urine stands for a long time, bacterial activity produces ammonia and the decomposition of urea with their characteristic pungent odors.

URINE pH ●

Normal Values

Average pH range: 4.6–8
Average pH is about 6 (acid)
(The pH of normal urine can vary widely.)

Background

The symbol "pH" expresses the urine as a dilute acid or a base solution and measures the free hydrogen ion concentration (H^+) in the urine: "7" is the point of neutrality on the pH scale. The lower the pH, the greater the acidity; the higher the pH, the greater the alkalinity. The pH, therefore, is an indicator of the renal tubules' ability to maintain normal hydrogen ion concentration in the plasma and extracellular fluid. The kidneys maintain normal acid–base balance primarily through the reabsorption of sodium and the tubular secretion of hydrogen and ammonium ions. Secretion of an acid or alkaline urine by the kidneys is one of the most important mechanisms of the body for maintaining a constant body pH.

Urine becomes increasingly acidic as the amount of sodium and excess acid retained by the body increases. Alkaline urine, usually containing bicarbonate–carbonic acid buffer, is normally excreted when there is an excess of base or alkali in the body.

Ingestion of different foods and sodium bicarbonate also affects urinary pH. The usual diet, rich in animal protein, produces an acidic urine. A diet high in citrus fruits and vegetables produces an alkaline urine.

Control of pH

Control of urinary pH is important in the management of several diseases. These include bacteriuria, renal calculi, and drug therapy in which streptomycin or methenamine mandelate is being administered.

A. *Renal calculi*

Renal stone formation partially depends on the pH of urine. Patients being treated for renal calculi are frequently given diets or medication to change the pH of the urine so that kidney stones will not form.

1. Calcium phosphate, calcium carbonate, and magnesium phosphate stones develop in alkaline urine. In such instances the urine must be kept acidic (see Diet).
2. Uric acid, cystine, and calcium oxalate stones precipitate in acidic urines. Therefore, as part of treatment, the urine should be kept alkaline (see Diet).

B. *Drug treatment*

1. Streptomycin, neomycin, and kanamycin are effective for treating genitourinary tract infections, provided the urine is *alkaline*.
2. During sulfonamide therapy, an *alkaline* urine should help prevent formation of sulfonamide crystals.
3. Urine should also be kept persistently *alkaline* in the presence of salicylate intoxication (excretion is enhanced) and during blood transfusions.

C. *Clinical conditions*

1. The urine should be kept *acidic* during treatment of urinary tract infections, persistent bacteriuria, and during management of urinary calculi that develop in alkaline urine.
2. An accurate measurement of urinary pH can be done only on a freshly voided specimen. If the urine must be kept for any length of time before analysis, it should be refrigerated.
3. Vegetarian diets, citrus fruits, milk, and other dairy products produce alkaline urine.
4. Highly concentrated urine, such as that formed in hot, dry environments, is strongly acidic and may produce irritation.
5. During sleep, decreased pulmonary ventilation causes respiratory acidosis; as a result, urine becomes highly acidic.
6. Chlorothiazide diuretic administration will cause acid urine to be excreted.
7. Bacteria of urinary tract infection or bacterial contamination of the specimen will produce alkaline urine. Urea will be converted to ammonia.

D. *Diet*

1. A diet that emphasizes citrus fruits and most vegetables, particularly legumes, will help keep the urine alkaline. Alkaline urine after meals is a normal response to the secretions of HCl in gastric juice.
2. A diet high in meat and cranberry juice will keep the urine acidic.

Explanation of Test

Urine pH is an important screening test for the diagnosis of renal disease, respiratory disease, and certain metabolic disorders. It can also monitor specific medication regimens or diet regimens when acidic or alkaline urine is desired. Maintenance of the urine at a consistent pH level requires frequent urine pH testing.

Procedure

1. *Dipstick measurement:* Reagent strips produce a spectrum of color changes from orange to green-blue to identify pH ranges from 5 to 9.
2. The dipstick is dipped into a freshly voided urine specimen, and the color change is compared with a standardized color chart on the bottle that correlates color results with pH values.

Clinical Implications

If urine pH is to be useful, it is necessary to use the pH information in conjunction with other diagnostic information. For example, in renal tubular necrosis, the kidney is not able to excrete a urine that is strongly acidic. Therefore, if a urine pH of 5 (quite acidic) is measured, renal tubular necrosis is eliminated as a possible diagnosis.

1. *Acidic urine* (pH less than 7) occurs in
   a. Acidosis, uncontrolled diabetes, pulmonary emphysema, diarrhea, starvation, dehydration
   b. Rarely, in severe alkalosis
   c. Respiratory diseases in which CO_2 retention occurs and acidosis develops
2. *Alkaline urine* (pH greater than 7) occurs in
   a. Urinary tract infections, pyloric obstruction, salicylate intoxications, renal tubular acidosis, chronic renal failure
   b. Rarely, during severe acidosis
   c. Respiratory diseases that involve hyperventilation ("blowing off" CO_2 and development of alkalosis).

Interfering Factors

1. With prolonged standing, the pH of a urine specimen will become alkaline because bacteria split urea and produce ammonia (a base).
2. Ammonium chloride and mandelic acid may produce acidic urine.

3. Sodium bicarbonate, potassium citrate, and acetazolamide may produce alkaline urine.

Patient Preparation

1. Explain test purpose and specimen collection procedure.
2. Follow guidelines in Chapter 1 for safe, effective, informed *pretest* care.

Patient Aftercare

1. Interpret test outcomes and monitor patient appropriately (see control of urine pH).
2. Follow guidelines in Chapter 1 for safe, effective, informed *posttest* care.

URINE BLOOD OR HEMOGLOBIN (Heme) ●

Normal Values

Negative/none

Background

The presence of free hemoglobin in the urine is referred to as *hemoglobinuria*. Hemoglobinuria is usually related to conditions outside the urinary tract and occurs when there is such extensive or rapid destruction (hemolysis) of circulating erythrocytes that the reticuloendothelial system cannot metabolize or store the excess free hemoglobin. Blood may appear as intact red cells or as free hemoglobin.

When intact red blood cells are present in the urine, the term *hematuria* is used to indicate bleeding somewhere in the urinary tract. Usually, both red blood cells and hemoglobin mark this disorder. Therefore, hematuria can be distinguished from hemoglobinuria by a microscopic examination of the sediment from a fresh urine specimen.

Explanation of Test

This test detects blood or hemoglobin in urine. Blood in urine is an important indicator of damage to the kidney or urinary tract.

The use of both a urine dipstick and microscopic examination of urine provides a complete clinical evaluation of hemoglobinuria and hematuria. Newer forms of dipsticks contain a lysing reagent that reacts with occult blood urea and detects intact as well as lysed red blood cells.

When urine sediment gives a positive result for occult blood, but no red blood cells are microscopically seen, *myoglobinuria* can be suspected. Myoglobinuria is the result of the excretion of myoglobin, a muscle protein, into the urine as a result of: (1) traumatic muscle injury, such as may occur in automobile accidents, football injuries, or electric shock; (2) a muscle disorder, such as an arterial occlusion to a muscle or muscular dystrophy; (3) certain kinds of poisoning, such as carbon monoxide or fish poisoning; or (4) in malignant hyperthermia, related to administration of certain anesthetic agents. Myoglobin must be distinguished from free hemoglobin in the urine by certain chemical tests.

Procedure

1. *Hemoglobin in urine—hemoglobinuria*
   a. Dipsticks are dipped into the urine and the color change on the dipstick is correlated with a standardized color chart specifically used with that particular type of dipstick.
   b. The color chart indicates color gradients for negative, moderate, and large amounts of hemoglobin.
2. *Hematuria*—red blood cells in urine
   a. This dipstick method allows detection of intact red blood cells when the number is greater than 10/μl. The color change appears stippled on the dipstick.
   b. To verify the presence of red blood cells, the urine sample is centrifuged, and the sediment is examined microscopically (see page 190).

Clinical Implications

1. *Hematuria* is found in
   a. Lower urinary tract infections
   b. Lupus erythematosus
   c. Urinary tract or renal cancers
   d. Urinary calculi
   e. Hemophilia
   f. Glomerulonephritis
   g. Heavy smokers
   h. Trauma
   i. Strenuous exercise
   j. Benign familial or recurrent hematuria (asymptomatic hematuria without proteinuria; other clinical and laboratory data are normal)
   k. Treatment with anticoagulants
2. *Hemoglobinuria* is found in
   a. Extensive burns and crushing injuries
   b. Transfusion reactions with incompatible blood products
   c. Febrile intoxication
   d. Certain chemical agents and alkaloids (poisonous mushrooms, snake venom)
   e. Malaria
   f. Bleeding resulting from operative procedures on the prostate (can be difficult to control, especially in the presence of malignancies)
   g. Hemolytic disorders such as sickle cell anemia, thalassemia, and G6PD deficiency
   h. Paroxysmal hemoglobinuria (large quantities of hemoglobin appear in urine at irregular intervals)
   i. Kidney infarction
   j. Hematuria from other causes (with RBC lysis or hypotonic urine)
   k. Fava bean sensitivity
   l. Disseminated intravascular coagulation (DIC)
   m. Strenuous exercise "march hemoglobinuria"

Clinical Alert

One of the early indicators of possible renal or urinary tract disease is the appearance of blood in the urine. This does not mean that blood will be present in every voided specimen in every case of these diseases. It does mean, however, that in most cases of renal or urinary tract disease, occult blood will appear in the urine with a reasonable degree of frequency. Any positive test for hematuria should be rechecked on a new urine specimen. If hematuria still appears, the patient should be further evaluated.

Interfering Factors

1. Drugs that cause a positive result for blood or hemoglobin include
   a. Drugs toxic to the kidneys (eg, bacitracin or amphotericin).
   b. Drugs that alter blood clotting (coumarins).
   c. Drugs that cause hemolysis of red blood cells (aspirin).
   d. Drugs that may give a false-positive result; these include bromides, copper, iodides, and oxidizing agents.
2. High doses of ascorbic acid or vitamin C may give false-negative results. (Ascorbic acid may be used as a preservative for antibiotics such as tetracycline.)
3. High specific gravity or elevated protein reduces sensitivity (see Chap. 1 concerning sensitivity.)
4. Myoglobin produces a false-positive result.
5. Highly alkaline urine tends to cause hemolysis of red cells.
6. Menstrual blood may contaminate the specimen and alter results.

Patient Preparation

1. Explain test purpose and procedure for urine specimen collection.
2. Follow guidelines in Chapter 1 for safe, effective, informed *pretest* care.

Patient Aftercare

1. Interpret test outcomes and explain possible need for follow-up testing.
2. Follow guidelines in Chapter 1 for safe, effective, informed *posttest* care.

URINE PROTEIN (ALBUMIN); **QUALITATIVE AND 24-HR**

Normal Values

Adult: 10–140 mg/L or 1–14 mg/dl in 24 hours
Child < 10 years: 10–100 mg/L or 1–10 mg/dl in 24 hours

Explanation of Test

Detection of protein in urine (proteinuria), combined with a microscopic examination of urinary sediment, provides the basis for differential diagnosis of renal disease. In a healthy renal and urinary tract system, the urine contains no protein or only slight trace amounts of protein. These consist of albumin (one-third of normal urine protein is albumin) and globulins from the plasma. Because albumin is filtered more readily than the globulins, it is usually very abundant in pathologic conditions. Therefore, the term *albuminuria* is often used synonymously with *proteinuria*.

Normally, the glomerules prevent passage of protein from the blood to the glomerular filtrate. Thus, the persistent presence of protein in the urine is the single most important indication of renal disease. Therefore, if more than a trace of protein is found in the urine, a quantitative 24-hour evaluation of protein excretion is necessary.

Procedure

QUALITATIVE PROTEIN COLLECTION

1. Collect random urine in a clean container and test it as soon as possible.
2. Use a protein reagent dipstick and compare the test result color with the color comparison chart provided on the reagent strip bottle. Protein can also be detected by turbidiometric methods using sulfosalicylic acid (SSA).
3. If one of these methods produces positive results, a 24-hour urine test for protein may be ordered. However, a new second specimen should be tested for positive results before the 24-hour specimen is collected.

24-HOUR URINE PROTEIN COLLECTION

1. Label a 24-hour urine container with the name of the patient, test, and the date and time the test is started.
2. Refrigerate the specimen as it is being collected.
3. See general instructions for 24-hour urine collection listed on page 154.
4. Record the exact start and end of the 24-hour collection on the specimen container and the patient's record (usual start and end times are 0700 to 0700).

Clinical Implications

1. Proteinuria is usually the result of increased glomerular filtration of protein because of some kind of glomerular damage. A follow-up to the 24-hour urine test for protein is indicated to arrive at a specific diagnosis.
2. Persistent proteinuria of any amount, in an apparently healthy person, usually indicates some renal disease.
3. In pathologic states, the level of proteinuria is rarely constant; thus, not every sample of urine will be abnormal in patients with renal disease.
4. Proteinuria occurs in the following renal diseases:
   - **a.** Nephritis/glomerulonephritis
   - **b.** Nephrosis
   - **c.** Renal vein thrombosis
   - **d.** Malignant hypertension
   - **e.** Polycystic kidney disease
   - **f.** Chronic urinary tract obstruction
5. Proteinuria may occur in the following nonrenal diseases and conditions:

a. Fever, acute infection
b. Trauma
c. Leukemia, multiple myeloma
d. Toxemia, preeclampsia of pregnancy
e. Diabetes mellitus
f. Vascular disease (hypertension)
g. Waldenstrom's macroglobulinemia
h. Systemic lupus erythematosus (SLE)
i. Poisoning from turpentine, phosphorus, mercury, sulfosalicylic acid, lead, phenol, opiates, or other drugs

6. Large numbers of leukocytes accompanying proteinuria usually indicate infection at some level in the urinary tract. Large numbers of both leukocytes and erythrocytes indicate a noninfectious inflammatory disease of the glomerulus. Proteinuria associated with pyelonephritis may have as many red blood cells as white cells.
7. Proteinuria does not always accompany renal disease. Pyelonephritis, urinary tract obstructions, nephrolithiasis, tumors, and congenital malformations can cause severe illness without the occurrence of protein leakage.
8. Proteinuria is associated with the finding of casts on the sediment examination because protein is necessary for cast formation.
9. Postural proteinuria results from the excretion of protein by patients who are standing or moving about all day (or night!). This type of proteinuria is intermittent and disappears when the person lies down. Postural proteinuria occurs in 3% to 15% of healthy young adults. It is also known as *orthostatic proteinuria*.

Collecting the Specimen for Orthostatic Proteinuria

1. The patient is instructed to void at bedtime and to discard this urine.
2. The next morning, a urine specimen is collected immediately after the patient awakes and before he or she has been in an upright position for more than 1 minute. This may involve the use of a bedpan or urinal.
3. A second specimen is collected after the patient has been standing or walking at least 2 hours.

Differentiation from other types of proteinuria is accomplished by testing for protein in the two urine specimens: the one collected before rising, and the other collected after the person has been standing or walking for more than 2 hours. With postural proteinuria, the first specimen contains no protein, whereas the second one is positive for protein.

The urine looks microscopically normal. No RBCs or WBCs are apparent. Orthostatic proteinuria is considered a benign condition and slowly disappears with time. Progressive renal impairment usually does not occur.

Clinical Alert

1. Proteinuria > 2000 mg/24 hr in adults and ≥ 40 mg/24 hr in children usually indicates glomerular etiology.
2. Proteinuria of > 3500 mg/24 hr points to a nephrotic syndrome.

Interfering Factors for Qualitative Protein Test

1. Because of renal vasoconstriction, the presence of a functional, mild, and transitory protein in the urine is associated with
   a. Strenous exercise
   b. Severe emotional stress, seizures
   c. Cold baths or exposure to very cold temperatures
2. Increased protein in urine occurs
   a. After eating large amounts of protein
   b. During pregnancy or immediately following delivery
   c. In newborn infants (first week)
   d. In the premenstrual state of the monthly cycle
3. False or accidental proteinuria may occur because of a mixture of pus and red blood cells in the urinary tract related to infections or the menstrual flow.
4. False-positive results can occur from incorrect use and interpretation of the color reagent strip test.
5. Alkaline urine can produce false-positive results on the dipstick reagent strip test because of alkaline, highly buffered urine.
6. Very dilute urine may give a falsely low protein value.
7. Certain drugs may cause false-positive or false-negative urine protein tests.
8. X-ray contrast substances may produce false-positive results with turbidiometric measurements.

Patient Preparation

1. Instruct patient about the purpose and collection of the 24-hour urine specimen. Emphasize the importance of compliance with the procedure.
2. Food and fluids are permitted; however, fluids should not be forced because very dilute urine can produce false-negative values.
3. Follow guidelines in Chapter 1 for safe, effective, informed *pretest* care.

Patient Aftercare

1. Interpret test outcomes and explain possible need for follow-up testing and treatment.
2. See guidelines in Chapter 1 for safe, effective, informed *posttest* care.

URINE BENCE JONES PROTEIN ●

Normal Values

Negative for Bence Jones protein.

Background

Bence Jones proteins are free (not attached to immunoglobulin) light chains that may be present in either serum or urine. Because these proteins are very small and soluble, the greatest concentrations are found in the urine.

Explanation of Test

This test is helpful in the diagnosis of multiple myeloma, lymphoma, macroglobunemia, leukemia, osteogenic sarcoma, amyloidosis, and other malignancies.

Screening for Bence Jones protein can be done by a turbidemetric test, such as sulfosalicylic acid, or by the heat precipitation test. Bence Jones protein will precipitate on heating between 45° and 60°C, and will then redissolve with further heating to the boiling point. When a screening test is positive, confirmatory testing must be done because the screening tests, in themselves, are not diagnostic. The best confirmatory tests are urine protein electrophoresis (UPE) and immunoelectrophoresis of the urine (see Chap. 8).

Procedure

1. Collect a 24-hour urine specimen (see page 154 for instructions).
2. Refrigerate the specimen during collection; no preservative is needed.
3. Blood in urine will cause unreliable results.

Clinical Implications

A positive Bence Jones protein (free light chains) test result is found in

1. 50%–80% multiple myeloma cases (malignant proliferation of plasma cells)
2. Waldenstrom's macroglobulinemia
3. Cryoglobulinemia
4. Primary amyloidosis
5. Adult Fanconi's syndrome
6. Hyperparathyroidism
7. Benign monoclonal gammopathy
8. Lymphatic leukemia
9. Lymphoma
10. Other malignant B-cell diseases
11. Light chain disease

Interfering Factors

Conditions that may produce a false-positive result include

1. Connective tissue disorders, (eg, systemic lupus erythematosis [SLE], rheumatoid arthritis)
2. Chronic renal insufficiency
3. Metastatic carcinoma of lung, GI, and GU tract
4. High doses of penicillin or aspirin
5. X-ray contrast media

Clinical Alert

1. The protein dipstick does not detect Bence Jones protein and, therefore, cannot be used for screening.
2. The dipstick method for detecting protein will give a false-negative result for Bence Jones protein—the protein dipstick reacts mainly with albumin. Bence Jones is a globulin.

Clinical Alert

When significant amounts of free kappa- and lambda-light chains are detected by electrophoresis, they should be confirmed by urine immunofixation for early diagnosis and assessment of this type of light chain disease.

Patient Preparation

1. Explain test purpose and specimen collection procedure.
2. See Chapter 1 guidelines for safe, effective, informed *pretest* care.

Patient Aftercare

1. Interpret test outcomes and monitor appropriately.
2. Follow Chapter 1 guidelines for safe, effective, informed *posttest* care.

URINE BETA$_2$-MICROGLOBULIN ●

Normal Values

< 1 mg/24 hr
0–160 μg/L

Background

Beta$_2$-microglobulin is a cell membrane–associated peptide, a component of the lymphatic human lymphocyte antibody (HLA) complex. It is structurally related to immunoglobulins.

Explanation of Test

This test measures beta$_2$-microglobulin, which is nonspecifically increased in inflammatory conditions and in active chronic lymphatic leukemia. It may be used to differentiate glomerular from tubular dysfunction. In glomerular disease, beta$_2$-microglobulin is increased in serum and decreased in urine, whereas in tubular disorders, it is decreased in serum and increased in urine. In amino glycoside toxicity, beta$_2$-microglobulin levels become abnormal before creatinine levels begin to show abnormal values.

Procedure

1. Collect a 10-ml random fresh urine sample or a 24-hour specimen.
2. Keep the pH neutral.
3. Either specimen must be frozen if not analyzed immediately.

Clinical Implications

Increased beta$_2$-microglobulins occur in

1. Tubular disorders
2. Heavy-metal poisoning—mercury, cadmium

3. Drug toxicity—amino glycosides, cyclosporine
4. Fanconi's syndrome
5. Pyelonephritis
6. Renal allograft rejection
7. Lymphoid malignancies

Interfering Factors

1. Highly acidic urine
2. Certain antibiotics (eg, gentamicin, tobramycin)
3. Recent radioactive scan

Patient Preparation

1. Instruct patient concerning the purpose and procedure of test.
2. See 24-hour urine collection, page 154.
3. See Chapter 1 for guidelines for safe, effective, informed *pretest* care.

Patient Aftercare

1. Interpret test outcomes and monitor appropriately.
2. See Chapter 1 guidelines for safe, effective, informed *posttest* care.

URINE GLUCOSE (SUGAR)

Normal Values

Random specimen: negative
24-hour specimen: < 0.3 g/24 hr

Background

Glucose is present in glomerular filtrate but is reabsorbed by the proximal tubule. However, should the blood glucose level exceed the reabsorption capacity of the tubules, glucose will spill into the urine.

Sugar in the urine (*glucosuria* or *glycosuria*) is not necessarily abnormal. It may appear in urine after a heavy meal or during times of emotional stress. For some persons, a low tubular reabsorption rate may account for glycosuria in the presence of normal blood glucose levels. This is a benign condition.

Explanation of Test

Urine glucose tests are used to screen for diabetes, to confirm a diagnosis of diabetes, or to monitor the degree of diabetic control. Diabetes mellitus is the main cause of glycosuria.

Nonetheless, a random-sample positive test for urine sugar is not adequate for a diagnosis of diabetes. A postprandial blood sugar test provides more accurate information in diabetes detection programs than does a urine sugar test. A urine glucose combined with a blood glucose test gives even better information. Moreover, an abnormal postprandial urine glucose test is more effective for recognizing diabetes than a fasting urine glucose test.

Types of Glucose Test

A. *Reduction tests* (Clinitest)

1. These are based on reduction of cupric ions by glucose. When these compounds are added to urine, a heat reaction takes place. This results in precipitation and a change in the color of the urine if glucose is present.
2. These are nonspecific for glucose because the reaction can also be caused by other reducing substances in the urine such as
   - **a.** Creatinine, uric acid, ascorbic acid;
   - **b.** Other sugars, such as galactose, lactose, fructose, pentose, and maltose

B. *Enzyme tests* (Clinistix, Diastix, Tes-Tape)

1. These are based on interaction between glucose oxidase (an enzyme) and glucose. When dipped into urine, the enzyme-impregnated strip changes color according to the amount of glucose in the urine. The manufacturer's color chart provides a basis for comparison of colors between the sample and the manufacturer's control.
2. These are specific for glucose only.

Procedure

1. Use a freshly voided specimen.
2. Follow exact directions on the test container. Timing must be exact; the color reaction must be compared with the closest matching control color on the manufacturer's color chart to ascertain accurate results.
3. Record results on the patient's record.
4. If a 24-hour urine specimen is also ordered, the entire urine sample must be refrigerated or iced during collection. See Table 3-1 for proper preservative.

Clinical Alert

1. Determine exactly what drugs the patient is taking and whether the metabolites of these drugs can affect the urine glucose results. Frequent updating about the effect of drugs on blood glucose levels is necessary in light of the many new drugs introduced and prescribed.
2. Test results can be reported as "plus (+)" or percentages. Percentages are more accurate.
3. When screening for galactose (galactosuria) in infants, the reduction test must be used. The enzyme tests do not react with galactose.

Clinical Implications

1. Increased glucose levels occur in
   a. Diabetes mellitus; pituitary diseases, such as thyrotoxicosis, Cushing's syndrome, acromegaly
   b. Central nervous system (CNS) diseases (brain injury)
   c. Renal tubule disease associated with lowered urine threshold (positive urine glucose with normal blood glucose and normal glucose tolerance test (GTT)
   d. Fanconi's syndrome
   e. Inflammatory renal disease
2. Increase of other sugars (react only with reduction tests)
   a. Lactose: increase seen in pregnancy, lactation, and lactose intolerance
   b. Galactose: increased in heredity galactosuria (severe enzyme deficiency in infants—must be treated promptly)
   c. Xylose: increase due to excessive ingestion of fruit
   d. Fructose: increased in hereditary fructose intolerance and hepatic disorders
   e. Pentose: certain drug therapies and rare hereditary conditions cause increases

Interfering Factors

1. Interfering factors for reduction test that produce false-positive results include
   a. Presence of non–sugar-reducing substances, such as ascorbic acid, homogentistic acid, creatinine
   b. Phenylketonuria, tyrosine
   c. Nalidixic acid, cephalosporins, probenecid, and penicillin
   d. Large amounts of urine protein (slows reaction)
2. Interfering factors for dipstick enzyme tests
   a. Ascorbic acid, in large amounts, may cause a false-negative result
   b. Large amount of ketones: false-negative result
3. Stress, excitement, myocardial infarct, testing after a heavy meal, and testing soon after the administration of intravenous glucose, all may cause false-positive results; most frequently trace reactions.
4. Contamination of the urine sample with bleach or hydrogen peroxide may invalidate results.

Patient Preparation

1. Instruct the patient about the test purpose the procedure, and the second-voiding technique.
   a. Discard the first-voided morning specimen, then void 30 to 45 minutes later for the test specimen. This second specimen reflects the immediate state of glucosuria more accurately because the first specimen is urine present in the bladder over a period of several hours.
   b. Advise the patient not to drink liquids between the first and second voiding so that the glucose present in the specimen is not diluted.

2. Instruct the patient about the 24-hour glucose procedure when applicable.
3. Follow Chapter 1 guidelines for safe, effective, informed *pretest* care.

Patient Aftercare

1. Interpret test outcomes and counsel appropriately.
2. See Chapter 1 guidelines for safe, effective, informed *posttest* care.

URINE KETONES (ACETONE; KETONE BODIES) ●

Normal Value

Negative

Background

Ketones, which result from the metabolism of fatty acid and fat, consist mainly of three substances: acetone, β-hydroxybutyric acid, and acetoacetic acid. The last two substances readily convert to acetone, in essence, making acetone the main substance being tested. However, some testing products measure only acetoacetic acid.

In healthy individuals, ketones are formed in the liver and are completely metabolized so that only negligible amounts appear in the urine. However, when carbohydrate metabolism is altered, excessive amounts of ketones are formed (acetosis) because fat becomes the predominant body fuel instead of carbohydrates. When the metabolic pathways of carbohydrates are disturbed, carbon fragments from fat and protein are diverted to form abnormal amounts of ketone bodies. Thus, the body's alkaline reserves become depleted and acidosis occurs.

Explanation of Test

The excess presence of ketones (ketonuria) in the urine is associated with diabetes or altered carbohydrate metabolism. Some "fad" diets, low in carbohydrates and high in fat and protein, also produce ketones in the urine. Testing for urine ketones in patients with diabetes may provide the clue to early diagnosis of ketoacidosis and diabetic coma.

Indications for Ketone Testing

GENERAL

Screening for ketonuria is frequently done for hospitalized patients, presurgical patients, pregnant women, children, and individuals with diabetes.

GLYCOSURIA—DIABETES

1. Testing for ketones is indicated for any patient showing elevated levels of urine and blood sugars.
2. When treatment is being switched from insulin to oral hypoglycemic agents, the development of ketonuria within 24 hours after the with-

drawal of insulin usually indicates a poor response to the oral hypoglycemic agents.
3. The urine of diabetic patients treated with oral hypoglycemic agents should be tested regularly for glucose and ketones because oral hypoglycemic agents, unlike insulin, do not control diabetes when acute complications such as infection develop.
4. Testing is indicated to differentiate between diabetic coma and insulin shock.

ACIDOSIS

1. Ketone testing is used to judge the severity of acidosis and to track the response to treatment.
2. Urine ketone measurement frequently provides a more reliable indicator of acidosis than blood testing (it is especially useful in emergency room situations).
3. Ketones appear in the urine before there is any significant increase of ketones in the blood.

PREGNANCY

During pregnancy, the early detection of ketones is essential because ketoacidosis is a prominent factor that contributes to intrauterine death.

Procedure

1. Dip the ketone reagent strip in fresh urine, tap off excess urine, time the reaction accurately, and then compare the strip with the control color chart on the time container.
2. If procedure differs from preceding technique, follow the manufacturer's directions exactly.
3. Do not use dipsticks to test for ketones in blood. Special testing products are designed for blood.

Clinical Implications

1. Ketosis and ketonuria may occur whenever increased amounts of fat are metabolized, carbohydrate intake is restricted, or the diet is rich in fats, either "hidden" or obvious. This state can occur in the following:
   a. Metabolic conditions
      (1) Diabetes mellitus
      (2) Renal glycosuria
      (3) Glycogen storage disease
   b. Dietary conditions
      (1) Starvation, fasting
      (2) High-fat diets
      (3) Prolonged vomiting
      (4) Anorexia
      (5) Low-carbohydrate diet
   c. Increased metabolic states caused by
      (1) Hyperthyroidism
      (2) Fever
      (3) Pregnancy or lactation
2. In nondiabetics, ketonuria will occur frequently during acute illness or se-

vere stress. Approximately 15% of hospitalized patients will have ketones in their urine, even though they do not have diabetes.

3. Children are particularly prone to developing ketonuria and ketosis.
4. Following anesthesia.

Interfering Factors

Drugs that may cause a false-positive result include

1. Levodopa
2. Phthalein compounds: bromosulfophthalein (BSP) or phenolsulfonphthalein (PSP)
3. Ether
4. Insulin
5. Isopropyl alcohol
6. Metformin
7. Paraldehyde
8. Phenazopyridine (Pyridium)
9. Phenformin

Clinical Alert

Urine ketones signal a need for caution, rather than crisis intervention, in either a diabetic or a nondiabetic patient. This, however, does not mean that this condition should be taken lightly.

1. In the diabetic patient, ketone bodies in the urine suggest that the patient is not adequately controlled and that adjustments of either the medication or the diet should be made promptly.
2. In the nondiabetic patient, ketone bodies indicate a reduced carbohydrate metabolism and excessive fat metabolism.

Patient Preparation

1. Explain test purpose and procedure.
2. Follow guidelines in Chapter 1 for safe, effective, informed *pretest* care.

Patient Aftercare

1. Interpret test outcomes and monitor appropriately.
2. See Chapter 1 guidelines for safe, effective, informed *posttest* care.

URINE NITRATE/BACTERIA

Normal Value

Negative for bacteria

Background

This test is an indirect method for detecting bacteria in the urine. Significant urinary tract infections may be present in patients who do not experience any symptoms. These urinary tract infections are serious and need prompt treatment because they can potentially cause severe kidney damage.

Physicians frequently request the urine nitrate test to screen high-risk patients who include pregnant women, school-aged children (especially girls), diabetic patients, elderly patients, and patients with a history of urinary tract infections.

Explanation of Test

Microscopic examination and chemical testing are used to detect bacteria in the urine during routine urinalysis. The sediment, when examined microscopically, can reveal the presence of bacteria. With chemical dipstick testing, the nitrite area in a multiple reagent strip is calibrated so that any shade of pink that develops within 30 seconds indicates nitrite from nitrate-producing organisms. Thus, a pink positive test indicates significant bacteremia.

Procedure

1. A first morning specimen is preferred because urine that has been in the bladder for several hours is more likely to yield a positive nitrite test than a random urine sample that may have been in the bladder for only a short time. A clean-catch or midstream urine specimen is needed to minimize bacterial contamination from adjacent areas.
2. Follow the exact testing procedure according to prescribed guidelines for reliable test results.
3. Comparing the used dipstick-reacted reagent area against a white background may aid in the detection of a faint pink hue that might otherwise be missed.

Clinical Implications

1. Twenty or more bacteria per high-powered microscopic field may indicate a urinary tract infection. Untreated bacteriuria can lead to very serious kidney disease.
2. The presence of a few bacteria suggests a urinary tract infection that cannot be confirmed or excluded until more definitive studies, such as culture and sensitivity tests, are performed. Again, this finding merits serious consideration for treatment.
3. A positive nitrite test is a reliable indicator of significant bacteriuria and is a cue for performing urine culture.
4. A negative result should *never* be interpreted as indicating absence of bacteriuria for the following reasons:
   a. If an overnight urine sample is not used, there may not have been enough time for the nitrate to convert to nitrite in the bladder.
   b. Some urinary tract infections are caused by organisms that do not convert nitrate to nitrite (eg, *Staphylococcus* or *Streptococcus* species).
   c. Sufficient dietary nitrate may not be present for the nitrate to nitrite reaction to occur.

Interfering Factors

1. Azo dye metabolites can produce false-positive results.
2. Ascorbic acid can produce false-negative results.

> **Clinical Alert**
>
> A negative urine nitrate test should never be interpreted as indicating the absence of bacteria.

Patient Preparation

1. Explain test purpose and urine specimen collection procedure. Instruct the patient in the procedure necessary for a midstream or clean-catch specimen.
2. Follow guidelines in Chapter 1 for safe, effective, informed *pretest* care.

Patient Aftercare

1. Interpret test outcomes and monitor appropriately.
2. See Chapter 1 guidelines for safe, effective, informed *posttest* care.

URINE LEUKOCYTE ESTERASE

Normal Value

Negative

Background

Usually, white cells (leukocytes) in the urine indicate a urinary tract infection. The leukocyte esterase test detects esterase released by the leukocytes into the urine.

Explanation of Test

Microscopic examination and chemical testing are used to determine the presence of leukocytes (white blood cells) in the urine. The second of these, the chemical test, employs a leukocyte esterase dipstick. The dipstick is calibrated so that the intensity of the reactive purple color is proportional to the concentration of white blood cells in the urine sample. This test can also detect intact leukoctyes, lysed leukocytes, and white blood cell casts.

Procedure

1. Collect a fresh, random urine specimen in a clean-catch or midstream technique.
2. Directions for dipstick use must be followed exactly. Timing is critical for accurate results.

Interfering Factors

Vaginal discharge or bleeding, trichomonas, parasites, or heavy mucus can cause false-positive results.

Clinical Implications

1. Normal urine is negative for WBCs.
2. Positive results are clinically significant and indicate pyuria.
3. Urine with positive results from the dipstick should be examined microscopically for WBCs and bacteria.

> **Clinical Alert**
>
> A urine sample that tests positive for both nitrate and leukocyte esterase should be cultured for pathogenic bacteria.

Patient Preparation

1. Explain test purpose and procedure.
2. See Chapter 1 guidelines for safe, effective, informed *pretest* care.

Patient Aftercare

1. Interpret test outcomes and monitor appropriately.
2. Follow Chapter 1 guidelines for safe, effective, informed *posttest* care.

URINE BILIRUBIN

Normal Values

Negative (0–0.02 mg/dl)

Background

Bilirubin is formed in the reticuloendothelial cells of the spleen and bone marrow, as a result of the breakdown of hemoglobin, and is then transported to the liver. Urinary bilirubin levels will be elevated to significant levels in the presence of any disease process that increases the amount of conjugated bilirubin in the bloodstream (see Chemistry Studies, Chap. 6). Normally, even though there is a small amount of urobilinogen in the urine, no more than 0.02 mg/dl of bilirubin is normal.

Explanation of Test

Urine bilirubin aids in the diagnosis and monitoring of treatment for hepatitis and liver dysfunction. In persons exposed to certain toxins and drugs, a positive test for bilirubinuria can be an early indicator of liver damage.

Urine bilirubin is an early sign of hepatocellular disease or intrahepatic or extrahepatic biliary obstruction. It should be a part of every urinalysis because bilirubin may often appear in the urine before other signs of liver dysfunction become apparent (eg, jaundice, weakness).

Procedure

1. Examine the urine within 1 hour of collection because urine bilirubin is unstable, especially when exposed to light.
2. Chemical strip testing:
   a. Dip a chemically reactive dipstick into the urine sample according to manufacturer's directions.
   b. Close comparison of color changes on the dipstick with control colors on the color chart is an absolute must. Failure to make a close approximation of color may result in failure to recognize urine bilirubin. Good lighting is absolutely necessary.
   c. Interpret results as "negative" to "3+" or as "small, moderate, or large" amounts of bilirubin.
3. When it is crucial to detect even very small amounts of bilirubin in the urine, as in the earliest phase of viral hepatitis, Icotest tablets are preferred for testing because they are more sensitive to urinary bilirubin. When elevated amounts of urinary bilirubin are present, a blue to purplish color forms on the absorptive mat. The rapidity and the intensity of the color are directly proportional to the amount of bilirubin in the urine.

Clinical Implications

1. Even trace amounts of bilirubin are abnormal and warrant further investigation. Normally, there is no detectable bilirubin in the urine.
2. *Increased levels* occur in
   a. Hepatitis and liver diseases caused by infections or exposure to toxic agents
   b. Obstructive biliary tract diseases

NOTE: *Urine bilirubin is negative in hemolytic disease.*

Interfering Factors

1. Drugs may cause false-positive or false-negative results.
2. Bilirubin rapidly decomposes when exposed to light; therefore, urine should be tested immediately.

Clinical Alert

Pyridiumlike drugs or urochromes may give the urine an amber or reddish color and can mask the bilirubin reaction or result in typical reactions.

Patient Preparation

1. Explain test purpose and procedure.
2. See Chapter 1 guidelines for safe, effective, informed *pretest* care.

Patient Aftercare

1. Interpret test outcomes and monitor appropriately.
2. Follow Chapter 1 guidelines for safe, effective, informed *posttest* care.

URINE UROBILINOGEN (RANDOM, TIMED) ●

Normal Values

2-hour specimen: 0.1–1.0 Ehrlich unit/ml/2 hr
24-hour specimen: 1–4 mg/ml/24 hr
Random: 0.1–1 Ehrlich unit/ml

Background

Bilirubin formed from the breakdown of hemoglobin and metabolism of hemoglobin enters the intestine in the bile; *bilirubin* is transformed through the action of bacterial enzymes into *urobilinogen*. Some of the urobilinogen formed in the intestine is excreted as part of the feces; another portion is absorbed into the portal bloodstream and carried to the liver, where it is metabolized and excreted in the bile. Traces of urobilinogen in the blood that escape removal by the liver are carried to the kidneys and excreted in the urine. This is the basis of the urine urobilinogen test. Unlike bilirubin, *urobilinogen* is colorless.

Explanation of Test

Urine urobilinogen is one of the most sensitive tests available to determine impaired liver function. Urinary urobilinogen is *increased* by any condition that causes an increase in the production of bilirubin and by any disease that prevents the liver from normally removing the reabsorbed urobilinogen from the portal circulation. An *increased* urobilinogen level is one of the earliest signs of acute liver cell damage.

Procedure

1. Follow instructions for collecting either a timed 24-hour or 2-hour specimen. Check with laboratory for specific protocols.
2. The 2-hour–timed collection is best done from 1:00 PM to 3:00 PM or 2:00 PM to 4:00 PM because peak excretion occurs during this time. No preservatives are necessary. Record total amount of urine voided. Protect the collection receptacle from light. Test immediately after specimen collection is completed.

Clinical Implications

1. Urinary urobilinogen is *increased*
   a. Whenever there is increased destruction of red blood cells, as in
      (1) Hemolytic anemias
      (2) Pernicious anemia
      (3) Malaria
   b. When hemorrhage into tissues occurs, as in
      (1) Pulmonary infarct
      (2) Excessive bruising
   c. When hepatic damage occurs as a result of
      (1) Biliary disease
      (2) Cirrhosis—viral or chemical
      (3) Acute hepatitis
   d. When cholangitis is present

2. Urinary urobilinogen is *decreased* or absent when normal amounts of bilirubin are not excreted into the intestinal tract. This usually indicates partial or complete obstruction of the bile ducts, such as may occur in
   a. Cholelithiasis
   b. Severe inflammation of the biliary ducts
   c. Cancer of the head of the pancreas

3. During antibiotic therapy, suppression of normal gut flora may prevent the breakdown of bilirubin to urobilinogen; therefore, urine levels will be lowered or absent.

4. More comprehensive information is obtained when the tests for urobilinogen and bilirubin are correlated (see the following comparisons).

Comparison of Urine Urobilinogen and Urine Bilirubin Values

	In Health	*In Hemolytic Disease*	*In Hepatic Disease*	*In Biliary Obstruction*
Urine Urobilinogen	Normal	Increased	Increased	Low or absent
Urine Bilirubin	Negative	Negative	Positive or negative	Positive

Clinical Alert

Urine urobilinogen rapidly decomposes at room temperature or when exposed to light.

Interfering Factors

1. Drugs that may affect urobilinogen levels include those that cause cholestasis and those that reduce the bacterial flora in the gastrointestinal tract (eg, chloramphenicol, neomycin, ammonium chloride, and ascorbic acid).
2. Peak excretion is known to occur from noon to 4:00 PM. The amount of urobilinogen in the urine is subject to diurnal variation.
3. Strongly alkaline urine will show a higher urobilinogen level, and strongly acidic urine will show a lower urobilinogen level.
4. Drugs that may cause *increased* urobilinogen include those that cause hemolysis, acetazolamide, and sodium bicarbonate.

Patient Preparation

1. Explain test purpose and urine collection procedures.
2. See Chapter 1 guidelines for safe, effective, informed *pretest* care.

Patient Aftercare

1. Interpret test outcomes and monitor appropriately. Advise concerning need for follow-up testing.
2. Follow Chapter 1 guidelines for safe, effective, informed *posttest* care.

● MICROSCOPIC EXAMINATION OF URINE SEDIMENT

Background

In health, the urine contains small numbers of cells and other formed elements from the entire genitourinary tract: casts and epithelial cells from the nephron; epithelial cells from the kidney, pelvis, ureters, bladder, and urethra; mucous threads and spermatozoa from the prostate; possibly red or white blood cells and an occasional cast (see page 191 for cast formation). In renal parenchymal disease, the urine usually contains increased numbers of cells and casts discharged from an organ that is otherwise accessible only by biopsy or surgery. (See the following list of elements and their significance.) Urinary sediment provides information useful for both diagnosis and prognosis. It provides a direct sampling of urinary tract morphology.

The urinary sediment is obtained by pouring 10 ml of well-mixed urine into a conical tube and centrifuging the sample at a specific speed for 10 minutes. The supernatant is poured off and 1 ml of sediment is mixed in a coverslip on a slide and examined under the microscope.

The urine sediment can be broken down into cellular elements (red and white blood cells and epithelial cells), casts, crystals, and bacteria. These may originate anywhere in the urinary tract. When casts do occur in the urine, they may indicate tubular or glomerular disorders.

Microscopic Examination of Urine Sediment

Urine Sediment Component	*Clinical Significance*
Bacteria	Urinary tract infection
Casts	Tubular or glomerular disorders
Broad casts	Formation occurs in collecting tubules; serious kidney disorder
Epithelial (renal) casts	Tubular degeneration
Fatty casts	Nephrotic syndrome
Granular or waxy casts	Renal parenchymal disease
Hyaline casts	Acidic urine—high salt content
Red cell casts	Acute glomerulonephritis
White cell casts	Pyelonephritis
Epithelial cells	Damage to various parts of urinary tract
Renal cells	Tubular damage
Squamous cells	Normal or contamination
Erythrocytes (red blood cells)	Most renal disorders; menstruation; strenuous exercise
Fat bodies (oval)	Nephrotic syndrome
Leukocytes (white blood cells)	Most renal disorders; urinary tract infection; pyelonephritis

Cast width is significant in determining the site of origin and may indicate the extent of renal damage. The width of the cast indicates the diameter of the tubule responsible for its formation. Cast width is described as *narrow* (one to two red blood cells in width), *medium broad* (three to four red blood cells in width), and *broad* (five red blood cells in width). The broad cast forms in the collecting tubule and may be of any composition. It usually indicates a marked reduction in the functional capacity of the nephron and suggests severe renal damage or "end-stage" renal disease.

Clinical Alert

Microscopic examination of urine sediment can provide the following information:

1. Evidence of renal disease as opposed to lower urinary tract infection.
2. The type and status of a renal lesion or disease.

URINE RED BLOOD CELLS AND RED BLOOD CELL CASTS

Normal Values

Red blood cells: 0–3/HPF (high-power field)
Red cell casts: 0/LPF (low-power field)

Explanation of Test

In health, red blood cells (RBCs) occasionally appear in the urine. However, *persistent* findings of even small numbers of erythrocytes, or RBCs, should be thoroughly investigated because these cells come from the kidney and may signal serious renal disease. They are usually diagnostic of glomerular disease.

Procedure for Microscopic Urine Examination

1. Collect a random urine specimen.
2. Urinary sediment is microscopically examined under low and high microscopic power. Low power is used to find and count casts; RBCs, WBCs, and bacteria show up and are counted under high power. Amounts present are defined in terms of: few, moderate, packed, packed solid, or 1+, 2+, 3+, and 4+. Crystals and other elements are also noted.

Clinical Implications

A. *Red cell casts* indicate hemorrhage and are always pathologic.
   1. Red blood cell casts are found in three forms:
      a. Free red cells
      b. Degenerating cells within a protein matrix
      c. Homogenous blood casts ("hemoglobin casts")
   2. Red blood casts indicate acute inflammatory or vascular disorders in the glomerulus. Their presence in urine may be the only manifestation of
      a. Acute glomerulonephritis
      b. Renal infarction
      c. Collagen disease
      d. Kidney involvement in subacute bacterial endocarditis
   3. Red blood cell casts and epithelial cell casts are usually associated with systemic lupus erythematosus (SLE).

B. *Red blood cells*
   1. The finding of more than one or two RBCs per high-powered microscopic field is abnormal and can indicate
      a. Renal or systemic disease
      b. Trauma to the kidney
   2. Increased RBCs occur in
      a. Pyelonephritis
      b. SLE
      c. Renal stones
      d. Cystitis
      e. Prostatitis
      f. Tuberculosis
      g. Genitourinary tract malignancies
      h. Hemophilia
      i. Malaria
      j. Polyarteritis nodosa
      k. Malignant hypertension
   3. Greater numbers of RBCs versus WBCs indicates bleeding into the urinary tract as may occur with
      a. Trauma
      b. Tumor
      c. Aspirin ingestion or overdose

d. Anticoagulant therapy overdose
e. Thrombocytopenia

Clinical Alert

1. In health, RCBs are occasionally found in the urine. However, persistent findings of even small numbers of RBCs should be thoroughly investigated, the first step being to request a fresh urine specimen for repeat testing.
2. Rule out possible presence of menstrual blood, vaginal bleeding, or trauma to perineal area in the female patient.

Interfering Factors

1. Increased numbers of RBCs may be found following a traumatic catheterization or passage of urinary tract or kidney stones.
2. Alkaline urine hemolyzes red cells and dissolves casts.
3. Some drugs can cause increased numbers of RBCs in the urine.
4. Red cell casts may appear after very strenuous physical activity or participation in contact sports.
5. Heavy smokers show small numbers of RBCs in the urine.

Patient Preparation

1. Explain test purpose and procedure for random urine sample collection.
2. See Chapter 1 guidelines for safe, effective, informed *pretest* care.

Patient Aftercare

1. Interpret test outcomes and counsel appropriately.
2. Follow Chapter 1 guidelines for safe, effective, informed *posttest* care.

URINE WHITE BLOOD CELLS AND WHITE BLOOD CELL CASTS

Normal Values

White blood cells: 0–4/HPF (high-powered field)
White blood cell casts: 0 (negative)/LPF (low-powered field)

Background

Leukocytes (WBCs) may originate from anywhere in the genitourinary tract. However, white cell casts always come from the kidney tubules.

Procedure

1. Collect a random urine specimen.
2. Urinary sediment is microscopically examined under high-power for cells and under low-power for casts.

Clinical Implications

A. *Leukocytes* (white blood cells)

1. Large numbers of WBCs (50 cells or more per high-powered field) usually indicate acute bacterial infection within the urinary tract.
2. Increased leukocytes are seen in
   a. All renal disease
   b. Urinary tract disease (eg, cystitis, prostatitis)
   c. Fever
   d. Strenuous exercise
   e. Chronic pyelonephritis
   f. Bladder tumors
   g. Tuberculosis
3. In kidney infections, white cells tend to be associated with bacteria, epithelial cells, and relatively few red cells.
4. Large numbers of lymphocytes in the presence of a kidney transplant may indicate early tissue rejection.

> **Clinical Alert**
>
> A urine culture (see section on urine cultures in Chap. 7) should be done in the presence of elevated leukocyte counts.

B. *White cell casts*

1. White cell casts indicate renal parenchymal infection.
2. They may occur in
   a. Pyelonephritis—most common cause
   b. Acute glomerulonephritis
   c. Interstitial inflammation of the kidney
3. It can be very difficult to differentiate between white blood cell casts and epithelial cell casts.

Interfering Factors

Vaginal discharge can contaminate a specimen with WBCs. Either a clean-catch urine specimen or a catheterized urine specimen should be obtained to rule out contamination as the cause for WBCs in the urine.

> **Clinical Alert**
>
> Pyelonephritis may remain completely asymptomatic, even though renal tissue is being progressively destroyed. Therefore, careful examination (using low power) of urinary sediment for leukocyte casts is vital.

Patient Preparation

The *pretest* care is the same as for red cells.

Patient Aftercare
The *posttest* care is the same as for red cells.

URINE EPITHELIAL CELLS AND EPITHELIAL CASTS ●

Normal Values
None to two renal epithelial cells.
Squamous epithelial cells are common in normal urine samples.

Background
Renal epithelial cell casts are formed from cast-off tubule cells that slowly degenerate, first into coarse and, then, progress to fine granular material. Urine epithelial cells can be one of three kinds:

1. Renal tubule epithelial cells are round and slightly larger than leukocytes (WBCs). Each cell contains a single large nucleus. These are the types of epithelial cells associated with renal disease. However, the presence of an occasional renal epithelial cell is not unusual because renal tubules are continually regenerating.
2. Bladder epithelial cells are larger than renal epithelials. They range in shape from flat, to cuboidal, to columnar.
3. Squamous epithelial cells are large, flat cells with irregular borders, a single, small nucleus and abundant cytoplasm. The majority of these cells are urethral and vaginal in origin.

Procedure
1. Collect a random urine specimen.
2. Examine the urine sediment microscopically.

Clinical Implications
1. Larger numbers of epithelial casts are found when the following diseases have damaged tubule epithelium:
   - **a.** Nephrosis
   - **b.** Amyloidosis
   - **c.** Poisoning from heavy metals or other toxins
   - **d.** Glomerulonephritis
   - **e.** Acute tubular necrosis
2. Renal epithelium cells are found in
   - **a.** Acute tubular damage
   - **b.** Acute glomerulonephritis
   - **c.** Salicylate overdose
   - **d.** Impending allograft rejection

Patient Preparation and Patient Aftercare
Same as for white blood cells and white blood cell casts.

URINE HYALINE CASTS ●

Normal Values
None to two hyaline casts per low-power field (LPF).

Background

Hyaline casts are clear, colorless casts formed when a specific protein (Tamm–Horsfall) within the tubules precipitates and gels. Their presence in urine depends on the rate of urine flow, urine pH, and the degree of proteinuria.

Procedure

Urinary sediment is microscopically examined for casts under low power. Casts are best seen when light intensity is reduced.

Clinical Implications

1. Hyaline casts indicate possible damage to the glomerular capillary membrane, which permits leakage of proteins through the glomerular filter system. These casts show up in
   - **a.** Nephritis
   - **b.** Malignant hypertension
   - **c.** Chronic renal disease
   - **d.** Congestive heart failure
   - **e.** Diabetic nephropathy
2. Hyaline casts may be a temporary phenomenon in the presence of
   - **a.** Fever
   - **b.** Postural orthostatic lordotic strain
   - **c.** Emotional stress
   - **d.** Strenuous exercise
   - **e.** Traumatic palpation of the kidney
3. Nephrotic syndrome may be suspected when large numbers of hyaline casts appear in the urine, together with significant proteinuria, fine granular casts, fatty casts, oval fat bodies, or fat droplets.
4. In cylindruria, large numbers of casts may be present, but protein in the urine may be absent.

Clinical Alert

Casts may not be found even if proteinuria is significant or if urine is dilute (1.010 specific gravity) or alkaline. In these cases, the casts are dissolved as soon as they are formed.

Patient Preparation

Same as for white blood cell casts.

Patient Aftercare

Same as for white blood cell casts.

URINE GRANULAR CASTS

Normal Values

Occasional granular casts are found: 0–2/low-power field (LPF).

Background

Granular casts appear homogenous, coarsely granular, colorless, and very dense. Coarse, granular casts may represent the first stage of epithelial cell cast degeneration. They then further degenerate into finely granular casts and terminate as waxy or fatty casts.

Procedure

1. Collect a random urine specimen.
2. Examine urinary sediment microscopically under low power.

Clinical Implications

Granular casts are found in

1. Acute tubular necrosis
2. Advanced glomerulonephritis
3. Pyelonephritis
4. Malignant nephrosclerosis
5. Chronic lead poisoning

Patient Preparation and Patient Aftercare

Same as for white blood cells and white blood cell casts.

URINE WAXY CASTS OR BROAD CASTS (RENAL FAILURE CASTS) ●

Normal Value

Negative for waxy or renal failure casts

Background

Broad, waxy casts are formed in the collecting tubules when the urine flow through them is reduced and renal failure progresses. Waxy casts may occur from cell casts, hyaline casts, or renal failure casts. In normal subjects, granular casts are probably the result of irregular precipitation of Tamm–Horsfall protein.

Explanation of Test

Waxy casts are composed of homogen201
ous, yellowish material. They are relatively broad and appear very brittle. Broad, waxy casts are from two to six times the width of ordinary casts and appear waxy and granular.

Procedure

Urine sediment is microscopically examined under low power.

Clinical Implications

Waxy casts are found in

1. Chronic renal disease
2. Tubular inflammation and degeneration
3. Localized nephron obstruction

Clinical Alert

The presence of broad, waxy casts signals very serious renal disease.

Patient Preparation
Same as for urine white blood cells and casts.

Patient Aftercare
Same as for urine white blood cells and casts.

URINE OVAL FAT BODIES AND FATTY CASTS

Background
In the presence of nephrotic syndrome, fat accumulates in the tubular cells and eventually sloughs off and forms oval, fat bodies. This fat is probably a cholesterol ester. Fatty casts are usually composed of individual fat droplets. The presence of fat droplets, oval, fat bodies, or fatty casts is the hallmark sign of nephrotic syndrome.

Clinical Implications
Fatty casts appear in chronic renal disease and indicate tubular inflammation and degeneration.

Patient Preparation
Same as for white blood cells and casts.

Patient Aftercare
Same as for white blood cells and casts.

URINE CRYSTALS

Background
A variety of crystals may appear in the urine. They can be identified by their specific appearance and solubility characteristics. Crystals in the urine may present no symptoms, or may be associated with the formation of urinary tract calculi and give rise to clinical manifestations associated with partial or complete obstruction of urine flow.

Explanation of Test
The type and quantity of crystalline precipitates vary with the pH of the urine. Amorphous crystalline material has no significance and forms as normal urine cools.

Procedure

1. Collect a random urine specimen.
2. Examine the urinary sediment microscopically under a high-power field.

Clinical Implications

See table entitled Clinical Implications of Urine Crystals.

> **Clinical Alert**
>
> Specific drugs may cause increased levels of their own crystals. Unless toxicity is suspected, they are of little clinical significance.

Patient Preparation

Same as for white blood cells and casts.

Patient Aftercare

Same as for white blood cells and casts.

URINE SHREDS

Background

Shreds consist of a mixture of mucus, pus, and epithelial (squamous) cells. They can be seen on gross examination.

Procedure

1. Examine a fresh urine specimen by visually checking for a hazy mass.
2. Centrifuge the specimen and examine the sediment microscopically to verify the presence of formed elements.

Clinical Implications

1. When mucus predominates, the shreds float on the surface.
2. When epithelial cells predominate, the shreds occupy the midzone.
3. When pus (white blood cells) predominates, the shreds are drawn to the bottom of the specimen.
4. Other findings in urine caused by specimen contamination include microscopic yeast, trichomonas, spermatozoa, vegetable fibers, parasites, and meat fibers. These should be reported because they have clinical significance.
   - **a.** Yeast may indicate urinary moniliasis or vaginal moniliasis (*Candida albicans*).
   - **b.** Parasites: usually from fecal or vaginal contamination.
   - **c.** Spermatozoa: seen following sexual intercourse, nocturnal emissions, or in the presence of prostatic disease.
   - **d.** Vegetable fibers, meat fibers: from fecal contamination.

Clinical Implications of Urine Crystals

Type of Urine Crystal	*Color*	*Shape*	*Clinical Implications*
ACIDIC URINE			
Amorphous urates	Pink to brick red	Granules	Normal
Uric acid	Yellow-brown	Polymorphous—whetstones, rosettes, or prisms, rhombohedral prisms, hexagonal plate	Normal or increased purine metabolism, gout
Sodium urate	Colorless to yellow	Fan of slender prisms	
Cystine (rare)	1. Colorless 2. Highly refractile	Flat hexagonal plates, with well-defined edges; singly or in clusters	Cystinuria—cystine stones in kidney; crystals also in spleen and eyes
Cholesterol (rare)	Colorless	"Broken window panes" with notched corners	Elevated cholesterol chyluria
Leucine (rare)	1. Yellow or brown 2. Highly refractile	Spheroids, with striations; pure form hexagonal	Protein breakdown, severe liver disease
Tyrosine (rare)	Colorless or yellow	Fine silky needles in sheaves or rosettes	Protein breakdown, severe liver disease
Bilirubin	Reddish brown	Cubes, rhombic plates, amorphous needles	Elevated bilirubin

ACID, NEUTRAL, OR SLIGHTLY ALKALINE URINE			
Calcium oxalate	Colorless	Octahedral; dumbbells often small: use high-power	Normal, large amounts in fresh urine may indicate severe chronic renal disease
Hippuric acid (rare)	Colorless	Rhombic plates; four-sided prisms	No significance
ALKALINE, NEUTRAL, OR SLIGHTLY ACIDIC URINE			
Triple phosphate	Colorless	"Coffin lids," 3 to 4 to 6-sided prism; occasional fern-leaf like	Urine stasis and chronic infection
ALKALINE URINE			
Calcium carbonate	Colorless	Needles, spheres, dumbbells	Normal
Ammonium biurate	Yellow, opaque, brown	"Thorn apple" spheres, dumbbells, sheaves of needles	Normal
Calcium phosphate	Colorless	Prisms, plates, needles	Normal; large amounts in chronic cystitis or prostatic hypertrophy
Amorphous phosphates	White	Granules	Normal

Patient Preparation and Patient Aftercare
Same as for white blood cells and white blood cell casts.

● URINE DRUG INVESTIGATION SPECIMENS

When screening for unknown drugs, the most valuable samples are obtained from (1) urine, (2) gastric contents, and (3) blood. Urine drug screening is preferred for several reasons:

1. Specimens are easily procured.
2. It is not an invasive procedure (unless bladder catheterization is involved).
3. Drug concentrations are more elevated in urine or may not be detectable in blood (Table 3-2).
4. Drug metabolites are excreted for a longer time period through urine (shows time of days or weeks past).
5. Test procedures are more easily done and are more economical.

NOTE: *Blood is the preferred medium for ethyl alcohol testing because the alcohol concentration is more elevated and, therefore, more reliable in a blood sample (see Chap. 6).*

Indications for Toxicology Screening
1. To confirm clinical or after-death diagnosis
2. To differentiate drug-induced disease from other causes, such as trauma, metabolic, or infectious disease processes
3. To identify contributing diagnosis such as ethanol abuse, trauma, presence of other drugs, or underlying psychoses

TABLE 3-2
Common Urine Drug Tests*†

Amphetamines	Phencyclidine (PCP)
Alcohol	Lysergic acid diethylamide (LSD)
Barbiturates	Analgesics
Benzodiazepines	Sedatives
Cocaine, "Crack"	Major tranquilizers†
Cyanide	Stimulants
Opiates	Sympathomimetics
Marijuana (THC)	

*Many of these drugs are detectable in urine but are not detectable in blood serum. However, all drugs detectable in blood serum are also detectable in urine, except for glutethimide.
†Because minor tranquilizers are almost completely metabolized, they are not likely to be detected in urine unless an overdose is taken.

4. Test results are used as basis for high-risk interventions, such as hemodialysis
5. To test for drug abuse in the workplace, especially when public safety is at risk or concern
6. As part of preemployment screening for drug use or abuse
7. To randomly test prisoners and parolees to deter or detect drug use

Clinical Alert

When reporting drug test results for substance abuse, healthcare workers and patients must be aware of the psychological, social, economic, and legal implications and the potential liabilities associated with the reporting or mismanagement of incorrectly reported results. Documented procedures should be established and followed to ensure that, before a result is reported, corroborating evidence exists to support that result. Confirmation of all positive results must be done through an equally sensitive and specific methodology that uses a different chemical principle to "cross-check" initial results. Keep in mind that problems associated with incorrect test results are directly proportional to the volume of drug abuse testing being done.

Urine screening is not a "cure-all" for preventing substance abuse in the workplace. When properly implemented, however, it can support a well-thoughtout substance abuse rehabilitation program. Screening can detect a problem that the employee may not admit to having. However, sure knowledge that an employee abuses drugs allows an employer to move with confidence toward handling the problem.

WITNESSED URINE SAMPLING FOR SUSPECTED SUBSTANCE ABUSE

Procedure

1. A trained individual must witness the actual procurement or delivery of a 50-ml random urine sample. After collection, tag the sample with a numerical code. (Check institutional protocols.)
2. Normally, obtain a signed consent form from the testee (patient).
3. Place the sample in a plastic, sealed sack, and mark it with a notary-style seal or with tamper-proof tape to protect against tampering.
4. Originate a "chain of custody" document at the time of the sample collection. The person who provides the urine specimen must sign the document, as does every other person who handles the sample.
5. After both initial and confirmatory testing, mark the sample, reseal it, marked, securely store it for a minimum of 30 days.
6. One must carefully maintain records of all tests done, together with the chain of custody report.

7. Confirm all positive test results by a second, different test method, because a false-negative result can misrepresent the danger a drug abuser poses to those around them; a false-positive result can seriously violate the civil and occupational rights of the testee, for which the testing laboratory can be held accountable.
8. Release the results of the test data only to predesignated, authorized persons because this lessens the risk of false or speculative information being spread about an individual.

Clinical Implications

Certain drugs can be detected in the urine for hours to several days after ingestion. A partial list includes

1. Amphetamines (4 hr)
2. Barbiturates (24 hr to 7 days)
3. Benzodiazapines (3 days)
4. Cannabenoids (21 hr to 3 days)
5. Cocaine as metabolites (2–3 days)
6. Codeine (4 hr)
7. Methadone (3 days)
8. Methaqualone (7 days)
9. Morphine (4 hr)
10. Phencyclidine (7 days)
11. Propoxyphene (6 hr)

Interfering Factors

Factors associated with incorrect test results for urine drug screens include the presence of the following:

1. Detergents
2. Sodium chloride (table salt)
3. Low specific gravity (dilute urine)
4. High pH (acidic urine)
5. Low pH (basic or alkaline urine)
6. Blood in the urine

Patient Preparation

1. Explain test purpose and procedure for specimen collection.
2. Follow Chapter 1 guidelines for safe, effective, informed *pretest* care.

Patient Aftercare

1. Interpret test outcomes and monitor appropriately.
2. See Chapter 1 guidelines for safe, effective, informed *posttest* care.

● OTHER URINARY CONSTITUENT TESTS

URINE CHLORIDES (CL); QUANTITATIVE (24-HR) ●

Normal Values

Adult: 140–250 mEq/L
Child: > 6 yr, 15–40 mEq/L; 10–14 yr, 64–176 mEq/L
(Children's values are much lower than adult values.)
Vary greatly with salt intake and perspiration.

It is rather difficult to talk about "normal" and "abnormal" ranges because test findings have meaning only in relation to salt intake and output.

Background

The amount of chloride excreted in the urine in 24 hours is an indication of the state of electrolyte balance. Chloride is most often associated with sodium balance and fluid change.

Explanation of Test

The measurement of urine chloride may be a useful means of diagnosing dehydration, or as a guide in adjusting fluid and electrolyte balance in postoperative patients. It also serves as a means of monitoring the effects of reduced salt diets, which are of great therapeutic importance in patients with cardiovascular disease, hypertension, liver disease, and kidney ailments.

Urine chloride is often ordered, along with sodium and potassium, as a 24-hour urine test. The urinary ion gap (Na + KCl) is useful for initial evaluation of metabolic alkalosis.

Procedure

1. Collect a 24-hour urine specimen.
2. Record the exact start and end times on the specimen container and the healthcare record.
3. The complete specimen should be sent to the laboratory for refrigeration until it can be analyzed.

> **Clinical Alert**
>
> Because electrolyte and water balance are so closely related, evaluate the patient's state of hydration by checking daily weight, recording accurate intake and output, and by observing and recording skin turgor, the appearance of the tongue, and the appearance of the urine sample.

Clinical Implications

1. Decreased urinary chlorides occur in
   - **a.** Chloride-depleted patients (< 10 mEq/L); these patients have low serum chloride levels and are chloride-responsive; they respond to chloride therapy so that serum and urine levels return to normal.
     - **(1)** SIADH (syndrome of inappropriate santidiuretic hormone [ADH])
     - **(2)** Vomiting, diarrhea
     - **(3)** Gastric suction
     - **(4)** Addison's disease
     - **(5)** Metabolic alkalosis
     - **(6)** Diuretic therapy
     - **(7)** Villous tumors of colon
   - **b.** Chloride is decreased by endogenous or exogenous corticosteroids

(> 20 mEq/L). This type of decreased urinary chloride is not responsive to the administration of chloride. Diagnosis of a chloride-resistant metabolic alkalosis helps identify a corticotropin (ACTH) or aldosterone-producing neoplasm.

(1) Cushing's syndrome
(2) Conn's syndrome
(3) Mineralocorticoid therapy
(4) Bartter's syndrome

2. Increased urinary chloride occurs in
   a. Dehydration
   b. Renal tubular acidosis
   c. Potassium depletion

Interfering Factors

1. Decreased chloride is associated with carbinicillin therapy, reduced dietary intake of chloride, ingestion of large amounts of licorice, and alkali ingestion.
2. Increased chloride is associated with ammonium chloride administration; excessive infusion of normal saline; sulfides, cyanides, halogens, bromides, and sulfhydryl compounds.

Patient Preparation

1. Instruct the patient about the test purpose and method for collecting a 24-hour specimen.
2. See Chapter 1 guidelines for safe, effective, informed *pretest* care.

Patient Aftercare

1. Interpret test outcomes and monitor appropriately for fluid imbalances.
2. See Chapter 1 guidelines for safe, effective, informed *posttest* care.

URINE SODIUM (Na); QUANTITATIVE (24-HR)

Normal Values

> 40–220 mEq/L per 24 hr or 40–220 mmol/day, diet-dependent
Child: 41–115 mEq/L

Background

Sodium is a primary regulator for retaining or excreting water and maintaining acid–base balance. The body has a strong tendency to maintain a total base content; on a relative scale, only small shifts are found, even under pathologic conditions. As the preponderant base substance in the blood, sodium helps regulate acid–base balance because of its ability to combine with chloride and bicarbonate. Sodium also promotes the normal balance of electrolytes in the intracellular and extracellular fluids by acting in conjunction with potassium (sodium–potassium pump). Sodium and potassium also influence nerve conduction and muscle irritability.

Explanation of Test

This test measures one aspect of electrolyte balance by determining the amount of sodium excreted in a 24-hour period. It is done for diagnosis of renal, adrenal, water, and acid–base imbalances.

Procedure

1. Properly label a 24-hour urine container.
2. The urine container must be refrigerated or kept on ice.
3. Follow general instructions for 24-hour urine collections.
4. Record exact start and ending times on the specimen container and in the healthcare record.
5. Transfer the specimen to the laboratory for proper storage when the test is completed.

Clinical Implications

1. *Increased urinary sodium levels* occur in
   - **a.** Adrenal failure (Addison's disease)
   - **b.** Salt-losing nephrites
   - **c.** Renal tubular acidosis
   - **d.** SIADH (syndrome of inappropriate antidiuretic hormone)
   - **e.** Diuretic therapy
   - **f.** Diabetes mellitus
   - **g.** Hypothyroidism
   - **h.** Vomiting
2. *Decreased urinary sodium levels* occur in
   - **a.** Dehydration
   - **b.** Congestive heart failure
   - **c.** Liver disease
   - **d.** Nephrotic syndromes
   - **e.** Prerenal azotemia
   - **f.** Stress syndrome diuresis
   - **g.** Acute oliguria

Interfering Factors

1. *Increased* sodium levels are associated with caffeine intake, diuretic therapy, dopamine, postmenstrual diuresis, and increased sodium intake.
2. *Decreased* sodium levels are associated with intake of corticosteroids, epinephrine, propranolol, low sodium intake, premenstrual sodium and water retention, and stress diuresis.

Patient Preparation

1. Instruct the patient about the purpose of the test, method of collection, and specimen refrigeration or icing. Written instructions can be helpful.
2. Encourage intake of food and fluids.
3. Follow Chapter 1 guidelines for safe, effective, informed *pretest* care.

Clinical Alert

Because electrolyte and water balance are so closely related, determine the patient's state of hydration by checking and recording daily weights, accurate intake and output, and observations about skin turgor and the appearance of the tongue and the urine.

Patient Aftercare

1. Interpret test outcomes and monitor as necessary for fluid and electrolyte state.
2. Follow Chapter 1 guidelines for safe, effective, informed *posttest* care.

URINE POTASSIUM (K); QUANTITATIVE (24-HR) ●

Normal Values

25–125 mEq/24 hr or 25–125 mmol/24 hr
Varies with diet
Child: 22–57 mmol/24 hr

Background

Potassium acts as a part of the body's buffer system and serves a vital function in the body's overall electrolyte balance. Because the kidneys cannot conserve potassium, this balance is regulated by the excretion of potassium through the urine.

Explanation of Test

This test provides insight into electrolyte balance by measuring the amount of potassium excreted in 24 hours. This measurement is useful in the study of renal and adrenal disorders and water and acid–base imbalances. An evaluation of urinary potassium can be helpful in determining the origin of abnormal potassium levels.

Procedure

1. Label a 24-hour urine container properly.
2. Refrigerate the urine container or keep it on ice during the collection.
3. Follow general instructions for 24-hour urine collection.
4. Record exact start and ending times on the container and in the health-care record.
5. Transfer the specimen to the laboratory for proper storage.

Clinical Implications

1. *Elevated levels* of urine potassium occur in

   a. Primary renal diseases
   b. Diabetic and renal tubule disease
   c. Albright-type renal disease
   d. Starvation (onset)
   e. Primary and secondary aldosteronism
   f. Cushing's disease
   g. During treatment with ACTH, hydrocortisone
   h. Fanconi's syndrome
   i. Bartter's syndrome
2. *Decreased levels* of urine potassium occur in
   a. Addison's disease
   b. Severe renal disease (eg, pyelonephritis, glomerulonephritis)
3. In patients with potassium deficiency, regardless of the cause, the urine pH tends to fall (becomes more acidic). This occurs because hydrogen ions are released in exchange for sodium ions, given that both potassium and hydrogen are excreted by the same mechanism.

> **Clinical Alert**
>
> In the presence of excessive vomiting or gastric suctioning, the resulting alkalosis maintains urinary potassium excretion at levels inappropriately high for the degree of actual potassium depletion that occurs.

Interfering Factors

1. *Increased urinary potassium levels* are associated with the ingestion of
   a. Acetazolamide and other diuretics
   b. Cortisone
   c. Sulfates
   d. EDTA anticoagulant
   e. Penicillin, carbenicillin
   f. Thiazides
   g. Licorice
   h. Sulfates
   i. Insulin
2. *Decreased urinary potassium levels* are associated with the ingestion of
   a. Amiloride
   b. Diazide
   c. Epinephrine
   d. Glucose
   e. Prolactin

Patient Preparation

1. Instruct the patient about the purpose of the test, collection procedure, and need for refrigeration or icing of 24-hour urine specimen. Written instructions can be helpful.
2. Food and fluids are permitted and encouraged.
3. Follow Chapter 1 guidelines regarding safe, effective, informed *pretest* care.

Clinical Alert

1. Because electrolyte and water balance are so closely related, determine the patient's state of hydration by checking and recording daily weights, accurate intake and output, and observations about skin turgor and the appearance of the tongue and urine.
2. Observe for signs of muscle weakness, tremors, changes in electrocardiographic tracings, and dysrhythmias. The degree of hypokalemia or hyperkalemia at which these symptoms occur varies with each person.

Patient Aftercare

1. Interpret test outcomes and monitor appropriately for signs and symptoms of electrolyte imbalances and kidney disorders.
2. See Chapter 1 guidelines regarding safe, effective, informed *posttest* care.

URINE URIC ACID; QUANTITATIVE (24-HR)

Normal Values

250–750 mg/24 hr or 1.48–4.43 mmol/day with normal diet
120 mg/24 hr or 2.48 mmol/day with purine-free diet
1000 mg/24 hr or 5.90 mmol/day with high-purine diet

Background

Uric acid is formed from the metabolic breakdown of nucleic acids. Purines are the principal source of this breakdown.

Explanation of Test

This test evaluates uric acid metabolism in gout and renal calculus formation. Evaluation of excess uric acid excretion is an important aid in diagnosing genetic defects, in minimizing stone formation, and in evaluating nephrolithiasis. It also reflects the effects of treatment with uricosuric agents by measuring the total amount of uric acid excreted within a 24-hour period.

Procedure

1. Properly label a 24-hour urine container to which the appropriate preservative has been added.
2. Follow general instructions for 24-hour urine collection.
3. Record exact start and end times on the specimen container and in the healthcare record.
4. When completed, send the specimen to the laboratory.

Clinical Implications

1. *Increased urine uric acid* levels (uricosuria) occur in

- **a.** Gout
- **b.** Chronic myelogenous leukemia
- **c.** Polycythemia vera
- **d.** Lesch–Nyhan syndrome
- **e.** Wilson's disease
- **f.** Viral hepatitis
- **g.** Sickle cell anemia
- **h.** May occur in pregnancy with salt-loading
- **i.** Cytotoxic drugs to treat lymphoma and leukemia
- **j.** High uric acid concentration plus low urine pH may produce uric acid stones in the urinary tract. (These patients do not have gout.)

2. *Decreased urine uric acid levels* are found in
- **a.** Chronic kidney disease
- **b.** Xanthinuria
- **c.** Folic acid deficiency
- **d.** Lead toxicity

Interfering Factors

1. Many drugs affect uric acid levels including
- **a.** Salicylates (aspirin) and other anti-inflammatory drugs
- **b.** Thiazide diuretics decrease uric acid excretion
- **c.** Vitamin C
- **d.** Warfarin

2. Other factors increasing uric acid urine levels include
- **a.** Presence of x-ray contrast medium
- **b.** Strenuous exercise
- **c.** Diet high in purines (kidney, sweetbreads) (See Chap. 6, Blood Chemistry).

Patient Preparation

1. Instruct the patient about the test purpose, interfering factors, collection process, and refrigeration or icing of 24-hour urine specimen. A written reminder may be helpful.
2. Encourage food and fluids. In some situations, a diet high or low in purines may be ordered during and before the test period.
3. Follow Chapter 1 guidelines for safe, effective, informed *pretest* care.

Patient Aftercare

1. Resume usual diet.
2. Interpret test outcomes and counsel appropriately concerning prescribed treatment and possible need for further testing.
3. See Chapter 1 guidelines for safe, effective, informed *posttest* care.

URINE CALCIUM; QUANTITATIVE (24-HR) SULKOWITCH ●

Normal Values

100–300 mg or 2.50–7.50 mmol/day normal diet
50–150 mg or 1.25–3.75 mmol/day low-calcium diet

Background

The bulk of calcium discharged is excreted in the stool. However, a small quantity of calcium is normally excreted in the urine. This amount varies with the quantity of dietary calcium ingested.

Explanation of Test

This 24-hour test is most often ordered to determine parathyroid gland function, which maintains the balance between calcium and phosphorus by means of parathyroid hormone produced by the parathyroid glands. Hyperparathyroidism is a generalized disorder of calcium, phosphate, and bone metabolism that results from increased secretion of parathyroid hormones and increased excretion of urinary calcium. On the other hand, in hypoparathyroidism, the urinary calcium excretion decreases.

Procedure

1. Properly label a 24-hour urine container.
2. Procure an acid-washed bottle. See Table 3-1 on page 152 for 24-hour urine collection data.
3. Follow general instructions for 24-hour urine collection. Refrigerate during collection.
4. Record exact start and ending times of the collection on the specimen container and the healthcare record.
5. Send the specimen to the laboratory when collection is completed.

Clinical Implications

1. *Increased urine calcium levels* are found in
   - **a.** Hyperparathyroidism (results in constant 3+ to 4+ Sulkowitch tests)
   - **b.** Sarcoidosis
   - **c.** Primary cancers of breast and bladder
   - **d.** Osteolytic bone metastases
   - **e.** Multiple myeloma
   - **f.** Paget's disease
   - **g.** Renal tubular acidosis
   - **h.** Glucocorticoid excess
   - **i.** Fanconi's syndrome
   - **j.** Vitamin D intoxication
   - **k.** Idiopathic hypercalciuria
   - **l.** Diabetes mellitus
   - **m.** Crohn's disease and some cases of ulcerative colitis
   - **n.** Thyrotoxicosis
2. Increased urinary calcium levels almost always accompany elevated blood calcium levels.
3. Calcium excretion levels greater than calcium intake levels are always excessive; urine excretion values above 400 to 500 mg/24 hours are reliably abnormal.
4. Increased calcium excretion occurs whenever calcium is mobilized from the bone, as in metastatic cancer or prolonged skeletal immobilization.
5. When calcium is excreted in increasing amounts, the situation creates the potential for nephrolithiasis or nephrocalcinosis.
6. *Decreased urine calcium levels* are found in

- **a.** Hypoparathyroidism (hypocalcemia caused by hypoparathyroidism is usually associated with negative reaction)
- **b.** Familial hypocalciuria, hypercalcemia
- **c.** Vitamin D deficiency (rickets)
- **d.** Preeclampsia
- **e.** Acute nephrosis, nephritis
- **f.** Renal osteodystrophy
- **g.** Malignant bone neoplasm
- **h.** Metastatic carcinoma of prostate
- **i.** Malabsorption syndrome—celiac–sprue disease

Interfering Factors

1. *Falsely elevated levels* may be due to
   - **a.** Excess milk intake
   - **b.** Some drugs (eg, growth hormone, PTH, vitamin D)
   - **c.** Urine procured immediately after meals in which high calcium intake has occurred
   - **d.** Corticosteroids
   - **e.** Increased exposure to sunlight
   - **f.** Immobilization (especially in children)
2. *Falsely decreased levels* may be found with
   - **a.** Increased phosphate, bicarbonate, antacid ingestion
   - **b.** Alkaline urine
   - **c.** Thiazide diuretics (can be used to therapeutically lower calcium levels)

Patient Preparation

1. Instruct the patient about the test purpose and procedure. Written instructions may be helpful.
2. Encourage food and fluids.
3. If the urine calcium test is done because of a metabolic disorder, the patient should eat a low-calcium diet and be receiving calcium medication restrictions for 1 to 3 days before specimen collection.
4. If the patient has a history of renal stone formation, urinary calcium results will be more meaningful if the patient is receiving his or her usual diet for 3 days before the test. Do **not** stop medications.
5. See Chapter 1 guidelines for safe, effective, informed *pretest* care.

Clinical Alert

1. Observe patients with very low urine calcium levels for signs and symptoms of tetany (muscle spasms, twitching, hyperirritable nervous system).
2. The first sign of calcium imbalance presents as a pathologic fracture that can be related to calcium excess.
3. The Sulkowitch test can be used in an emergency, especially when hypercalcemia is suspected because hypercalcemia is life-threatening. A fasting, first morning specimen is examined for turbidity. Normal levels: 8 to 12 mg/dl.

Patient Aftercare

1. Interpret test outcomes, monitor, and counsel accordingly.
2. Follow Chapter 1 guidelines regarding safe, effective, informed *posttest* care.

URINE MAGNESIUM; QUANTITATIVE (24-HR) ●

Normal Values

6.0–10.0 mEq/24 hr or 3.00–5.00 mmol/24 hr

Background

Magnesium excretion controls serum magnesium balance. Urinary magnesium excretion is diet dependent.

Explanation of Test

This test evaluates magnesium metabolism, investigates electrolyte status, and is a component of a workup for nephrolithiasis.

Procedure

1. Collect a 24-hour urine specimen in a metal-free and acid-rinsed container.
2. Record exact start and end times.
3. See page 152 for 24-hour urine collection guidelines.

Clinical Implications

1. *Increased urinary magnesium excretion* is associated with
   a. Increased blood alcohol
   b. Bartter's syndrome
2. *Decreased urinary magnesium* excretion is associated with
   a. Malabsorption
   b. Long-term chronic alcoholism
   c. Long-term parenteral therapy
   d. Magnesium deficiency
   e. Chronic renal disease

Interfering Factors

1. Increased magnesium levels are associated with:
   a. Corticosteroids
   b. Cisplatin therapy
   c. Thiazide diuretics
   d. Aldosterone
   e. Blood in urine
2. Decreased magnesium levels are found in hypercalciuria.

Patient Preparation

1. Explain purpose of test and collection procedures.
2. Instruct that the specimen will be unacceptable if it comes in contact with any type of metal.
3. See Chapter 1 guidelines concerning safe, effective, informed *pretest* care.

Patient Aftercare

1. Interpret test outcomes and monitor appropriately.
2. Follow Chapter 1 guidelines concerning safe, effective, informed *posttest* care.

URINE OXALATE; QUANTITATIVE (24-HR)

Normal Values

Male: 7–44 mg/24 hr or 228–684 μmol/24 hr
Female: 4–31 mg/24 hr or 228–627 μmol/24 hr
Child: 13–38 mg/24 hr

Background

Normal oxalate is derived from dietary oxalic acid (10%) and the metabolism of ascorbic acid (35%–50%) and glycine (40%). Patients who form calcium oxalate kidney stones appear to absorb and excrete a higher proportion of dietary oxalate in the urine.

Explanation of Test

Twenty-four hour urine collections for oxalate are indicated in patients with surgical loss of the distal small intestine, especially those with Crohn's disease. The incidence of nephrolithiasis in patients who have inflammatory bowel disease is 2.6% to 10%. Hyperoxaluria is regularly present after jejunoileal bypass for morbid obesity; such patients may develop nephrolithiasis.

Oxaluria is also a characteristic of ethylene glycol intoxication. Additionally, vitamin C increases oxalate excretion and may be a risk factor for calcium oxalate nephrolithiasis. Such ingestion can usually be determined through the patient's history. If oxalate excretion becomes normal after reducing vitamin C intake, additional therapy to prevent stones may not be required.

Procedure

1. Collect and refrigerate or ice a 24-hour urine specimen according to protocols. Do not acidify.
2. See page 152 for directions for 24-hr collection.

Clinical Implications

1. *Increased urine oxalate values* are associated with
   - **a.** Ethylene glycol poisoning (> 150 mg/day or > 1710 μmol/day)
   - **b.** Primary hyperoxaluria (a rare genetic disorder) (100–600 mg/day or 1140–6840 μmol/day [nephrocalcinosis])
   - **c.** Diabetes mellitus and other pancreatic disorders
   - **d.** Cirrhosis
   - **e.** Vitamin B_6 deficiency

   f. Sarcoidosis
   g. Roan's disease
   h. Biliary diversion
   i. Small-intestine stasis
   j. Gout
   k. Celiac disease (sprue)
   l. Jejunoileal bypass for treatment of morbid obesity
2. *Decreased urine oxalate values* occur in
   a. Renal failure
   b. Hypercalciuria

Interfering Factors

1. Foods such as rhubarb, strawberries, beans, beets, spinach, tomatoes, gelatin, chocolate, cocoa, and tea contain oxalates.
2. Ethylene glycol
3. Vitamin C (ascorbic acid)
4. Calcium
5. Methoxyflurane anesthesia

Patient Preparation

1. Explain test purpose and procedure.
2. Advise the patient to avoid foods that promote oxalate excretion before the test. A list of such foods is helpful.
3. Vitamin C should not be taken within 24 hours of beginning the test nor during the test.
4. Follow Chapter 1 guidelines for safe, effective, informed *pretest care.*

Patient Aftercare

1. Resume normal diet and exercise.
2. Interpret test outcomes and counsel appropriately.
3. See Chapter 1 guidelines for safe, effective, informed *posttest* care.

URINE FOLLICLE-STIMULATING HORMONE (FSH); LUTEINIZING HORMONE (LH) (24-HR) ●

Normal Values

FOLLICLE-STIMULATING HORMONE (FSH)

Men: 1–20 IU/24 hr
Women: 5–20 IU/24 hr
Postmenopausal: 30–440 IU/24 hr
Midcycle peak: 15–30 IU/24 hr

LUTEINIZING HORMONE (LH)

Men: 5–20 IU/24 hr
Women: 5–15 IU/24 hr follicular phase
Postmenopausal: 50–100 IU/24 hr
Midcycle peak: 30–95 IU/24 hr

See your laboratory references for values in infants and children.

Background

FSH and LH are glycoprotein pituitary hormones produced and stored in the anterior pituitary. They are under complex regulation by hypothalamic gonadotropin-releasing hormone and by gonadal sex hormones (estrogen and progesterone in females and testosterone in males); FSH acts on granulosa cells of the ovary and the Sertoli cells of testis; LH acts on Leydig (interstitial) cells of the gonads. Normally, FSH increases occur at earlier stages of puberty, 2 to 4 years before LH reaches comparable levels. In males, FSH and LH are necessary for spermatozoa development and maturation. In females, follicular formation in the early stages of the menstrual cycle is stimulated by FSH. Then, the midcycle surge of LH causes ovulation of the FSH-ripened ovarian follicles to occur.

Explanation of Test

This 24-hour urine test measures the gonadotropic hormones FSH and LH and may help determine whether a gonadal deficiency is of primary origin or is due to insufficient stimulation by the pituitary hormones.

Evaluation of FSH supports other studies related to determining causes of hypothyroidism in women and endocrine dysfunction in men. In primary ovarian failure or testicular failure, FSH levels are increased. Measuring urine FSH and LH are of value for children with endocrine problems related to precocious puberty. Urine essays also are used to monitor ovulatory cycles of *in vitro* fertilization patients.

Procedure

1. Label a 24-hour urine collection container properly. The 24-hour urine collection minimizes problems with episodic secretion spikes that occur with blood serum specimens.
2. Collect urine into the correct container; it may contain a preservative or may need to be refrigerated. Check with your laboratory concerning protocols.
3. The completed 24-hour urine specimen is sent to the laboratory.

Clinical Alert

A blood sample of at leat 3 ml also may be ordered at this time. Sometimes multiple blood specimens are necessary because of episodic releases of FSH from the pituitary gland. An isolated sample may not indicate what the actual activity is.

In the case of anovulatory fertility problems, the presence or absence of a midcycle peak can be established through a series of daily blood specimens.

Clinical Implications

1. *Decreased urinary FSH levels* occur in
   - **a.** Feminizing and masculinizing ovarian tumors when FSH production is inhibited because of increased estrogen secretion
   - **b.** Failure of pituitary or hypothalamus to function properly
   - **c.** Anorexia nervosa
   - **d.** Neoplasm of testes or adrenal glands that influences secretion of estrogens or androgens
   - **e.** Polycystic ovarian disease
   - **f.** Hemochromatosis
   - **g.** Pregnancy
2. *Increased urinary FSH levels* occur in
   - **a.** Turner's syndrome (ovarian dysgenesis). Approximately 50% of patients with primary amenorrhea have Turner's syndrome.
   - **b.** Hypopituitarism
   - **c.** Sheehan's syndrome
   - **d.** Precocious puberty, either idiopathic or secondary to a central nervous system lesion
   - **e.** Klinefelter's syndrome
   - **f.** Castration
   - **g.** Alcoholism
   - **i.** Menopause and menstrual disorders
3. *Both FSH and LH are increased* in
   - **a.** Hypogonadism
   - **b.** Complete testicular feminization syndrome
   - **c.** Gonadal failure
   - **d.** Congenital absence of testicle(s)
   - **e.** Menopause
4. *Decreased FSH and LH* occur in pituitary or hypothalamic failure.

Interfering Factors

1. Recently administered radioisotopes
2. Hemolysis of blood sample
3. Estrogens or oral contraceptives
4. Corticosteroids
5. Various drugs
6. Hematuria

Patient Preparation

1. Instruct the patient about the purpose and procedure of 24-hour urine specimen collection. A written reminder may be helpful.
2. For females, record date of last menstrual period.
3. See Chapter 1 guidelines for safe, effective, informed *pretest* care.

Patient Aftercare

1. Interpret test outcomes and counsel appropriately.
2. See Chapter 1 guidelines for safe, effective, informed *posttest* care.

URINE PREGNANEDIOL (24-HR)

Normal Values

This test is difficult to standardize; it varies with age, sex, and length of existing pregnancy.

Men: 0–1 mg/24 hr
Women: Pregnancy: 1st trimester, 10–30 mg/24 hr
2nd trimester, 35–70 mg/24 hr
3rd trimester, 70–100 mg/24 hr
Postmenopausal: 0.2–1 mg/24 hr
Follicular: 0.5–1.5 mg/24 hr

Explanation of Test

This test measures ovarian and placental function. Specifically, it measures the hormone progesterone and its principal excreted metabolite, pregnanediol. Progesterone exerts its main effect on the endometrium by causing the endometrium to enter the secretory phase and to become ready for implantation of the blastocyte, should fertilization take place.

Pregnanediol excretion is elevated in pregnancy and decreased in luteal deficiency or placental failure.

Procedure

1. Label a 24-hour urine container properly.
2. Refrigeration of the specimen or a boric acid preservative may be required. Check laboratory policy.
3. Follow general instructions for 24-hour urine collection.
4. Record exact start and end times on the specimen container and the healthcare record.
5. Send the completed specimen to the laboratory.

Clinical Implications

1. *Increased levels* are associated with
   - **a.** Luteal cysts of ovary (ovarian cyst)
   - **b.** Arrhenoblastoma of the ovary
   - **c.** Congenital hyperplasia of adrenal gland
   - **d.** Malignant neoplasm of trophoblasts
2. *Decreased levels* are associated with
   - **a.** Amenorrhea (ovarian hypofunction)
   - **b.** Threatened abortion (of < 15 mg/24 hr), abortion is imminent
   - **c.** Fetal death, intrauterine death
   - **d.** Toxemia, eclampsia
   - **e.** Benign neoplasm of ovary
   - **f.** Granulosa cell tumor of ovary
   - **g.** Lutein cell tumor of ovary
   - **h.** Theca cell tumor of ovary
   - **i.** Hydatidiform mole

Interfering Factors

Decreased values occur during estrogen or progesterone therapy and with the use of oral contraceptives.

Patient Preparation

1. Instruct the patient about the test purpose and 24-hour urine specimen collection process. A written reminder may be helpful.
2. Allow food and fluids.
3. See Chapter 1 guidelines for safe, effective, informed *pretest* care.

Patient Aftercare

1. Interpret test outcomes and counsel appropriately.
2. Follow Chapter 1 guidelines for safe, effective, informed *posttest* care.

URINE PREGNANETRIOL (24-HR) ●

Normal Values

Male: 0.4–2.5 mg/24 hr
Female: Follicular phase, 0.1–1.8 mg/24 hr
Luteal phase, 0.9–2.2 mg/24 hr
Children: 0.3–1.1 mg/24 hr
Infants: < 0.02 mg/24 hr

Background

Pregnanetriol is a compound substance reflecting one segment of adrenocortical activity. Pregnanetriol should not be confused with pregnanediol, despite the similarity of name. Pregnanetriol is a precursor in adrenocorticoid synthesis and arises from 17-hydroxyprogesterone, not from progesterone.

Explanation of Test

This 24-hour urine test is done to diagnose adrenocortical dysfunction, adrenogenital syndrome, or a defect in 21-hydroxylation. The diagnosis of adrenogenital syndrome is indicated in

1. Adult women who show signs and symptoms of excessive androgen production, with or without hypertension
2. Craving for salt
3. Sexual precocity in boys
4. Infants who exhibit signs of failure to thrive
5. Presence of external genitalia in females (pseudohermaphroditism). In males, differentiation must be made between a virilizing tumor of the adrenal gland, neurogenic and constitutional types of sexual precocity, and interstitial cell tumor of the testes.

Procedure

1. Label a 24-hour urine container properly.
2. Refrigerate the specimen if necessary; some laboratories may require a boric acid preservative in the collection receptacle.
3. Follow general instructions for 24-hour urine collection.
4. Record exact start and end times on the specimen container and in the healthcare record.
5. Send the completed specimen to the laboratory.

Clinical Implications

1. *Elevated urinary pregnanetriol levels* occur in
   a. Congenital adrenocortical hyperplasia
   b. Stein–Leventhal syndrome
   c. Ovarian and adrenal tumors
2. *Decreased urinary pregnanetriol levels* occur in
   a. Hydroxylase deficiency
   b. Ovarian failure

Patient Preparation

1. Instruct the patient about the test purpose and procedure for collection of a 24-hour urine specimen. A written reminder may be helpful.
2. Allow food and fluids.
3. Avoid muscular exercise before and during test.
4. See Chapter 1 guidelines for safe, effective, informed *pretest* care.

Patient Aftercare

1. Interpret test outcomes and counsel appropriately.
2. Follow Chapter 1 guidelines for safe, effective, informed *posttest* care.

URINE 5-HYDROXYINDOLEACETIC ACID (5-HIAA) (5-HYDROXY-3, SEROTONIN, INDOLEACETIC ACID) (24-HR) ●

Normal Values

Qualitative: negative
Quantitative: 2–6 mg/24 hr, or 10.4–31.2 μmol/24 hr

Background

Serotonin is a vasoconstricting hormone normally produced by the argentaffin cells of the GI tract. The principal function of the cells is to regulate smooth-muscle contraction and peristalsis. 5-HIAA is the major urinary metabolite of serotonin.

Explanation of Test

This urine test is conducted to diagnose the presence of a functioning carcinoid tumor that can be shown by significant elevations of 5-HIAA, a product of serotonin. Excess amounts of 5-HIAA are produced by most carcinoid tumors. Carcinoid tumors produce symptoms of flushing, hepatomegaly, diarrhea, bronchospasm, and heart disease.

Procedure

1. Caution patient not to eat any bananas, pineapple, tomatoes, eggplants, plums, or avocados for 48 hours before and also during the 24-hour test because these foods contain serotonin.
2. Properly label a 24-hour urine container that contains the preservative.
3. Follow general instructions for 24-hour urine collection.

4. Record exact start and end times of the collection on the specimen container and in the healthcare record.
5. Send the completed specimen to the laboratory.

Clinical Implications

1. Levels over 100 mg/24 hr indicate large carcinoid tumors, especially when metastatic.
   - **a.** Ilial tumors
   - **b.** Pancreatic tumors
   - **c.** Duodenal tumors
   - **d.** Biliary tumors
2. *Increased 5-HIAA levels* are found in
   - **a.** Cystic fibrosis
   - **b.** Ovarian carcinoid tumor
   - **c.** Tropical sprue
   - **d.** Severe pain of sciatica or skeletal and smooth-muscle spasm
   - **e.** Bronchial adenoma, carcinoid type
   - **f.** Malabsorption
   - **g.** Celiac disease
   - **h.** Whipple's disease
   - **i.** Stasis syndrome
   - **j.** Chronic intestinal obstruction
   - **k.** Oat cell cancer of respiratory system
3. *Decreased 5-HIAA levels* are found in
   - **a.** Depressive illness
   - **b.** Small-intestinal resection
   - **c.** Phenylketonuria (PKU)
   - **d.** Hartnup's disease
   - **e.** Mastocytosis

Interfering Factors

1. *False-positive* results occur with
   - **a.** Ingestion of banana, pineapple, plum, walnut, eggplant, tomato, chocolate, and avocado, which may increase the 5-HIAA levels, because of their serotonin content.
   - **b.** Some drugs
2. *False-negative* results can be caused by specific drugs that depress 5-HIAA production.

Patient Preparation

1. Instruct the patient about test purpose and procedures for collection of the 24-hour urine specimen. Written instructions may be helpful.
2. Encourage intake of food and water. Foods high in serotonin content must not be eaten for 48 hours before or during the test.
3. If possible, no drugs should be taken for 72 hours before the test nor during the test.
4. See Chapter 1 guidelines for safe, effective, informed *pretest* care.

Patient Aftercare

1. Resume normal diet and medications when test is completed.
2. Follow Chapter 1 guidelines for safe, effective, informed *posttest* care.

> **Clinical Alert**
>
> A serum serotonin assay may detect some carcinoids missed by the 5-HIAA urine assay.

URINE VANILLYLMANDELIC ACID (VMA) (CATECHOLAMINES, 3-METHOXY-4-HYDROXYMANDELIC ACID) (24-HR) ●

Normal Values—Adults

Vanillylmandelic acid: up to 2–7 mg/24 hr
Catecholamines: Total 14–110 μg/2 hr, 270 μg/24 hr
Epinephrine: 0–20 μg/24 hr
Norepinephrine: 15–80 μg/24 hr
Dopamine: 65–400 μg/24 hr
Children's levels are different from adult levels. Check with your laboratory for child values.

NOTE: *Different laboratories report values in different units—this should be kept in mind when analyzing results.*

Background

The principal substances formed by the adrenal medulla and excreted in urine include VMA, epinephrine, norepinephrine, metanephrine, and normetanephrine. These substances contain a catechol nucleus together with an amine group and, thus, are referred to as *catecholamines*. The major portions of these hormones are changed into metabolites, the principal one being 3-methoxy-4-hydroxymandelic acid, or VMA.

Vanillylmandelic acid is the primary urinary metabolite of the catecholamine group, and has a urine concentration much greater than the other amines (10 to 100 times). It is also fairly simple to detect. Methods used for catecholamine determination are much more complex.

Explanation of Test

This 24-hour urine test of adrenomedullar function is primarily done when a person with hypertension is suspected of having a pheochromocytoma, a tumor of the chromaffin cells of the adrenal medulla.

The assay for pheochromocytoma is most valuable when a urine specimen is collected during a hypertensive episode. Because a 24-hour urine collection represents a longer sampling time than a random urine sample or a symptom-directed serum sample, the 24-hour urine test may detect a pheochromocytoma that might be missed by a single blood level.

Procedure

1. Properly label a 24-hour urine container with preservative and refrigerate the container or keep it on ice.
2. Follow general instructions for 24-hour urine collection.
3. Record exact start and end time of the collection on the specimen container and in the healthcare record.
4. Send the specimen to the laboratory.

Clinical Implications

1. *Elevated urinary levels of VMA* occur as follows:
   a. High levels found in pheochromocytoma
   b. Slight to moderate elevations in
      (1) Neuroblastomas
      (2) Ganglioneuromas
      (3) Ganglioblastomas
      (4) Carcinoid tumors (some cases)
2. *Elevated urinary catecholamines* are found in
   a. Pheochromocytoma
   b. Neuroblastomas
   c. Ganglioneuromas
   d. Myocardial infarction
   e. Hypothyroidism
   f. Diabetic acidosis
   g. Long-term manic–depressive states

Interfering Factors

A. *Increased levels of VMA* and catecholamines are caused by
   1. Hypoglycemia (for this reason, the test should *not* be scheduled while the patient is NPO).
   2. Many foods, such as the following:
      a. Tea
      b. Coffee
      c. Cocoa
      d. Vanilla
      e. Fruit, especially bananas
      f. Fruit juice
      g. Chocolate
      h. Cheese flavoring or coloring
      i. Cider vinegar
      j. Gelatin foods
      k. Salad dressing
      l. Carbonated drinks, except gingerale
      m. Jelly and jam
      n. Candy and mints
      o. Cough drops
      p. Chewing gum
      q. Foods containing artificial flavoring or coloring
      r. Licorice
   3. Many drugs will cause increased VMA levels.

B. *False decreased levels of VMA* and catecholamines are caused by
   1. Alkaline urine
   2. Uremia (causes toxicity and impaired excretion of VMA)
   3. X-ray contrast agents (for this reason, an intravenous pyelogram should not be scheduled before a VMA test).
   4. Certain drugs

Patient Preparation

1. Instruct the patient about the test purpose and procedure for collection of the 24-hour urine specimen. A written reminder may be helpful, especially for restricted foods.
2. Explain diet and drug restrictions. Diet restrictions will vary among laboratories, but coffee, tea, bananas, cocoa products, vanilla products, and aspirin are always excluded for 3 days (2 days before testing and the day of the test).
3. Many laboratories require that all drugs be discontinued for 4 to 7 days before testing.
4. Encourage adequate rest, food, and fluids.
5. Stress and strenuous exercise should be avoided during the test.
6. See Chapter 1 guidelines for safe, effective, informed *pretest* care.

Patient Aftercare

1. Resume pretest diet, drugs, and activity when the test is completed.
2. Interpret test outcomes and counsel appropriately.
3. Follow Chapter 1 guidelines for safe, effective, informed *posttest* care.

URINE 17-KETOSTEROIDS (17-KS); **17-HYDROXYCORTICOSTEROIDS** (17-OHCS); **17-KETOGENIC STEROIDS** (17-KGS) (24-HR) ●

Normal Values

17-KETOSTEROIDS (17-KS)

Age (yr)	*mg/24 hr*
0–1	0–1 females
1–4	0–2 females
4–8	0–3 females
8–16	5–12 females
16–21	9–22 males
	6–15 females
>21	8–20 males
	6–15 females

17-HYDROXYCORTICOSTEROIDS (17-OHCS)

Men: 3–10 mg/24 hr
Women: 2–6 mg/24 hr
Child: 1–5 mg/24 hr

17-KETOGENIC STEROIDS (17-KGS)

Men: 5–24 mg/24 hr
Women: 5–15 mg/24 hr

Background

Urinary steroids can be divided into three main groups: *17-ketosteroids* (17-KS)—adrenal hormones and metabolites of testicular androgens. In men, the adrenals produce two-thirds of 17-KS, and the testes produce the remainder. In women the adrenals produce all of these hormones. In both sexes, 17-KS declines with age, and *17-ketogenic steroids* (17-KGS) reflect adrenal cortex activity (corticosteroids); *17-hydroxycorticosteroids* (17-OHCS) are also known as Porter–Silber chromogens.

Explanation of Test

These 24-hour tests of adrenal function measure the urinary excretion of steroids and are used to diagnose endocrine disturbances of the adrenal androgens.

For the most part, this test has been replaced by serum immunoassays. This test does not detect the major androgens, testosterone and dihydrotestosterone. If low androgens are suspected, a serum testosterone determination is the test of choice.

Procedure

1. Properly label a 24-hour urine container that contains preservative.
2. Follow general instructions for 24-hour urine collection.
3. Record exact start and end times of the collection on the specimen container and the healthcare record.
4. Send the completed specimen to the laboratory.

Clinical Implications

1. *Increased urinary 17-KS* occurs in
   - **a.** Adrenal carcinomas and adenomas
   - **b.** Third-trimester pregnancy
   - **c.** Pituitary tumor or hyperplasia
   - **d.** ACTH-producing tumors
   - **e.** Testicular interstitial cell tumors
   - **f.** Cushing's syndrome
   - **g.** Stein–Leventhal syndrome
   - **h.** Androgenic arrenoblastoma
   - **i.** Luteal cell ovarian tumors
   - **j.** Female pseudohermaphroditism
   - **k.** Congenital adrenal hyperplasia
2. *Decreased urinary 17-KS* occurs in
   - **a.** Addison's disease
   - **b.** Panhypopituitarism
   - **c.** Myxedema (hypothyroidism)
   - **d.** Nephrosis
   - **e.** Castration
   - **f.** Hypogonadism (Klinefelter's syndrome)
   - **g.** Secondary female hypogonadism
   - **h.** Primary ovarian agenesis
3. *Increased urinary 17-OHCS* occurs in
   - **a.** Any acute illness or stress state
   - **b.** Cushing's disease
   - **c.** Pregnancy, third-trimester
   - **d.** Virilism
   - **e.** Ectopic ACTH syndrome
   - **f.** Severe hypertension
   - **g.** Obesity
   - **h.** Thyrotoxicosis

4. *Decreased urinary 17-OHCS* occurs in
   a. Addison's disease
   b. Congenital adrenal hyperplasia
   c. Hypopituitarism
   d. Hypothyroidism
5. *Increased urinary ketogenic steroids* occurs in
   a. Adrenal hyperplasia
   b. Adrenal adenoma
   c. Adrenal carcinoma
   d. Cushing's syndrome
   e. ACTH therapy
6. *Decreased urinary ketogenic steroid* levels occur in
   a. Addison's disease
   b. Hypopituitarism
   c. Cretinism
   d. Cessation of corticosteroid therapy

Interfering Factors

1. Severe stress and obesity will cause increased levels of ketosteroids and hydroxycorticosteroids.
2. Ketosteroid levels are often increased in the third trimester of pregnancy, and slightly increased in early pregnancy.
3. Many drugs affect test outcomes, especially
   a. ACTH
   b. Cortisone, prednisone
   c. Testosterone

Patient Preparation

1. Instruct the patient about the test purpose and 24-hour urine specimen collection. A written reminder may be helpful.
2. Encourage food and fluids.
3. Caution the patient to avoid stressful situations.
4. Follow Chapter 1 guidelines for safe, effective, informed *pretest* care.

Patient Aftercare

1. Resume normal diet and exercise.
2. Interpret test outcomes and counsel appropriately.
3. See Chapter 1 guidelines for safe, effective, informed *posttest* care.

URINE PORPHYRINS AND PORPHOBILINOGENS (24-HR AND RANDOM) **DELTA-AMINOLEVULINIC ACID** (ALA, ΔALA) ●

Normal Values

PORPHOBILINOGENS

Random: 0–2.0 mg/L or negative
24-hour: 0–2.5 mg/24 hr

DELTA AMINOLEVULINIC ACID (ΔALA)

Random: 0–4.5 mg/L
24-hour: 0–7.5 mg/24 hr

PORPHYRINS

Random: negative

24-hour (units are μg/24 hr)

Porphyrin	*Male*	*Female*
Uroporphyrin	8–44	4–22
Coproporphyrin	10–109	3–56
Heptacarboxyporphyrin	0–12	0–9
Pentacarboxyporphyrin	0–4	0–3
Hexacarboxyporphyrin	0–5	0–5
Total porphyrin	8–149	3–78

Background

Porphyrins are cyclic compounds formed from delta-aminolevulinic acid (ΔALA or ALA), which plays a role in the formation of hemoglobin and other hemoproteins that function as carriers of oxygen in the blood and tissues. In health, insignificant amounts of porphyrin are excreted in the urine. However, in certain conditions, such as porphyria (disturbance in metabolism of porphyrin), liver disease, lead poisoning, and pellagra, increased levels of porphyrins, as well as ALA are found in the urine. Disorders in porphyrin metabolism also result in increased amounts of porphobilinogen. The most common signs and symptoms of acute intermittent porphyria are abdominal pain and tachycardia. Patients with the phorphyrias may pass urine the color of port wine.

When the urine is tested for the presence of porphyrins, porphobilinogen, or ALA, or a combination thereof, it is also given the black light screening test (porphyrins are fluorescent when exposed to black or ultraviolet light; Wood's light tests). See Chapter 2 for other tests for porphyria.

Explanation of Test

This test is used to diagnose porphyrias and lead poisoning. The following is a summary of laboratory findings for various porphyrias.

CONGENITAL ERYTHROPOIETIC PORPHYRIA. Elevations of urinary uroporphyrin and coproporphyrin occur, with the former exceeding the latter.

ACUTE, INTERMITTENT PORPHYRIA. Porphobilinogen and delta-aminolevulinic acid are elevated in acute attacks, and small increases of urinary uroporphyrin and coproporphyrin may be found.

HEREDITARY COPROPORPHYRIA. Urine coproporphyrin and porphobilinogen and markedly increased during acute attacks, increases of urinary uroporphyrin may also be found.

VARIEGATE PORPHYRIA. In acute attacks, results are similar to those of acute, intermittent porphyria. Porphobilinogen and ALA usually return to normal between attacks. Urine coproporphyrin exceeds uroporphyrin excretion during acute attacks.

CHEMICAL PORPHYRIAS. Porphyrinogenic chemicals include certain halogenated hydrocarbons that cause increased uroporphyrin levels in the urine.

LEAD POISONING. Delta-aminolevulinic acid levels exceed those of porphobilinogen, which may remain normal.

Procedure

1. Properly label a 24-hour clean-catch urine container.
2. Provide refrigeration or icing. The specimen needs to be kept protected from exposure to light. Check with laboratory about need for preservatives.
3. Follow general instructions for 24-hour urine collection.
4. Record exact start and end times on the specimen container and the healthcare record.
5. Send the specimen to the laboratory.
6. For random tests, midmorning or midafternoon specimens are best because it is more likely that the patient will excrete porphyrins at those times. Transport to lab immediately. Protect the specimen from light.
7. Observe and record the urine color. If porphyrins are present, the urine may appear amber red or burgundy, or it may vary from pale pink to almost black. Some patients will excrete normal-colored urine that turns dark after standing in the light.

Clinical Implications

1. *Increased urinary porphobilinogen* levels occur in
   - **a.** Porphyria—acute, intermittent type
   - **b.** Variegate porphyria
   - **c.** Hereditary coproporphyria
   - **d.** Also, see explanation of test for others

> **Clinical Alert**
>
> Porphobilinogen is not increased in lead poisoning.

2. *Increased fractionated porphyrin* levels occur in
   - **a.** Acute, intermittent porphyria
   - **b.** Congenital erythropoietic porphyria
   - **c.** Hereditary coproporphyria
   - **d.** Varigate porphyria
   - **e.** Chemical porphyria caused by heavy metal poisoning or carbon tetrachloride
   - **f.** Lead poisoning
   - **g.** Viral hepatitis
   - **h.** Cirrhosis (alcoholism)
   - **i.** Newborn of mother with porphyria
   - **j.** Congenital hepatic porphyria

3. *Increased delta-aminolevulinic acid* can occur in
   a. Acute, intermittent porphyria (in acute phase)
   b. Variegate porphyria during crisis
   c. Hereditary coproporphyria
   d. Lead poisoning, increases early and may remain elevated for several months after control of lead exposure
   e. Diabetic acidosis
   f. Third trimester of pregnancy
   g. Chronic liver diseases associated with alcoholism

Interfering Factors

1. Oral contraceptives and diazepam can cause acute porphyria attacks in susceptible patients.
2. Alcohol ingestion
3. Many other drugs, especially phenazopyridine, procaine sulfamethoxazole, and the tetracyclines.

Patient Preparation

1. Instruct the patient about the purpose and procedure of collecting a 24-hour urine specimen. A written reminder may be helpful.
2. Allow food and fluids, but avoid alcohol and excessive fluid intake during the 24-hour collection.
3. If possible, discontinue all drugs for 2–4 weeks before test so that results will be accurate.
4. See Chapter 1 guidelines for safe, effective, informed *pretest* care.

Patient Aftercare

1. Resume normal activities and medications.
2. Interpret test outcomes and counsel appropriately.
3. Follow Chapter 1 guidelines for safe, effective, informed *posttest* care.

> **Clinical Alert**
>
> This test should not be ordered for patients receiving Donnatal or other barbiturate preparations. However, if intermittent porphyria is being tested for, the patient should take those medications according to prescribed protocols because these drugs may provoke an attack of porphyria.

URINE AMYLASE EXCRETION/CLEARANCE
(TIMED URINE AND BLOOD)

Normal Values

Amylase/creatinine clearance: 1%–4%
Amylase 2-hr: 2–34 units/2 hr

Amylase 24-hr: 24–408 units/24 hr
Values may vary according to laboratory methods used.

Background

Amylase is an enzyme that changes starch to sugar. It is produced in the salivary glands, pancreas, liver, and fallopian tubes, and is normally excreted in small amounts in the urine. If the pancreas or salivary glands are inflamed, much more of the enzyme enters the blood; therefore, more amylase is excreted in the urine.

Explanation of Test

This test of blood and urine indicates pancreatic function and is done to differentiate acute pancreatitis from other causes of abdominal pain, epigastric discomfort, or nausea and vomiting. The timed urine and amylase test (2 hours or 24 hours) can be done to detect inflammation of the salivary glands or pancreas, to monitor treatment of acute pancreatitis, and to pinpoint recurrent attacks of acute pancreatitis.

The 2-hour urine amylase excretion is a more sensitive test than either the serum amylase or lipase test. In patients with acute pancreatitis, the urine often shows a prolonged elevation of amylase compared with the short-lived peak in the blood. Moreover, urine amylase may be elevated when blood amylase is within normal range and, conversely, the blood amylase may be elevated when urine amylase is within normal range. The 24-hour urine level may be normal even when some of the 1- or 2-hour specimens show increased values. The advantage of the amylase creatinine clearance test is that the test can be done on a single random urine specimen and a single serum sample instead of having to wait for a 2- or 24-hour urine collection to be done.

Procedure

For the amylase clearance test, a venous blood sample of 4 ml must be collected at the same time a random urine specimen is obtained.

1. A 1-hour, 2-hour, or 24-hour timed specimen will be ordered. A 2-hour specimen is usually collected.
2. Refrigerate the specimen.
3. Follow general instructions for a timed or a 24-hour urine collection.
4. Record exact start and end times on the specimen container and on the healthcare record.
5. Send the specimen to the laboratory.

Clinical Implications

1. Amylase/creatine clearance is *increased* in
   - **a.** Pancreatitis
   - **b.** Diabetic ketoacidosis
   - **c.** Burns
   - **d.** Renal insufficiency
2. Urinary amylase is *increased* in

a. Pancreatitis
b. Parotitis
c. Intestinal obstruction
d. Diabetic ketoacidosis
e. Strangulated bowel
f. Pancreatic cyst
g. Peritonitis
h. Renal failure

3. Urinary amylase levels are *decreased* in
   a. Pancreatic insufficiency
   b. Advanced cystic fibrosis
   c. Severe liver disease

Interfering Factors

1. High levels of glucose interfere with the amylase excretion test.
2. Some drugs produce increased amylase and possibly pancreatitis.

Patient Preparation

1. Instruct the patient about the test purpose and procedure for urine specimen collection. A written instruction sheet may be helpful.
2. Encourage fluids if not restricted.
3. See Chapter 1 guidelines for safe, effective, informed *pretest* care.

Patient Aftercare

1. Interpret test outcomes and monitor appropriately.
2. Follow Chapter 1 guidelines for safe, effective, informed *posttest* care.

Clinical Alert

Follow-up calcium levels should be checked in fulminating pancreatitis because extremely low calcium levels can occur.

URINE PHENYLKETONURIA (PKU) AND BLOOD

Normal Values

Blood: < 2 mg/dl (2–5 days after birth)
Urine: negative dipstick; no observed color change indicative of PKU.

Background

Routine blood and urine tests are done on newborns to detect PKU, a genetic disease that can lead to mental retardation and brain damage if untreated. This disease is characterized by a lack of the enzyme that converts phenylalanine, an amino acid, to tyrosine, which is necessary for normal metabolic function. If tyrosine accumulates in the tissues, phenylpyruvic acid, a metabolite of phenylalanine, will be produced and cause brain damage.

Explanation of Test

This test is used for newborns to detect the metabolic disorder hyperphenylalaninemia. If untreated, this disorder can lead to mental retardation or even death. Cord blood cannot be used for analysis.

Procedure

COLLECTING BLOOD SAMPLE

1. Cleanse the skin with an antiseptic and pierce the infant's heel with a sterile disposable lancet.
2. If bleeding is slow, support the infant so blood flows by means of gravity while spotting the blood on the filter paper.
3. The circles on the filter paper must be completely filled. This can best be done by placing one side of the filter paper against the infant's heel and watching for the blood to appear on the other side of the paper until it completely fills the circle.

COLLECTING URINE SAMPLE IN NURSERY OR AT HOME

1. Dip the reagent strip into a fresh sample of urine or press it against a wet diaper.
2. After exactly 30 seconds, compare the strip with a color chart, according to manufacturer's directions.

Clinical Implications

Increased levels of phenylalanine are found in

1. Hyperphenylalaninemia. In a positive test for PKU, the blood phenylalanine is greater than 15 mg/dl. Blood tyrosine is less than 5 mg/dl. It is never increased in PKU. The urine test is positive in PKU.
2. Sepsis
3. Severe burns
4. Transient tyrosinemia of newborn

Interfering Factors

1. Premature infants (infants weighing less than 11 kg [5 lb]) may have elevated phenylalanine and tyrosine levels without having the genetic disease. This is a result of delayed development of appropriate enzyme activity in the liver (liver immaturity).
2. Antibiotics will interfere with the assay.

Instructions to Mothers

1. Inform the mother about the purpose of the test and the method of collecting the specimens.
2. Most parents would be interested in knowing that PKU (a genetic disease in which a defective gene is passed on from each parent) was first recognized about 40 years ago by a young mother of two mentally retarded children. She was aware that the urine of these children had a peculiar

odor and, on the basis of this, was able to have a biochemist study the urine and identify phenylpyruvic acid. About 10 years later, the first successful dietary treatment (restriction of phenylalanine, as in milk) of those newborn babies identified as having PKU was started and resulted in normal mental development of these children.

3. Interpret test outcomes and counsel appropriately.

Clinical Alert

1. The blood test must be performed at least 3 days after birth or after the child has ingested protein (milk) for at least 24 to 48 hours.
2. Urine testing is usually done at the 4- or 6-week checkup if a blood test was not done.
3. The PKU studies should be done on all infants who weigh 11 kg (5 lb), or more, before they leave the hospital.
4. Sick or premature infants should be tested within 7 days after birth, regardless of protein intake, weight, or antibiotic therapy.

URINE TUBULAR REABSORPTION PHOSPHATE
(TRP) (TIMED URINE AND BLOOD)

Normal Values
82%–95% or 0.82–0.95 reabsorbed with a normal diet.

Background
The TRP is a rough estimate of parathyroid hormone levels in the blood. The test is based on the fact that excessive parathyroid hormone increases renal tubular reabsorption of phosphate. However, the test has limited value. Determination of increased calcium levels in the blood is still essential for an accurate diagnosis of hyperparathyroidism.

Explanation of Test
This test is done to detect hyperparathyroidism. A fasting blood sample for a 24-hour or a 4-hour urine sample is obtained and analyzed for levels of phosphorus and creatinine. Test results are based on the ratio of creatinine clearance to phosphate clearance.

Procedure
1. Overnight fasting from food is usually necessary, but water is encouraged to promote hydration and formation of urine.
2. Obtain early-morning venous blood sample at the end of the test.
3. Properly label 24-hour urine container (also used for 4-hour test) with preservatives.

4. Follow general instructions for 24-hour or 4-hour urine collection.
5. Record exact start and end times on the specimen container and the healthcare record.
6. Send the specimen to the laboratory.

Clinical Implications

1. Urinary TRP is *increased* in
   a. *Hypo*parathyroidism
   b. Pseudohypoparathyroidism
2. Urinary TRP is *decreased* in
   a. *Hyper*parathyroidism
   b. When successful parathyroid surgery is performed, TRP levels will rise to 95% to 100% of normal within 18 to 24 hours after the procedure.

Interfering Factors

Low results may occur in the presence of uremia, renal tubular disease, osteomalacia, or sarcoidosis.

Patient Preparation

1. Instruct the patient about the purpose and procedure of the test, collection of 24-hour or 4-hour urine specimen, overnight fast if ordered, and blood sampling. A written reminder is helpful.
2. Encourage the patient to drink water, especially the morning of the test.
3. The patient must eat a normal calcium and phosphorus diet for 5 days preceding the test.
4. See Chapter 1 guidelines for safe, effective, informed *pretest* care.

Patient Aftercare

1. Interpret test outcomes and monitor appropriately.
2. Follow Chapter 1 guidelines for safe, effective, informed *posttest* care.

URINE D-XYLOSE ABSORPTION (TIMED) ●

Normal Values

60-minute serum/plasma: 0–5 months, > 15 mg/dl; 6 months to 16 years, > 20 mg/dl; 17 years and older, 21–57 mg/dl

120-minute serum/plasma: 0–5 months, > 25 mg/dl; 6 months to 16 years, > 20 mg/dl; 17 years and older, 32–58 mg/dl

Urine xylose 5-hour (%) *reference range:* 0–64 years, > 16% of dose; 65 years and older, > 14% of dose

Urine xylose 5-hour (g) *reference range:* 0–64 years, > 4.0 g/5 hr; 65 years and older, > 3.5 g/5 hr

Background

The D-xylose test is a diagnostic measure for evaluating malabsorptive conditions and intestinal absorption of D-xylose, a pentose not normally present in the blood in significant amounts. It is partially absorbed when ingested and is excreted in the urine. Little is metabolized.

Explanation of Test

This test directly measures intestinal absorption and is used in the differential diagnosis of steatorrhea. The usual problem is differentiating pancreatic from enterogenous steatorrhea. When D-xylose (which is not metabolized by the body) is administered orally, blood and urine levels are checked for absorption rates. Absorption is normal in pancreatic steatorrhea but will be impaired in enterogenous steatorrhea.

Procedure

1. Do not allow food or liquids by mouth for at least 8 hours before the start of the test.
2. The patient should void at the beginning of the test. Discard this urine.
3. Administer the oral dose of D-xylose after it has been dissolved in water. (Dosage is 0.5 g/lb body weight for child and up to 25 g in 100 ml H_2O for adult.) Additional water up to 250 ml should be taken at this time. Record these times on the patient's healthcare record. Give no further fluids or food until the test is completed.
4. Within 60 to 120 minutes later, draw a 3-ml sample of venous blood.
5. The patient must rest quietly and remain stationary until the test is completed.
6. Five hours from the start of the test the patient should void. Save all urine voided during the test.

Clinical Implications

1. *Decreased* levels of urinary D-xylose are found in
   a. Tropical and nontropical sprue
   b. Adult celiac disease
   c. Amyloidosis
   d. Small bowel ischemia
   e. Whipple's disease
   f. Nongranulomatous jejunitis
   g. Bacterial overgrowth in small intestine
2. The D-xylose test is normal when malabsorption is due to pancreatic insufficiency.

Interfering Factors

1. Many drugs and antibiotics
2. Nonfasting state or treatment with hyperalimentation
3. Foods rich in pentose (fruits and preserves)

Patient Preparation

1. Explain purpose and procedure of the test and urine collection process. The entire 5-hour specimen must be collected.
2. Patient must fast at least 8 hours before the start of the test.
3. Children under 9 years of age should fast for only 4 hours.
4. Water may be taken at any time.

5. Weigh patient to determine proper dose of D-xylose.
6. Patient must not ingest contraindicated drugs for 1 week before the test.
7. See Chapter 1 guidelines for safe, effective, informed *pretest* care.

Patient Aftercare

1. Normal food, fluids, and activities can be resumed.
2. See Chapter 1 guidelines for safe, effective, informed *posttest* care.

> **Clinical Alert**
>
> Nausea, vomiting, and diarrhea may result from the D-xylose. If vomiting occurs, the test is invalid and must be repeated.

URINE CREATININE/CREATININE CLEARANCE (TIMED URINE AND BLOOD)

Normal Values

Urine creatinine
  Men: < 0.8–1.8 g/24 hr
  Women: 0.6–1.6 g/24 hr
Blood creatinine
  0.4–1.5 mg/dl
Creatinine clearance: (ml/min/1.73 m^2)

Age (yr)	*Males*	*Females*
< 20	88–146	81–134
20–30	88–146	81–134
30–40	82–140	75–128
40–50	75–133	69–122
50–60	68–126	64–116
60–70	61–120	58–110
70–80	55–113	52–105

Background

Creatinine is a substance that, in health, is easily excreted by the kidney. It is the by-product of muscle energy metabolism and is produced at a constant rate, according to the muscle mass of the individual. Endogenous creatinine production is constant as long as muscle mass remains intact. Because all creatinine filtered by the kidneys in a given time interval is excreted into the urine, creatinine levels are equivalent to the glomerular filtration rate (GFR). Disorders of kidney function prevent maximum excretion of creatinine. The creatinine clearance test is frequently part of every battery of quantitative urine tests. Creatinine clearance is measured together with other urinary components and to interpret the overall excretion rate of the various urinary components.

Explanation of Test

The creatinine clearance test is a specific measurement of kidney function, primarily glomerular filtration. It measures the rate at which the kidneys clear creatinine from the blood. In a broad sense, clearance of a substance may be defined as the imaginary volume (ml/min) of plasma from which the substance would have to be completely extracted for the kidney to excrete that amount in 1 minute. This test is used to evaluate renal function in slightly built or debilitated individuals, to follow the treatment response and progression of renal disease, and to adjust medication dosage.

Procedure

1. Properly label a 12-hour or 24-hour urine container.
2. Refrigerate or ice the specimen.
3. Follow general instructions for 24-hour urine collection.
4. Record exact start and end times on the specimen container and the healthcare record.
5. Send the entire specimen to laboratory.
6. Also contain a 5-ml venous blood sample when the test begins.
7. Record the patient's height and weight on the container and in the healthcare record because creatinine clearance values are based on the patient's surface area.

Clinical Implications

1. *Decreased* creatinine clearance is found in
   - **a.** Impaired kidney function, intrinsic renal disease, glomerulonephritis, pyelonephritis, nephrotic syndrome, acute tubular dysfunction, amyloidosis
   - **b.** Shock
   - **c.** Hemorrhage
   - **d.** Congestive heart failure
   - **e.** Hepatic failure
2. *Increased* creatinine clearance is found in
   - **a.** State of high cardiac output
   - **b.** Pregnancy
   - **c.** Burns
   - **d.** Carbon monoxide poisoning
3. *Increased* urine creatinine levels are found in
   - **a.** Acromegaly
   - **b.** Gigantism
   - **c.** Diabetes mellitus
   - **d.** Hypothyroidism
4. *Decreased* urine creatinine levels are found in
   - **a.** Hyperthyroidism
   - **b.** Anemia
   - **c.** Muscular dystrophy
   - **d.** Polymyositis, neurogenic atrophy
   - **e.** Inflammatory muscle disease
   - **f.** Advanced renal disease, renal stenosis
   - **g.** Leukemia

Interfering Factors

1. Exercise may increase creatinine clearance.
2. Pregnancy substantially increases creatinine clearance.
3. Many drugs decrease creatinine clearance.
4. The creatinine clearance overestimates the GFR when serum creatinine is elevated.
5. A diet high in meat may elevate urine creatinine levels.

Clinical Alert

Determination of urine creatinine is of little value for evaluating renal function unless done as part of a creatinine clearance test.

Patient Preparation

1. Instruct the patient about the purpose, procedure of the test, and urine specimen collection. A written reminder may be helpful.
2. Allow food and encourage fluids for good hydration. Large urine volumes assure optimal test results.
3. Avoid vigorous exercise during the test.
4. Drugs affecting the results should be stopped beforehand (especially cephalosporins). Check with physician.
5. Avoid eating large amounts of meat. Check with physician.
6. See Chapter 1 guidelines for safe, effective, informed *pretest* care.

Patient Aftercare

1. Resume normal food, fluids, and activity.
2. Interpret test outcomes and monitor appropriately.
3. Follow Chapter 1 guidelines for safe, effective, informed *posttest* care.

URINE CYSTINE (24-HR AND RANDOM) ●

Normal Values

Qualitative: Negative
Quantitative: Children, 5–31 mg/24 hr
Adults, < 38 mg/24 hr

Explanation of Test

These urine tests are useful for differential diagnosis of cystinuria, an inherited disease characterized by bladder calculi (cystine has low solubility). Patients with cystine stones face recurrent urolithiasis and repeated urinary infections.

Procedure

1. Obtain a random 20-ml urine specimen for a quantitative screen.
2. When collecting a 24-hour urine specimen, the container needs a preservative. Follow general procedures for a 24-hour urine specimen.

Clinical Implications

1. *Cystine values are increased* in
   a. Cystinuria (up to 20 times normal) in which there is excess urinary excretion of lysine, ornithine, arginine, and cystine
2. *Cystine values are decreased* in burn patients.

Clinical Alert

1. Cystinosis, a different entity from cystinuria, is not detected by cystine studies. A majority of patients with infantile nephropathic cystinosis have renal defects that become apparent in infancy. Failure to thrive and renal tubular dysfunction are evidence of this disease.
2. Patients with cystinosis have a defect in renal tubular reabsorption (Fanconi syndrome), which leads to a generalized amino aciduria. The urinary cystine is elevated in the same proportion as all amino acids. They never have a high enough concentration of cystine in their urine to form cystine stones. The plasma cystine concentration is normal. However, these patients do have an elevated cystine content in all of their tissues. For purposes of diagnosis, this measurement is usually done in white blood cells. Normal individuals have cystine content of less than 0.2 nmol 1/2 cystine/mg protein in peripheral leukocytes, whereas patients with cystinosis have a value greater than 2. The mean value is much higher, approximately 7. This is an autosomal recessive condition, and heterozygotes have a white blood cell cystine content four to five times greater than normal. This is best seen in polymophonuclear cells.

Patient Preparation

1. Explain test purpose and procedure for timed urine collection.
2. See Chapter 1 guidelines for safe, effective, informed *pretest* care.

Patient Aftercare

1. Interpret test outcomes and counsel appropriately.
2. Follow Chapter 1 guidelines for safe, effective, informed *posttest* care.

URINE HYDROXYPROLINE (TIMED URINE AND BLOOD) ●

Normal Values

Total: 0–6 mg/24 hr, or 38–500 µmol/24 hr
Free: 0–2 mg/24 hr, or < 30 µmol/24 hr

Background

Hydroxyproline is an amino acid found only in collagen that increases during periods of rapid growth, with bone diseases, and in some endocrine disorders. Less than 10% of hydroxyproline is normally free; almost all is peptide-bound. In adults, hydroxyproline excretion reflects bone resorption (breakdown). Diurnal rhythms of hydroxyproline excretion show greater excretion levels during the night.

Explanation of Test

This test indicates the presence of bone collagen reabsorption in various disorders, as well as evaluates the degree of destruction from primary or secondary bone tumors. It measures the severity of Paget's disease and indicates the response to treatment.

Procedure

1. Obtain a 2-hour specimen after the patient has fasted overnight.
2. Notify the laboratory of the patient's age and sex.
3. If ordered, collect a 24-hour urine specimen. No preservative is required, but the specimen needs to be refrigerated or iced.
4. Follow 24-hour collection procedures. The laboratory will record the total 24-hour volume.
5. The preferred method of testing in the first few months of life is through blood sampling.

Clinical Implications

1. *Free hydroxyproline is increased* in
   - **a.** Hydroxyprolinemia, a hereditary autosomal recessive condition (rare)
   - **b.** Familial aminoglycinuria, also inherited
2. *Total hydroxyproline levels are increased* in
   - **a.** Hyperparathyroidism
   - **b.** Paget's disease
   - **c.** Marfan syndrome
   - **d.** Hypothyroidism
   - **e.** Osteoporosis (osteomyelitis)
   - **f.** Bone tumors (neoplasia)
   - **g.** Growth spurts
   - **h.** Acromegaly
3. *Total hydroxyproline is decreased* in
   - **a.** Hypopituitarism
   - **b.** Hypothyroidism
   - **c.** Hypoparathyroidism
   - **d.** Malnutrition
   - **e.** Chronic muscular dystrophy

Interfering Factors

Meat and gelatin may affect test results (false-positives).

Patient Preparation

1. Explain test purpose and process for timed urine collection. Fasting and special fluid requirements before testing are often required for 2-hour timed procedure. Check with laboratory.
2. Avoid gelatin foods for several days before test.
3. See Chapter 1 guidelines for safe, effective, informed *pretest* care.

Patient Aftercare

1. Resume normal diet and activity.
2. Interpret test outcomes and counsel appropriately.
3. Follow Chapter 1 guidelines for safe, effective, informed *posttest* care.

URINE LYSOZYME (24-HR, RANDOM URINE AND BLOOD) ●

Normal Values

Blood plasma: 4–13 μg/ml
Urine: 0–2 μg/ml/24 hr

Background

Lysozyme (muramidase) in blood or urine is a bacteriolytic enzyme that comes from degradation of granulocytes and monocytes.

Explanation of Test

This blood and urine test differentiates acute myelogenous or monocytic leukemia from acute lymphatic leukemia.

Procedure

1. Collect a 10-ml venous blood sample or a urine specimen.
2. Follow general instructions for random urine collection or 24-hour urine collections. **Transport sample to lab immediately following collection.**

Clinical Implications

1. *Levels are elevated* in
   - **a.** Acute myelogenous leukemia
   - **b.** (Granulocytic) acute monocytic leukemia
2. *Levels may be elevated* in
   - **a.** Renal disorders and transplant rejection
   - **b.** Tuberculosis
   - **c.** Sarcoidosis (sarcoid lymph nodes)
   - **d.** Crohn's disease
3. Levels are normal in acute lymphatic leukemia.

URINE MYOGLOBIN

Normal Values

Urine: < 20 ng/dl
Negative for myoglobin
Increases slightly with age

Background

Myoglobin is the oxygen-binding protein of striated muscle. It resembles hemoglobin. However, it is unable to release oxygen except at extremely low oxygen tensions. Injury to skeletal or cardiac muscle releases myoglobin. It is rapidly excreted from the blood into the urine. There is a threshold level of 2 mg/dl.

Explanation of Test

Urine myoglobin tests help to evaluate a variety of conditions, including some metabolic disorders and those caused by trauma.

Procedure

1. Collect and refrigerate a 1-ml urine sample.
2. The urine must test positive for hemoglobin before the test can be carried out.

Clinical Implications

Increased urinary myoglobin values are associated with

1. Myocardial infarction
2. Other muscle injury (eg, sports, auto accidents)
3. Phosphorylase deficiency (hereditary myoglobinuria)
4. Unknown metabolic defects
5. Renal failure
6. Metabolic myoglobinuria
7. Mechanical crushing injuries (crush syndrome)
8. Progressive muscular dystrophy
9. Hyperthermia or malignant hyperthermia (anesthetic complication)
10. Electric shock, convulsions seizures
11. Viral and bacterial infections
12. Cocaine-induced renal artery vasoconstriction
13. Drug and chemical poisoning

> **Clinical Alert**
>
> If large amounts of myoglobin are presented to the kidney, anuria may result from renal damage caused by myoglobins.

Interfering Factors

1. Many drugs and chemicals
2. Illicit drugs: cocaine, heroin, methadone, amphetamines

Patient Preparation

1. Explain test purpose and urine collection procedure.
2. See Chapter 1 guidelines for safe, effective, informed *pretest* care.

Patient Aftercare

1. Interpret test outcomes and counsel appropriately.
2. Follow Chapter 1 guidelines for safe, effective, informed *posttest* care.

URINE PREGNANCY TESTS ●

Normal Values

Positive in urine: pregnancy exists
Negative in urine: nonpregnant state

Background

From the earliest stage of development (9 days old), the placenta produces hormones, either on its own or in conjunction with the fetus. The very young placental trophoblast produces appreciable amounts of the hormone human chorionic gonadotropin (hCG) that is excreted in the urine. Human chorionic gonadotropin is not found in the urine of normal, young, nonpregnant women.

Explanation of Test

Increased urinary hCG levels form the basis of most tests for pregnancy and for trophoblastic tumors in males. All pregnancy tests are designed to detect hCG. Human chorionic gonadotropin is present in blood and urine whenever there is living chorionic/placental tissue. Human chorionic gonadotropin can be further identified as alpha- or beta-HCG. Human chorionic gonadotropin can be detected in the urine of pregnant women 26 to 36 days after the first day of the last menstrual period (8 to 10 days after conception). Pregnancy tests should return to negative 3 to 4 days after delivery.

Procedure

1. Collect an early-morning urine specimen. The first morning specimen generally contains the greatest concentration of hCG. However, a random specimen may be used, but the specific gravity must be at least 1.005.
2. Do not use grossly bloody specimens. If necessary, a catheterized specimen should be used.

Clinical Implications

1. A positive result usually indicates pregnancy. Only two-thirds of women with ectopic pregnancies will have positive pregnancy tests.
2. Positive results also occur in
   - **a.** Choriocarcinoma
   - **b.** Hydatidiform mole
   - **c.** Testicular tumors
   - **d.** Chorioepithelioma
   - **e.** Chorioadenoma destruens
   - **f.** About 65% of ectopic pregnancies

3. Negative or decreased results occur in
   a. Fetal death
   b. Abortion (test remains positive after procedure)

Interfering Factors

1. *False-negative tests* and false low levels of hCG may be caused by very dilute urine (low specific gravity) or by using a specimen obtained too early in pregnancy.
2. *False-positive tests* are associated with
   a. Proteinuria
   b. Hematuria
   c. In the presence of excess pituitary gonadotropin (luteinizing hormone; cross-reaction is minimal)
   d. Certain drugs, especially methadone

URINE ESTROGEN; TOTAL AND FRACTIONS, ESTRADIOL (E_2), ESTRIOL (E_3) (24-HR URINE AND BLOOD) ●

Normal Values

Vary widely between women and men; also, the presence of pregnancy, the menopausal state, or follicular, ovulatory, and luteal stage of menstrual cycle.

ESTRADIOL—URINE

Male: 0–6 μg/24 hr
Female:
  Follicular: 0–3 μg/24 hr
  Ovulatory Peak: 4–14 μg/24 hr
  Luteal: 4–10 μg/24 hr
  Postmenopausal: 0–4 μg/24 hr

ESTRIOL—URINE:

Male: 1–11 μg/24 hr
Female:
  Follicular phase: 0–14 μg/24 hr
  Ovulatory phase: 13–54 μg/24 hr
  Luteal phase: 8–60 μg/24 hr
  Postmenopausal: 0–11 μg/24 hr
  Pregnancy:
    1st trimester: 0–800 μg/24 hr
    2nd trimester: 800–12,000 μg/24 hr
    3rd trimester: 5000–50,000 μg/24 hr

TOTAL ESTROGEN—URINE

Male: 4–25 μg/24 hr
Female:
  Nonpregnant: 4–60 μg/24 hr

Pregnant:
- 1st trimester: 0–800, μg/24 hr
- 2nd trimester: 800–5000 μg/24 hr
- 3rd trimester: 5000–50,000 μg/24 hr

Background

Estradiol is the most active of the endogenous estrogens. The test evaluates female menstrual and fertility problems. In males, estradiol is useful for evaluating estrogen-producing tumors. Estriol is the prominent urinary estrogen in pregnancy. Serial measurements reflect the integrity of the fetal–placental complex.

Total estrogens evaluate ovarian estrogen-producing tumors in premenarcheal or postmenopausal females. During pregnancy, a different total estrogen test is used. This must be communicated. During pregnancy, serial estrogen tests are more meaningful for pregnancy evaluation.

Explanation of Test

These measurements, together with gonadotropins, are useful in evaluating menstrual and fertility problems, male feminization characteristics, estrogen-producing tumors, and pregnancy. Estradiol (E_2) is the most active of the endogenous estrogens. Estriol (E_3) levels in both plasma and urine rise as pregnancy advances; significant amounts are produced in the third trimester. Total estrogens may be helpful to establish time of ovulation and optimum time for conception.

Procedure

1. Obtain a venous blood sample.
2. Collect a 24-hour urine specimen and use boric acid preservative for all estrogen tests. Refrigerate or ice during collection.
3. Follow general collection procedures for 24-hour specimen.
4. Record the age and sex of the patient.
5. The number of gestational weeks must be communicated if patient is pregnant.
6. The days into the menstrual cycle must be documented for the nonpregnant female.

Clinical Implications

1. Urinary estradiol (E_2 levels) are *increased* in
   - **a.** Feminization in children (testicular feminization syndrome)
   - **b.** Estrogen-producing tumors
   - **c.** Precocious puberty related to adrenal tumors
   - **d.** Hepatic cirrhosis
   - **e.** Hyperthyroidism
   - **f.** In females, estradiol increases during menstruation, preovulation, and during the 23rd to 41st weeks of pregnancy.

2. Urinary estradiol levels are *decreased* in
   a. Primary and secondary hypogonadism
   b. Kallman syndrome
   c. Anorchia; primary testicular failure
   d. Hypofunction or dysfunction of pituitary and adrenal glands
   e. Menopause

Clinical Alert

Estradiol may be used for Pergonal monitoring. Serial measurements of E_2 during ovulation induction enable the physician to minimize high E_2 levels from ovarian overstimulation and thereby decrease side effects.

3. *Increased* levels of estriol (E_3) are found in pregnancy—sharp rise if delivery is imminent

4. Urinary estriol (E_3) is *decreased* in
   a. Placental insufficiency
   b. Fetal distress—an abrupt drop of 40% or more on 2 consecutive days.

5. Serial monitoring of estriol for 4 consecutive days is recommended to evaluate fetal distress.

Clinical Alert

Normal values are guidelines and must be interpreted in conjunction with clinical findings.

6. Total urinary estrogens are *increased* in
   a. Malignant neoplasm of adrenal gland
   b. Malignant neoplasm of testis
   c. Benign neoplasm of ovary
   d. Granulosa cell tumor of ovary
   e. Lutein cell tumor of ovary
   f. Theca cell tumor of ovary
   g. Benign neoplasm of testis
   h. Acute and subacute necrosis of liver
   i. Pregnancy and following administration of acetazolamide during pregnancy

7. Total urinary estrogens are *decreased* in
   a. Ovarian hypofunction (ovarian agenesis; primary ovarian malfunction)
   b. Intrauterine death
   c. Preeclampsia
   d. Hypopituitarism
   e. Hypofunction of adrenal cortex
   f. Menopause
   g. Anorexia nervosa

Patient Preparation

1. Explain the test purpose and procedure.
2. Stress test compliance. The patient must be able to adjust daily activities to accommodate urine collection protocols.
3. Do not administer radioisotopes for 48 hours before test.
4. Discontinue all medications for 48 hours before the test (with physician's approval). Drugs deemed necessary must be documented and communicated.
5. See Chapter 1 guidelines for safe, effective, informed *pretest* care.

Patient Aftercare

1. Resume medications and activity.
2. Interpret test outcomes, monitor, and counsel appropriately.
3. Follow Chapter 1 guidelines for safe, effective, informed *posttest* care.

URINE AMINO ACIDS (TOTAL/FRACTIONS) (URINE 24-HR, RANDOM AND BLOOD) ●

Normal Values

Urine and blood amino acid values are age dependent.

Background

Many abnormalities in amino acid transport or metabolism can be detected by physiologic fluid analysis (urine, plasma, spinal fluid). Free amino acids are found in urine or acid filtrates of protein-containing fluids. Urine is used for initial screening of inborn metabolic errors. Both transport and metabolic errors can be detected by changes in observed amino acid patterns. In many cases, metabolic errors are detected when the amino acid or metabolite exceeds its renal threshold. Many intermediary metabolites have low renal thresholds.

Explanation of Test

This test is the initial screen for inborn errors of metabolism and transport in cases of suspected genetic abnormalities, such as mental retardation, reduced growth, or other unexplained symptoms. More than 50 aminoacidopathies are now recognized.

Procedure

1. A fasting blood specimen may need to be obtained.
2. Collect random or 24-hour timed urine specimens and keep refrigerated or ice the samples.

Clinical Implications

1. *Total serum amino acids are increased* in
   a. Specific aminoacidopathies (see urine section)

b. Secondary causes
   (1) Diabetes with ketosis
   (2) Malabsorption
   (3) Hereditary fructose intolerance
   (4) Conditions with severe brain damage
   (5) Reye's syndrome
   (6) Acute and chronic renal failure
   (7) Eclampsia
   (8) Specific aminoacidopathies

2. *Total serum amino acids are decreased* in
   a. Adrenocortical hyperfunction
   b. Huntington's chorea
   c. Phlebotomus fever
   d. Nephritic syndrome
   e. Rheumatoid arthritis
   f. Hartnup disease
   g. Fever
   h. Malnutrition

3. *Total urine amino acids are increased* in specific aminoacidurias, as described below:

Aminoacidurias Disease	*Amino Acids Increased in Urine and Blood*	*Presence of Abnormal Enzymes*
Phenylketonuria	Phenylalanine	Phenylalanine hydroxylase
Tyrosinosis	Tyrosine	*p*-Hydroxyphenylpyruvic acid oxidase
Histidinemia	Histidine	Histidase
Maple-syrup urine disease	Valine, leucine, and isoleucine	Branched-chain keto acid decarboxylase
Hypervalinemia	Valine	Probably valine transaminase
Hyperglycinemia	Glycine (lysine on high-protein diet)	Associated with CP synthetase deficiency and other disorders
Hyperprolinemia		
Type I Type II	Proline	Proline oxidase pyrrolin-5-carboxylate dehydrogenase
Hydroxyprolinemia	Hydroxyproline	Hydroxyproline oxidase
Homocystinuria	Methionine, homocystine	Cystathionine synthetase
Hyperlysinemia	Lysine	Lysine-α-ketoglutarate reductase
Citrullinemia	Citrulline	Argininosuccinic acid synthetase

(continued)

Aminoacidurias Disease	Amino Acids Increased in Urine and Blood	Presence of Abnormal Enzymes
Alcaptonuria	Homogentisic acid (2:5-dihydroxyphenylacetic acid). No abnormal amino acid	Homogentisic acid oxidase
Oasthouse urine disease	Methionine, phenylalanine, valine, leucine, isoleucine, and tyrosine; also α-hydroxybutyric acid in urine	Possibly methionine malabsorption syndrome

4. Absence of aminoacidurias as in the following:

Disease	Amino Acids in Urine	Presence of Abnormal Enzyme
Argininosuccinic aciduria	Argininosuccinic acid (also citrulline)	Argininosuccinase
Cystathion–cystathioninuria		Cystathioninase
Homocystin–homocystinuria		Cystathionine synthetase
Hypophosphatasia	Phosphoethanolamine	Serum alkaline phosphate

5. Renal transport aminoacidurias, as in the following:

Disease	Amino Acids in Urine	Abnormality
Cystinuria (cystine stones)	Cystine; lysine; arginine, ornithine (basic amino acids)	Incomplete absorption of cystine, lysine, arginine, ornithine
Hartnup disease	Monoaminomonocarboxylic (neutral) amino acids (proline, glycine, hydroxyproline, and methionine not increased)	Incomplete absorption of monoaminomonocarboxyamino acids
Glycinuria—renal type	Glycine—proline, hydroxyproline	Membrane transport defect
Familial iminogycinuria		

6. Secondary aminoacidouria, as follows:

a. Viral hepatitis
b. Multiple myeloma
c. Hyperparathyroidism
d. Rickets (vitamin D-resistant)
e. Osteomalacia
f. Hereditary fructose intolerance

g. Galactosemia
h. Uric disease
i. Renal failure
j. Wilson's disease
k. Muscular dystrophy

Interfering Factors

1. Dilute urine (> 1.010) affects test.
2. Hyperalimentation and IVs affect outcome.
3. Drugs, such as amphetamines, norepinephrine, levodopa, and all antibiotics, affect results.

Patient Preparation

1. Instruct the patient regarding test purpose, collection process and need for refrigeration. A written reminder may be helpful.
2. Allow foods and moderate amounts of fluids (do not overhydrate).
3. It may be necessary to consume proteins or carbohydrates for a challenge load to produce certain amino acid metabolites.
4. See Chapter 1 guidelines for safe, effective, informed *pretest* care.

Patient Aftercare

1. Interpret test outcomes and counsel appropriately.
2. Follow Chapter 1 guidelines regarding safe, effective, informed *posttest* care.

BIBLIOGRAPHY

Ashcroft KW (ed): Pediatric Urology. Philadelphia, WB Saunders, 1990

Brady S: Urodynamics: An overview. Urological Nursing 9(1): 837–841, January/March 1990

Everett WD, London M: Drug testing in the work place: What primary care physicians need to know. Postgraduate Medicine 91:287, 1992

Fischbach F: Analyzing urinalysis results. Dimensions of Critical Care Nursing 2(4): 225–232. August 1983

Graff L: A Handbook of Routine Urinalyses. Philadelphia, JB Lippincott, 1983

Henry JB (ed): Todd–Sanford–Davidsohn Clinical Diagnosis and Management by Laboratory Methods, 18th ed. Philadelphia, WB Saunders, 1990

Jacobs A, Winslow AH: Working smart. Myth of the clean catch. AJN 20, August 1993

Krane RJ, Siroky M, Fitzpatrick J (eds): Clinical Urology. Philadelphia, JB Lippincott, 1994

Leavelle DE (ed): Mayo Medical Laboratories: Interpretive Handbook. Rochester, MN, Mayo Medical Laboratories, 1990

Morris A et al: Current issues in the laboratory diagnosis of urinary tract infections. New Zealand Journal of Medical Laboratory Technology 44(3): 67–70, August 1990

Pappas P: Laboratory in the diagnosis and management of urinary tract infections. Medical Clinics of North American 75 (2): 313–323, March 1991

Sacher RA, McPherson RA: Widmann's Clinical Interpretation of Laboratory Tests, 10th ed. Philadelphia, FA Davis, 1991

Sultan JM: Evaluation of hematuria in adults. JAMA, 263(18): 2475–2479, May 9, 1990

Tietz NW (ed): Clinical Guide to Laboratory Tests, 3rd ed. Philadelphia, WB Saunders, 1995

U.S. Preventive Task Force: Screening for asymptomatic bacteruria, hematuria, and proteinuria. Washington, DC: National Health Information Center, August 1990

Wallach J: Interpretation of Diagnostic Tests, 5th ed. Little, Brown & Company, 1992

Wrenn KD et al: The syndrome of alcoholic ketoacidosis. American Journal of Medicine 91: 119, 1991

4

Stool Studies

OVERVIEW OF STOOL STUDIES

Formation and Composition of Feces

The elimination of digestive waste products from the body is essential to health. These excreted waste products are known as *stool* or *feces.* Stool examination is often done for evaluation of gastrointestinal (GI) disorders. These studies are helpful in detecting gastrointestinal bleeding, gastrointestinal obstruction, obstructive jaundice, parasitic disease, dysentery, ulcerative colitis, and increased fat excretion.

An adult excretes 100 to 300 g of fecal matter a day. Of this, as much as 70% may be water. The feces are what remains of the 8 to 10 L of digested fluidlike material that enters the intestinal tract each day, and oral food and fluids, saliva, gastric secretions, pancreatic juice, and bile add to the formation of feces.

Feces are composed of

1. Waste residue of indigestible material, such as cellulose from food eaten during the previous 4 days.
2. Bile (pigments and salts); stool color is normally due to bile pigments that have been altered by bacterial action.
3. Intestinal secretions, including mucus.
4. Leukocytes that migrate from the bloodstream (normally very few).
5. Epithelial cells that have been shed.
6. Large numbers of bacteria that can make up to one-third of the total solids.
7. Inorganic material (10%–20%), chiefly calcium and phosphates.
8. Undigested or unabsorbed food (normally present in very small quantities).

The output of feces depends on a complex series of absorptive, secretory, and fermentative processes. Normal function of the colon involves three physiologic processes: (1) absorption of fluid and electrolytes; (2) contractions that churn and expose the contents to the GI tract mucosa and transport the contents to the rectum; and (3) defecation.

The small intestine is approximately 23 feet (7 m) long and the large intestine 4 to 5 feet (1.2–1.5 m) long. The small intestine degrades ingested fats, proteins, and carbohydrates to absorbable units and then absorbs them. Pancreatic, gastric, and biliary secretions exert their effects upon the GI contents to prepare this material for active mucosal transport. Other active substances absorbed in the small intestine include fat-soluble vitamins, iron, and calcium. Vitamin B_{12}, after combining with intrinsic factors, is absorbed in the ileum. The small intestine also absorbs as much as 9.5 L of water and electrolytes for return to the bloodstream. Small intestine contents (chyme) begin to enter the rectum as soon as 2 to 3 hours after a meal, but the process is not complete until 6 to 9 hours postprandial.

The large intestine performs less complex functions than the small intestine. The proximal or right colon absorbs most of the water remaining after the GI contents have passed through the small intestine. Colonic absorption of water, sodium, and chloride is a passive process. Fecal water excretion is only about 100 ml/day. The colon mainly moves the luminal contents to and fro by seemingly random contractions of circular smooth muscle. Increased propulsive activity (peristalsis) occurs after eating. Peristaltic waves are caused by the gastrocolic and duodenocolic reflexes, which are initiated after meals and stimulated by the emptying of the stomach into the duodenum. The muscles of the colon are innervated by the autonomic nervous system. Additionally, the parasympathetic nervous system stimulates movement and the sympathetic system inhibits movement. Massive peristalsis usually occurs several times a day. Resultant distention of the rectum initiates the urge to defecate. In persons with normal motility and with a mixed dietary intake, normal colon transit time takes 24 to 48 hours.

● STOOL ANALYSIS

Stool analysis determines the various properties of the stool for diagnostic purposes. Some of the more frequently ordered tests on feces include tests for blood, bile, parasites, and parasite eggs (ova). Stool is also examined by *chromatographic* analysis for the presence of gallstones. The recovery of a gallstone from feces provides the only proof that a common bile duct stone has been dislodged and excreted. Stool testing also screens for colon cancer and asymptomatic ulcerations or other masses of the GI tract and evaluates GI diseases in the presence of diarrhea or constipation.

Patients and health personnel may dislike collecting and examining fecal material. However, this natural aversion must be overcome in the light of the value of a stool examination for diagnosing disturbances and diseases of the GI tract, the liver, and the pancreas.

RANDOM COLLECTION OF STOOL SPECIMENS ●

1. Observe universal precautions (Appendix IX) when handling specimens.
2. Collect feces in a dry, clean, urine-free container that has a properly fitting cover.
3. The specimen should be uncontaminated with urine or other body secretions, such as menstrual blood.
4. Collect the entire stool specimen and transfer to a container with a clean tongue blade or similar object.
5. For best results, cover specimens and deliver to the laboratory immediately after collection. Depending on the examination to be performed, the specimen either should be refrigerated or kept warm. If unsure of how to handle specimen, contact the laboratory for *detailed instructions* concerning the disposition of the fecal specimen.

6. Post signs in bathrooms that say "DO NOT DISCARD STOOL" or "SAVE STOOL" to serve as remainders that fecal specimen collection is in progress.

OVA AND PARASITES COLLECTION

1. Wear gloves. Observe universal precautions (Appendix IX).
2. Warm stools are best for detecting ova and parasites. Do *not* refrigerate specimens for ova and parasites.
3. Special vials for ova and parasites stool samples that contain 10% formalin and PVA fixative may be used. In this case, timing and specimen storage temperature is not critical.
4. Because of the cyclic life cycle of parasites, three separate random stool specimens for analysis are recommended.

ENTERIC PATHOGENS COLLECTION

1. Some coliform bacilli produce antibiotic substances that destroy enteric pathogens. Refrigerate specimen immediately.
2. A diarrheal stool will usually give accurate results.
3. A freshly passed stool is the specimen of choice.
4. Preferably, stool specimens should be collected before antibiotic therapy is initiated, as early in the course of the disease as possible.
5. It is recommended that the entire stool evacuated be sent for examination. If mucus or blood is present, it definitely should be included with the specimen because pathogens are more likely to be found in these substances. If only a small amount of stool is available, a walnut-sized specimen is usually adequate.
6. Accurately label all stool specimens with the patient's name, date, and tests ordered on the specimen. Keep the outside of the container free from contamination and send the sealed container to the laboratory at once.

Interfering Factors For All Types of Stool Collection

1. Stool specimens from patients receiving tetracyclines, antidiarrheal medications, barium, bismuth, oil, iron, or magnesium may not yield accurate results.
2. Bismuth found in paper towels and toilet tissue interferes with accurate results.
3. Do not collect or retrieve stool from the toilet bowl or that has been contaminated with urine or water. A clean, dry bedpan may be the best receptacle for defecation.
4. Inaccurate test results may result if the sample is not representative of the entire stool evacuation.
5. Lifestyle, personal habits, travel, home and work environments, and bathroom accessibility are some of the factors that may interfere with proper sample procurement.

Patient Preparation

1. Explain the purpose, procedure of the test, and interfering factors in language the patient understands. Because the specimen cannot be obtained on demand, it is important to provide detailed instructions before the test so that the specimen is collected when the opportunity presents itself. Provide written instructions if necessary.
2. Provide proper containers and other collection supplies. Instruct the patient to defecate in a clean bedpan or large-mouthed plastic container. Provide for and respect patient's privacy.
3. Instruct the patient *not to urinate* into the bedpan or collecting container.
4. No toilet paper should be placed in the bedpan or container because it interferes with testing.
5. If the patient has diarrhea, a large plastic bag attached by adhesive tape to the toilet seat may be helpful in the collection process. After defecation, the bag can be placed into a gallon container.
6. Specimens for most tests can be produced by a warm saline enema or Fleet Phospho-Soda enema.
7. The physician may order both ova and parasite testing and cultures. In this case, the specimen should be divided into two samples: one portion refrigerated (for culture testing) and one portion kept at room temperature (for ova and parasite testing). There are commercial collection kits that require the stool to be divided and placed into separate vials for better recovery of ova and parasites and enteric pathogens. (See Chap. 7 for microbiologic analysis of feces.)
8. See Chapter 1 guidelines for safe, effective, informed *pretest* care.

Patient Aftercare

1. Provide patient privacy and the opportunity to cleanse perineal area and hands. Assist as necessary.
2. See Chapter 1 guidelines for safe, effective, informed *posttest* care.

Clinical Alert

1. Any stool collected may harbor highly infective pathogens. Use extreme caution and proper handling techniques at all times.
2. Instruct patients in proper handwashing techniques after each use of the bathroom.

STOOL CONSISTENCY, SHAPE, FORM, AND AMOUNT

Normal Values

100–200 g/day

Plastic, soft, formed; soft and bulky on a high-fiber diet; small and dry on a high-protein diet; seeds and visible undigested fiber and indigestible fiber present (Table 4-1).

TABLE 4-1
Normal Values in Stool Analysis

Macroscopic Examination	***Normal Value***
Amount	100–200 g/day
Color	Brown
Odor	Varies with pH of stool and depends on bacterial fermentation and putrefaction
Consistency	Plastic; not unusual to see fiber, vegetable skins, and seeds; soft and bulky in high-vegetable diet; small and dry in high-meat diet
Size, shape	Formed
Gross blood	None
Mucus	None
Pus	None
Parasites	None
Microscopic Examination	***Normal Values***
Fat	Colorless, neutral fat (18%) and fatty acid crystals and soaps.
Undigested food, meat fibers, starch, trypsin	None to small amount
Eggs and segments of parasites	None
Yeasts	None
Leukocytes	None
Chemical Examination	***Normal Values***
Water	Up to 75%
pH	Neutral to weakly alkaline (6.5–7.5)
Occult blood	Negative
Urobilinogen	50–300 µg/24 hr
Porphyrins	Coporphyrins: 400–1200 µg/24 hr Uroporphyrins: 10–40 mg/24 hr
Nitrogen	< 2.5 g/24 hr
Bile	Negative in adults; positive in children
Trypsin	20–950 units/g (positive in small amounts in adults; present in greater amounts in normal children)
Osmolality, used with serum osmolality to calculate osmotic gap	200–250 mOsm 5.8–9.8 mEq/24 hr
Sodium	2.5–3.9 mEq/24 hr
Chloride	15.7–20.7 mEq/24 hr*
Potassium	0–6 g/24 hr
Lipids (fatty acids)	

*Reference values for electrolytes differ greatly from laboratory to laboratory.

Explanation of Test

Normally evacuated feces reflect the shape and caliber of the colonic lumen as well as the colonic motility. The normal consistency is somewhat plastic, neither fluid, mushy, nor hard. Consistency also can be described as formed, soft, mushy, frothy, or watery.

Procedure

Collect random stool specimen in plastic container (see page 255).

Clinical Implications

1. Fecal consistency may be altered in various disease states.

- **a.** Diarrhea mixed with mucus and red blood cells is associated with
  - **(1)** Typhus
  - **(2)** Typhoid
  - **(3)** Cholera
  - **(4)** Amebiasis
  - **(5)** Large bowel cancer
- **b.** Diarrhea mixed with mucus and white blood cells is associated with
  - **(1)** Ulcerative colitis
  - **(2)** Regional enteritis
  - **(3)** Shigellosis
  - **(4)** Salmonellosis
  - **(5)** Intestinal tuberculosis
- **c.** "Pasty" stool is associated with a high-fat content in the stool:
  - **(1)** A significant increase of fat is usually detected on gross examination.
  - **(2)** With common bile duct obstruction, the fat gives the stool a putty-like appearance.
  - **(3)** In sprue and celiac disease, the stool often resembles aluminum paint owing to the presence of fatty acid.
  - **(4)** In cystic fibrosis, the increase of neutral fat gives a greasy, "butter stool" appearance.
- **d.** A bulky, frothy stool is associated with sprue and celiac disease.

2. Alterations in size or shape indicate altered motility or colon wall abnormalities.

- **a.** A narrow, ribbonlike stool suggests the possibility of spastic bowel, rectal narrowing or stricture, decreased elasticity, or a partial obstruction.
- **b.** Excessively hard stools are usually due to increased fluid absorption because of prolonged contact of luminal contents with colon mucosa during delayed transit time through the colon.
- **c.** A very large-circumference stool indicates dilation of the viscus.
- **d.** Small, round, hard stools (scybala) accompany habitual, moderate constipation.
- **e.** Severe fecal retention can produce huge, firm, impacted stool masses, with a small amount of liquid stool as overflow. These must be removed manually or, occasionally, under light anesthesia.

Patient Preparation

ASSESSMENT OF DIARRHEA AND CONSTIPATION

1. In the presence of diarrhea or constipation, it is important to obtain and record:
   a. An estimate of volume and frequency of fecal output
   b. Stool consistency and presence of blood, pus, mucus, oiliness, or bad odor in specimen; evaluate through direct observation
   c. Decrease or increase in frequency of defecation
   d. Sensations of rectal fullness with incomplete stool evacuation
   e. Painful defecation
2. Assess the patient's emotional state. In many instances, psychological stress may be the major reason for altered bowel habits.
3. Assess dietary habits.
4. Follow guidelines in Chapter 1 concerning diverse patient needs and principles of safe, effective, informed pretest care.

STOOL ODOR ●

Normal Values

Characteristic odor: varies with the pH of stool and with diet.

Explanation of Test

Substances called indole and skatole, formed by intestinal bacterial putrefaction and fermentation are primarily responsible for the odor of normal stools. Fecal odor should be assessed whenever a stool specimen is collected.

Procedure

Collect and refrigerate random stool specimen in plastic container.

Clinical Implications

1. A foul odor is caused by degradation of undigested protein.
2. A foul odor is produced by excessive carbohydrate ingestion.
3. A sickly sweet odor is produced by volatile fatty acids and undigested lactose.

Patient Preparation

1. Barium procedures and laxative preparations should be avoided for 1 week before stool specimen collection.
2. Advise patient of purpose of test and instruct in collection techniques and refrigeration of specimen.
3. Follow guidelines in Chapter 1 for safe, effective, informed pretest care.

Patient Aftercare

Evaluate outcome and record findings. If abnormal odors are detected, assess dietary patterns. Counsel appropriately.

STOOL pH

Normal Values
Neutral to slightly acid or alkaline

Explanation of Test
The stool pH is diet dependent and based on bacterial fermentation in the small intestine. Carbohydrate fermentation changes the pH to acid; protein breakdown changes the pH to alkaline.

Procedure
Collect a fresh, random stool specimen in a plastic container with tight-fitting lid. Refrigerate specimen.

Clinical Implications.
1. Increased pH (alkaline)
   a. Protein breakdown
   b. Colitis
   c. Villous adenoma
   d. Antibiotic use

2. Decreased pH (acid)
   a. Carbohydrate malabsorption
   b. Fat malabsorption
   c. Disaccharidase deficiency

Interfering Factors
Barium procedures and laxatives affect outcomes. They should be avoided for 1 week before stool sample collection.

Patient Preparation
1. Explain purpose and procedure following general guidelines in Chapter 1 concerning safe, effective, informed *pretest* care.
2. Advise patient that laxatives and barium procedures should be avoided for 1 week before stool sampling.
3. Schedule barium procedures after test or at least 1 week before.

Patient Aftercare
Interpret pH outcome and record findings. If abnormal pH is found, assess dietary patterns and antibiotic use. Monitor as appropriate for malabsorption syndrome.

STOOL COLOR

Normal Values
Brown

Explanation of Test
The color of the feces should be assessed and recorded because it can provide information about pathologic conditions, organic dysfunction, bleeding,

diet, or intake of drugs. Color abnormality may aid the clinician to select appropriate diagnostic chemical and microbiologic stool tests.

The brown color of normal feces is probably due to stercobilin (urobilin), a bile pigment derivative, which results from the action of reducing bacteria in bilirubin and other undetermined factors.

Procedure

Collect random stool specimen (see page 255).

Clinical Implications

1. The color of feces changes in some disease states.
   a. Yellow to yellow-green: severe diarrhea
   b. Green: severe diarrhea
   c. Black, "tarry" consistency: usually the result of bleeding into the upper gastrointestinal tract (> 100 ml blood)
   d. Tan or clay colored: blockage of the common bile duct; pancreatic insufficiency produces a pale, greasy, acholic stool. In these instances, reduced amounts of bile pigments enter the intestine because of intrinsic hepatobiliary disease or obstruction.
   e. Maroon-to-red-to-pink: possible result of bleeding from the lower gastrointestinal tract (eg, tumors, hemorrhoids, fissures, inflammatory process).
2. Grossly visible blood always indicates an abnormal state.
   a. Blood streaked on the outer surface usually indicates hemorrhoids or anal abnormalities.
   b. Blood present in stool can also arise from abnormalities higher in the colon. If transit time is sufficiently rapid, blood from the stomach or duodenum can appear as bright or dark red or maroon in stool.

Interfering Factors

1. Stool darkens on standing.
2. Color is influenced by diet (certain foods), food dyes, and drugs.
   a. Yellow to yellow-green color occurs in the stool of breast-fed infants who lack normal intestinal flora.
   b. Green color occurs in diets high in chlorophyll-rich vegetables, such as spinach or in antibiotic therapy.
   c. Black may be due to foods such as cherries, to an unusually high proportion of dietary meat, or artificially colored foods such as black jelly beans.
   d. Light-colored stool with little odor may be due to diets high in milk and low in meat.
   e. Claylike color may be due to a diet with excessive fat intake, bile duct obstruction.
   f. Red may be due to a diet high in beets or tomatoes.
   g. Certain color changes may result from drugs.

(1) Black: iron salts, bismuth salts, charcoal
(2) Green: mercurous chloride, indomethacin, calomel
(3) Green to blue: dithiazanine
(4) Brown staining: anthraquinones
(5) Red: phenolphthalein, pyrvinium pamoate, tetracyclines in syrup, Bromsulphalein
(6) Yellow: santonin, antibiotics
(7) Yellow to brown: senna
(8) Light to whitish: barium, antacids
(9) Orange-red: phenazo-pyridine
(10) Pink to red to black: anticoagulants (excessive dose), salicylates, NSAIDs (may cause internal GI bleeding)

Clinical Alert

A complete dietary and drug history will help differentiate significant abnormalities from interfering factors.

Patient Preparation

1. Advise patient of purpose of test. Follow guidelines in Chapter 1 for safe, effective, informed *pretest* care.
2. Record dietary and drug history.
3. No laxatives or barium procedures for 1 week before collection.

Patient Aftercare

Interpret and document abnormal appearance and colors; counsel patient appropriately.

BLOOD IN STOOL

Normal Values

Negative for blood

Explanation of Test

The normal person passes 2.0 to 2.5 ml of blood into the gastrointestinal tract daily. Passage of more than 2.8 ml of blood in 24 hours is an important sign of GI disease. Blood is most commonly seen when hemorrhoids and anal fissures are present. Detection of occult (hidden) blood in the stool is very useful in detecting or localizing disease of the GI tract. This test demonstrates the presence of blood in upper GI bleeding, as in the presence of gastric ulcer. This test also screens for colonic carcinoma and other sources of occult bleeding.

Procedure

1. Obtain a random stool specimen free of interfering factors. Tests for detecting fecal blood use substances that depend on peroxidase content as

an indication of hemoglobin content to cause a color change in the stool specimen being tested. The sensitivities are adjusted to detect blood loss greater than 5 ml/day. Hematest is more sensitive, but also produces more false-positive results. Hemoccult (guaiac) is less sensitive, but produces more false-negative results.
2. Use a portion from two different areas of the stool sample.
3. Protect Hemoccult slide from heat, sunlight, and fluorescent light.
4. Transport to laboratory without delay.

Clinical Implications

1. Stool that appears dark red to tarry black indicates a loss of 0.50 to 0.75 ml of blood from the upper GI tract. Smaller quantities of blood in the GI tract can produce similar stools or appear as bright red blood.
2. A stool should be considered grossly bloody only after chemical testing for presence of blood. This will eliminate the possibility that coloring caused by diet or drugs may be mistaken for bleeding in the GI tract (see section on color).
3. Positive testing for occult blood may be caused by
   - **a.** Carcinoma of colon
   - **b.** Ulcerative colitis
   - **c.** Adenoma
   - **d.** Diaphragmatic hernia
   - **e.** Gastric carcinoma
   - **f.** Diverticulitis
   - **g.** Ulcers

Clinical Alert

1. To be accurate, the test employed must be repeated three to six times on different stool samples.
2. The patient's diet should be free of meat and vegetable sources of peroxidase activity (eg, turnips, horseradish). Only after following this regimen can a positive series of tests be considered as an indication for further evaluation and testing of the patient.

Interfering Factors

1. Drugs such as salicylates, steroids, indomethacin, NSAIDs, anticoagulants, colchicine, iron (when used in very large doses), and rauwolfia derivatives are associated with increased GI blood loss in normal persons and with more pronounced bleeding when disease is present. Gastrointestinal bleeding can also follow parenteral administration of the aforementioned drugs.
2. Drugs that may cause a false-positive test for occult blood include
   - **a.** Boric acid
   - **b.** Bromides
   - **c.** Colchicine
   - **d.** Iodine
   - **e.** Inorganic iron
   - **f.** Oxidizing agents

3. Foods that may cause false-positive results for occult blood testing include
   a. Meat, which in the diet contains hemoglobin, myoglobin, and certain enzymes that can give false-positive tests for up to 4 days after eating them.
   b. Vegetables with peroxidase activity (eg, turnips, horseradish).

   Vitamin C (ascorbic acid) taken in quantities greater than 500 mg/day may cause a false-negative test for occult blood in the stool.
4. The testing method must be followed exactly or the results are not reliable. Liquid stools may cause false-negative results with filter paper methods of collection.
5. Other factors affecting the test include
   a. Bleeding hemorrhoids
   b. Collection of specimen during menstrual period
   c. Long-distance runners (23%) have positive outcomes for occult blood

Patient Preparation

1. Explain purpose, procedure, interfering factors, and the need to follow appropriate stool collection protocols.
2. It is recommended that the patient consume a high-residue diet, starting 2 days before and continuing throughout the collection period. *Diet may include*
   a. Meats: only small amounts of chicken, turkey, and tuna
   b. Vegetables: generous amounts of both raw and cooked vegetables, including lettuce, corn, spinach, carrots, and celery. Avoid those with high peroxidase activity (see foods that should be avoided).
   c. Fruits: plenty of fruits, especially prunes and apples
   d. Cereals: bran and bran-containing cereals
   e. Moderate amounts of peanuts and popcorn daily. If any of the foregoing foods are known to cause discomfort, the patients should consult with the physician.
3. *The following foods should be avoided*:
   a. Fruits and vegetables containing high peroxidase activity, such as turnip, cauliflower, broccoli, cantaloupe, horseradish, and parsnip.
   b. Meat: no red or rare cooked meat.
4. No alcohol, aspirin, or vitamin C 2 days before and during the test period. Check with physician if unsure about other drugs.

Patient Aftercare

1. Patient may resume normal diet.
2. Interpret occult blood test results and record findings. Counsel and monitor patient as necessary. Advise that further testing and follow-up may be necessary.
3. Follow guidelines in Chapter 1 regarding safe, effective, informed patient care.

Clinical Alert

1. Blood in the stool is abnormal and should be reported and recorded.
2. The Hemoccult test is usually positive when fecal leukocytes are present.

MUCUS IN STOOL

Normal Values

Negative for mucus

Explanation of Test

The mucosa of the colon secretes mucus in response to parasympathetic stimulation. Recognizable mucus in a stool specimen is abnormal and should be reported and recorded.

Procedure

Collect a random stool specimen (see page 255).

Clinical Implications

1. Presence of recognizable mucus is abnormal.
2. Translucent gelatinous mucus clinging to the surface of formed stool occurs in
   a. Spastic constipation
   b. Mucous colitis
   c. Emotionally disturbed patients
   d. Excessive straining at stool
3. Bloody mucus clinging to the feces suggests
   a. Neoplasm
   b. Inflammation of the rectal canal
4. In villous adenoma of the colon, copious quantities of mucus may be passed (up to 3–4 L in 24 hours).
5. Mucus with pus and blood is associated with
   a. Ulcerative colitis
   b. Bacillary dysentery
   c. Ulcerating cancer of colon
   d. Acute diverticulitis
   e. Intestinal tuberculosis

Patient Preparation

1. Advise patient of purpose of test. Follow guidelines in Chapter 1 for safe, effective, informed *pretest* care.
2. No laxatives or barium test procedures for 1 week before test.

Patient Aftercare

1. Report and record presence, type, and amount of mucus.
2. Interpret meaning of abnormal mucus. Counsel patient appropriately. Monitor bowel habits. Explain that further testing and follow-up monitoring may be necessary.

COLLECTION OF 24-, 48- AND 72-HOUR STOOL SPECIMENS ●

This method is used to test for fat, porphyrins, urobilinogen, nitrogen, and electrolytes.

Special Instructions for Submitting Individual Specimens

1. Collect all stool specimens for 1 to 3 days. The entire stool should be collected.
2. Label specimens *Day 1, Day 2, Day 3,* time of day collected, patient's name, and tests ordered.
3. Submit individual specimens to the laboratory as soon as they are collected.

Special Instructions for Submitting Timed/Total Specimens

1. Obtain a 1-gallon container from the laboratory (1 gal paint tin or covered plastic pail is preferred).
2. Save all stool and place in the container. Keep refrigerated or in a container with canned ice. Replace ice as needed.
3. At the end of the collection period, transfer the properly labeled container to the laboratory.
4. Record dates, duration of collection time period, tests to be performed, patient's name, and other vital information on the collection receptacle.

FAT IN STOOL ●

Normal Values

In a normal diet, fat in stool will account for up to 20% of total solids.
Lipids are measured as fatty acids: (0–6.0 g/24 hr)

Explanation of Test

This test is the gold standard in diagnosing steatorrhea, which supports the diagnosis of one of the malabsorption syndromes.

Procedure

1. Collect a 48-hour to 72-hour specimen. Each individual stool specimen is collected and identified with the name of the patient, time, date, and test

and sent immediately to the laboratory. Also, indicate the length (actual time frame) of the collection period.

2. Follow the procedure for the collection of 24-, 48-, or 72-hour specimens.

Clinical Implications

1. Increases in fecal fat and fatty acids are associated with the malabsorption syndrome:
   - **a.** Nontropical sprue
   - **b.** Crohn's disease
   - **c.** Whipple's disease
   - **d.** Cystic fibrosis

   A high fat value is indicative of steatorrhea and excessive fat loss through stools.
2. Increases are also found in
   - **a.** Enteritis and pancreatic diseases when there is a lack of lipase (as in chronic pancreatitis)
   - **b.** Surgical removal of a section of the intestine
3. Fecal test does not provide a diagnostic explanation for the presence of steatorrhea.

Interfering Factors

1. Increased neutral fat may occur under the following nondisease conditions:
   - **a.** Use of rectal suppositories or oily creams applied to the perineum
   - **b.** With the ingestion of castor oil or mineral oil
   - **c.** With the ingestion of dietetic low-calorie mayonnaise
   - **d.** Ingestion of a high-fiber diet (> 100 g/24 hr) or Metamucil.
   - **e.** Use of psyllium-based stool softeners (Metamucil)
2. Barium and bismuth interfere with test results.
3. Urine contaminates the specimen.
4. A random stool specimen is not an acceptable sample.

Patient Preparation

1. Explain the purpose of the test, interfering factors, and the procedure for the collection of specimens. Follow guidelines in Chapter 1 concerning diverse patient needs and safe, effective, informed *pretest* care.
2. For a 72-hour stool collection, a diet containing 60 to 100 g of fat, 100 g of protein, and 180 g of carbohydrate is eaten for 6 days before and also during the test.
3. Follow the procedure for the actual collection of 72-hour stool specimens.

Patient Aftercare

1. Resume normal diet.
2. Record appearance, color, and odor of all stools in persons suspected of having steatorrhea. The typical stool is foamy, greasy, soft, pasty, and foul-smelling.

3. Counsel patient concerning test outcome and possible need for further testing.
4. Follow guidelines in Chapter 1 for safe, effective, informed *posttest* care.

MEAT FIBERS IN STOOL

Normal Values

Negative: no meat fibers are present in the normal stool.

Explanation of Test

The presence of undigested meat fibers (muscle fibers) in stool implies impaired intraluminal digestion. There is a substantial correlation with the amount of fat excretion in the stool.

Procedures for Meat Fibers

1. The patient must eat an adequate amount of red meat for 24 to 72 hours before testing.
2. Specimens obtained with a warm saline enema or Fleet Phospho-Soda are acceptable. Specimens obtained after use of mineral oil, bismuth, or magnesium compounds cannot be used. See collection of random stool specimens, page 255.
3. Record method/type of stool procurement.

Clinical Implications

Increased amounts of meat fibers are found in

1. Malabsorption syndromes
2. Pancreatic exocrine dysfunction
3. Gastrocolic fistula

Interfering Factors

1. Specimens should not be obtained with purgatives other than saline or Fleet Phospho-Soda.
2. Barium procedures or laxatives should be avoided for 1 week before collection.

Patient Preparation

1. Explain purpose of test and interfering factors. Follow guidelines in Chapter 1 regarding safe, effective, informed *pretest* care.
2. Patient must eat high meat diet for 72 hours before test.

Patient Aftercare

1. Resume normal diet.
2. Interpret test outcomes. See Chapter 1 guidelines for safe, effective, informed *posttest* care.

UROBILINOGEN IN STOOL

Normal Values

125–400 Ehrlich units/24 hr, or
75–350 Ehrlich units/100 g

Explanation of Test

This test investigates hemolytic diseases to determine if there is excess production of urobilinogen. Determination of this substance estimates the total excretion of bile pigments, which are the breakdown products of hemoglobin. Increased destruction of red blood cells, as in hemolytic anemia, increases the amount of urobilinogen excreted. Liver disease, in general, reduces the flow of bilirubin to the intestine and, thereby, decreases the fecal excretion of urobilinogen. In addition, complete obstruction of the bile duct reduces urobilinogen to very low levels.

Procedure

See "Random Collection of Stool Specimens," page 255. Protect from light. Send the specimen to the laboratory at once.

Clinical Implications

1. *Increased values* are associated with hemolytic anemias.
2. *Decreased values* are associated with
   - **a.** Complete biliary obstruction
   - **b.** Severe liver disease, infectious hepatitis
   - **c.** Oral antibiotic therapy that alters intestinal bacterial flora
   - **d.** Infants are negative up to 6 months of age

Patient Preparation

1. Explain purpose of test. Follow guidelines in Chapter 1 for safe, effective, informed *pretest* care.
2. Patient should not be receiving oral antibiotic therapy for 1 week before test.
3. Patient should not have laxatives or barium procedures 1 week before test.

Patient Aftercare

Interpret test outcomes. Counsel patient appropriately concerning further testing. Monitor for liver disease and biliary obstruction.

BILE IN STOOL

Normal Values

Adults: negative for unaltered bile
Children: positive

Explanation of Test

A test for bile in the stool helps determine the presence and degree of biliary tract obstruction in jaundiced patients. Normally, unaltered bile is never found in feces.

Procedure

Obtain a random stool specimen.

Clinical Implications

1. Bile may be present in diarrheal stools.
2. Increased bile levels occur in hemolytic jaundice.
3. Decreased levels closely follow urobilinogen in the stool (see page 270).

Patient Preparation

1. Explain purpose of test. Follow guidelines in Chapter 1 for safe, effective, informed *pretest* care.
2. Patient should not be receiving oral antibiotic therapy for 1 week before test.
3. Patient should not have laxatives or barium procedures 1 week before test.

Patient Aftercare

1. Interpret test outcomes. Counsel patient appropriately concerning further testing. Monitor for liver disease and biliary obstruction.
2. Follow guidelines in Chapter 1 for safe, effective, informed *posttest* care.

TRYPSIN IN STOOL ●

Normal Values

Positive for small amounts in 95% of normal persons. Present in greater amounts in the stools of normal children. In older children and adults, trypsin is destroyed by bacteria in the GI tract.

Explanation of Test

This test is used as an indicator for pancreatic function and for evaluating the ability of trypsin to split carbohydrates, protein, and fats by this pancreatic enzyme. This test is more useful in evaluating malabsorption in children under age 4.

Procedure

1. Collect random specimens and send to the laboratory. Three separate fresh stools are usually collected. See random stool collection procedures, page 255.

2. In older children, a cathartic is given before obtaining a specimen (saline or Fleet only).

Interfering Factors

1. No trypsin activity is detectable in constipated stools owing to the prolonged exposure to intestinal bacteria.
2. Barium and laxatives used less than 1 week before test affect results.
3. In adults, the test is unreliable owing to trypsin inactivation by intestinal flora.

Clinical Implications

Decreased amounts occur in

1. Pancreatic deficiency
2. Malabsorption syndromes
3. Screen for cystic fibrosis (sweat chloride test is preferred)

Patient Preparation

1. Explain purpose of test and interfering factors. Follow guidelines in Chapter 1 for safe, effective, informed *pretest* care.
2. Avid barium and laxatives for 1 week before stool collection.

Patient Aftercare

Interpret abnormal test results and counsel concerning possible need for follow-up testing.

Clinical Alert

1. Diagnosis of pancreatic insufficiency should not be made until three separate specimens exhibit no trypsin activity.
2. Bacterial protease may produce positive reactions when no trypsin is present; therefore, both positive and negative reactions should be carefully interpreted.

LEUKOCYTES IN STOOL

Normal Values

Negative for leukocytes

Explanation of Test

Microscopic examination of the feces for white blood cells is helpful in differentiating between certain bacterial diseases in which white blood cells are absent or ulcerative colitis in which there are increased leukocytes (see following lists). Persons with localizing abscesses or fistulas communicating with the bowel lumen will also have increased fecal leukocytes. Recognizable pus is seldom seen in stools unless there is a draining rectal infection, ulceration, or fungating process.

Procedure

See "Random Collection of Stool Specimens," page 255. Mucus or liquid stool specimen can be used.

Clinical Implications

1. Large amounts of leukocytes accompany
   - **a.** Chronic ulcerative colitis
   - **b.** Chronic bacillary dysentery
   - **c.** Localized abscesses
   - **d.** Fistulas of sigmoid rectum or anus
2. Primary mononuclear leukocytes appear in typhoid.
3. Primary polymorphonuclear leukocytes appear in
   - **a.** Shigellosis
   - **b.** Salmonellosis
   - **c.** Yersinia
   - **d.** Invasive *Escherichia coli* diarrhea
   - **e.** Ulcerative colitis
4. Absence of leukocytes is associated with
   - **a.** Cholera
   - **b.** Nonspecific diarrhea
   - **c.** Viral diarrhea
   - **d.** Amebic colitis
   - **e.** Noninvasive *E. coli* diarrhea
   - **f.** Toxigenic bacteria—*Staphylococcus* spp., *Clostridium* cholera
   - **g.** Parasites—*Giardia, Entamoeba*

Patient Preparation

1. Explain purpose of test and collection procedure. Follow guidelines in Chapter 1 regarding safe, effective informed *pretest* care.
2. Barium procedures and laxatives should be avoided for 1 week before test.
3. Withhold antibiotic therapy until after collection.

Patient Aftercare

1. Interpret abnormal test results. Monitor for diarrhea and rectal and colon infections. Counsel concerning need for follow-up tests and treatment.
2. See Chapter 1 guidelines for safe, effective, informed *posttest* care.

PORPHYRINS IN STOOL ●

Normal Values

Coproporphyrin: 400–1200 μg/24 hr
Uroporphyrin: 10–40 μg/24 hr

> **NOTE:** *Reference values vary widely from lab to lab, depending on testing method used.*

Explanation of Test

Analysis of fecal porphyrins is especially helpful in the differential diagnoses of coproporphyria, porphyria variegata, or protoporphyria. The pattern of porphyrin excretion in feces and urine and accumulation within the red blood cells provides the basis for detecting and differentiating the porphyrias (see "Porphyrins and Porphobilinogens," p. 227, and red cells, p. 76.

Procedure

1. Collect a 24- to 72-hour stool specimen. Contact laboratory for specific protocols.
2. Protect specimen from heat and light.
3. If specimen cannot be transferred to lab immediately, it must be frozen.
4. Label each container with date and time interval of collection.

Clinical Implications

1. *Increased fecal coproporphyrin* is associated with
   - **a.** Coproporphyria, persistently high (hereditary)
   - **b.** Porphyria variegata
   - **c.** Protoporphyria
   - **d.** Hemolytic anemia
2. *Increased fecal protoporphyrin* is associated with
   - **a.** Porphyria variegata
   - **b.** Protoporphyria
   - **c.** Acquired liver disease

Patient Preparation

1. Explain purpose and procedure of 24- to 72-hour stool collection.
2. Barium and laxatives should be withheld for 1 week before specimen collection.
3. Avoid alcohol intake during the collection period.
4. Follow guidelines in Chapter 1 for safe, effective, informed *pretest* care.

Patient Aftercare

1. Interpret outcomes. Monitor as appropriate for porphyria. Follow guidelines in Chapter 1 for safe, effective, informed *posttest* care.
2. Explain need for possible follow-up testing.

STOOL ELECTROLYTES: SODIUM, CHLORIDE, POTASSIUM ●

Normal Values

Sodium: 5.8–9.8 mEq/24 hr
Chloride: 2.5–3.9 mEq/24 hr
Potassium: 15.7–20.7 mEq/24 hr

> **NOTE:** *Reference values vary from laboratory to laboratory. Check with your laboratory for normal values.*

Explanation of Test
Stool electrolytes are used to assess electrolyte imbalance in persons with diarrhea. The stool electrolytes must be evaluated along with the serum and urine electrolytes, as well as interpreting clinical findings in the patient.

Procedure
Collect random or 24-hour stool specimen. See page 267 for collection protocols. Keep specimen covered and refrigerated.

Interfering Factors
The stool cannot be contaminated with urine.

Clinical Implications
1. Abnormalities occur in
   a. Idiopathic proctocolitis: *Increased* sodium (Na) and chloride (Cl), *normal* potassium (K).
   b. Ileostomy: *Increased* sodium (Na) and chloride (Cl), *low* potassium (K).
   c. Cholera: *Increased* sodium (Na) and chloride (Cl).
2. Chloride is greatly increased in stool in the following conditions:
   a. Congenital chloride diarrhea
   b. Acquired chloride diarrhea
   c. Secondary chloride diarrhea
   d. Idiopathic protocolitis
   e. Cholera

Patient Preparation
1. Explain purpose of test, procedure for stool collection, and interfering factors.
2. Withhold barium and laxatives for 1 week before collection of specimen.
3. Follow safe, effective, informed, *pretest* care guidelines in Chapter 1.

Patient Aftercare
1. Interpret abnormal test outcomes. Monitor diarrhea episodes and record findings. Assess for electrolyte imbalances.
2. Follow safe, effective, informed *posttest* care guidelines in Chapter 1.

BIBLIOGRAPHY

Bakerman, S: in ABCs of Interpretive Laboratory Data, 2nd ed, Greenville, NC, Interpretive Laboratory Data, 1984

Blair ER et al (eds): Damon Clinical Laboratories Handbook. Stow, OH, Lexi-Comp, 1991

Boucher A et al: Gastroenterology: Clinical Science and Practice, 2nd ed. Philadelphia: WB Saunders, 1994

Helena Laboratories: Color Screen Self-Test: A Technical Overview. Beaumont, TX, Helena Laboratories, 1992

Henry JB: Todd–Sanford–Davidsohn Clinical Diagnosis and Management by Laboratory Methods, 18th ed. Philadelphia, WB Saunders, 1990

Krom FA et al: Clinitesting neonatal stools. Neonatal Network 8(2):37–40, October 1989

Matzen RN: Fecal occult blood testing: Guidelines for follow-up after positive findings. Postgraduate Medicine 90:181–191, 1991

Medical Science Laboratories: Laboratory Handbook. Hudson, OH, Lexi-Comp, 1992

Ming SC, Goldman H: Pathology of the Gastrointestinal Tract. Philadelphia, WB Saunders, 1992

Sacker RA, McPherson RA: Widmann's Clinical Interpretation of Laboratory Tests, 10th ed. Philadelphia, FA Davis, 1991

Siegel DL, Edelstein PH, Nachomken I: Inappropriate testing for diarrheal diseases in the hospital. JAMA 263: 979, 1990

Speicher CE: The Right Test, a Physician's Guide to Laboratory Medicine, 2nd ed. Philadelphia, WB Saunders, 1993

Wallach J. Interpretation of Laboratory Tests, Synopsis of Laboratory Medicine, 5th ed. Boston, Little, Brown & Co, 1992

5

Cerebrospinal Fluid Studies

DESCRIPTION, FORMATION, AND COMPOSITION OF CEREBROSPINAL FLUID (CSF)

Background

Cerebrospinal fluid (CSF) is a clear, colorless fluid formed within the cavities or ventricles of the brain by the choroid plexus and diffused blood plasma. Approximately 500 ml of CSF fluid is formed per day, although only 120 to 150 ml is present in the system at any one time. The CSF is completely replaced about three times a day.

Circulating slowly from the ventricular system into the spaces surrounding the brain and spinal cord, CSF serves as an hydraulic shock absorber, diffusing external forces to the skull that might otherwise cause severe injury. The CSF also helps to regulate intracranial pressure and to transport nutrients and waste products. This fluid is believed to influence other control mechanisms, such as glucose levels on the hypothalamus, hunger sensations, and eating behaviors.

Most CSF constituents are present in the same or in lower concentrations than in the blood plasma, except for chloride concentrations, which are usually higher. Thus, similar to blood plasma, CSF contains few cells and little protein. Disease, however, can cause elements ordinarily restrained by the blood–brain barrier to enter the spinal fluid. Erythrocytes and leukocytes can enter the CSF from the rupture of blood vessels or from meningeal reaction to irritation. Bilirubin can be found in the spinal fluid after intracranial hemorrhage. In such cases, the arachnoid granulations and the nerve root sheaths will reabsorb the bloody fluid. Normal CSF pressure will consequently be maintained by the absorption of CSF in amounts equal to production. Blockage will cause an increase in the amount of CSF, resulting in hydrocephalus in infants or increased intracranial pressure in adults. Of the many factors that regulate the level of CSF pressure, venous pressure is the most important because the reabsorbed fluid ultimately drains into the venous system.

Despite the continuous production (about 0.3 ml/min) and reabsorption of CSF and the exchange of substances between the CSF and the blood plasma, considerable pooling occurs in the lumbar sac. The lumbar sac at L-4 to L-5 is the usual site for puncture because damage to the nervous system is less likely to occur in this area. In infants, the spinal cord is situated more caudally than in adults (L-3 to L-4 until 9 months of age, when the cord ascends to L-1 to L-2); therefore, a low lumbar puncture should be made.

LUMBAR PUNCTURE

Explanation of Test

Cerebrospinal fluid is obtained by lumbar puncture. A lumbar puncture is done for the following reasons:

1. To examine the spinal fluid (for example, suspected meningitis or intracranial hemorrhage).
2. To determine the level of CSF pressure, to document impaired CSF flow, or to lower the pressure by removing a volume of fluid. (Fluid removal can be dangerous because the brain stem can dislocate.)
3. To introduce anesthetics, drugs, or contrast media used for x-ray studies into the spinal cord.

Certain observations are made each time lumbar puncture is performed (Table 5-1):

1. The general appearance, consistency, and tendency of the CSF to clot are noted.
2. The CSF pressure is measured.
3. The CSF cell count is performed to distinguish types of cells present; this must be done within 2 hours of obtaining the CSF sample.
4. The CSF protein, chloride, and glucose concentrations are determined.
5. Other clinical serologic and bacteriologic tests are done when the patient's condition warrants (for example, culture for aerobic and anaerobic bacteria or for tuberculosis).
6. There are tumor markers in CSF that are useful as supplements to CSF cytological analysis (Table 5-2).

Clinical Alert

1. Blood levels for specific substances should always be measured simultaneously with the CSF determinations for meaningful interpretation of results.
2. Before the lumbar puncture, check eyegrounds for evidence of papilledema, because its presence may signal potential problems or complications of lumbar puncture.

PROCEDURE FOR STERILE LUMBAR PUNCTURE (SPINAL TAP)

1. The patient is usually placed in a side-lying position with head flexed onto the chest, and the knees drawn up to, but not compressing, the abdomen to "bow" the back. This position helps increase the space between the lower lumbar vertebrae so that the spinal needle can be inserted more easily between the spinal processes. However, a sitting position with head flexed to chest can be used. The patient is helped to relax and instructed to breathe slowly and deeply with mouth open.
2. The puncture site is selected, usually between L-4 and L-5 or lower. There is a little bone landmark at the L5-S interspace ("surgeon's delight") that helps locate the puncture site. The site is thoroughly cleansed with

TABLE 5-1
Normal CSF Values

Volume	90–150 ml; child: 60–100 ml		
Appearance	Crystal clear, colorless		
Pressure	50–180 mm H_20		
Total cell count	RBCs: 0		
		Adults	***Newborn (0–14 d)***
	WBCs	0–5 cells	0–30 cells
	Diff		
	Lymphs	40%–80%	5%–35%
	Monos	15%–45%	50%–90%
	Polys	0%–6%	0%–8%
Specific gravity	1.006–1.008		
Osmolality	280–290 mOsm/kg		
CLINICAL TESTS			
Glucose	40–70 mg/dl		
Protein			
Lumbar	Neonates		15–100 mg/dl
	3 mo–60 yr		15–45 mg/dl
	> 60 yr		15–60 mg/dl
Cisternal			15–25 mg/dl
Ventricular			15–16 mg/dl
Lactic acid	10–24 mg/dl		
Glutamine	0.4–1.1 μmol/ml		
Albumin	10–30 mg/dl		
Urea nitrogen	5–25 mg/dl		
Creatinine	0.5–1.2 mg/dl		
Cholesterol	0.2–0.6 mg/dl		
Uric acid	0.5–4.5 mg/dl		
Bilirubin	0 (none)		
LDH	1/10 that of serum LDH		
ELECTROLYTES AND pH			
pH	7.30–7.40		
Chloride	118–132 mEq/L		
Sodium	144–154 mEq/L		
Potassium	2.0–3.5 mEq/L		
CO_2 content	25–30 mEq/L (mmol)		
Pco_2	42–53 mm Hg		
Po_2	40–44 mm Hg		
Calcium	2.1–2.7 mEq/L		
Magnesium	2.4 mEq/L		
SEROLOGY AND MICROBIOLOGY			
VDRL	Negative		
Bacteria	None present		
Viruses	None present		

TABLE 5-2
Tumor Markers in CSF

Determination	*For Diagnosis of*	*Normal Values*
alpha-Fetoprotein (AFP)	CNS dysgerminomas and meningeal carcinomas	<1.5 mg/ml
beta-Glucuronidase	Possible meningeal carcinomatosis	<49 mU/L Indeterminate 49–70 mU/L Suspicious >70 mU/L
Carcinoembryonic antigen (CEA)	Meningeal carcinomatosis: intradural or extradural or brain parenchymal metastasis from adenocarcinoma. Although the assay appears to be specific for adenocarcinoma and squamous cell carcinoma, increased CEA values in CSF are not seen in all such tumors of the brain.	<0.6 mg/ml
Human chorionic gonadotropin (HCG)	Adjunct for determining CNS dysgerminomas and meningeal carcinomatosis	<0.21 U/L
Lysozyme (muramidase)	CNS tumors, especially myoclonal and monocytic leukemia	4–13 µg/ml

an antiseptic solution, and the surrounding area is draped with sterile towels in such a way that the drapes do not obscure important landmarks.

3. A local anesthetic is then injected slowly into the dermis around the intended puncture site.
4. A spinal needle with stylet is inserted into the midline between the spines of the lumbar space and slowly advanced until it enters the subarachnoid space. The patient may feel the entry ("pop") of the needle through the dura mater. Once this happens, the patient can be helped to straighten the legs slowly to relieve abdominal compression.
5. With the needle remaining in the subarachnoid space, the stylet is removed and a pressure manometer is attached to the needle to record the opening CSF pressure.

NOTE: *If the initial pressure is normal, the Queckenstedt's test may be done. (This test is not done if a central nervous system [CNS] tumor is suspected.) In this test, pressure is placed on both jugular veins to occlude them temporarily and to produce an acute rise in CSF pressure. Normally, pressure rapidly returns to average levels after jugular vein occlusion is re-*

moved. Total or partial spinal fluid blockage is diagnosed if the lumbar pressure fails to rise when both jugular veins are compressed, or if the pressure requires more than 20 seconds to fall after compression is released.

6. A specimen of 10 to 20 ml of CSF is removed. Usually three samples of 2- to 3-ml each are taken, placed in separate, sterile vials, and labeled sequentially: No. 1 is used for chemistry and serology; No. 2 is used for microbiology studies; No. 3 is used for hematology cell counts. A closing pressure reading may be taken before the needle is withdrawn. In cases of increased intracranial pressure (ICP), very little fluid is withdrawn because of the risk that the brain stem may shift out of place.
7. A small sterile dressing is applied to the puncture site.
8. Tubes should be correctly labeled with the proper sequential number (1, 2, or 3), the patient's name, and date. Specimens of CSF must be immediately delivered to the laboratory, where they should be given to a lab person with specific instructions regarding the testing. The spinal fluid samples should never be placed in the refrigerator, because refrigeration will alter test results if bacteriologic and fungal studies are ordered. Analysis should be started immediately. If viral studies are to be done, a portion of specimen should be frozen.
9. Record the procedure start and completion times, patient's status, the CSF appearance, and the pressure readings.

Patient Preparation

1. Explain the purpose, benefits and risks of the lumbar puncture and explain tests to be performed on CSF specimen; present a step-by-step description of the actual procedure. Emphasize the need for patient cooperation. Assess for contraindications or impediments, such as arthritis.
2. Help the patient relax by having them breathe slowly and deeply. The patient needs to refrain from breath-holding, straining, moving, and talking during the procedure.
3. Follow the guidelines in Chapter 1 for safe, effective, informed *pretest* care.

Patient Aftercare

1. The patient should lie prone (flat or horizontal, or on the abdomen) for approximately 4 to 8 hours. Turning from side to side is permitted as long as the body is kept in a horizontal position.
2. Women may have difficulty voiding in this position. The use of a "fracture bedpan" may help.
3. Fluids are encouraged to help prevent or to relieve possible headache.
4. Interpret test outcomes. Assess and monitor for abnormal outcomes and complications, such as paralysis (or progression of paralysis, as with spinal tumor), hematoma, meningitis, asphyxiation of infants owing to tracheal obstruction from pushing the head forward, and infection. Institute infection control precautions if test outcomes reveal an infectious process.
5. Observe for neurologic changes in level of consciousness, change in

pupils, temperature, increased blood pressure, irritability, numbness and tingling sensations, especially the lower extremities.

6. If headache should occur, administer ordered analgesics and encourage a longer period of flat bed rest. If headache persists, a "blood patch" may need to be done. When the practitioner performs a blood patch, a small amount of the patient's own blood is introduced into the spinal canal at the same level that the canal was previously entered. For reasons not totally understood, this blood patch very effectively stops spinal headaches within a very short time.
7. Check the puncture site for leakage.
8. Document the procedure completion and any problems encountered or complaints voiced.
9. Follow guidelines in Chapter 1 for safe, effective, informed *posttest* care.

Clinical Alert

1. Extreme caution should be used when performing lumbar puncture if ICP is elevated, especially in the presence of papilledema or split cranial sutures. However, with some cases of increased ICP, such as with a coma, intracranial bleeding, or suspected meningitis, the need to establish a diagnosis is absolutely essential and outweighs the danger of the procedure.
2. Other contraindications to lumbar puncture are
   - Suspected epidural infection
   - Infection or severe dermatologic disease in the lumbar area, which may be introduced into the spinal canal
   - Severe psychiatric or neurotic problems; chronic back pain
   - Anatomic malformations, scarring in puncture site areas, or previous spinal surgery at site
3. If there is CSF leakage at the puncture site, notify the physician immediately. Document findings.
4. Observe universal precautions (Appendix IX) when handling CSF specimens.

CSF PRESSURE

Normal Values

50–180 mm H_2O (in the lateral recumbent position).

This value is height-dependent and will change with the horizontal or sitting posture.

Background

The CSF pressure is directly related to pressure in the jugular and vertebral veins that connect with the intracranial dural sinuses and the spinal dura. In conditions such as congestive heart failure or obstruction of the superior vena cava, CSF pressure is increased, but in circulatory collapse, it is decreased.

Explanation of Test

Pressure measurement is done to detect impairment of CSF flow or to lower the CSF pressure by removing a small volume of CSF fluid. Provided initial pressure is not elevated and there is no marked fall in pressure when fluid is removed, from 10 to 20 ml of CSF may be removed without danger to the patient.

Procedure

1. The CSF pressure should be measured before any CSF fluid is withdrawn.
2. Usually three samples of 2- to 3-ml each are taken and placed in separate, sterile vials and labeled sequentially:
   No. 1 is used for chemistry and serology.
   No. 2 is used for microbiology studies.
   No. 3 is used for hematology cell counts.

Clinical Implications

1. *Increases* in CSF pressure can be a significant finding in:
   - **a.** Intracranial tumors; abscess
   - **b.** Pyogenic or tuberculous meningitis
   - **c.** Inflammation of meninges
   - **d.** Hypoosmolality owing to hemodialysis
   - **e.** Congestive heart failure
   - **f.** Acute obstruction of superior vena cava
   - **g.** Subarachnoid hemorrhage
   - **h.** Cerebral hemorrhage
   - **i.** Subdural hematoma
   - **j.** Uremia
2. *Decreases* in pressure can be a significant finding in:
   - **a.** Circulatory collapse
   - **b.** Severe dehydration
   - **c.** Hyperosmolality
   - **d.** Leakage of spinal fluid
   - **e.** Complete subarachnoid block
3. *Significant variations* between opening and closing CSF pressures can be found in
   - **a.** Tumors or spinal blockage when there is a large pressure drop indicative of a small CSF pool
   - **b.** Hydrocephalus when there is a small pressure drop that is indicative of a large CSF pool

Clinical Alert

If initial CSF pressure is near 200 mm, only 1 to 2 ml of fluid should be removed. Spinal cord compression or cerebellar or brain stem herniation could result. See **Note** in spinal tap procedure for Queckenstedt's test.

Interfering Factors

1. Slight elevations of pressure may occur in an anxious patient who holds the breath or tenses muscles.
2. If a patient's knees are flexed too firmly against the abdomen, venous compressions will cause an elevation in pressure. This can occur in patients of either normal weight or who are obese.

Patient Preparation

1. See page 282 for care before lumbar puncture.
2. Follow guidelines in Chapter 1 for safe, effective, informed *pretest* care.

Patient Aftercare

1. Interpret abnormal pressure levels, monitor and intervene appropriately to prevent complications.
2. See pages 282–283 for care after lumbar puncture.
3. Follow guidelines in Chapter 1 for safe, effective, informed *posttest* care.

CSF COLOR AND APPEARANCE ●

Normal Values

Clear and colorless

Background

Normal CSF is crystal clear, with the appearance and viscosity of water. Abnormal CSF may appear hazy, cloudy, smokey, or bloody. Clotting of CSF is abnormal and indicates increased protein or fibrinogen present in CSF.

Explanation of Test

Inflammatory diseases, hemorrhage, tumors, and trauma bring about elevated cell counts and corresponding changes in appearance.

Procedure

The CSF should be compared with a test tube of distilled water held against a white background. If there is no turbidity, newsprint can be read through the CSF in the tube.

Clinical Implications

1. Abnormal colors (see Table 5-3)—their causes and indications:
   a. Blood (the blood is evenly mixed in all three tubes in subarachnoid and cerebral hemorrhage). (See Chart 5-1 on page 286 for differentiation of bloody spinal tap versus cerebral hemorrhage.) Clear CSF fluid does not rule out intracranial hemorrhage.
   b. Turbidity is graded from 1+ to 4+ and may be caused by:
      (1) Leukocytes (pleocytosis)
      (2) Red blood cells

TABLE 5-3
Color Changes in CSF Suggestive of Disease States

Appearance	*Condition*
Opalescent, slightly yellow with delicate clot	Tuberculous meningitis
Opalescent to purulent, slightly yellow with coarse clot	Acute pyogenic meningitis
Slightly yellow; may be clear or opalescent with delicate clot	Acute anterior poliomyelitis
Bloody; purulent; may be turbid	Primary amebic meningoencephalitis
Generally clear, but may be xanthochromic	Tumor of brain or cord
Xanthochromic	Toxoplasmosis

CHART 5-1
Differentiation of Bloody CSF Caused by Subarachnoid Hemorrhage Versus Traumatic Lumbar Puncture

CSF FINDINGS	SUBARACHNOID HEMORRHAGE	TRAUMATIC LUMBAR PUNCTURE
CSF pressure	Often increased	Low
Blood in CSF collection tubes	Mix with blood is uniform in all tubes	First tubes more bloody than subsequent tubes
CSF clotting	Does not clot	Often clots
Xanthochromia	Present if >8–12 hours since cerebral hemorrhage	Absent unless patient is jaundiced
Immediate repeat of lumbar puncture at higher level	CSF same as initial puncture	CSF clear (if atraumatic)

Clinical Alert

Spinal fluid should be cultured for bacteria, fungi, and tuberculosis. In children, *Haemophilus influenzae*, type B, is the most common cause of bacterial meningitis; for adults, the most common bacterial pathogens for meningitis are meningococci and pneumococci.

(3) Microorganisms, such as fungus and bacteria
(4) Radiologic contrast media
(5) Epidural fat aspirated (pale pink to dark yellow)

c. Xanthochromia (pale pink to dark yellow) caused by:
(1) Oxyhemoglobin from lysed RBCs present in CSF before lumbar puncture
(2) Methemoglobin
(3) Bilirubin
(4) Increased protein (> 150 mg/dl)
(5) Melanin (meningeae melanocarcinoma)
(6) Carotene (systemic carotenemia)

Interfering Factors

1. The CSF can look xanthochromic from contamination by methylate used to disinfect skin.
2. If the blood in the specimen is due to a traumatic spinal tap, the CSF in the third tube should be clearer than that in tube 1 or 2; a traumatic tap makes interpretation of results difficult.

Patient Preparation

1. Observations of color and appearance of CSF are always noted.
2. See page 282 for care before lumbar puncture.

Patient Aftercare

1. Recognize abnormal color and presence of turbidity and monitor appropriately. Notify physician if necessary.
2. See pages 282–283 for care after lumbar puncture.

CSF MICROSCOPIC EXAMINATION OF CELLS; TOTAL CELL COUNT; DIFFERENTIAL CELL COUNT ●

Normal Values

Adults: 0–5 WBC/μg/L or 0–5×10^6 WBC/L
Newborn: 0–30×10^6 WBC/L

Differential	*Adults*	*Newborn (0–14 days)*
Lymphocytes	40%–80%	5%–35%
Monocytes	15%–45%	50%–90%
Polys	0%–6%	0%–8%

Background

Normal CSF is essentially free of cells. An increase in the number of white blood cells (WBCs) in CSF is termed *pleocytosis.* Disease processes may lead to abrupt increases or decreases of cells.

Explanation of Test

The CSF is examined for the presence of RBCs and WBCs. The cells are counted and identified by cell type; the percentage of cell type is compared with the total number of white or red cells present. In general, inflammatory disease, hemorrhage, neoplasms, and trauma will cause an elevated WBC cell count.

Procedure

Tube No. 3 is used for counting the cells present in the CSF sample. The cells are counted by either a manual counting chamber or by electronic means. A CSF smear is made and counted for differentiation of cells.

Clinical Implications

A. *White cell counts*

1. White cell counts above 500 usually arise from a purulent infection and are preponderantly granulocytes (neutrophils). Neutrophilic reaction classically suggests meningitis caused by a pyogenic organism, in which case the WBC count can exceed 1000×10^6 and can reach $20{,}000 \times 10^6$.
   - **a.** Increases in neutrophils are associated with
     - **(1)** Bacterial meningitis
     - **(2)** Early viral meningitis
     - **(3)** Early tuberculosis
     - **(4)** Fungal mycositic meningitis
     - **(5)** Amebic encephalomyelitis
     - **(6)** Early stages of meningovascular syphilis
     - **(7)** Aseptic meningitis
     - **(8)** Systemic lupus erythematosus (SLE)
   - **b.** Noninfectious causes of neutrophilia are
     - **(1)** Reaction to central nervous system hemorrhage
     - **(2)** Injection of foreign materials into subarachnoid space (for example, x-ray contrast medium or anticancer drugs)
     - **(3)** Pneumoencephalogram
     - **(4)** Metastatic tumor
     - **(5)** Chronic granulocytic leukemia involving the central nervous system

Clinical Alert

Neutrophilic reaction classically suggests meningitis caused by a pyogenic organism.

2. White counts of 300 to 500 with preponderantly lymphocytes are indicative of
   - **a.** Viral and aseptic meningitis
   - **b.** Syphilis of CNS
   - **c.** Tuberculous meningitis
   - **d.** Brain tumor or abscess
   - **e.** Partially treated bacterial meningitis
   - **f.** Multiple sclerosis (33% of cases)
   - **g.** Encephalopathy caused by drug abuse
   - **h.** Guillain-Barré syndrome (15%)
   - **i.** Acute disseminated encephalomyelitis

j. Sarcoidosis of meninges
k. HTLV III
l. Atypical bacterial meningitis such as Lyme disease
m. Fungal meningitis
n. Parasitic meningitis

3. White cell counts with 40% or more monocytes are seen after
   a. Subarachnoid hemorrhage
   b. Toxoplasmosis
4. Malignant cells (lymphocytes or histiocytes) may be present with primary and metastatic brain tumors, especially with meningeal extension.
5. Increased numbers of plasma cells may occur in association with lymphocytic reactions.
   a. Subacute and chronic inflammatory processes
   b. Multiple sclerosis
   c. Leukoencephalitis
   d. Delayed hypersensitivity responses
   e. Subacute viral encephalitis
   f. Meningitis (tuberculous or fungal)
   g. Certain brain tumors

   Plasma cells are responsible for an increase in IgG and altered patterns in immunoelectrophoresis.
6. Macrophages are present in traumatic and ischemic cranial infarcts, tuberculous or mycotic meningitis, reaction to erythrocytes, foreign substances, or lipids in the CSF.
7. Glial, ependymal, and plexus cells may be present after surgical procedures or trauma to the CNS.
8. Leukemic cells appear in CSF after several remissions have been achieved by chemotherapy. Leukemic cells also may appear in CSF during apparent remission and after chemotherapy has been discontinued.
9. The WBC count may increase owing to a contaminated lumbar puncture.
10. The WBCs may increase owing to repeated lumbar punctures.

Patient Preparation

1. See page 282 for care before lumbar puncture.
2. Follow guidelines in Chapter 1 for safe, effective, informed *pretest* care.

Patient Aftercare

1. Interpret abnormal cell counts. Monitor and intervene as appropriate for infection and malignancy.
2. See pages 282–283 for care after lumbar puncture.
3. Follow guidelines in Chapter 1 for safe, effective, informed *posttest* care.

CSF CHLORIDE ●

Normal Values

Adult: 120–130 mEq/L
Child: 111–130 mEq/L

Explanation of Test

Any condition that alters the blood plasma chloride level will also affect the CSF chloride level. Chlorides in CSF are normally higher (1.2–1) than in blood plasma. The measurement of CSF chloride is most useful in the diagnosis of tuberculous meningitis.

Clinical Implications

Decreased levels are associated with

1. Tuberculous meningitis
2. Bacterial meningitis

Interfering Factors

1. Concurrent intravenous administration of chloride will alter test results.
2. Test values are invalidated if blood, as from a traumatic tap, is mixed with the CSF specimen.

Patient Preparation

1. See page 282 for care before lumbar puncture.
2. Follow guidelines in Chapter 1 for safe, effective, informed *pretest* care.

Patient Aftercare

1. Interpret abnormal chloride levels; monitor and intervene appropriately to prevent complications.
2. See pages 282–283 for care after lumbar puncture.
3. Follow guidelines in Chapter 1 for safe, effective, informed *posttest* care.

CSF GLUCOSE ●

Normal Values

Adult: 40–70 mg/dl
Child: 60–80 mg/dl
CSF/plasma glucose ratio = 0.4 to 0.80
CSF = 40%–80% of blood glucose levels

Background

The CSF glucose level varies with the blood glucose levels. It is usually about 60% of blood glucose. A blood glucose specimen should be obtained at least 60 minutes before lumbar puncture for comparisons. Any changes in blood sugar are reflected in the CSF 1 to 3 hours later.

Explanation of Test

This measurement is helpful in determining impaired transport of glucose from plasma to CSF and increased use of glucose by the CNS, leukocytes, and microorganisms.

Procedure

One milliliter (1 ml) of CSF is put in a sterile tube. The glucose test should be done on tube No. 1 when three tubes of CSF are taken. Accurate evaluation of CSF glucose requires a simultaneous plasma glucose measurement.

Clinical Implications

1. *Decreased* levels are associated with
   a. Acute bacterial meningitis (CSF levels of 25% to 40% of blood glucose is almost diagnostic)
   b. Tuberculosis, fungal, and amebic meningitis
   c. Subarachnoid hemorrhage
   d. Neoplasia
   e. Insulinoma (hypoglycemia)
2. *Uncommonly decreased* in
   a. Lymphomas with meningeal spread
   b. Leukemia with meningeal spread
   c. Mumps meningoencephalitis
   d. Sarcoidosis and neurosyphilis
3. *Increased* levels are associated with diabetes and diabetic coma.

Interfering Factors

1. False decreased levels may be due to cellular and bacterial metabolism if the test is not performed immediately.
2. Hemolyzed samples may give misleading results.

Clinical Alert

1. *All types* of organisms consume glucose; therefore, decreased glucose reflects bacterial activity.
2. Panic value is less than 20 mg/dl.

Patient Preparation

1. See page 282 for care before lumbar puncture.
2. Explain the need for a blood specimen test for glucose.
3. Follow guidelines in Chapter 1 for safe, effective, informed *pretest* care.

Patient Aftercare

1. Interpret abnormal glucose levels and correlate with presence of meningitis, cancer, hemorrhage, and diabetes. Monitor and intervene appropriately to prevent complications.
2. See pages 282–283 for care after lumbar puncture.

CSF GLUTAMINE

Normal Values
0.4–1.1 μmol/ml
Reference values vary.

Background
Glutamine is synthesized in brain tissue from ammoniac and glutamic acids. Production of glutamine provides a mechanism for removing ammonia from the CNS.

Explanation of Test
This test is used to determine hepatic encephalopathy and aids in evaluation of its severity. It also is used for evaluation of coma.

Procedure
Two milliliters (2 ml) of CSF is needed for the glutamine test. Tube No. 1 is used for the chemistry test. If cells are present, the samples must be centrifuged to remove the cells.

Clinical Implications
Increased levels are associated with

1. Hepatic coma
2. Reye's syndrome
3. Some cases of meningitis
4. Hepatic encephalopathy
5. CSF pleocytosis

Patient Preparation
1. See page 282 for care before lumbar puncture.
2. Follow guidelines in Chapter 1 for safe, effective, informed *pretest* care.

Patient Aftercare
1. Interpret abnormal glutamine levels and correlate with presence of liver disease or coma. Monitor and intervene appropriately to prevent complications.
2. See pages 282–283 for care after lumbar puncture.
3. Follow guidelines in Chapter 1 for safe, effective, informed *posttest* care.

CSF LACTIC ACID

Normal Values
< 24 mg/dl (reported reference values vary)
Adult: 10–25 mg/dl or 0–2.8 mmol/L
Newborn: up to 45 mg/dl

Background
The source of CSF lactic acid is probably CNS anaerobic metabolism. Lactic acid in CSF may vary independently of the level in the blood. It appears that diffusion of lactic acid across the blood–CSF barrier is very slow.

Explanation of Test

Measurement of CSF lactate may be useful as a screening test to detect CNS disease and in the differential diagnosis of bacterial meningitis versus viral meningitis (nonbacterial meningitis).

Procedure

Two milliliter (2 ml) of CSF is needed in a sterile test tube (tube No. 1). Do not refrigerate the sample.

Clinical Implications

Increased levels are associated with

1. Bacterial meningitis
2. Hypocapnia
3. Hydrocephalus
4. Brain abscess or tumor
5. Cerebral ischemia
6. Traumatic brain injury
7. Seizures
8. Stroke (cerebral infarct)
9. Pleocytosis

Patient Preparation

1. See page 282 for care before lumbar puncture.
2. Follow guidelines in Chapter 1 for safe, effective, informed *pretest* care.

Patient Aftercare

1. Interpret test outcomes; monitor and intervene appropriately to detect CNS disease and prevent complications.
2. See pages 282–283 for care after lumbar puncture.
3. Follow guidelines in Chapter 1 for safe, effective, informed *posttest* care.

Clinical Alert

Increases in lactic acid must be interpreted in light of the clinical findings and in conjunction with glucose, protein, and cell count of the CSF. Equivocal results in some instances of aseptic meningitis may lead to erroneous diagnosis of a bacterial etiology.

CSF LACTATE DEHYDROGENASE (LD/LDH); CSF LDH ISOENZYMES

Normal Values

One-tenth that of serum

Background

Although many different enzymes have been measured in CSF, only lactate dehydrogenase (LDH) appears useful clinically. Sources of LDH in normal CSF include diffusion across the blood–CSF barrier, diffusion across the brain–CSF barrier, and LDH activity in cellular elements of CSF such as leukocytes, bacteria, and tumor cells. Because the brain tissue is rich in LDH, damaged CNS tissue can cause increased levels of LDH in the CSF.

Explanation of Test

High levels of LDH occur in about 90% of bacterial meningitis cases and in only 10% of viral meningitis cases. When high levels of LDH do occur in viral meningitis, the condition is usually associated with encephalitis and a poor prognosis. Tests of LDH isoenzymes have been used to improve the specificity of LDH measurements and are useful for differential diagnoses of viral versus bacterial meningitis (see Chap. 6 for a complete description of isoenzymes).

Procedure

One milliliter (1 ml) of CSF is needed and taken to the laboratory as quickly as possible. Tube No. 1 is used for LDH examination.

Clinical Implications

1. *Increased* LDH levels are associated with
   - **a.** Bacterial meningitis (90% of cases)
   - **b.** Viral meningitis (10% of cases) (cerebrovascular accident)
   - **c.** Leukemia or lymphoma with meningeal infiltration
   - **d.** Metastatic carcinoma of the CNS
2. In viral meningitis, the presence of LDH isoenzyme 1, 2, or 3 reflects a combined CNS lymphocytic reaction.
3. In bacterial meningitis, the LDH isoenzyme pattern reflects a granulocytic reaction with LDH 4 and 5 present.
4. High levels of LDH 1 and 2 isoenzymes in either viral or bacterial meningitis suggest extensive CNS damage and a poor prognosis.

Interfering Factors

For the test to be valid, CSF must not be contaminated with blood. A bloody tap will make results difficult to interpret.

Patient Preparation

1. See page 282 for care before lumbar puncture.
2. Follow guidelines in Chapter 1 for safe, effective, informed *pretest* care.

Patient Aftercare

1. Interpret abnormal LDH test patterns; monitor and intervene appropriately to detect and prevent complications.
2. See pages 282–283 for care after lumbar puncture.
3. Follow guidelines in Chapter 1 for safe, effective, informed *posttest* care.

CSF TOTAL PROTEIN

Normal Values

Adults: 15–45 mg/dl (lumbar)
Adults: 15–25 mg/dl (cisternal)
Adults: 5–15 mg/dl (ventricular)
Neonates: 15–100 mg/dl (lumbar)
3 mo–60 yr: 15–45 mg/dl (lumbar)
> 60 yr: 15–60 mg/dl (lumbar)

Background

The CSF normally contains very little protein because the protein in blood serum is in the form of large molecules that do not easily cross the blood–brain barrier.

Explanation of Test

The CSF protein is useful as a nonspecific but reliable indication of CNS pathology, such as meningitis, brain abscess, neoplastic diseases, multiple sclerosis, and other degenerative processes causing neurologic disease.

Procedure

One milliliter (1 ml) of CSF is needed for protein analysis. Tube No. 1 should be used for protein examination.

Clinical Implications

1. *Moderate to marked increases* in total protein level are caused by increased permeability of the blood–CSF barrier, obstructions in circulation of CNS, or increased synthesis of protein within the central nervous system.
2. *Increased* CSF protein occurs in

a. Increased plasma protein	Slightly increased CSF protein owing to diffusion across blood–CSF barrier.
b. Traumatic tap	Normal pressure; CSF initially streaked with blood, clearing in subsequent tubes.
c. Increased permeability of blood–CSF barrier	CSF protein 100–500 mg/dl
d. Infectious conditions	
(1) Bacterial meningitis	Gram stain usually positive; culture may be negative if antibiotics have been administered
(2) Tuberculous	CSF protein 50–300 mg/dl; mixed cellular reaction typical
(3) Fungal meningitis	CSF protein 50–300 mg/dl; special stains helpful.

(4) Viral meningoencephalitis	CSF protein usually less than 100 mg/dl
e. Noninfectious conditions	
(1) Subarachnoid hemorrhage	Xanthochromia 2–4 hours after onset
(2) Intracerebral hemorrhage	CSF protein 20–200 mg/dl; marked fall in pressure after removing small amounts of CSF; xanthochromia
(3) Cerebral thrombosis	Slightly increased CSF protein in 40% of cases (usually under 100 mg/dl)
f. Endocrine, metabolic, and toxic endocrine conditions: diabetic neuropathy, myxedema, hyperadrenalism, hypoparathyroidism	CSF protein 50–150 mg/dl in about 50% of cases
g. Metabolic conditions: uremia, hypercalcemia, hypercapnia, dehydration	CSF protein slightly elevated (usually less than 100 mg/dl)
h. Toxic conditions: ethanol, isopropanol, heavy metals, phenytoin	CSF protein slightly elevated in about 40% of cases (usually less than 200 mg/dl)
i. Obstruction to circulation of CSF	
(1) Mechanical obstruction (tumor, abscess)	Rapid fall in pressure (yellow CSF; contains excess protein)
(2) Loculated effusion of CSF	Repeated taps may show progressive increase in CSF protein; diagnosis by myelography
j. Increased permeability of blood–CSF barrier	
(1) Meningitis	Increased CSF protein
(2) Guillain-Barré syndrome (infectious polyneuritis)	CSF protein usually 100–400 mg/dl
(3) Collagen diseases (eg, periarteritis, lupus)	CSF protein usually less than 400 mg/dl
k. Multiple sclerosis	CSF protein slightly increased
l. Subacute sclerosing panencephalitis	Increased CSF protein
m. Neurosyphilis	CSF protein normal or slightly increased < 100 mg/dl

2. *Decreased* CSF protein

a. Leakage of CSF
b. Removal of large volume CSF
c. Intracranial hypertension
d. Hyperthyroidism

Clinical Alert

More than 1000 mg/dl protein suggests subarachnoid block. In a complete spinal block, the lower the tumor location, the higher the CSF protein value.

Interfering Factors

1. Hemolyzed or xanthochromic drugs may falsely depress results.
2. Traumatic tap will invalidate the protein results.
3. See Patient Preparation and Aftercare on page 282.

Patient Preparation

1. See page 282 for care before lumbar puncture.
2. Follow guidelines in Chapter 1 for safe, effective, informed *pretest* care.

Patient Aftercare

1. Interpret abnormal CSF protein levels; monitor for both infectious and noninfectious conditions and intervene appropriately to prevent and detect complications.
2. See pages 282–283 for care after lumbar puncture.
3. Follow guidelines in Chapter 1 for safe, effective, informed *posttest* care.

CSF ALBUMIN AND IMMUNOGLOBULIN G (IgG) ●

Normal Values

Albumin: 11–48 mg/dl
IgG: 0–4.5 mg/dl (< 10% of total CSF protein)
IgG/albumin ratio: 0.15–3.8 ratio
IgG index: 0.77

Background

Because albumin and IgG are present normally in CSF, increased levels of both are indicative of damage to the CSF–blood barrier.

Explanation of Test

The measurement of albumin and IgG is used to evaluate the integrity and permeability of the blood–CSF barrier and to measure the synthesis of IgG within the CNS. The IgG/albumin index is a sensitive method to determine local CNS synthesis of IgG, and to detect increased permeability of the blood–CNS barrier.

$$\text{IgG index} = \frac{\text{CSF IgG/plasma IgG}}{\text{CSF albumin/plasma albumin.}}$$

The IgG index method is superior to the IgG/albumin ratio or measurement of IgG only.

Procedure

One-half milliliter (1/2 ml) of CSF in a sterile tube is needed for this test. It must be frozen if the determination is not done immediately.

Clinical Implications

1. *Increased albumin* occurs in

   a. Lesions of choroid plexus
   b. Blockage of CSF flow
   c. Bacterial meningitis
   d. Guillain-Barré syndrome
   e. Many infectious diseases such as typhoid fever, tularemia, diphtheria, septicemia
   f. Malignant neoplasms
   g. Polycythemia
   h. Hypothyroidism
   i. Diabetes mellitus
   j. Glomerulonephritis and other nephrotic syndromes
   k. Systemic lupus erythematosus
   l. Mercury poisoning and other toxic substances
   m. Electric shock
2. *Increased IgG/albumin index* (increased IgG, normal albumin) occurs in
   a. Subacute sclerosing leukoencephalitis
   b. Multiple sclerosis
   c. Neurosyphilis
   d. Chronic phases of CNS infections (subacute sclerosing panencephalitis [SSPE])
   e. Some patients with meningitis
   f. Some with Guillain-Barré syndrome

Interfering Factors

A traumatic tap will invalidate the results.

Patient Preparation

1. See page 282 for care before lumbar puncture.
2. Follow guidelines in Chapter 1 for safe, effective, informed *pretest* care.

Patient Aftercare

1. Interpret test outcomes; monitor and intervene appropriately to prevent and detect complications.
2. See pages 282–283 for care after lumbar puncture.
3. Follow guidelines in Chapter 1 for safe, effective, informed *posttest* care.

CSF PROTEIN ELECTROPHORESIS; ALBUMIN AND IMMUNOGLOBULIN G (IgG); OLIGOCLONAL BANDS; MULTIPLE SCLEROSIS PANEL ●

Normal Values

Albumin: 11–48 mg/dl
Oligoclonal banding: none present
IgG: 0–4.5 mg/dl
IgG/albumin: 0.15–3.8
Prealbumin: 2%–7%
Albumin: 52%–72%
$alpha_1$: 1%–7%
$alpha_2$: 3%–12%
beta: 7%–23%
A/G ratio: 2:1
gamma: 3%–13%

Background

Abnormalities of CSF in multiple sclerosis (MS) include an increase in total protein, primarily from IgG. The IgG protein in MS (and other neuropathies) migrates as a *diffuse* band. Abnormal immunoglobulins migrate as *discrete, sharp* bands called oligoclonal bands. This is the pattern observed in MS, a pattern of discrete bands within the gamma globulin portion of the electrophoretic pattern. However, oligoclonal bands are found in the CSF of patients with other types of inflammatory disease.

Explanation of Test

Fractionation (electrophoresis) of CSF protein is used to evaluate bacterial and viral infections and tumors of the CNS. However, the most important application of CSF protein electrophoresis is detection and diagnosis of MS.

Procedure

1. Three milliliters (3 ml) of CSF in tube No. 1 is used. The sample is frozen if test is not run immediately.
2. Cerebral spinal fluid is concentrated approximately 80-fold by selective permeability. A sample of the CSF concentrate is applied to a thin layer of agarose gel, and the patient's blood serum is positioned adjacent to the CSF sample. The agarose gel is then subjected to electrophoresis. A serum electrophoresis must be done at the same time for interpretation of the bands.

Clinical Implications

1. *Increases* in IgG or IgG/albumin index occur in
   - **a.** Infectious disease
   - **b.** Subacute sclerosing leukoencephalitis
   - **c.** Multiple sclerosis
   - **d.** Neurosyphilis
   - **e.** Chronic phases of CNS infections
   - **f.** Some patients with meningitis, Guillain-Barré syndrome, lupus erythematosus involving CNS, and other neurologic conditions
2. IgG is normally absent; it may be abnormally present in
   - **a.** Tumors of brain and meninges
   - **b.** Meningitis
   - **c.** Multiple sclerosis
3. *Increased* levels of albumin are associated with
   - **a.** Lesions to choroid plexus
   - **b.** Blockage of CSF flow
   - **c.** Damage to blood and CNS
4. *Increased* levels of gamma globulin in the presence of normal albumin level are associated with
   - **a.** Multiple sclerosis
   - **b.** Neurosyphilis

   c. Subacute sclerosing panencephalitis
   d. Chronic phase of CNS infections
5. Oligoclonal bands are found in
   a. Multiple sclerosis
   b. Cryptococcal meningitis
   c. Idiopathic polyneuritis
   d. Neurosyphilis
   e. Chronic rubella panencephalitis
   f. Subacute sclerosing panencephalitis
   g. Burkitt's lymphoma

Clinical Alert

1. A serum electrophoresis must be done at the same time as the CSF electrophoresis. An abnormal result is the finding of two or more bands in the CSF that are *not* present in the serum specimen.
2. Oligoclonic bands are not specific for MS; however, the sensitivity is 80%–94% for MS.

Interfering Factors

A traumatic tap will invalidate the results.

Patient Preparation

1. See page 282 for care before lumbar puncture.
2. Follow guidelines in Chapter 1 for safe, effective, informed *pretest* care.

Patient Aftercare

1. Interpret test outcome; monitor for MS and other CNS disorders and intervene appropriately to prevent and detect complications.
2. See pages 282–283 for care after lumbar puncture.
3. Follow guidelines in Chapter 1 for safe, effective, informed *posttest* care.

CSF SYPHILIS SEROLOGY

Normal values are negative (nonreactive). Neurosyphilis is characterized by an increase in protein, an increase in the number of lymphocytes, and a positive test for syphilis (see Chap. 8).

BIBLIOGRAPHY

Bakerman S: ABC's of Interpretive Laboratory data, 2nd ed. Greenville, NC, Interpretive Laboratory Data, 1984

Bishop ML, Duben-Engelkirk JL, Fody EP: Clinical Chemistry, Principles, Procedures, Correlation, 2nd ed. Philadelphia, JB Lippincott, 1992

Fishman RA: Cerebrospinal fluid in diseases of the nervous system, 2nd ed. Philadelphia, WB Saunders, 1992

Harrer AF (ed): DeJong's. The Neurologic Examination, 5th ed. Philadelphia, JB Lippincott, 1992

Henry JB (ed): Todd, Sanford, Davidsohn: Clinical Diagnosis and Management by Laboratory Methods, 18th ed. Philadelphia, WB Saunders, 1990

Laboratory Handbook, Medical Science Laboratories, Hudson, OH, LexiComp, Inc, 1992

Leavelle, DE (ed): Interpretive Handbook: Interpretive Data for Diagnostic Laboratory Tests. Rochester, MN, Mayo Medical Laboratories, 1990

Mason-Bastnagal PJ: Neurodiagnostic testing in critically injured adults. Critical Care Nurse 64-75, August 1992

Sacher RA, McPherson RA: Widmann's Clinical Interpretation of Laboratory Tests, 10th ed. Philadelphia, FA Davis, 1991

Smith S, Forman D: Laboratory analysis of cerebrospinal fluid. Clinical Laboratory Science 7(4): 32-38, Jan/Feb 1994

Swash M, Schwartz MS: Neurology, a Concise Clinical Text. Philadelphia, WB Saunders (Bailliere Tindall), 1990

Tietz NB (ed): Clinical Guide to Laboratory Tests, 3rd ed. Philadelphia, WB Saunders, 1995

Wallach J: Interpretation of Diagnostic Tests, 5th ed. Little, Brown & Co, 1992

Weiner WJ: Emergent and Urgent Neurology: Philadelphia, JB Lippincott, 1992

6

Chemistry Studies

Frances Fischbach: A MANUAL OF LABORATORY & DIAGNOSTIC TESTS, Fifth Edition.

OVERVIEW OF CHEMISTRY STUDIES ●

Blood chemistry testing identifies many chemical blood constituents. It is often necessary to measure several blood chemicals to establish a pattern of abnormalities. A wide range of tests can be grouped under the headings of enzymes, electrolytes, blood sugar, lipids, hormones, vitamins, minerals, and drug investigation. Other tests have no common denominator. Selected tests serve as screening devices to identify target-organ damage.

GENERAL BIOCHEMICAL PROFILES ●

Profiles are a group of select tests that screen for certain conditions. Some of the more common profiles or panels are listed here:

Disorder	***Tests Suggested***
Cardiac enzymes	CPK, AST, LDH, SGOT
Kidney functions/disease	BUN, phosphorus, LDH, creatinine, creatinine clearance, uric acid, total protein, A/G ratio, albumin, globulins, calcium, glucose, cholesterol
Lipids	Cholesterol, triglycerides, lipoprotein electrophoresis (LDL, VLDL, HDL)
Liver function/disease	Total bilirubin, alkaline phosphatase, cholesterol, GGT, total protein, A/G ratio, albumin, globulins, AST, LDH, viral hepatitis panel, prothrombin time (PT), partial thromboplastin time (PTT)
Thyroid function	T_3 uptake, free T_4, total T_4, T_7 (free thyroxine index [FTI]), TSH

USE OF THE AUTOANALYZER

Sophisticated automated instrumentation makes it possible to conduct a wide variety of chemical tests on a single sample of blood and to report results in a timely manner. Computerized interfaces allow direct transmission between laboratory and clinical settings. "Hard copy" printouts can then become a permanent part of the healthcare record.

Not only does this method provide a baseline for future comparisons but it has also uncovered unsuspected diseases and led to early diagnosis when symptoms are vague or absent.

> **NOTE:** *Normal or reference values for any chemistry determination vary with the method or assay employed. For example, differences in substrates or temperature at which the assay is run will alter the "normal range." Thus, normal ranges will vary between laboratories.*

The more commonly ordered chemistries include

Albumin, globulin
Alkaline phosphatase
Aspartate transaminase (AST)
Blood urea nitrogen (BUN)
Calcium (Ca^{2+})
Cholesterol
Creatinine
Glucose
Inorganic phosphorus
Total bilirubin
Total protein (TP) (discussed in Chap. 8)
Triglycerides
Uric acid
Electrolytes, sodium, potassium, and chloride

Patterns of abnormal values provide data for arriving at a definitive diagnosis.

Use of Multiple Laboratories
Certain tests may be sent out to reference or commercial laboratories. A certain percentage of these tests will fall into the category of being too sophisticated or of too low a volume to obtain reliable results. This is one of the reasons why test results may not immediately be available for interpretation.

● ELECTROLYTE TESTS

CALCIUM (Ca^{2+}) ●

Normal Values

Calcium Total			*Calcium Ionized*		
Age	*mg/dl*	*mmol/L*	*Age*	*mg/dl*	*mmol/L*
0–10 d	7.6–10.4	1.90–2.60	Newborn	4.20–5.48	1.05–1.37
10 d–2 yr	9.0–11.0	2.25–2.75	1–18 yr	4.80–5.52	1.20–1.38
2 yr–12 yr	8.8–10.8	2.20–2.70	Adult	4.65–5.28	1.16–1.32
12 yr–18 yr	8.9–10.2	2.10–2.55			
Adult	8.6–10.0	2.15–2.50			

Background
The bulk of body calcium (98%–99%) is stored in the skeleton and teeth, which act as huge reservoirs for maintaining the blood levels of calcium. About 50% of blood calcium is ionized; the rest is protein bound. However, only ionized calcium can be used by the body in such vital processes as muscular contraction, cardiac function, transmission of nerve impulses, and blood clotting. Thus, ionized calcium values are more accurate indicators in open-heart, renal, and long operative procedures.

The amount of protein in the blood also affects calcium levels because 50% of the blood calcium is protein bound. Thus, a decrease in serum albumin will result in a profound decrease in total serum calcium. The decrease, however, does not alter the concentration of the ionized form. *Measurement of ionized calcium* is done during open-heart operations, liver transplants, and other operations in which large volumes of blood, anticoagulated with citrate, are given. It is also used to monitor renal disease, renal transplantation, or hemodialysis; hyperparathyroidism or hypoparathyroidism; pancreatitis, or malignancy. Parathyroid hormone, calcitonin, vitamin D, estrogens, androgens, carbohydrates, and lactose are all factors that influence calcium levels.

Explanation of Test

This test measures the concentration of total and ionized calcium in the blood to reflect parathyroid function, calcium metabolism, and malignant activity.

> **Clinical Alert**
>
> Hyperparathyroidism and cancer are the most common causes of hypercalcemia. Hypoalbuminemia is the most common cause of decreased total calcium.

Procedure

A 5-ml venous blood sample provides serum for this test. Observe universal precautions. Citrated EDTA and oxalated blood give falsely low values. Heparinized samples are preferred for ionized calcium studies.

Clinical Implications

1. *Normal levels of total blood calcium,* combined with other findings:
- **a.** Normal calcium levels with overall normal results in other tests indicate no problems with calcium metabolism.
- **b.** Normal calcium and abnormal phosphorus values indicate impaired calcium absorption owing to alteration of parathyroid hormone activity or secretion (eg, in rickets, the calcium level may be normal or slightly lowered and the phosphorus level depressed).
- **c.** Normal calcium and elevated blood urea nitrogen (BUN) levels indicate
  - **(1)** Possible secondary hyperparathyroidism. Initially, a lowered serum calcium results from uremia and acidosis. The lower calcium level stimulates the parathyroid to release parathyroid hormone, which acts on bone to release more calcium.
  - **(2)** Possible primary hyperparathyroidism. Excessive amounts of parathyroid hormone cause elevation in calcium levels, but secondary kidney disease would cause retention of phosphate and concomitant lower calcium.
  - **(3)** Normal calcium and decreased serum albumin indicates hypercalcemia. (Normally, a decrease in calcium should be associated with a decrease in albumin.)

2. *Hypercalcemia (increased total calcium levels)* is caused by or associated with
- **a.** Hyperparathyroidism caused by parathyroid adenoma, hyperplasia of parathyroid glands, or associated with hypophosphatemia
- **b.** *Cancer*
  - **(1)** Metastatic bone cancers; cancers of lung, breast, thyroid, kidney, liver, and pancreas

(2) Hodgkin's disease, lymphomas, leukemia
(3) Multiple myeloma, with extensive bone destruction
(4) Primary squamous cell carcinoma of lung, neck, and head

c. Granulomatous disease (eg, tuberculosis, sarcoidosis)
d. Hyperthyroidism
e. Paget's disease of bone (also accompanied by high levels of alkaline phosphatase)
f. Prolonged immobilization
g. Bone fractures, combined with bed rest
h. Excessive intake of vitamin D
i. Renal transplant
j. Milk–alkali syndrome (excessive intake of milk and antacids)

3. *Hypocalcemia (decreased total calcium levels)* is commonly caused by or associated with

a. Pseudohypocalcemia, which reflects reduced albumin levels (the reduced protein is responsible for the low calcium level because 50% of the calcium total is protein-bound.)

NOTE: *Excessive intravenous fluids will decrease albumin levels and, thus, decrease calcium. Total serum protein and albumin should be measured at the same time as calcium for the proper interpretation of calcium levels.*

b. Hypoparathyroidism (primary is very rare) may be due to accidental surgical removal of parathyroid glands, irradiation, hypomagnesemia, gastrointestinal (GI) disorders, renal wasting.
c. Hyperphosphatemia caused by renal failure, laxative intake, cytotoxic drugs
d. Malabsorption caused by sprue, celiac disease, pancreatic dysfunction (fatty acids combine with calcium and are precipitated and excreted in the feces)
e. Acute pancreatitis
f. Alkalosis (calcium ions become bound to protein)
g. Osteomalacia
h. Renal failure
i. Vitamin D deficiency
j. Malnutrition
k. Alcoholism, hepatic cirrhosis

Clinical Alert

Panic values for total calcium:

< 6 mg/dl (1.50 mmol/L) may produce tetany and convulsions.
> 13 mg/dl (3.25 mmol/L) may cause cardiotoxicity, arrhythmias, and coma.

Rapid treatment of hypercalcemia with calcitonin solution is indicated.

4. *Increased ionized calcium levels* occur in
   a. Hyperparathyroidism
   b. Ectopic parathyroid hormone-producing tumors
   c. Increased vitamin D intake, malignancies
5. *Decreased ionized calcium levels* occur in
   a. Hyperventilation to control increased intracranial pressure (total Ca^{2+} may be normal)
   b. Administration of bicarbonate to control metabolic acidosis
   c. Acute pancreatitis (eg, diabetic acidosis and sepsis)
   d. Hypoparathyroidism
   e. Vitamin D deficiency
   f. Toxic shock syndrome
   g. Fat embolism

Clinical Alert

Panic values for ionized calcium

< 2.0 mg/dl (0.78 mmol/L) tetany, life-threatening complications
2.0–3.0 mg/dl (< 1.00 mmol/L) in cases of multiple blood transfusions (this is an indication to administer calcium)
> 7.0 mg/dl (> 1.58 mmol/L) coma

Interfering Factors

1. Thiazide diuretics may impair urinary calcium excretion and result in hypercalcemia.
2. For patients with renal insufficiency undergoing dialysis, a calcium–ion-exchange resin is sometimes used for hyperkalemia. This resin may increase calcium levels.
3. Increased magnesium and phosphate uptake and excessive use of laxatives may lower blood calcium level because of increased intestinal calcium loss.
4. When decreased calcium levels are due to magnesium deficiency (as in poor bowel absorption), the administration of magnesium will correct the calcium deficiency.
5. If a patient is known to have, or suspected of having, a pH abnormality, a concurrent pH with ionized calcium should be requested.
6. Many drugs may cause increased or decreased levels of calcium. Calcium supplements taken shortly before specimen collection will cause falsely high values.

Patient Preparation

1. Explain purpose and procedure. Encourage relaxation.
2. Tourniquet application should be as brief as possible when drawing ionized calcium to prevent venous stasis.

3. Calcium supplements should not be taken within 8 to 12 hours before the blood sample is drawn.
4. See Chapter 1 guidelines for safe, effective, informed *pretest* care.

Patient Aftercare

1. Resume normal activities.
2. Interpret test results and monitor appropriately for calcium abnormalities.
3. Follow Chapter 1 guidelines for safe, effective, informed *posttest* care.

CHLORIDE (Cl^-)

Normal Values

Newborn:	98–113 mmol/L or mEq/L
Adult:	98–106 mmol/L or mEq/L

Background

Chloride, a blood electrolyte, is an anion that exists predominantly in the extracellular spaces as a combination in sodium chloride or hydrochloric acid. Chloride maintains cellular integrity through its influence on osmotic pressure and acid–base and water balance. It has the reciprocal power of increasing or decreasing in concentration in response to concentrations of other anions. In metabolic acidosis, there is a reciprocal rise in chloride concentration when the bicarbonate concentration drops. Similarly, when aldosterone directly causes an increase in the reabsorption of sodium (the positive ion), the indirect effect is an increase in the chloride (the negative ion) absorption.

Chlorides are excreted with cations (positive ions) during massive diuresis from any cause and are lost from the GI tract when vomiting, diarrhea, or intestinal fistulas occur.

Explanation of Test

Alteration of sodium chloride is seldom a primary problem. Measurement of chlorides is usually done for inferential value and is helpful in diagnosing disorders of acid–base and water balance. Because of the relatively high chloride concentrations in the gastric juices, prolonged vomiting may lead to considerable chloride loss and lowered serum chloride levels.

In an emergency, chloride is the least important electrolyte to measure. However, it is especially important in the correction of hypokalemic alkalosis. If potassium is supplied without chloride, hypokalemic alkalosis may persist.

Procedure

Obtain a 2-ml venous blood sample in a heparinized syringe. Observe universal precautions.

Clinical Implications

1. Whenever serum chloride levels are much lower than 100 mEq/L, urinary excretion of chlorides is also low.
2. Plasma chloride can remain at near normal levels in the presence of severe renal failure.
3. *Decreased blood chloride levels* occur in
   - **a.** Severe vomiting
   - **b.** Gastric secretion
   - **c.** Chronic respiratory acidosis
   - **d.** Burns
   - **e.** Metabolic alkalosis
   - **f.** Diabetes
   - **g.** Addison's disease
   - **h.** Salt-losing diseases
   - **i.** Overhydration
   - **j.** Select diuretic therapy
4. *Increased blood chloride levels* occur in
   - **a.** Dehydration
   - **b.** Cushing's syndrome
   - **c.** Hyperventilation (causes respiratory alkalosis)
   - **d.** Metabolic disorders
   - **e.** Hyperparathyroidism
   - **f.** Select kidney disorders (renal tubular acidosis)
   - **g.** Diabetes insipidus

Interfering Factors

1. The plasma chloride concentration in infants is usually higher than in children and adults.
2. Certain drugs may alter chloride levels.
3. Increases are associated with excessive saline IV infusions.

Clinical Alert

Panic values for serum chloride: < 70 or > 120 mEq/L (mmol/L).

Patient Preparation

1. Explain test purpose and blood collection procedure.
2. If possible, patient should be fasting at least 8–12 hours before the test.
3. See Chapter 1 guidelines for safe, effective, informed *pretest* care.

Patient Aftercare

1. Resume normal activities and diet.
2. Interpret test results and monitor appropriately.
3. If an electrolyte disorder is suspected, daily weight and accurate fluid intake and output should be recorded.
4. Follow Chapter 1 guidelines for safe, effective, informed *posttest* care.

PHOSPHATE (P)/INORGANIC PHOSPHORUS (PO_4)

Normal Values

Adults:	2.5–4.5 mg/dl or 0.87–1.45 mmol/L
Children:	4.5–5.5 mg/dl or 1.45–1.78 mmol/L
Newborn:	4.5–9.0 mg/dl or 1.45–2.91 mmol/L

Background

The body's total phosphorus content is combined with calcium in the bone (85%); the remainder is within the cells. Most of the phosphorus in the blood exists as phosphates or esters. Phosphate is required for generation of bony tissue and functions in the metabolism of glucose and lipids, in the maintenance of acid–base balance, and in the storage and transfer of energy from one site in the body to another. Phosphorus enters the cell with glucose and is lowered after carbohydrate ingestion.

Explanation of Test

Phosphate levels are always evaluated in relation to calcium levels because there is an inverse relation between the two. When calcium levels are decreased, phosphorus levels increase; when phosphorus levels decrease, calcium levels increase. An excess in serum levels of one electrolyte causes the kidneys to excrete the other. Many of the causes of elevated calcium are also causes of lower phosphorus levels. As with calcium, the controlling factor is parathyroid hormone.

Procedure

Obtain a fasting 5-ml venous blood sample. Serum is preferred, but heparinized blood is acceptable. Observe universal precautions.

Clinical Implications

1. *Hyperphosphatemia* (increased blood phosphorus levels) is most commonly found in association with kidney dysfunction and uremia. This is because phosphate is so closely regulated by the kidneys.
   - **a.** Renal insufficiency and severe nephritis (accompanied by elevated BUN and creatinine), renal failure
   - **b.** Hypoparathyroidism (accompanied by elevated phosphorus, decreased calcium, and normal renal function), pseudohypoparathyroidism
   - **c.** Hypocalcemia
   - **d.** Excessive intake of alkali (possible history of peptic ulcer), milk–alkali syndrome
   - **e.** Excessive intake of vitamin D
   - **f.** Fractures in the healing stage
   - **g.** Bone tumors, bone metastases
   - **h.** Addison's disease
   - **i.** Acromegaly
   - **j.** Liver disease, cirrhosis
   - **k.** Cardiac resuscitation

2. *Hypophosphatemia* (decreased phosphorus levels) occurs in
   - **a.** Hyperparathyroidism
   - **b.** Rickets (childhood) or osteomalacia (adult), vitamin D deficiency
   - **c.** Diabetic coma (increased carbohydrate metabolism)
   - **d.** Hyperinsulinism
   - **e.** Continuous administration of intravenous glucose in a nondiabetic patient (phosphorus follows glucose into the cells)
   - **f.** Liver disease
   - **g.** Dialysis
   - **h.** Vomiting

i. Severe malnutrition
j. Gram-negative septicemia

Interfering Factors

1. Normally high in children.
2. Falsely increased by hemolysis of blood; therefore, separate serum from cells as soon as possible.
3. Drugs can be the cause of decreases.
4. The use of laxatives or enemas containing large amounts of sodium phosphate will cause increased phosphorus levels. With the oral intake of the laxative, the blood level may increase as much as 5 mg/dl 2 to 3 hours after the dose. This increased level is only temporary (5–6 hours), but this factor should be considered when abnormal levels are seen that cannot otherwise be explained.
5. Seasonal variation—maximum levels in May and June and lowest in winter.

Patient Preparation

1. Explain test purpose and blood sampling procedures. Patient should be fasting.
2. Note on requisition if any catastrophic stressful events have taken place that may cause high levels.
3. Note time of day test is drawn—levels are highest in the morning and lowest in the evening.
4. See Chapter 1 guidelines for safe, effective, informed *pretest* care.

Patient Aftercare

1. Resume normal activities.
2. Interpret test outcomes and monitor as appropriate for calcium imbalances. When phosphorus rises rapidly, calcium drops—watch for arrhythmias and muscle twitching.
3. See Chapter 1 guidelines for safe, effective, informed *posttest* care.

Clinical Alert

Panic value: < 1.0 mg/dl

MAGNESIUM (Mg^{2+})

Normal Values

Adult:	1.3–2.1 mEq/L or 0.65–1.05 mmol/L
Newborn:	1.2–1.8 mEq/L or 0.6–0.9 mmol/L
Child:	1.4–1.7 mEq/L or 0.71–0.78 mmol/L

Background

Magnesium in the body is concentrated in the bone, cartilage, and within the cell itself, and is required for the use of adenosine triphosphate (ATP) as a source of energy. Therefore, it is necessary for the action of numerous enzyme systems, such as carbohydrate metabolism, protein synthesis, nucleic acid synthesis, and contraction of muscular tissue. Along with sodium, potassium, and calcium ions, magnesium also regulates neuromuscular irritability and the clotting mechanism.

Magnesium and calcium are intimately tied together in their body functions, and deficiency of either one has a significant effect on the metabolism of the other. This is because of magnesium's importance in the absorption of calcium from the intestines and in calcium metabolism. A magnesium deficiency will result in the drift of calcium out of the bones, possibly resulting in abnormal calcification in the aorta and the kidney in the absence of a calcium pump mechanism. This condition responds to administration of magnesium salts. Normally, 95% of the magnesium that is filtered through the glomerulus is reabsorbed in the tubule. When there is decreased kidney function, greater amounts of magnesium are retained, resulting in increased blood serum levels.

Explanation of Test

Magnesium measurement is used as an index for metabolic activity in the body and to evaluate renal function and electrolyte status.

Procedure

Obtain a fasting 4-ml venous blood sample. Avoid hemolysis and separate serum from cells as soon as possible. Observe universal precautions.

Clinical Implications

1. *Reduced blood magnesium levels* occur in
- **a.** Blood transfusions
- **b.** Chronic diarrhea
- **c.** Hemodialysis
- **d.** Chronic renal disease
- **e.** Hepatic cirrhosis
- **f.** Chronic pancreatitis
- **g.** Abuse of diuretics
- **h.** Severe burns
- **i.** Ulcerative colitis
- **j.** Hyperaldosteronism
- **k.** Toxemia of pregnancy
- **l.** Hyperthyroidism and hypoparathyroidism
- **m.** Excessive loss of body fluids (eg, sweating, lactation)
- **n.** Malabsorption syndromes
- **o.** Chronic alcoholism
- **p.** Prolonged gastric drainage
- **q.** Long-term hyperalimentation

In magnesium deficiency states, *urinary magnesium decreases* before the serum does.

2. *Increased blood magnesium levels* occur in
- **a.** Renal failure or reduced renal function
- **b.** Dehydration
- **c.** Hypothyroidism

d. Addison's disease
e. Adrenalectomy
f. Diabetic acidosis—severe
g. Use of antacids containing magnesium (eg, Milk of Magnesia), administration of magnesium salts

Interfering Factors

1. Prolonged salicylate therapy, lithium, and magnesium products (antacids, laxatives) will cause falsely increased magnesium levels, particularly if there is renal damage.
2. Calcium gluconate, as well as a number of other drugs, can interfere with testing methods and cause falsely decreased results.
3. Hemolysis will invalidate results because about three-fourths of the magnesium in the blood is found intracellularly in the red blood cells.

Patient Preparation

1. Explain test purpose and blood-drawing procedure.
2. Patient should be fasting, if possible, and be in a prone position when blood is drawn.
3. See Chapter 1 guidelines for safe, effective, informed *pretest* care.

Patient Aftercare

1. Interpret test results and monitor as appropriate. Treatment of diabetic coma often results in low plasma magnesium levels. This change occurs because magnesium moves with potassium into the cells after insulin administration.
2. Magnesium deficiency may cause apparently unexplained hypocalcemia and hypokalemia. In these instances, patients may have neurologic or GI symptoms.
3. Observe for signs of too much magnesium (which acts as a sedative):
   a. Lethargy, flushing, nausea, vomiting, slurred speech
   b. Weak or absent deep tendon reflexes
   c. Electrocardiogram: prolonged PR and Q-T intervals, widened QRS; bradycardia
   d. Hypotension, drowsiness, and respiratory depression
4. Measure serum magnesium in persons receiving aminoglycosides and cyclosporine. There is a known association between these therapies and hypermagnesemia. Treatment of hypermagnesemia involves withholding source of magnesium excess, promoting excretion, giving calcium salts, and hemodialysis.
5. Observe for signs of insufficient magnesium, which include
   a. Muscle tremors, twitching, tetany
   b. Hypocalcemia
   c. Hyperactive deep tendon reflexes
   d. Electrocardiogram: prolonged P-R and Q-T intervals; broad, flat T waves; premature ventricular contractions; ventricular tachycardia; and fibrillation
   e. Anorexia, nausea, and vomiting
   f. Lethargy and insomnia

6. Treatment of hypomagnesia involves administering magnesium salts and reducing auditory, mechanical, and visual stimuli.
7. See Chapter 1 guidelines for safe, effective *posttest* care.

Clinical Alert

Panic values for magnesium

< 1.0 mEq/L or < 0.50 mmol/L (tetany occurs)
> 5.0 mEq/L or 2.50 mmol/L
5.0–10.0 mEq/L—cardioconduction is retarded
10.0–13.0 mEq/L—deep tendon reflexes are lost
15.0 mEq/L—respiratory paralysis occurs
> 25.0 mEq/L—cardiac arrest

POTASSIUM (K^+)

Normal Values

Age	*mmol/L or mEq/L*
0–7 d	3.7–5.9
7 d–1 yr	4.1–5.3
1–18 yr	3.4–4.7
Adult	3.5–5.3

Background

Potassium is the principal electrolyte (cation) of intracellular fluid and the primary buffer within the cell itself. Ninety percent of potassium is concentrated within the cell; only small amounts are contained in bone and blood. A kilogram of tissue, such as red blood cells or muscle, contains about 90 mEq of potassium. Damaged cells release potassium into the blood.

The body is adapted to efficient potassium excretion. Normally, 80% to 90% of the cells' potassium is excreted in the urine by the glomeruli of the kidneys; the remainder in sweat and in the stool. Even when no potassium is taken into the body (as in a fasting state), 40 to 50 mEq are still excreted daily in the urine. The kidneys do not conserve potassium, and when an adequate amount of potassium is not ingested, a severe deficiency will occur. Potassium balance is maintained in adults on an average dietary intake of 80 to 200 mEq/day. The normal intake, minimal needs, and maximum tolerance for potassium are almost the same as those for sodium.

Potassium plays an important role in nerve conduction, muscle function, acid–base balance, and osmotic pressure. Along with calcium and magnesium, potassium controls the rate and force of contraction of the heart and, thereby, the cardiac output. Evidence of a potassium deficit can be noted on an electrocardiogram (ECG) by the presence of a U wave.

Potassium and sodium ions are particularly important in the renal regulation of acid–base balance because hydrogen ions are substituted for sodium and potassium ions in the renal tubule. Potassium is more important than sodium, because potassium bicarbonate is the primary intracellular inorganic buffer. In potassium deficiency, there is a relative deficiency of intracellular potassium bicarbonate, and the pH is relatively acidic. The respiratory center responds to the intracellular acidosis by lower PCO_2, through the mechanism of hyperventilation. Concentration of potassium is greatly affected by the adrenal hormones. A potassium deficiency will cause a significant reduction in protein synthesis.

Explanation of Test

This test evaluates changes in body potassium and diagnoses acid–base and water imbalances: not an absolute value, it varies with the circulatory volume and other factors. Because a totally unsuspected potassium imbalance can suddenly prove lethal, its development must be anticipated. Thus, it is important to check this value in severe cases of Addison's disease, uremic coma, intestinal obstruction, acute renal failure, GI loss with the administration of diuretics, steroid therapy, and in cardiac patients receiving digitalis.

Procedure

1. Obtain a 5-ml venous blood sample. Use serum or a heparinized syringe. Observe universal precautions. Avoid hemolysis in obtaining the sample.
2. The sample must be delivered to the laboratory and spun at once to separate cells from serum. Potassium leaks out of the cell and will be falsely elevated after 4 hours.

Clinical Implications

1. *Decreased blood potassium (hypokalemia)* levels are associated with shifting of K^+ into cells, K^+ loss from GI and biliary tracts, renal K^+ excretion, and reduced K^+ intake as in the following:
   - **a.** Diarrhea
   - **b.** Vomiting
   - **c.** Starvation
   - **d.** Malabsorption
   - **e.** Excessive sweating
   - **f.** Draining wounds
   - **g.** Cystic fibrosis
   - **h.** Severe burns
   - **i.** Primary aldosteronism
   - **j.** Excessive licorice ingestion
   - **k.** Osmotic hyperglycemia
   - **l.** Respiratory alkalosis
   - **m.** Renal tubular acidosis
   - **n.** Diuretic, antibiotic, and mineralocorticoid administration
   - **o.** Barium chloride poisoning
   - **p.** Treatment of megaloblastic anemia with vitamin B_{12} or folic acid
2. Potassium values of 3.5 mEq/L are more commonly associated with deficiency, rather than normality. A falling trend (0.1–0.2 mEq/day) is indicative of a developing potassium deficiency.
   - **a.** The most frequent cause of potassium deficiency is GI loss.
   - **b.** The most frequent cause of potassium depletion is IV fluid administration without adequate potassium supplements.

3. *Increased K^+ levels (hyperkalemia)* occur when K^+ shifts from cells to intracellular fluid, with inadequate renal excretion, and excessive K^+ intake as in
   a. Renal failure, dehydration, obstruction, and trauma
   b. Cell damage, as in burns, accidents, surgery, chemotherapy, and disseminated intravascular coagulation (damaged cells will release potassium into the blood)
   c. Acidosis (drives potassium out of the cells) metabolic, diabetic ketoacidosis
   d. Addison's disease
   e. Pseudohypoaldosteronism
   f. Uncontrolled diabetes, decreased insulin
   g. Primary acquired hyperkalemia, such as systemic lupus erythematosus (SLE), sickle cell, interstitial nephritis, and tubular disorders

Interfering Factors

1. Hemolyzed blood and forearm exercise. Hemolyzed blood may not be used; K^+ values are elevated up to 50% of normal with moderate hemolysis. Opening and closing the fist ten times with a tourniquet in place results in an increase of the potassium level by 10% to 20%. Consequently, it is recommended that the blood sample be obtained without a tourniquet, or that the tourniquet be released after the needle has entered the vein and 2 minutes are allowed to elapse before the sample is withdrawn.
2. Drug usage
   a. The IV use of *potassium penicillin* may cause hyperkalemia; *penicillin sodium* may cause an increased excretion of potassium.
   b. Glucose administered during tolerance testing, or the ingestion and administration of large amounts of glucose in patients with heart disease, may cause a decrease of as much as 0.4 mEq/L in potassium blood levels.
   c. A number of drugs interfere with potassium levels.
   d. Excessive intake of licorice interferes.

Patient Preparation

1. Explain test purpose and blood-drawing procedure. Do not have patient open and close fist.
2. See Chapter 1 guidelines for safe, effective, informed *pretest* care.

Clinical Alert

1. Panic values: < 2.5 mEq/L (ventricular fibrillation); > 7.0 mEq/L (muscle irritability including myocardial).

(continued)

(Clinical Alert continued)

2. The most common cause of hypokalemia in patients receiving IV fluids is water and sodium chloride administration without adequate replacement for K^+ lost in urine and drainage fluids. A patient receiving IV fluids needs K^+ every day. The minimum daily dose should be 40 mEq, but the optimum daily dose ranges between 60 and 120 mEq. Potassium needs are greater in tissue injury, wound infection, gastric, intestinal, or biliary drainage. If adequate amounts of potassium are not given in IV solution (40 mEq/day), hypokalemia will eventually develop.

   Patients receiving more than 10 mEq KCl in 100 ml of IV solution should be ECG-monitored for potential arrhythmia if the IV rate is 100 ml/hr or greater. Concentrated doses of IV potassium should always be administered by volume-controlled IV infusion devices. A burning sensation felt at the site of needle insertion may indicate that the concentration is toxic, and the IV rate can be reduced. Some physicians will order that a small dose of lidocaine (Xylocaine) be added to IV potassium to eliminate the "burning" sensation some patients experience. Always be sure to check for lidocaine allergies before administration of this local anesthetic.
3. Closely monitor patients taking digitalis and diuretics for hypokalemia, because cardiac arrhythmias can occur. Hypokalemia enhances the effect of digitalis preparations, creating the possibility of digitalis intoxication from even an average maintenance dose. Digitalis, diuretics, and hypokalemia are a potentially lethal combination.

Patient Aftercare

Interpret test results, monitor changes in body potassium, and intervene as appropriate. Recognizing signs and symptoms of hypokalemia and hyperkalemia is very important. Many of them originate in the nervous and muscular systems and are usually nonspecific and similar. The potassium blood level rises 0.6 mEq/L for every 0.1 decrease in blood pH.

HYPERKALEMIA (EXCESS K^+)

1. Record fluid intake and output. Check blood volume and venous pressure which will give a clue to dehydration or circulatory overload. Identify ECG changes. In *Hyperkalemia* these include
   a. Elevated T-wave heart block
   b. Flattened P wave
   c. Cardiac arrest may occur without warning other than ECG changes

2. Observe for slow pulse, oliguria, neuromuscular disorders, such as muscle weakness and impaired muscle function, flaccid paralysis, tremors, and twitching preceding actual paralysis.

HYPOKALEMIA (DEFICIENCY OF K^+)

1. Record fluid intake and output. Check blood volume and venous pressure, which will give a clue to circulatory overload or dehydration. Identify ECG changes. In *hypokalemia* these include
   a. Depressed T waves
   b. Peaking of P waves
2. Observe for dehydration caused by severe vomiting, hyperventilation, sweating, diuresis, nasogastric tube with gastric suction. Accurately record state of hydration or dehydration.
3. Observe for neuromuscular changes, such as fatigue, muscle weakness, muscle pain, flabby muscles, paresthesia; hypotension and rapid pulse; respiratory muscle weakness, leading to paralysis, cyanosis, and respiratory arrest; anorexia, nausea, vomiting, paralytic ileus; apathy, drowsiness, irritability, tetany, and coma.
4. Hyperkalemia can be treated with sodium bicarbonate, glucose, and insulin.
5. Diuretics, dialysis, and sodium polystyrene sulfonate (Kayexolate; a sodium–potassium exchange resin) can be administered orally, nasogastrically, or rectally.
6. Hypocalcemia may be treated with a K^+ rice diet, or K^+ sparing diuretics. Salt-substitute tests contain potassium chloride and IV or oral potassium chloride supplements.
7. Follow Chapter 1 guidelines for safe, effective, informed *posttest* care.

Clinical Alert

1. Be on the alert for these arrhythmias that may occur with hyperkalemia.
   (a) Sinus bradycardia
   (b) Sinus arrest
   (c) First-degree atrioventricular block
   (d) Nodal rhythm
   (e) Idioventricular rhythm
   (f) Ventricular tachycardia
   (g) Ventricular fibrillation
   (h) Ventricular arrest
2. Be on the alert for these arrhythmias that may occur with hypokalemia: ventricular premature beats, atrial tachycardia, nodal tachycardia, ventricular tachycardia, and ventricular fibrillation.

SODIUM (Na^+)

Normal Values

Adult:	135–145 mmol/L or 135–145 mEq/L
Premature infant:	140 mEq/L
Full-term infant:	133–142 mEq/L
Children aged 1–16 yr:	135–145 mEq/L

Background

Sodium is the most abundant cation (90% of the electrolyte fluid) and the chief base of the blood. Its primary functions in the body are to chemically maintain osmotic pressure, acid–base balance, and to transmit nerve impulses. The body has a strong tendency to maintain a total base content, and only slight changes are found, even under pathologic conditions. Mechanisms for maintaining a constant sodium level in the plasma and extracellular fluid include *renal blood flow, carbonic anhydrase enzymatic activity, aldosterone, action of other steroids* the plasma level of which is controlled by the anterior pituitary gland, *renin enzymatic secretion,* and *antidiuretic hormone (ADH)* and *vasopressin secretion*.

Explanation of Test

Determinations of plasma sodium levels detect gross changes in water and salt balance with *urinary* sodium a more sensitive indicator of altered sodium balance than the *blood*.

Procedure

Obtain a 5-ml venous blood sample. Heparinized blood can be used. Avoid hemolysis. Observe universal precautions.

Clinical Implications

1. *Hyponatremia* (a decreased level) reflects a relative excess of body water, rather than a low total body sodium level. *Reduced* sodium levels (hyponatremia) are associated with
   - **a.** Severe burns
   - **b.** Congestive heart failure (predictor of cardiac mortality)
   - **c.** Excessive fluid loss (eg, severe diarrhea, vomiting, sweating)
   - **d.** Excessive IV induction of nonelectrolyte fluids (glucose)
   - **e.** Addison's disease (lack of adrenal steroids impairs sodium reabsorption)
   - **f.** Severe nephritis (nephrotic syndrome)
   - **g.** Pyloric obstruction
   - **h.** Malabsorption syndrome
   - **i.** Diabetic acidosis
   - **j.** Drugs such as diuretics
   - **k.** Edema (dilutional hyponatremia)
   - **l.** Large amounts of water by mouth
   - **m.** Stomach suction accompanied by water or ice chips by mouth
   - **n.** Hypothyroidism

2. *Hypernatremia* (an increased sodium level) is uncommon, but when it does occur it is associated with
   a. Dehydration and insufficient water intake
   b. Conn's syndrome
   c. Primary aldosteronism
   d. Coma
   e. Cushing's disease
   f. Diabetes insipidus
   g. Tracheobronchitis

Clinical Alert

Panic values for sodium:

< 120 mEq/L (mmol/L)—weakness
90–105 mEq/L—severe neurologic symptoms
> 155 mEq/L (mmol/L)—cardiovascular and renal symptoms
> 160 mEq/L—heart failure

Interfering Factors

1. Many drugs affect levels of blood sodium.
   a. Anabolic steroids, corticosteroids, calcium, fluorides, and iron can cause increases.
   b. Heparin, laxatives, sulfates, and diuretics can cause decreases.
2. High triglyceride or low protein levels cause artificially low sodium values.

Patient Preparation

1. Explain test purpose and procedure.
2. See Chapter 1 guidelines for safe, effective, informed *pretest* care.

Patient Aftercare

1. Interpret test outcomes and monitor for fluid and sodium imbalances.
2. IV therapy considerations are as follows:
   a. Sodium balance is maintained in adults with an average dietary intake of 90 to 250 mEq/day. The maximum daily tolerance to an acute load is 400 mEq/day. If a patient is given 3 L of isotonic saline in 24 hours, he or she will receive 465 mEq of sodium. This amount exceeds the average, healthy adult's tolerance level. It will take a *healthy* person 24 to 48 hours to excrete the excess sodium.
   b. After surgery, trauma, or shock, there is a decrease of extracellular fluid volume. Replacement of extracellular fluid is essential if water and electrolyte balance is to be maintained. The ideal replacement IV solution should have a sodium concentration of 140 mEq/L.
3. Monitor for signs of edema or hypertension, record and report if present.
4. Follow Chapter 1 guidelines for safe, effective, informed *posttest* care.

OSMOLALITY AND WATER-LOAD TEST (WATER-LOADING ANTIDIURETIC HORMONE SUPPRESSION TEST) ●

Normal Values

Serum Osmolality

Adult:	275–295 mOsm/kg
Newborn:	as low as 266 mOsm/kg

Urine Osmolality

24-hr:	+300–900 mOsm/kg
Random:	50–1200 mOsm/L
After 12-hr fluid restriction:	> 850 mOsm/L
Ratio of urine/serum osmolality:	0.2–4.7 average 1.0–3.0
After fluid restriction:	3.0–4.7

Background

Osmolality, the measure of the number of dissolved solute particles in solution, increases with dehydration and decreases with overhydration. In general, the same conditions that reduce or increase serum sodium affect the osmolality.

Explanation of Test

This test is used as an evaluation of water and electrolyte balance. It is helpful in assessing hydration status, seizures, liver disease, ADH function, coma, and in toxicology workups, including ethanol, ethylene glycol, isopropanol, and methanol ingestions.

Clinical Alert

1. Simultaneous determination of urine and serum osmolalities facilitates interpretation of results. A high urinary/serum (U/S) ratio is seen in concentrated urine. Normal ranges for the U/S ratio are approximately 0.2–4.7, and > 93 with overnight dehydration. With poor-concentrating ability the ratio is low, but still > 91. In SIADH urine, the sodium and urine osmolalities are high for serum osmolality.
2. Determination of the urine osmolar gap is used to characterize metabolic acidosis. The *urine osmolar gap* is described as the sum of urinary concentrations of sodium, potassium, bicarbonate, chloride, glucose, and urea, compared with measured urine osmolality. The gap is normally 80–100 mOsm/kg/H_2O.

Procedure for Osmolality

1. Obtain a 5-ml venous blood sample. Serum or green top (heparinized) plasma is acceptable. Observe universal precautions.

2. A 24-hour urine may be collected at the same time and kept on ice.
3. The osmolality is determined in the laboratory using the freezing-point depression method for both serum and urine.

Procedure for Water-Loading Antidiuretic Hormone Suppression

1. The ideal position during testing period is the recumbent position, because in an upright position the response to water-loading is reduced.
2. One hour before testing, the patient is given 300 ml of water to replace fluid lost during the overnight fast. This water is not counted as part of the test load.
3. The patient drinks a test load of water (calculated as 20 ml/kg of body weight) within 30 minutes.
4. After water is consumed, all urine is collected for the next 4 to 5 hours, and each voiding is checked for its volume osmolality and specific gravity. When the test is completed, a blood sample is obtained for osmolality, and the entire volume of urine obtained is checked for osmolality.
5. Normal values for water-loading antidiuretic hormone suppression test is excretion of greater than 90% of the water load within 4 hours. Urine osmolality falls to < 100 mOsm/kg. Specific gravity falls to 1.003.

Clinical Implications of Water Loading Test

1. In *decreased renal function,* < 80% of fluid is excreted and the urine's specific gravity may not fall below 1.010. This phenomenon occurs in
   - **a.** Adrenocortical insufficiency
   - **b.** Malabsorption syndrome
   - **c.** Edema
   - **d.** Ascites
   - **e.** Obesity
   - **f.** Hypothyroidism
   - **g.** Dehydration
   - **h.** Congestive heart failure
   - **i.** Cirrhosis
2. Disorders with *increased ADH secretion (SIADH)* give inadequate response.

Patient Preparation for Water Loading Test

1. Explain the test purpose and procedure. The test takes 5 to 6 hours to complete.
2. No food, alcohol, medications, or smoking for 8 to 10 hours before testing. No muscular exercise during test.
3. The patient may experience nausea, abdominal fullness, fatigue, and desire to defecate.
4. Discard first morning urine specimen.
5. See Chapter 1 guidelines for safe, effective, informed *pretest* care.

Patient Aftercare for Water Loading Test

1. Observe for adverse reactions to water-load testing, such as extreme abdominal discomfort, shortness of breath, or chest pain.

2. If water clearance is impaired, the water load will not induce diureses and maximum urinary dilution will not occur.
3. Accurate results may not be obtained if nausea, vomiting, or diarrhea occur, or if disturbance in bladder emptying is present. Note on chart if any of these effects occur.
4. Follow Chapter 1 guidelines for safe, effective, informed posttest care.

Clinical Alert

In patients with impaired ability to tolerate a water load, seizures or fatal hyponatremia may occur.

Clinical Implications of Osmolality

1. *Increased values (hyperosmolality)* are associated with
   - **a.** Dehydration
   - **b.** Diabetes insipidus, central or nephrogenic
   - **c.** Hypercalcemia
   - **d.** Diabetes mellitus, hyperglycemia
   - **e.** Hypernatremia
   - **f.** Cerebral lesions
   - **g.** Alcohol ingestion
   - **h.** Mannitol therapy
   - **i.** Azotemia
2. *Decreased values (hypoosmolality)* are associated with
   - **a.** Loss of sodium with diuretics and low-salt diet
   - **b.** Hyponatremia
   - **c.** Adrenocortical insufficiency
   - **d.** Inappropriate secretion of ADH, as in trauma and lung cancer
   - **e.** Excessive water replacement (overhydration; water intoxication)
   - **f.** Panhypopituitarism

Interfering Factors

1. Decreases are associated with altitude, diurnal variation with water retention at night, and some drugs.
2. Some drugs also cause increases.

Patient Preparation for Osmolality

1. Explain test purpose and procedure.
2. No alcohol for 24 hours before test.
3. See Chapter 1 guidelines for safe, effective, informed *pretest* care.

Patient Aftercare for Osmolality

1. Interpret test results and monitor appropriately. The patient receiving IV fluids should have a normal osmolality. If the osmolality increases, the fluids contain relatively more electrolytes than water. If it falls, relatively more water than electrolytes is present.

2. If the ratio of serum sodium to serum osmolality falls below 0.43, the outlook is guarded. This ratio may be distorted in drug intoxication.
3. Follow Chapter 1 guidelines for safe, effective, informed *posttest* care.

Clinical Alert

1. *Panic serum values* are results that are less than 240 or greater than 321. A value of 385 relates to stupor in hyperglycemia. Values of 400 or 420 are associated with grand mal seizures; values greater than 420 are fatal.
2. A water-loading antidiuretic hormone suppression test may be ordered to investigate impaired renal excretion of water.

SWEAT TEST

Normal Values

Sweat Sodium	
Normal:	16–46 mmol/L or mEq/L
Cystic fibrosis:	75–145 mmol/L or mEq/L
Sweat Chloride	
Normal:	8–43 mmol/L
Cystic fibrosis:	79–148 mmol/L
Potassium Sweat	
Normal:	6–17 mEq/L or mmol/L
Cystic fibrosis:	14–30 mEq/L or mmol/L

Explanation of Test

This test is done to diagnose cystic fibrosis. Abnormally high concentrations of sodium and chloride appear in the secretions of eccrine sweat glands in cystic fibrosis. The abnormality is present at birth and persists throughout life. This study uses sweat-inducing techniques stimulated by pilocarpine iontophoresis, followed by chemical analysis to determine sodium, chloride, and potassium content.

Procedure

1. The forearm is the preferred site for stimulation of sweating, but in thin or small babies, the thigh, back, or leg may be a better area to use. It may be necessary to stimulate sweating in two places to obtain enough sweat, especially in young infants. At least 100 µl of sweat is necessary. In cold weather, or if the room is cold, a warm covering should be placed over the arm or site of sweat collection.
2. Sweat production is stimulated by skin application of gauze pads or filter

paper saturated with a measured amount of pilocarpine and attachment of electrodes through which a current of 4 to 5 milliamps is delivered at intervals for a total of 5 minutes.

3. The electrodes and pad are removed and the area is thoroughly washed with distilled water and carefully dried.
4. Successful iontophoresis is indicated by a red area about 1 in. (2.4 cm) in diameter that appears where the electrode was placed.
5. The skin is scrubbed thoroughly with distilled water and dried carefully. The area for sweat collection must be completely dry, free from contamination by powder or antiseptic, and the skin must be free of any area that might ooze.
6. Collection of sweat occurs by applying preweighed filter or sweat collection cups that are taped securely over the red spot. The inside surfaces of the collecting device should never be touched.
7. The paper is left on for at least 1 hour before removal and is then placed on a preweighed flask to avoid evaporation. The flask is again weighed. The desired volume of sweat is 200 mg; mineral volume is 100 mg.
8. If the cup is used, it is left on for 1 hour, then carefully removed by scraping it across the iontophoresed area. This "puddles" the sweat in the cup to reduce evaporation and to redissolve any salts left by the evaporation. Suction capillary tubes are used to take sweat out of the collection cups.

Clinical Implications

1. Children with cystic fibrosis will have sodium and chloride values above 60 mEq/L (mmol/L).
2. Borderline or gray-zone cases are those with values between 40 and 60 mEq/L for both sodium and chloride and require retesting. Potassium values do not assist in differentiating these borderline cases.
3. In adolescence and adulthood, chloride levels over 80 mEq/L usually indicate cystic fibrosis.
4. Elevated sweat electrolytes can be associated with
    a. Addison's disease
    b. Congenital adrenal hyperplasia
    c. Vasopressin-resistant diabetes insipidus
    d. Glucose-6-phosphatase deficiency
    e. Glycogen storage disease

Interfering Factors

1. The sweat test is not valuable after puberty because levels may vary over a very wide range.
2. Dehydration and edema, particularly of areas where sweat is collected, may interfere with test results.
3. A gap of more than 30 mmol/L between sodium and chloride values indicates a calculation or analysis error, or contamination.
4. Sweat testing is not considered accurate until the third or fourth week of life. Infants younger than 6 weeks may not sweat enough.

Clinical Alert

1. The test should always be repeated if the result, the clinical features, or other diagnostic tests do not fit together.
2. The test can be used to exclude the diagnosis of cystic fibrosis in siblings of patients with this diagnosis.
3. There have been reports of cystic fibrosis patients with normal sweat electrolyte levels.
4. Sweat potassium is not diagnostically valuable.

Patient Preparation

1. Explain test purpose and procedure. The sweat test is indicated for the following:
   a. *Infants* who pass initial meconium late, with intestinal obstruction in newborn, failure to thrive, steatorrhea, chronic diarrhea, rapid respiration and retraction with chronic cough, asthma, hypoproteinemia (especially on soy bean formula), atelectasis or hyperaeration on x-ray, hyperprothrombinemia, rectal prolapse, who taste salty, of a CF parent (the obligate heterozygote).
   b. Persons suspected of having cystic fibrosis or celiac disease, all siblings of patients with cystic fibrosis, disaccharide intolerance, recurrent pneumonia, chronic atelectasis, chronic pulmonary disease, bronchiolectasis, chronic cough, nasal polyposis, cirrhosis of liver, and hypertension.
   c. Any parents who request a sweat test on their child.
2. Inform the patient that a slight stinging sensation is usually experienced, especially in fair-skinned persons.
3. See Chapter 1 guidelines for safe, effective, informed *pretest* care.

Patient Aftercare

1. After the cup is removed, carefully wash the skin and dry to prevent irritation from collection cups.
2. Resume normal activities.
3. Interpret test results, counsel and monitor as appropriate. Provide genetic counseling. Cystic fibrosis is transmitted as an autosomal recessive trait; white carrier rate is 1:20; black carrier rate is 1:60 to 1:100.
4. Follow Chapter 1 guidelines for safe, effective, informed *posttest* care.

● BLOOD GLUCOSE AND RELATED TESTS

C PEPTIDE ●

Normal Values

Fasting:	0.5–3.0 ng/ml or 0.17–0.99 mmol/L
30- to 60-minute postglucose load:	5–12 ng/ml

Background

The C peptide is formed in the beta cells of the pancreas and is secreted into the blood serum in concentrations almost equal to insulin. Normally, there is a strong correlation between insulin and C peptide levels, except, possibly, in the presence of obesity and islet cell tumors.

Explanation of Test

The C peptide levels provide reliable indicators for pancreatic, beta-cell, and secretory functions, and for insulin secretion. In the patient with insulin-dependent diabetes mellitus (IDDM), C peptide measurements can mark endogenous beta-cell activity. It can also be used to confirm suspected surreptitious insulin injections (factitious hypoglycemia). Findings in these patients reveal that insulin levels are usually high, insulin antibodies may be high, but C peptide levels are low or undetectable. This test also monitors the patient's recovery after excision of an insulinoma: a rising C peptide levels suggest insulinoma tumor recurrence or metastasis.

Procedure

1. A fasting, 1-ml venous blood sample is drawn.
2. The blood is separated in a 4° centrifuge or frozen if tested later.

Clinical Implications

1. *Increased C peptide* values occur in
   - **a.** Endogenous hyperinsulinism
   - **b.** Oral hypoglycemic drug ingestion
   - **c.** Pancreas or beta-cell transplant
   - **d.** Renal failure
2. *Decreased C peptide* levels occur in
   - **a.** Factitious hypoglycemia caused by surreptitious insulin administration
   - **b.** Radical pancreatectomy
3. Normal C peptide levels are found in
   - **a.** Diabetes mellitus remission
   - **b.** Non–insulin-dependent diabetes (type II)

> **Clinical Alert**
>
> C peptide measurements before and after glucagon stimulation may be valuable for assessing diabetic insulin therapy. The glucagon-stimulated C peptide test delineates insulin-dependent (type I) from non–insulin-dependent (type II) diabetes.

Patient Preparation

1. Explain the test purpose and blood-drawing procedure.
2. The patient must fast from food, except for water, for 8 to 12 hours before the blood draw.

3. Radioisotope testing should take place *after* blood is drawn for C peptide levels.
4. If the C peptide stimulation test is done, IV glucagon needs to be given after a baseline value blood sample is drawn.
5. See Chapter 1 guidelines for safe, effective, informed *pretest* care.

Patient Aftercare

1. Resume normal activities.
2. Interpret test results and monitor as appropriate.
3. Follow Chapter 1 guidelines for safe, effective, informed *posttest* care.

GLUCAGON ●

Normal Values

50–200 pg/ml or ng/L plasma

Also, during a glucose tolerance test in healthy persons, glucagon levels will decline significantly (as compared with baseline, fasting levels), as normal hyperglycemia takes place during that first hour of testing.

Background

Glucagon is a peptide hormone that originates in the alpha-cells of the pancreatic islets of Langerhans. This hormone promotes glucose production in the liver. Normally, insulin opposes this action. Glucagon provides a sensitive coordinated control mechanism for glucose production and storage. For example, low blood glucose levels cause glucagon to stimulate glucose release into the bloodstream, whereas elevated blood glucose levels reduce the amount of circulating glucagon to approximately 50% of that found in the fasting state. The kidneys also affect glucagon metabolism. Elevated fasting glucagon levels in the presence of renal failure return to normal levels following successful renal transplantation. Abnormally high glucagon levels drop toward normal once insulin therapy controls diabetes. However, when compared with a "normal" person, glucagon secretion in the person with diabetes does not decrease after eating carbohydrates. Moreover, in healthy persons, an arginine infusion will cause increased glucagon secretion.

Explanation of Test

This test measures glucagon production and metabolism. A glucagon deficiency reflects pancreatic tissue loss. Failure of glucagon levels to rise during arginine infusion confirms glucagon deficiency. Hyperglucagonemia (elevated glucagon levels) occurs in diabetes, acute pancreatitis, and in those situations in which catecholamine secretion is stimulated (eg, pheochromocytoma or infection).

Procedure

A fasting 5-ml blood sample is drawn into an EDTA Vacutainer tube containing aprotinin (Trasyol) proteinase inhibitor. Special handling is required because glucagon is very prone to enzymatic degradation. Blood-drawing tubes must be chilled and iced, and plasma must be frozen as soon as possible after centrifuging. Observe universal precautions.

Clinical Implications

1. *Increased glucagon levels* are associated with
   - **a.** Acute pancreatitis (eg, pancreatic alpha-cell tumor)
   - **b.** Diabetes mellitus. Persons with severe diabetic ketoacidosis are reported to have fasting glucagon levels five times normal, despite marked hyperglycemia.
   - **c.** Glucagonoma (familial): Glucagonoma may be manifested by three different syndromes. The first syndrome exhibits a characteristic skin rash, necrolytic migratory erythema, diabetes mellitus or impaired glucose tolerance, weight loss, anemia, and venous thrombosis. This form usually shows elevated glucagon levels > 1000 pg/ml; the second syndrome occurs with severe diabetes. The third form is associated with multiple endocrine neoplasia syndrome and can show relatively lower glucagon levels, compared with the other two.
   - **d.** Chronic renal failure
   - **e.** Hyperlipidemia
   - **f.** Stress
   - **g.** Uremia
   - **h.** Hepatic cirrhosis
   - **i.** Hyperosmolality
   - **j.** Burns
   - **k.** Trauma
   - **l.** Surgery
2. *Reduced glucagon levels* are associated with
   - **a.** Loss of pancreatic tissue
     - **(1)** Pancreatic neoplasms
     - **(2)** Pancreatectomy
   - **b.** Chronic pancreatitis
   - **c.** Cystic fibrosis

Patient Preparation

1. Explain test purpose and blood-drawing procedure. A minimum 8-hour fast is necessary.
2. Promote relaxation in a low-stress environment (stress alters normal glucagon levels).
3. No radioisotopes should be administered within 1 week before the test.
4. See Chapter 1 guidelines for safe, effective, informed *pretest* care.

Patient Aftercare

1. Resume normal activities.
2. Interpret test outcome and monitor as appropriate.
3. Follow Chapter 1 guidelines for safe, effective, informed *posttest* care.

FASTING BLOOD GLUCOSE (FBG); **FASTING BLOOD SUGAR** (FBS) ●

Normal Values

Age:	*mg/dl*	or	*nmol/L*
0–7 d	30–100		1.7–5.6
7 d–6 yr	74–127		4.2–7.0
6–18 yr	70–106		3.9–6.0
Adult	65–110		3.5–6.1

Background

Glucose is formed from carbohydrate digestion and conversion of glycogen to glucose by the liver. The two hormones that directly regulate blood glucose are glucagon and insulin. Glucagon accelerates glycogen breakdown in the liver and causes the blood glucose to rise. Insulin increases cell membrane permeability to glucose, transports glucose into cells (for metabolism), stimulates glycogen formation, and reduces blood glucose levels. Driving glucose into the cells requires insulin and insulin receptors. For example, after a meal, the pancreas releases insulin for glucose metabolism, provided there are enough insulin receptors. Insulin binds to these receptors on the surface of target cells, such as are found in fat and muscle. This opens the channels so that glucose can pass into cells where it can be converted to energy. As cellular glucose metabolism occurs, blood glucose levels fall. Adrenocorticosteroids, ACTH, epinephrine, and thyroxine also play key roles in glucose metabolism.

Explanation of Test

Fasting blood glucose is a vital component of diabetes management. Abnormal glucose metabolism may be caused by inability of pancreatic beta-islet cells to produce insulin, reduced numbers of insulin receptors, faulty intestinal glucose absorption, inability of the liver to metabolize glycogen, or altered levels of hormones that play a role in glucose metabolism (eg, ACTH).

Usually, significantly elevated fasting blood sugar levels (eg, > 140 mg/dl; hyperglycemia) are, in themselves, diagnostic for diabetes. However, mild "borderline" patients may present with normal fasting glucose values. If diabetes is suspected, a glucose tolerance test can confirm the diagnosis. Occasionally, other diseases may produce elevated blood sugar levels (eg, pheochromocytoma). Therefore, a comprehensive history, physical examination, and "workup" should be done before a definitive diagnosis of diabetes is established.

Procedure

1. A 5-ml, fasting venous blood sample is drawn. In known cases of diabetes, the drawing of blood should precede insulin or oral hypoglycemic administration. Observe universal precautions.

2. Self-monitoring of blood glucose by the person with diabetes can be done by finger-stick blood drop sampling, several times a day if necessary. Several devices are on the market for this process. They are relatively easy to use and have been established as a major component in satisfactory diabetes control.

Clinical Implications

1. *Elevated blood sugar (hyperglycemia)* occurs in
   - **a.** Diabetes mellitus. A fasting glucose > 140 mg/dl on more than one occasion is usually diagnostic for diabetes mellitus. An oral glucose tolerance test is not usually necessary in this instance.
   - **b.** Other conditions that produce elevated blood glucose levels include
     - **(1)** Cushing's disease (increased glucocorticoids cause elevated blood sugar levels)
     - **(2)** Acute emotional or physical stress situations (eg, myocardial infarction, or severe infection)
     - **(3)** Pheochromocytoma
     - **(4)** Pituitary adenoma (increased secretion of growth hormone causes elevated blood glucose levels)
     - **(5)** Glucagonoma
     - **(6)** Pancreatitis
     - **(7)** Brain trauma or brain hemorrhage, CVA, convulsions
     - **(8)** Chronic liver disease
     - **(9)** Chronic renal disease
     - **(10)** Vitamin B deficiency
     - **(11)** During pregnancy (may signal potential for onset of diabetes later in life)
2. *Decreased blood glucose (hypoglycemia)* levels occur in
   - **a.** Pancreatic islet cell carcinoma (insulinomas)
   - **b.** Extrapancreatic stomach tumors (carcinoma)
   - **c.** Addison's disease (adrenal insufficiency)
   - **d.** Hypopituitarism
   - **e.** Starvation
   - **f.** Liver damage (alcoholism)
   - **g.** Premature infant; infant delivered of a diabetic mother
   - **h.** Enzyme deficiency diseases (eg, galactosemia, inherited maple syrup disease)
   - **i.** Insulin overdose (accidental or deliberate)

Interfering Factors

1. Steroids, diuretics, other drugs
2. Pregnancy (normally a slight blood glucose elevation occurs)
3. Surgical procedures and anesthesia
4. Obesity or sedentary lifestyle
5. Parenteral glucose administration (eg, from total parenteral nutrition)

Patient Preparation

1. Explain test purpose and blood-drawing procedure.
2. The test requires at least a 12-hour fast; water is permitted. Instruct the patient to defer taking insulin or oral hypoglycemics until after the blood has been drawn (unless specifically instructed to do otherwise).
3. The last time the patient ate must be noted in the record and on the laboratory requisition.
4. See Chapter 1 guidelines for safe, effective, informed *pretest* care.

Patient Aftercare

1. The patient may eat and drink after the blood draw.
2. Interpret test results and monitor appropriately for hyper- and hypoglycemia. Counsel concerning needed lifestyle changes (diet, exercise, glucose monitoring, medication).
3. Persons with values of 200 mg/dl or greater should be placed on a strict intake and output regimen.
4. Follow Chapter 1 guidelines for safe, effective, informed *posttest* care.

Clinical Alert

1. If a person with known or suspected diabetes experiences headaches, irritability, dizziness, weakness, fainting, or impaired cognition, a blood glucose test or finger-stick test must be done before giving insulin. Similar symptoms may be present for both hypoglycemia and hyperglycemia. If a blood glucose cannot be obtained and one is uncertain about the situation, glucose may be given in the form of orange juice, sugar-containing soda, candy (eg, "Life-savers"). **Caution:** make certain the person is conscious enough to manage eating or swallowing. In the acute care setting, IV glucose may be given in the event of severe hypoglycemia. A glucose of "gel" is also commercially available and may be rubbed on the inside of the mouth by another, should the person with diabetes be unable to swallow or to respond properly. Instruct persons prone to hypoglycemia to carry sugar-type items on their person and to wear an ID necklace or bracelet that identifies the person as diabetic.
2. Frequent blood glucose monitoring, including self-monitoring, allows better control and management of diabetes than urine glucose monitoring.
3. When blood glucose values are greater than 300 mg/dl, urine output increases as does the risk of dehydration.
4. Panic values—critical values:

(continued)

(Clinical Alert continued)

- **a.** Less than 40 mg/dl—possible brain damage
- **b.** Greater than 470 mg/dl—possible coma

5. Diabetes is a "disease of the moment": the persons living with diabetes are continually affected by fluctuations in blood glucose levels and must learn to manage and adapt their lifestyle within this framework. For some, adaptation is relatively straightforward; for others, especially those identified as being "brittle," lifestyle changes and management are more complicated and require constant vigilance, attention, encouragement, and support.

NOTE: *Each person with diabetes may experience certain symptoms in their own unique way and pattern.*

2-HOUR POSTPRANDIAL BLOOD SUGAR/GLUCOSE (2-HR PPBS)

Normal Values

65–139 mg/dl or 3.5–7.7 mmol/L.

Explanation of Test

A *postprandial* test, is drawn *after* a meal. Glucose concentration in a 2-hour fasting blood specimen after a meal is rarely elevated in nondiabetic persons but is significantly increased in diabetic patients.

Procedure

Two hours after the patient eats, a 5-ml venous blood sample is obtained. Observe universal precautions.

Clinical Implications

1. *Elevated* levels

- **a.** 140–200 mg/dl indicates impaired glucose tolerance
- **b.** > 200 mg/dl (> 11.1 mmol/L) is diagnostic for diabetes mellitus
- **c.** Gestational diabetes > 150 mg/dl (> 8.3 mmol/L) should be followed-up with a 3-hour glucose tolerance to confirm
- **d.** Other:
  - **(1)** Advanced cirrhosis of liver
  - **(2)** Cushing's syndrome
  - **(3)** Acromegaly
  - **(4)** Hyperthyroidism
  - **(5)** Pheochromocytoma
  - **(6)** Lipoproteinemia
  - **(7)** Myocardial or cerebral infarction
  - **(8)** Chronic renal disease

2. *Decreased* levels

- **a.** Anterior pituitary insufficiency
- **b.** Islet cell adenoma
- **c.** Hypopituitarism
- **d.** Addison's disease

Interfering Factors

Vomiting, gum chewing, and snacking during the 2-hour test interval invalidates the test.

Patient Preparation

1. Fasting blood glucose determination and glucose 2-hour postprandial test are recommended to establish the diagnosis of diabetes mellitus. Glycosylated hemoglobin is recommended for monitoring diabetes control.
2. Explain purpose and procedure of test. The patient must fast at least 12 hours before the blood is drawn. Only water may be taken.
3. Ideally, the patient should be on a high carbohydrate diet 2 to 3 days before testing.
4. After fasting, a high carbohydrate meal is taken.
5. The test is timed from the beginning of the meal. Document time in patient's record.
6. The patient should rest during the 2-hour interval. Smoking is not permitted during this time.
7. See Chapter 1 guidelines for safe, effective, informed *pretest* care.

Patient Aftercare

1. After the blood is drawn, the patient may resume eating and activity.
2. Interpret test results and counsel appropriately.
3. Follow Chapter 1 guidelines for safe, effective, informed *posttest* care.

Clinical Alert

1. Blood glucose values of 140 to 200 mg/dl indicate decreased glucose tolerance and a follow-up glucose tolerance test should be done.
2. Test results are reliable only to the extent the patient is properly prepared.
3. The test is contraindicated in the presence of obvious diabetes mellitus.

GLYCOSYLATED HEMOGLOBIN (HbA_{1c}); GLYCOHEMOGLOBIN (G-Hb); DIABETIC CONTROL INDEX

Normal Values

Results are expressed as percentage of total hemoglobin.

Normal (nondiabetic):	5.5%–8.5%
Diabetes:	Good control, 7.5%–11.4%
	Moderate control, 11.5%–15%
	Poor control, >15%

Background

Glycohemoglobin is a normal minor type of hemoglobin. Hemoglobin A_1 undergoes change or glycosylation to hemoglobin A_{1a}, A_{1b}, and A_{1c} by a slow, nonenzymatic process within the red blood cells (RBCs) during their 120-day circulating lifespan. Simply, glycohemoglobin is blood glucose bound to hemoglobin. The RBC, as it circulates, combines some of the blood glucose with its own hemoglobin to form glycohemoglobin. The amount of glycosylated hemoglobin bound to the erythrocyte is directly proportional to the amount of glucose available to it over the 120-day RBC life. In the presence of hyperglycemia, an increase in glycohemoglobin is usually caused by an increase in HbA_{1c}. If the glucose concentration increases because of insulin deficiency, then glycosylation is irreversible.

Explanation of Test

Glycosylated hemoglobin reflects average blood sugar levels for the 2- to 3-month period before the test. This test provides information for evaluating diabetic treatment modalities, is useful in determining treatment for juvenile-onset diabetes with acute ketoacidosis, and tracks control of blood glucose in milder cases of diabetes. It can be a valuable adjunct in determining therapeutic choices and directions (oral antihypoglycemic agents, insulin, beta-cell transplants). A blood sample can be drawn at any time. The measurement is of particular value for specific groups of patients: diabetic children, diabetics in whom the renal threshold for glucose is abnormal, unstable insulin-dependent diabetics in whom blood sugars vary markedly from day to day, type II diabetics who become pregnant, and persons who, before their scheduled appointments, will change their usual habits, dietary or otherwise, so that their metabolic control appears better than it actually is.

Procedure

Obtain a 3-ml venous blood sample with EDTA anticoagulant additive. Serum may not be used. Observe universal precautions.

Clinical Implications

1. Values are frequently increased in poorly controlled and newly diagnosed diabetes, and HbA_{1c} levels may constitute greater than 15% of the total hemoglobin.
2. With optimal control, the HbA_{1c} moves toward normal.
3. A diabetic patient who recently comes under good control may still show higher concentrations of glycosylated hemoglobin. This level declines gradually over several months as nearly normal glycosylated hemoglobin replaces older RBCs with higher concentrations.
4. Values are also increased in iron-deficiency anemia, splenectomy, and alcohol and lead toxicity.
5. Decreases in glycosylated hemoglobin occur in
   - **a.** Hemolytic anemia
   - **b.** Chronic blood loss
   - **c.** Pregnancy
   - **d.** Chronic renal failure

Interfering Factors

1. Presence of Hb F, S + H causes falsely high values.
2. Hb S, C, E, D, G, and Lepore will cause falsely low values.

Patient Preparation

1. Explain test purpose and blood-drawing procedure. Observe universal precautions. Fasting is not required.
2. Note that this test is *not* meant for short-term diabetes mellitus management, rather, it assesses the efficacy of long-term management modalities over several weeks or months.
3. See Chapter 1 guidelines for safe, effective, informed *pretest* care.

Patient Aftercare

1. Interpret test outcome and counsel appropriately for management of diabetes. If test results are not consistent with clinical findings, check the patient for HbF, which raises the A_{1c} results.
2. Follow Chapter 1 guidelines for safe, effective, informed *posttest* care.

Clinical Alert

1. A number of different tests can determine glycosylated hemoglobin, each with their own values. The most specific of these measures hemoglobin A_{1c}. There are different expected values for each test. Keep in mind that hemoglobin A_1 is always 2% to 4% higher than A_{1c}. When interpreting, be certain of the specific test used.
2. Check with your laboratory for type of test and normal values.

INSULIN

Normal Values

Adult:	6–24 μU/ml or 42–167 pmol/L (immunoreactive)
Newborn:	3–20 μU/ml or 21–139 pmol/L

Background

Insulin, a hormone produced by the pancreatic beta-cells of the islets of Langerhans, regulates carbohydrate metabolism, together with contributions from the liver, adipose tissue, and other target cells. It is responsible for maintaining blood glucose levels constant within the defined range. The rate of insulin secretion is regulated primarily by the level of blood glucose perfusing the pancreas; however, it can also be affected by hormones, the autonomic nervous system, and nutritional status.

Explanation of Test

Insulin levels are valuable for establishing the process of an insulinoma (tumor of the islets of Langerhans), evaluating abnormal carbohydrate and lipid metabolism, and diagnosing diabetes when abnormal glucose tolerance values occur. It is valuable for investigating the causes of fasting hypoglycemic states and neoplasm differentiation.

The insulin study can be done in conjunction with a glucose tolerance test or fasting blood glucose.

Procedure

1. Obtain a 4-ml, fasting blood sample; serum is preferred. Observe universal precautions.
2. If done in conjunction with a glucose tolerance test, the specimens should be drawn before administering oral glucose and again at 30, 60, and 120 minutes after glucose ingestion (the same times as the GTT).

Clinical Implications

1. *Increased insulin values* are associated with
   - **a.** Insulinoma (pancreatic islet tumor). Diagnosis is based on
     - **(1)** The Association of Hyperinsulinemia and hypoglycemia
     - **(2)** Persistent hypoglycemia together with hyperinsulinemia 2 to 3 hours after tolbutamide injection
     - **(3)** Failed C peptide suppression with a plasma glucose value of 30 mg/dl or less and an insulin/glucose ratio greater than 0.3.
   - **b.** Non–insulin-dependent diabetes mellitus (type II) (NIDDM)
   - **c.** Acromegaly
   - **d.** Cushing's syndrome
   - **e.** Liver disease
   - **f.** Obesity (most common cause)
   - **g.** Familial galactose or fructose intolerance
2. *Decreased insulin values* are found in
   - **a.** Insulin-dependent (type II) diabetes mellitus
   - **b.** Hypopituitarism

Interfering Factors

1. Surreptitious insulin or oral hypoglycemic agent ingestion or injection causes elevated insulin levels.
2. Oral contraceptives and other drugs cause falsely elevated values.
3. Recently administered radioisotopes affect test results.

Patient Preparation

1. Explain test purpose and procedure.
2. The patient should fast from all food and fluid except water unless otherwise directed.
3. Because insulin release from an insulinoma may be erratic and unpre-

dictable, it may be necessary for the patient to fast for as long as 72 hours pretest.

4. See Chapter 1 guidelines for safe, effective, informed *pretest* care.

Patient Aftercare

1. Resume normal activity and diet.
2. Interpret test results and counsel appropriately. Obese patients may have insulin resistance and unusually high fasting and postprandial insulin levels.
3. Follow Chapter 1 guidelines for safe, effective, informed *posttest* care.

Clinical Alert

A potentially fatal situation may exist if the insulinoma secretes unpredictably high levels of insulin. In this case, the blood glucose may drop to such dangerously low levels that the person is rendered comatose and unable to self-administer oral glucose forms. Patients and their families need to learn how to deal with such an emergency and to be vigilant until the problem is treated.

GLUCOSE TOLERANCE TEST (GTT); ORAL GLUCOSE TOLERANCE TEST (OGTT)

Normal Values

FASTING

Adult:	70–110 mg/dl; 3.9–6.1 mmol/L
Child:	< 130 mg/dl; < 72 mmol/L

30 MINUTE

Adult:	110–170 mg/dl; 6.1–9.4 mmol/L

60 MINUTE (1 HR)

Adult:	120–170 mg/dl; 6.7–9.4 mmol/L
Child:	< 140 mg/dl

120 MINUTE (2 HR)

Adult:	70–120 mg/dl; 3.9–6.7 mmol/L
Child:	< 140 mg/dl; < 7.8 mmol/L

3 HOUR

Adult:	70–120 mg/dl; 3.9–6.7 mmol/L

All four blood values must fall within normal limits to be considered normal. All urine samples also should test negative for glucose.

Background

In a healthy individual, the insulin response to a large oral glucose dose is almost immediate. It peaks in 30 to 60 minutes and returns to normal levels within 3 hours. In this instance, sufficient insulin is present to metabolize the glucose ingested at the beginning of the test.

Explanation of Test

If fasting and postprandial glucose test results are borderline, the glucose tolerance test can support or rule out diabetes mellitus; it can also be a part of a workup for unexplained hypertriglyceridemia, neuropathy, impotence, diabeteslike renal diseases, or retinopathy. It may be ordered when there is sugar in the urine or when the fasting blood sugar or 2-hour postprandial blood sugar is significantly elevated. The glucose tolerance test is more definitive for diagnosing hypoglycemia, malabsorption syndrome, Cushing's syndrome, and acromegaly (see Table 6-1).

Indications for Test

The glucose tolerance test should be done on certain patients, particularly those with the following

1. Family history of diabetes
2. Obesity
3. Unexplained episodes of hypoglycemia
4. History of recurrent infections (boils and abscesses)
5. (In women) history of delivery of large infants, stillbirths, neonatal death, premature labor, and abortions.
6. Transitory glycosuria or hyperglycemia during pregnancy, surgery, trauma, stress, myocardial infarction, ACTH administration.

Procedure

This is a timed test. A 2-hour test is done for detecting diabetes in individuals, with the exception of pregnant women; the 3-hour test is done for pregnant women; the 5-hour test evaluates possible hypoglycemia.

1. A diet of 150 g of carbohydrates or greater should be eaten for 3 days pretest.
2. The following drugs may influence test results and should be discontinued 3 days before the test:
   - **a.** Hormones, oral contraceptives
   - **b.** Salicylates
   - **c.** Diuretic agents
   - **d.** Hypoglycemic agents
3. Insulin and oral hypoglycemics should be withheld until the test is completed.
4. Record the patient's weight.
   - **a.** Pediatric doses of the glucose are based on body weight calculated as 1.75 g up to 75 g of glucose.
   - **b.** Pregnant females: 100 g glucose.
   - **c.** Nonpregnant adult: 75 g of glucose.

5. A 5-ml sample of venous blood is drawn. The patient should fast 12 to 16 hours before testing. After the blood is drawn, the patient drinks all of a specially formulated glucose solution within a 5-minute time frame.
6. Blood and urine samples are then obtained at 30 minutes, 1 hour, 2 hours, 3, 4, and 5 hours after glucose ingestion.
7. The fifth hour specimens are significant for detecting hypoglycemia.
8. Tolerance tests can also be performed for pentose, lactose, galactose, and D-xylose.

Clinical Implications

1. The presence of abnormal glucose tolerance values (decreased tolerance to glucose) is based on the International Classification for Diabetes Mellitus and the glucose intolerance categories:
   - **a.** At least two GTT values must be abnormal for a diagnosis of diabetes mellitus to be validated.
   - **b.** In cases of overt diabetes, no insulin is secreted; abnormally high glucose levels persist throughout the test.
   - **c.** Glucose values that fall above normal values, but below the diagnostic criteria for diabetes or impaired glucose tolerance (IGT), should be considered as nondiagnostic conditions.
2. Interpretation of glucose tolerance levels:

Adult diabetes mellitus 1-hour glucose	> 200 mg/dl
and 2-hour glucose	> 200 mg/dl
Adult impaired glucose tolerance 1-hour glucose	> 200 mg/dl
and 2-hour glucose	> 140 mg/dl
Juvenile diabetes mellitus (fasting glucose)	> 140 mg/dl
and 1-hour glucose	> 200 mg/dl
and 2-hour glucose	> 200 mg/dl
Impaired glucose tolerance in children (fasting glucose	< 140 mg/dl
and 2-hour glucose	> 140 mg/dl

3. A diagnosis of *gestational diabetes* is based on the following blood glucose results *(two or more must be met and exceeded)*: Fasting, > 105 mg/dl; 1-hr, > 190 mg/dl; 2-hr, > 165 mg/dl; 3-hr, > 145 mg/dl.
   - **a.** If abnormal results occur during pregnancy, repeat GTT at the first postpartum visit.
   - **b.** Hb A_{1c} is not a reliable test for gestational diabetes.
   - **c.** During labor, maintain maternal glucose levels at 80–100 mg/dl; beware of markedly increased insulin sensitivity in the immediate postpartum period.
4. Decreased glucose tolerance occurs with high glucose values in
   - **a.** Diabetes mellitus
   - **b.** Postgastrectomy
   - **c.** Hyperthyroidism
   - **d.** Excess glucose ingestion
   - **e.** Hyperlipidemia, types III, IV, and V
   - **f.** Hemochromatosis
   - **g.** Cushing's disease (steroid effect) elevates glucose levels
   - **h.** CNS lesions
   - **i.** Pheochromocytoma

TABLE 6-1
International Classifications for Diabetes Mellitus and Other Glucose Intolerance Categories*

Five Major Clinical Classes					*Two Statistical Classes*	
Type 1	*Type 2*	*Type 3*	*Type 4*	*Type 5*	*No. 1*	*No. 2*
Insulin-dependent diabetes mellitus (IDDM)	Non–insulin-dependent diabetes mellitus (NIDDM) A. Nonobese B. Obese	Diabetes mellitus with other conditions or syndromes	Impaired glucose tolerance (IGT) A. Nonobese B. Obese C. Associated with other diseases or conditions	Gestational diabetes (GDM)	Previous abnormality of glucose tolerance (Prev AGT)	Potential abnormality of glucose tolerance (Pot AGT)

Diagnostic Criteria				
Types 1 & 2	*Type 3*	*Type 4*	*Type 5*	*Nos. 1 & 2*
Adults Classic symptoms and unequivocal elevation of plasma glucose *or* Fasting plasma glucose >140 mg/dl more than once *or* Oral glucose tolerance test (challenge dose 75 g) > 200 mg/dl at 1 and 2 hours, confirmed by repetition.	Same as for IDDM including associated conditions or syndromes	***Adults*** Fasting plasma glucose < 140 mg/dl; oral glucose tolerance test > 200 mg/dl at 1 hour; 140–199 mg/dl at 2 hours.	Two of the following minimum levels: Fasting plasma glucose > 105 mg/dl; oral glucose tolerance test (challenge dose 100 g) > 190 me/dl at 1	***Adults*** Fasting plasma glucose below 115 mg/dl; oral glucose tolerance test < 200 mg/dl at 1 hour < 140 mg/dl at 2 hours ***Children*** Fasting plasma glucose < 130 mg/dl; oral glucose tolerance < 140 mg/dl at 2 hours.

Children Classic symptoms and random plasma glucose > 200 mg/dl *or* Fasting plasma glucose > 140 mg/dl more than once *and* Oral glucose tolerance test (challenge dose 1.75 g/kg ideal body weight, up to a maximum of 75 g) > 200 mg/dl at 1 and 2 hours, confirmed by repetition.	***Children*** Fasting plasma glucose < 140 mg/dl; oral glucose tolerance test at 2 hours > 140 mg/dl	hour; > 165 mg/dl at 2 hours, or > 145 mg/dl at 3 hours

*National Diabetes Data Group, National Institutes of Health, Bethesda, MD.

5. Decreased glucose levels and hypoglycemia can be found in von Gierke's disease, severe liver damage, and increased epinephrine levels.
6. Increased glucose tolerance with flat curve (glucose does not increase, but may decrease to hypoglycemic levels) occurs in
   - **a.** Pancreatic islet cell hyperplasia or tumor
   - **b.** Poor intestinal absorption caused by diseases such as s prue, celiac disease, Whipple's disease
   - **c.** Hypoparathyroidism
   - **d.** Addison's disease
   - **e.** Liver disease
   - **f.** Hypopituitarism

Interfering Factors

1. Smoking increases glucose levels.
2. Altered diets (such as weight-reduction) before testing can diminish carbohydrate tolerance and suggest a "false diabetes."
3. Glucose levels normally tend to increase with aging.
4. Prolonged oral contraceptive use will present significantly higher glucose levels in the second hour or in later blood specimens.
5. Infectious diseases, illnesses, and operative procedures will affect glucose tolerance. Two weeks of recovery should be allowed before the test.
6. Certain drugs will impair glucose tolerance levels:
   - **a.** Insulin
   - **b.** Oral hypoglycemics
   - **c.** Large doses of salicylates
   - **d.** Thiazide diuretics
   - **e.** Oral contraceptives
   - **f.** Corticosteroids
   - **g.** Estrogens
   - **h.** Ferrous ascorbinate
   - **i.** Nicotinic acid
   - **j.** Phenothiazines
   - **k.** Lithium
   - **l.** Metyrapone (metopirone)

   If possible, these drugs should be held for at least 3 days before testing.
7. Prolonged bed rest will influence glucose tolerance results. If possible, the patient should be ambulatory and active.

Patient Preparation

1. Explain test purpose and procedure. A written reminder may be helpful.
   - **a.** A diet composed of high carbohydrates (150 g) should be eaten for 3 days preceding the test. Instruct the patient to abstain from alcohol.
   - **b.** The patient should fast for 12 hours, but not more than 16 hours before the test. Only water may be taken during fasting time and test time. Use of tobacco products is not permitted during testing.
   - **c.** Patients should rest quietly during the test period. They may feel weak or faint during the test. Also, exercise alters glucose values.
2. Collect urine and blood specimens at the prescribed times and record exact times collected. The patient should empty the bladder completely each time. A written reminder of collection times is usually helpful.
3. See Chapter 1 guidelines for safe, effective, informed *pretest* care.

Patient Aftercare

1. The patient may resume normal diet and activities at the end of the test. Encourage eating complex carbohydrates and protein if permitted.
2. Administer prescribed insulin or oral hypoglycemics when the test is done. Arrange for the patient to eat within a short (half hour) time after these medications are taken.
3. Interpret test results and counsel appropriately. Patients with a new diagnosis of diabetes will need diet, medication, and lifestyle modification instructions.
4. See Chapter 1 guidelines for safe, effective, informed *posttest* care.

Clinical Alert

1. Glucose tolerance testing is contraindicated for patients with a recent history of surgery, myocardial infarction, or labor and delivery; these conditions can produce invalid values.
2. If the fasting glucose is > 140 mg/dl on two separate occasions, or the 2-hour postprandial blood glucose is > 200 mg/dl on two separate occasions, this test is not necessary for a diagnosis of diabetes mellitus to be established.
3. The glucose tolerance test is of limited diagnostic value for children.
4. The test should be postponed if the patient becomes ill, even with the usual common illnesses, such as "flu" or a severe cold.
5. Record and report any reactions during the test. Weakness, faintness, and sweating may occur between the second and third hours of the test. If this occurs, a blood sample for a glucose level is drawn immediately, and the GTT test is aborted.
6. Should the patient vomit the glucose solution, the test is declared invalid; it can be repeated in 3 days (approx. 72 hours).

LACTOSE TOLERANCE; BREATH HYDROGEN TEST ●

Normal Values

A rise in glucose greater than 30 mg/dl, absence of abdominal symptoms such as pain or diarrhea.

Hydrogen (breath): less than 50 ppm hydrogen (H_2) increase from baseline.

Background

Lactose intolerance often begins in infancy, with symptoms of diarrhea, vomiting, failure to thrive, and malabsorption. The patient becomes asymptomatic when lactose is removed from the diet. This syndrome is caused by a deficiency of sugar-splitting enzymes (lactose) in the intestinal tract.

Explanation of Test

This is actually a glucose tolerance test done to diagnose intestinal disaccharidase (lactase) deficiency. Breath samples reveal increased hydrogen levels that are caused by lactose buildup in the intestinal tract.

Procedure

1. Follow instructions given for the glucose tolerance test.
2. A fasting blood specimen is drawn. The patient then drinks 100 g of lactose mixed in 200 ml of water.
3. Blood lactose samples are then drawn at 15-, 30- 60-, and 120-minute intervals.
4. Fasting hydrogen breath samples are taken at the same time intervals as the blood specimens. See your laboratory for collection procedures.

Clinical Implications

1. Lactose intolerance occurs as follows:
   - **a.** A "flat" lactose tolerance finding (no glucose rise) points to a deficiency of sugar-splitting enzymes, as in irritable bowel syndrome. Deficiency is more prevalent in American Indians, blacks, Oriental, and Jewish persons.
   - **b.** A monosaccharide tolerance test, such as glucose/galactose tolerance test, should be done as a follow-up.
     - **(1)** The patient ingests 25 g of both glucose and galactose.
     - **(2)** A normal increase in glucose indicates a lactose deficiency.
   - **c.** The hydrogen breath test is abnormal in the lactose deficiency test because
     - **(1)** Malabsorption causes hydrogen (H_2) production through the process of fermentation in the colon.
     - **(2)** The H_2 formed is directly proportional to the amount of test dose lactose ***not*** absorbed.
   - **d.** In diabetes, blood glucose values may show increases greater than 20 mg/dl, despite impaired lactose absorption.

Patient Preparation

1. Explain test purpose and procedure. The patient must fast for 12 hours before the test.
2. No dark bread, peas, beans, sugars, or high-fiber foods should be taken within 24 hours of the test.
3. Smoking is not permitted during the test and for 8 hours before testing.
4. No antibiotics should be taken for 2 weeks before test unless specifically ordered.
5. See Chapter 1 guidelines for safe, effective, informed *pretest* care.

Patient Aftercare

1. Resume normal diet and activity.

2. Interpret test results and counsel appropriately. Patients with irritable bowel syndrome with gas, bloating, abdominal pain, constipation, and diarrhea have lactase deficiency. Restricting milk intake relieves symptoms.
3. Follow Chapter 1 guidelines for safe, effective, informed *posttest* care.

● END PRODUCTS OF METABOLISM AND OTHER TESTS

AMMONIA (NH_3) ●

Normal Values

Neonate:	64–107 μmol/L	Child:	21–50 μmol/L
< 2 wk:	56–92 μmol/L	Adult:	9–33 μmol/L

Values test somewhat higher in capillary blood samples. Repeated values can vary greatly because of testing methods used.

Background

Ammonia, an end product of protein metabolism, is formed by bacteria acting on intestinal proteins, together with glutamine hydrolysis in the kidneys. The liver normally removes most of this ammonia through the portal vein circulation and converts the ammonia to urea. Because any appreciable level of ammonia in the blood affects the body's acid–base balance and brain function, its removal from the body is essential. The liver accomplishes this by synthesizing urea so that it can be excreted by the kidneys.

Explanation of Test

Blood ammonia levels are used to diagnose Reye's syndrome, to evaluate metabolism, and to determine the progress of severe liver disease and its response to treatment.

Procedure

1. Obtain a 3-ml, fasting, venous heparinized plasma sample. Observe universal precautions.
2. Place the sample in an iced container and perform test within 20 minutes.
3. Note all antibiotics the patient is receiving; these drugs lower ammonia levels.

Clinical Implications

1. *Increased ammonia levels* occur in
   - **a.** Reye's syndrome
   - **b.** Liver disease, cirrhosis
   - **c.** Hepatic coma (does not reflect degree of coma)
   - **d.** GI hemorrhage (with liver disease)
   - **e.** Eck's fistula
   - **f.** Shock

g. Asparagine intoxication
h. Some cases of congestive heart failure
i. GI tract infection with distention and stasis

2. *Decreased ammonia levels* occur in hyperornithinemia.

Interfering Factors

1. Ammonia levels vary with protein intake and many drugs.
2. Exercise may cause an increase in ammonia levels.
3. Levels may be increased by tight tourniquet or tightly clenched fist.

Patient Preparation

1. Explain test purpose and procedure. Instruct the patient to fast (if possible) for 8 hours before the blood test. Water is permitted.
2. See Chapter 1 guidelines for safe, effective, informed *pretest* care.

Patient Aftercare

1. Interpret test outcomes, monitor appropriately, and begin treatment.
2. In patients with impaired liver function demonstrated by elevated ammonia levels, the blood level can be lowered by reduced protein intake and by use of antibiotics to reduce intestinal bacterial counts.
3. Follow Chapter 1 guidelines for safe, effective, informed *posttest* care.

Clinical Alert

Ammonia should be measured in all cases of unexplained lethargy and vomiting, encephalitis, or any neonate with unexplained neurologic deterioration.

BILIRUBIN

Normal Values

Adult:	Total bilirubin, 0.2–1.0 mg/dl or 3.4–17.1 μmol/L
	Conjugated direct, 0.0–0.2 mg/dl or 0.0–3.4 μmol/L
	Unconjugated indirect: 0.2–0.8 mg/dl or 3.4–13.68 μmol/L
Newborn:	
Total:	1.0–10.0 mg/dl
Conjugated (direct):	0.0–0.8 mg/dl
Unconjugated (indirect):	0.0–10.0 mg/dl

Background

Bilirubin, resulting from the breakdown of hemoglobin in the red blood cells (RBCs), is a by-product of hemolysis (RBC destruction). It is produced by the reticuloendothelial system and removed from the body by the liver, which excretes it into the bile. It gives the bile its major pigmentation. Usually a small amount of bilirubin is found in the serum. A rise in serum levels will occur if there is an excessive destruction of RBCs or if the liver is unable to excrete the normal amounts of bilirubin produced.

There are two forms of bilirubin in the body: (1) indirect or unconjugated bilirubin (which is protein-bound); and (2) direct or conjugated bilirubin that circulates freely in the blood until it reaches the liver, where it is conjugated by glucuronosyltransferase and then excreted into the bile. An increase in protein-bound bilirubin (unconjugated bilirubin) is more frequently associated with increased destruction of RBCs (hemolysis); an increase in free-flowing bilirubin is more likely seen in dysfunction or blockage of the liver. A routine examination measures only the total bilirubin. A normal level of total bilirubin rules out any significant impairment of the excretory function of the liver or excessive hemolysis of red cells. Only when the levels are elevated will there be a call for differentiation of the bilirubin according to the conjugated and unconjugated levels.

Explanation of Test

The measurement of bilirubin evaluates liver function, hemolytic anemias, and hyperbilirubinemia (in newborns).

Procedure

1. Obtain a 5-ml, nonhemolyzed, fasting sample. Observe universal precautions.
2. Protect the sample from ultraviolet light (sunlight).
3. Avoid air bubbles and unnecessary shaking of the sample during blood collection.
4. If the specimen cannot be examined immediately; store in a refrigerator and in darkness.
5. In infants, blood can be collected from a heel puncture. Two full blood microsampling tubes are collected. (In newborns, the sample size is 0.3 ml).

Clinical Implications

1. *Bilirubin elevations accompanied by jaundice* may be due to hepatic, obstructive, or hemolytic causes:
   - **a.** *Hepatocellular jaundice* results from injury or disease of the parenchymal cells of the liver and can be caused by
     - **(1)** Viral hepatitis
     - **(2)** Cirrhosis
     - **(3)** Infectious mononucleosis
     - **(4)** Reactions of certain drugs such as chlorpromazine
   - **b.** *Obstructive jaundice* is usually the result of obstruction of the common bile or hepatic ducts caused by stones or neoplasms. The obstruction produces high, conjugated bilirubin levels owing to bile regurgitation.

c. *Hemolytic jaundice* is due to overproduction of bilirubin, resulting from hemolytic processes that produce high levels of unconjugated bilirubin. Hemolytic jaundice can be found in
   (1) Hemolytic disease of the newborn (erythroblastosis fetalis)
      (a) Rh incompatibility
      (b) ABO incompatibility (less severe hemolytic anemia)
   (2) Pernicious anemia
   (3) Sickle cell anemia
   (4) Transfusion reactions
   (5) Crigler–Najjar syndrome (a severe disease that results from a genetic deficiency of a hepatic enzyme needed for the conjugation of bilirubin).

2. *Elevated indirect* ***nonconjugate*** *bilirubin levels* occur in
   a. Hemolytic anemias
   b. Trauma in the presence of a large hematoma
   c. Hemorrhagic pulmonary infarcts
   d. Crigler–Najjar syndrome (rare)
   e. Gilbert's disease (rare; conjugated hyperbilirubinemia)
3. *Elevated direct* ***conjugate*** *bilirubin levels* occur in
   a. Cancer of the head of the pancreas
   b. Choledocholithiasis
   c. Dubin–Johnson syndrome

Interfering Factors

1. A 1-hour exposure of the specimen to sunlight or high-intensity artificial light at room temperature will decrease the bilirubin content.
2. No contrast medium administration 24 hours before measurement; a high-fat meal may also cause decreased bilirubin levels by interfering with the chemical reactions.
3. Air bubbles and shaking the specimen may cause decreased levels.
4. Foods (carrots, yams) and drugs increase the yellow hue in the serum, but do not increase bilirubin levels.
5. Prolonged fasting raises the bilirubin level.

Clinical Alert

1. In newborns, if total bilirubin approaches > 15 mg/dl, aggressive treatment has to be initiated immediately (exchange transfusion) or mental retardation may result.
2. Panic value in adults is > 12 mg/dl.

Patient Preparation

1. Explain test purpose and procedure and its relation to jaundice. **Jaundice/icterus:** Excessive amounts of bilirubin eventually seep into

the tissues, which then assume a yellow hue. The yellow color is a clinical sign of jaundice. In newborns, signs of jaundice may indicate hemolytic anemia or congenital icterus. If the bilirubin levels reach a critical point in the infant, damage to the central nervous system may occur in a condition known as *kernicterus*. Therefore, in these infants, it is the level of bilirubin that is the deciding factor in the decision to do an exchange transfusion. Total bilirubin must be > 2.5 mg/dl to detect jaundice.

2. The patient should be fasting, if possible.
3. See Chapter 1 guidelines for safe, effective, informed *pretest* care.

Patient Aftercare

1. Interpret test outcome and monitor appropriately.
2. Resume normal activities.
3. Follow Chapter 1 guidelines for safe, effective, informed *posttest* care.

BLOOD UREA NITROGEN (BUN)

Normal Values

Adult:	7–18 mg/dl, or 2.5–6.4 mmol/L
> 60 years:	8–20 mg/dl, or 2.9–7.5 mmol/L
Child:	5–18 mg/dl, or 1.8–6.4 mmol/L

Background

Urea forms in the liver and, along with CO_2, constitutes the final product of protein metabolism. The amount of excreted urea varies directly with the dietary protein intake, with increased excretion in fever, diabetes, and increased adrenal gland activity.

Explanation of Test

The test for BUN, measuring the nitrogen portion of urea, is used as a gross index of glomerular function and the production and excretion of urea. Rapid protein catabolism and impairment of kidney function will result in an elevated BUN. The rate at which the BUN rises is influenced by the degree of tissue necrosis, protein catabolism, and the rate at which the kidneys excrete the urea nitrogen. The BUN is less sensitive than creatinine clearance tests and may not be abnormal until the creatinine clearance is moderately abnormal.

Procedure

Obtain a 5-ml venous blood sample; serum is preferred. Observe universal precautions.

Clinical Implications

1. *Increased BUN levels (azotemia)* occur in
   - **a.** Impaired renal function
   - **b.** Congestive heart failure
   - **c.** Salt and water depletion
   - **d.** Shock

- **e.** Hemorrhage into GI tract
- **f.** Acute myocardial infarction
- **g.** Stress
- **h.** Excessive protein intake or protein catabolism

2. *Decreased BUN levels* are associated with
- **a.** Liver failure (severe liver disease) such as hepatitis, drugs, poisoning
- **b.** Acromegaly
- **c.** Malnutrition
- **d.** Anabolic steroid use
- **e.** IV feedings only (overhydration)
- **f.** Impaired absorption (celiac dis ease)
- **g.** Nephrotic syndrome (occasional)
- **h.** Syndrome of inappropriate secretion of antidiuretic hormone (SIADH)

Interfering Factors

1. A combination of a low-protein and a high-carbohydrate diet can cause a decreased BUN level.
2. The BUN is normally lower in children and women because they have a smaller muscle mass than adult men.
3. Increased BUN values normally occur in late pregnancy and infancy because of increased use of protein.
4. Older persons may have an increased BUN when their kidneys are not able to concentrate urine adequately.
5. Decreased BUN values may normally occur earlier in pregnancy because of physiologic hydremia.
6. Many drugs may cause increased and decreased BUN levels.

Clinical Alert

1. If a patient is confused, disoriented, or has convulsions, the BUN should be checked. If the level is high, it may help to explain these signs and symptoms.
2. Panic value of BUN is greater than 100 mg/dl.
3. In chronic renal disease, BUN correlates better with symptoms of uremia than does serum creatinine levels.

Patient Preparation

1. Explain BUN test purpose and blood-drawing procedure. Assess dietary history.
2. See Chapter 1 guidelines for safe, effective, informed *pretest* care.

Patient Aftercare

1. Interpret test outcome and monitor as appropriate for impaired kidney function.

2. In patients with an elevated BUN, fluid and electrolyte regulation may be impaired.
3. See Chapter 1 guidelines for safe, effective, informed *posttest* care.

CHOLINESTERASE (SERUM) AND CHOLINESTERASE (RBC)

Normal Values

Serum cholinesterase:	4.9–11.9 U/ml or kU/L
Dibucaine inhibition:	79%–84%
RBC cholinesterase:	6,700–10,000 U/L

Values vary with substrate and method. These are two different tests.

Background

The cholinesterase of serum is referred to as pseudocholinesterase to distinguish it from the true cholinesterase of the red blood cell (RBC). Both of these enzymes act on acetylcholine and other cholinesters. Alkylphosphates are potent inhibitors of both serum and RBC cholinesterase.

Patients who are homozygous for the atypical gene that controls serum cholinesterase activity have low levels of cholinesterase that are not inhibited by dibucaine. Those persons with normal serum cholinesterase activity show 70% to 90% inhibition by dibucaine.

Explanation of Test

These are two separate tests. The primary use of serum cholinesterase measurement (pseudocholinesterase) is to monitor the effect of muscle relaxants, such as succinylcholine, that are used in surgery. Patients for whom succinylcholine (suxamethonium) anesthesia is planned should be tested for the presence of atypical cholinesterase variants—which are incapable of hydrolyzing this widely used muscle relaxant—employing the dibucaine inhibition test.

The RBC cholinesterase test is used when poisoning by pesticides, such as parathion or malathion, is suspected. Severe insecticide poisoning causes headaches, visual distortions, nausea, vomiting, pulmonary edema, confusion, convulsions, respiratory paralysis, and coma.

Procedures

1. Serum cholinesterase: Obtain 5 ml of blood; 3 ml of serum is needed. The test must be performed within 48 hours. Observe universal precautions.
2. RBC cholinesterase: a blood sample is drawn using sodium heparin as an anticoagulant (serum cannot be used). Observe universal precautions.

Clinical Implications

1. *Decreased or no serum cholinesterase* occurs in
   a. Congenital inherited recessive disease. These patients will not be able

to hydrolyze drugs, such as muscle relaxants, in surgery. These patients may have a prolonged period of apnea if they are given succinylcholine (possibly fatal).

b. Poisoning from organic phosphate insecticides.

c. Liver diseases, hepatitis, cirrhosis with jaundice.

d. Conditions that may have decreased blood albumin, such as malnutrition, anemia, infections, skin diseases, and acute myocardial infarction.

e. Congestive heart failure.

2. *Decreased RBC cholinesterase levels* occur in

a. Congenital inherited recessive disease

b. Organic phosphate poisoning

c. Evaluation of paroxysmal nocturnal hemoglobinemia

d. Anemia

e. Tuberculosis

f. Hypoproteinemia

g. Uremia

h. Shock

3. *Increased serum cholinesterase* is found in

a. Type IV hyperlipidemia

b. Nephrosis

c. Obesity

d. Diabetes

4. *Increased RBC cholinesterase* is associated with reticulocytosis.

Patient Preparation

1. Explain test purpose and procedure.
2. Draw blood for serum cholesterinase 2 days before surgery.
3. Blood should not be drawn in recovery room; prior administration of surgical drugs and anesthesia invalidates the test.
4. See Chapter 1 guidelines for safe, effective, informed *pretest* care.

Patient Aftercare

1. Interpret test outcome and counsel appropriately.
2. Patients exhibiting < 70% inhibition should be considered as an atypical cholinesterase variant and the administration of succinylcholine or similar type drugs may pose a risk.
3. See Chapter 1 guidelines for safe, effective, informed *posttest* care.

Clinical Alert

1. In industrial exposure, workers should not return to work until values rise to 75% of normal. RBC cholinesterase regenerates at the rate of 1% per day. Plasma cholinesterase regenerates at the rate of 25% in 7 to 10 days and returns to baseline in 4 to 6 weeks.
2. Cholinesterase activity is completely and irreversibly inhibited by organophosphate pesticides.

CREATININE

Normal Values

Adult:		0.6–1.3 mg/dl, or 62–115 μmol/L
Child:	0–3 yr,	0.3–0.7 mg/dl, or 27–62 μmol/L
	3–18 yr,	0.5–1.0 mg/dl, or 44–88 μmol/L

Background

Creatinine is a by-product in the breakdown of muscle creatine phosphate, resulting from energy metabolism. It is produced at a constant rate, depending on the muscle mass of the person and is removed from the body by the kidneys. Production of creatinine is constant as long as muscle mass remains constant. A disorder of kidney function reduces excretion of creatinine, resulting in increased blood levels.

Explanation of Test

The test diagnoses impaired renal function. It is a more specific and sensitive indicator of kidney disease than BUN, although in chronic renal disease, BUN correlates more accurately with symptoms of uremia than does the blood creatinine.

Procedure

Obtain a 5-ml venous blood sample; serum preferred, but heparinized blood can be used. Observe universal precautions.

Clinical Implications

1. *Increased blood creatinine levels* occur in
- **a.** Impaired renal function
- **b.** Chronic nephritis
- **c.** Obstruction of the urinary tract
- **d.** Muscle disease
  - **(1)** Gigantism
  - **(2)** Acromegaly
  - **(3)** Myasthenia gravis
  - **(4)** Muscular dystrophy
  - **(5)** Poliomyelitis
- **e.** Congestive heart failure
- **f.** Shock
- **g.** Dehydration
- **h.** Rhabdomyolysis

2. *Decreases are not clinically significant.* Causes of *low creatinine* are small stature, decreased muscle mass, some complex cases of advanced and severe liver disease, and inadequate dietary protein.

Interfering Factors

1. High levels of ascorbic acid and cephalosporin antibiotics can cause a falsely increased level.

2. Drugs that influence kidney function plus other medications can cause a change in the blood creatinine.
3. A diet high in meat can cause increased levels.
4. Creatinine is falsely decreased by bilirubin, glucose, histidine, and quinidine compounds.

Clinical Alert

1. Panic value is 10 mg/dl in nondialysis patients.
2. Creatinine should always be checked before giving nephrotoxic chemotherapeutics, such as methotrexate, cisplatin, cyclophosphamide (Cytoxan), plicamycin (mithramycin), or semustine.

Patient Preparation

1. Explain test purpose and procedure.
2. Assess diet for meat intake.
3. See Chapter 1 guidelines for safe, effective, informed *pretest* care.

Patient Aftercare

1. Interpret test results and monitor as appropriate for impaired renal function.
2. See Chapter 1 guidelines for safe, effective, informed *posttest* care.

URIC ACID

Normal Values

Men:	3.5–7.2 mg/dl, or 0.21–0.42 mmol/L
Women:	2.6–6.0 mg/dl, or 0.154–0.35 mmol/L
Children:	2.0–5.5 mg/dl, or 0.12–0.32 mmol/L

Background

Uric acid is formed from the breakdown of nucleonic acids and is an end product of purine metabolism. A lack of the enzyme uricase allows this poorly soluble substance to accumulate in body fluids. Two-thirds of the uric acid produced daily is excreted by the kidneys, whereas the remaining one-third exits by the stool. The basis for this test is that an overproduction of uric acids occurs when there is excessive cell breakdown and catabolism of nucleonic acids (as in gout), excessive production and destruction of cells (as in leukemia), or an inability to excrete the substance produced (as in renal failure).

Explanation of Test

Measurement of uric acid is used most commonly in the evaluation of renal failure, gout, and leukemia. In hospitalized patients, renal failure is the most common cause of elevated uric acid levels, and gout is the least common cause. This test is also valuable in assessing the prognosis of eclampsia because of the uric acid level's ability to reflect the extent of liver damage in toxemia of pregnancy.

Procedure

Obtain a 5-ml venous blood sample. Serum is preferred; heparinized blood is acceptable. Observe universal precautions.

Clinical Implications

1. *Elevated uric acid levels (hyperuricemia)* occur in
   a. Gout (the amount of increase is not directly related to the severity of the disease)
   b. Renal diseases and renal failure
   c. Alcoholism
   d. Dehydration (prerenal azotemia)
   e. Lead poisoning
   f. Leukemia
   g. Lymphoma
   h. Starvation
   i. Metabolic acidosis
   j. Toxemia of pregnancy
   k. Infectious mononucleosis
   l. Hyperlipidemia
   m. Hypoparathyroidism
   n. Hemolytic anemia
   o. Following excessive cell destruction, as in chemotherapy and radiation treatment
2. *Decreased levels of uric acid* occur in
   a. Fanconi's syndrome
   b. Wilson's disease
   c. SIADH
   d. Heavy-metal poisoning
   e. Some malignancies (eg, Hodgkin's disease, multiple myeloma)
   f. Xanthinuria (deficiency of xanthine oxidase)

Interfering Factors

1. Stress and strenuous exercise will falsely elevate uric acid.
2. Many drugs cause increase or decrease of uric acid.
3. A purine-rich diet (liver, kidney, sweetbreads) increases uric acid levels.

Patient Preparation

1. Advise patient of test purpose and blood-drawing procedure.
2. Promote relaxation; avoid strenuous exercise.
3. See Chapter 1 guidelines for safe, effective, informed *pretest* care.

Patient Aftercare

1. Resume normal activities.
2. Interpret test results and monitor appropriately for renal failure, gout, or leukemia. Uric acid level should fall in patients who are treated with uricosuric drugs, such as allopurinol, probenecid, and sulfinpyrazone.
3. See Chapter 1 guidelines for safe, effective, informed *posttest* care.

Clinical Alert

1. Monitor uric acid levels during treatment of leukemia.
2. Acute dangerous levels may occur following cytotoxic drug administration.

HORMONE TESTS

ANDROSTANEDIONE

Normal Values

Child:	0.08–0.5 ng/ml
Male:	0.57–2.65 ng/ml
Female:	0.47–2.68 ng/ml
Postmenopausal female:	< 1.0 ng/ml

Background

Androstanedione is one of the major androgens produced by the ovaries in females, and, to a lesser extent, in the adrenal glands in both sexes. This hormone is converted to estrogens by hepatic enzymes.

Explanation of Test

This hormone measurement is helpful in the evaluation of conditions characterized by hirsutism and virilization.

Procedure

1. Obtain a 5-ml venous blood sample in the morning and place on ice. Observe universal precautions.
2. In females, collect this specimen 1 week before or after the menstrual period. Record date of last menstrual period on the laboratory form.

Clinical Implications

1. *Increased androstanedione values* are associated with
   a. Stein–Leventhal syndrome
   b. Cushing's syndrome
   c. Certain ovarian tumors
   d. Ectopic ACTH-producing tumor
   e. Late-onset congenitive adrenal hyperplasia
   f. Ovarian stromal hyperplasia
2. *Decreased androstanedione values* are found in sickle cell anemia and adrenal and ovarian failure.

Patient Preparation

1. Explain purpose of test and blood-drawing procedure.
2. Patient should be fasting and blood should be drawn at peak production (7:00 AM).
3. Collect 1 week before menstrual period in females.
4. See Chapter 1 guidelines for safe, effective, informed *pretest* care.

Patient Aftercare

1. Resume normal activities.
2. Interpret test results and counsel appropriately for ovarian and adrenal dysfunction.
3. See Chapter 1 guidelines for safe, effective, informed *posttest* care.

ALDOSTERONE ●

Normal Values

Plasma is taken with the patient in an upright position for 2 hours and with unrestricted salt intake.

Women:	5–30 ng/dl, or 0.14–0.83 nmol/L (two to three times higher in pregnancy)
Men:	6–22 ng/dl, or 0.17–0.61 nmol/L
Normal diet:	6–25 μg/24 hr
Low-salt diet:	17–44 μg/24 hr
High-salt diet:	0–6 μg/24 hr

Background

This hormone, derived from cholesterol, is the most potent of the mineralocorticoids. Aldosterone secretion causes the retention of sodium and chloride and the elimination of potassium and hydrogen. The second major effect is the maintenance of blood pressure and blood volume. Minute quantities will depress the urinary and salivary sodium/potassium ratio, primarily because of decreased sodium excretion.

Explanation of Test

This test is useful in detecting primary or secondary aldosteronism. Patients with primary aldosteronism characteristically have hypertension, muscular pains and cramps, weakness, tetany, paralysis, and polyuria.

Procedure

1. Obtain a 10-ml venous blood specimen, with heparin or EDTA added. The cells must be separated from plasma immediately. Obtain the specimen in the morning after the patient has been upright for at least 2 hours. Blood should be drawn with patient sitting. Observe universal precautions.

2. Specify and record the source of the specimen, as from a "peripheral vein."
3. A 24-hour urine specimen is obtained with boric acid preservative. Refrigerate during collection.

Clinical Implications

1. *Elevated aldosterone levels (primary aldosteronism)* occur in
   a. Aldosterone-producing adenoma (Conn's disease)
   b. Adrenal cortical hyperplasia (pseudoprimary aldosteronism)
   c. Indeterminate hyperaldosteronism
   d. Glucocorticoid remediable hyperaldosteronism
2. *Secondary aldosteronism* occurs when aldosterone output is elevated owing to external stimuli or because of greater activity in the renin–angiotensin system, as in
   a. Salt depletion
   b. Potassium loading
   c. Laxative abuse
   d. Cardiac failure
   e. Cirrhosis of liver with ascites
   f. Nephrotic syndrome
   g. Bartter's syndrome
   h. Diuretic abuse
   i. Hypovolemia and hemorrhage
   j. After 10 days of starvation
   k. Toxemia of pregnancy
3. *Decreased aldosterone levels* are found in
   a. Aldosterone deficiency
   b. Addison's disease
   c. Syndrome of renin deficiency (very rare)

Interfering Factors

1. Values are increased in pregnancy and by posture.
2. Recently administered radioactive medications will affect test outcomes.

Clinical Alert

1. The simultaneous measurement of aldosterone and renin is helpful in differentiating primary from secondary hyperaldosteronism. Renin is high in secondary aldosteronism, low in primary aldosteronism.
2. Potassium deficiencies should be corrected before testing for aldosterone.

Patient Preparation

1. Explain test purpose and procedures. If 24-hour urine specimen is required, follow protocols in Chapter 3.
2. Diuretic agents, progestational agents, estrogens, and licorice should be discontinued for 2 weeks before the test.
3. The patient's diet for 2 weeks before the test should be normal and in-

clude 3 g (135 mEq/L) of sodium per day. Check with your laboratory for special protocols.

4. See Chapter 1 guidelines for safe, effective, informed *pretest* care.

Patient Aftercare

1. Resume normal activities and diet.
2. Interpret test results and monitor appropriately for aldosteronism and aldosterone deficiency.
3. See Chapter 1 guidelines for safe, effective, informed *posttest* care.

ANTIDIURETIC HORMONE (ADH); ARGININE VASOPRESSOR HORMONE ●

Normal Values

0.0–4.7 pg/ml, or < 1.5 mg/L

Background

This hormone is excreted by the posterior pituitary gland. When ADH activity is present, small volumes of concentrated urine are excreted. When ADH is absent, large amounts of diluted urine are produced.

Explanation of Test

This measurement of the level of ADH is useful in the differential diagnosis of polyuric and hyponatremic states. ADH aids in diagnosis of urine concentration disorders, especially diabetes insipidus, the syndrome of inappropriate ADH (SIADH), psychogenic water intoxication, and syndromes of ectopic ADH production.

Procedure

1. Venous blood samples are drawn into prechilled tubes and put on ice. Observe universal precautions.
2. Patient should be in a sitting position and calm during blood collection.

Clinical Implications

1. *Increased secretion of ADH* is associated with
   - **a.** Syndrome of inappropriate ADH (SIADH) (relative to plasma osmolality)
   - **b.** Ectopic ADH production (systemic neoplasm)
   - **c.** Nephrogenic diabetes insipidus
   - **d.** Acute intermittent porphyria
   - **e.** Guillain–Barré syndrome
   - **f.** Brain tumor, diseases, injury, neurosurgery
   - **g.** Pulmonary diseases
2. *Decreased secretion of ADH* occurs in
   - **a.** Central diabetes insipidus (hypothalamic or neurogenic)
   - **b.** Psychogenic polydipsia (water intoxication)
   - **c.** Nephrotic syndrome

Interfering Factors

1. Recently administered radioisotopes cause spurious results.
2. Many drugs affect results.

Patient Preparation

1. Explain test purpose and procedure.
2. Encourage relaxation before and during blood drawing.
3. See Chapter 1 guidelines for safe, effective, informed *pretest* care.

Patient Aftercare

1. Resume normal activities.
2. Interpret test results and counsel appropriately for urine concentration disorders and polyuria.
3. See Chapter 1 guidelines for safe, effective, informed *posttest* care.

Clinical Alert

To distinguishm SIADH from other conditions that cause dilutional hyponatremia, other tests must be done such as plasma osmolality, plasma sodium, and water-loading test.

CHORIONIC GONADOTROPIN, HUMAN CHORIONIC GONADOTROPIN (hCG) β-SUBUNIT, PREGNANCY TEST ●

Normal Values

Qualitative (for routine pregnancy tests): urine or serum—negative (not pregnant)

Qualitative (for nonroutine detection of hCG):

Males:	< 2.5 IU/L, or mIU/ml
Nonpregnant females:	< 5.0 IU/L, or mIU/ml
Postmenopausal females:	< 9.0 IU/L, or mIU/ml
Pregnancy:	

Weeks Past Last Menstrual Period	*mIU/ml or IU/L*
3	0–5
4	3–426
5	18–7,340
6	1,080–56,500
7–8	7,650–229,000
9–12	25,700–288,000
13–16	13,300–253,000
17–24	4,060–65,400
25–40	3,640–117,000

Background

The glycoprotein hormones, hCG, luteinizing hormone, follicle-stimulating hormone, and TSH, are composed of two different subunits; α-subunit is similar in all of the glycoprotein hormones, the β-subunit is unique to each hormone. Highly specific assays allow hCG to be measured in the presence of other glycoprotein hormones. The increased sensitivity of the β-hCG test detects pregnancy as early as 6 to 10 days after implantation. In normal pregnancy hCG can be detected up to 4 to 6 weeks after termination. The β-subunit pregnancy tests can be positive up to 3 to 4 weeks after termination. The time interval for hCG to disappear after evacuation of a molar pregnancy, either by total hysterectomy or by suction and D and C is 73 to 76 days, with a large range of 11 to 219 days. A variety of poorly differentiated or undifferentiated neoplasms may produce ectopic chorionic gonadotropin. Assay for total hCG both α- and β-subunits, or β-hCG may detect ectopic tumors (eg, choriocarcinoma, hydatidiform mole, and germinal testicular tumors). In these neoplasms hCG is usually the product of syncytiotrophoblastic cells.

Explanation of Test

This qualitative test detects normal pregnancy. It is quicker, but less sensitive (sensitivity 20–50 mIU/ml), than the quantitative test. This test can be expected to become positive within 3 days of implantation; also, in a molar pregnancy or an ectopic pregnancy. The cross-reactivity with LH is low and false-positive tests are rare. Occasionally, a patient with very high LH levels will give a borderline reaction.

The qualitative hCG, β-subunit is used for nonroutine detection of hCG. It is sensitive down to 1 to 3 mIU/L. This test provides the most sensitive **and** specific test for the detection of early pregnancy, diagnosis of ectopic pregnancy, or threatened abortion. It is also useful in the workup and management of testicular tumors. High levels may be found with choriocarcinoma, embryonal cell carcinoma, and in the detection of ectopic pregnancy. The hCG levels are extremely useful in following germ cell neoplasms that produce hCG, especially trophoblastic neoplasms. In germ cell neoplasms in the male, β-hCG and alphafetoprotein are both useful tumor markers, and can be used to evaluate recurrence.

Procedure

Obtain a 5-ml venous blood sample. Serum is used for the test. Observe universal precautions.

Clinical Implications

1. *Increased hCG values* are found in

- **a.** Pregnancy
- **b.** Hydatidiform mole
- **c.** Choriocarcinoma
- **d.** Seminoma
- **e.** Ovarian and testicular teratomas

- **f.** Multiple pregnancy
- **g.** Neoplasms of stomach, pancreas, lung, colon, and liver
- **h.** Malignant melanoma and sarcoma

2. *Decreased hCG values* are found in threatened abortion and ectopic pregnancy.

Interfering Factors

Lipemia, hemolysis, and radioisotopes administered within 1 week affect results.

Patient Preparation

1. Explain test purpose and procedure.
2. Determine and record date of last menstrual period (for females).
3. See Chapter 1 guidelines for safe, effective, informed *pretest* care.

Patient Aftercare

1. Resume normal activities.
2. Interpret test results and counsel appropriately for pregnancy.
3. See Chapter 1 guidelines for safe, effective, informed *posttest* care.

CORTISOL (HYDROCORTISONE) ●

Normal Values for Cortisol

8:00 AM:	5–23 μg/dl, or 138–635 mmol/L
4:00 PM:	3–16 μg/dl, or 83–441 mmol/L
Newborn:	1–24 μg/dl, or 28–662 mmol/L

After first week of life cortisol levels attain adult values.

Normal Values for Suppression

8:00 AM:	5–23 μg/dl, or 138–635 mmol/L
4:00 PM:	3–16 μg/dl, or 83–441 mmol/L

8:00 AM following administration of dexamethasone: less than 5 μg/dl.

Normal Values for Stimulation

Baseline at least 5 μg/dl After cortrosyn rise of at least 10 μg/dl

Background

Cortisol, (hydrocortisone/compound F) is a glucocorticosteroid of the adrenal cortex and affects metabolism of proteins, carbohydrates, and lipids. Cortisol stimulates glucogenesis by the liver, inhibits the effect of insulin, and decreases the rate of glucose use by the cells. In health, the secretion rate of cortisol is higher in the early morning (6–8 AM) and lower in the evening (4–6 PM). This variation is lost in patients with Cushing's syndrome and in persons under stress.

Explanation of Test

The cortisol test evaluates adrenal hormone function. Cortisol is elevated in adrenal hyperfunction and decreased in adrenal hypofunction. Suppression and stimulation tests may also be done. Cortisol (dexamethasone) suppression test screens for Cushing's syndrome and identifies depressed persons who are likely to respond to antidepressants or electroshock therapy. It is based on the fact that ACTH production will be suppressed in healthy persons after a low dose of dexamethasone, whereas it is not in Cushing's syndrome or in some depressed persons.

Procedure

Obtain 5-ml venous blood samples at 8:00 AM and at 4:00 PM. Serum is preferred. Heparin anticoagulant may be used. Observe universal precautions.

Clinical Implications

1. *Decreased cortisol levels* are found in
  - **a.** Adrenal hyperplasia
  - **b.** Addison's disease
  - **c.** Anterior pituitary hyposecretion (pituitary destruction)
  - **d.** Hypothyroidism (hypopituitarism)
  - **e.** Hepatitis and cirrhosis

2. *Increased cortisol levels* are found in
  - **a.** Hyperthyroidism
  - **b.** Stress (trauma, surgery)
  - **c.** Carcinoma (extreme elevation in the morning and no variation later in the day)
  - **d.** Cushing's syndrome (high upon rising but no variation later in the day)
  - **e.** Overproduction of ACTH caused by tumors (oat cell cancers)
  - **f.** Adrenal adenoma
  - **g.** Obesity

Interfering Factors

1. Pregnancy will cause an increased value.
2. There is no normal diurnal variation in patients under stress.
3. Drugs, such as spironolactone and oral contraceptives, will give falsely elevated values.
4. Decreased levels found in therapy with dexamethasone, prednisone, and prednisolone (steroids).

Patient Preparation

1. Explain test purpose and blood-drawing procedure. Blood must be drawn at 8:00 AM and 4:00 PM.
2. Encourage relaxation.
3. No radioisotopes within 1 hour of test.
4. See Chapter 1 guidelines for safe, effective, informed *pretest* care.

Patient Aftercare

1. Resume normal activities.
2. Interpret test results and counsel appropriately for adrenal dysfunction.
3. See Chapter 1 guidelines for safe, effective, informed *posttest* care.

CORTISOL SUPPRESSION (DEXAMETHASONE SUPPRESSION; DST) ●

Normal Values

See foregoing Cortisol test for values.

Procedure

1. Obtain venous blood samples the day following administration of dexamethasone. Serum or heparinized plasma are acceptable. Observe universal precautions.
2. Late evening or bedtime, dexamethasone tablets are administered by mouth. The dosage varies according to weight. Usually 1 mg is given.

Clinical Implications

No diurnal variation or suppression will occur in Cushing's syndrome (> 10 μg/dl) and in endogenous depression (50% of cases).

Interfering Factors

False-positive suppression tests may occur in

1. Pregnancy
2. High doses of estrogens
3. Anorexia nervosa
4. Uncontrolled diabetes
5. Trauma, high stress
6. Fever
7. Dehydration
8. Acute withdrawal from alcohol
9. Phenytoin (Dilantin) administration
10. Failure to take dexamethasone

Patient Preparation

1. Explain suppression test purpose and procedure. Fasting is required for the 8 AM test.
2. Discontinue all medications for 24 to 48 hours before the study. Especially important are spironolactone (Aldactone), estrogens, birth control pills, cortisol, tetracycline, stilbestrol, and phenytoin (Dilantin). Check with physician.
3. Weigh the patient and record weight.
4. Have baseline blood cortisol drawn at 8:00 AM and 4:00 PM. Give dexamethasone at 11:00 PM the same day. Draw blood at 8:00 AM the next day.
5. No radioisotopes administered within 1 week before test.
6. See Chapter 1 guidelines for safe, effective, informed *pretest* care.

Patient Aftercare

1. Resume normal activities.
2. Interpret test results and counsel appropriately for Cushing's or depression.
3. See Chapter 1 guidelines for safe, effective, informed *posttest* care.

CORTISOL STIMULATION (COSYNTROPIN; CORTROSYN STIMULATION); **ACTH STIMULATION** ●

Explanation of Test

This detects adrenal insufficiency after cosyntropin (Cortrosyn) administration. Cosyntropin (Cortrosyn) is a synthetic subunit of ACTH that exhibits the full corticosteroid-stimulating effect of ACTH in healthy persons. Failure to respond is an indication of adrenal insufficiency. See foregoing Cortisol test for values.

Procedure

1. Obtain a 4-ml fasting venous blood sample at 8:00 AM. Observe universal precautions.
2. Administer Cortrosyn intramuscularly.
3. Obtain additional 4-ml blood specimens 30 and 60 minutes after administration of Cortrosyn. Serum or heparinized blood is acceptable.

Clinical Implications

Absent or blunted response to cortisol stimulation occurs in adrenal insufficiency and hypopituitarism.

Interfering Factors

Prolonged steroid administration and recently administered radioisotopes affect stimulation results.

Patient Preparation

1. Explain stimulation test purpose and procedure. Fasting during test is required. Blood specimens are obtained before or after intramuscular injection of Cortrosyn.
2. See Chapter 1 guidelines for safe, effective, informed *pretest* care.

Patient Aftercare

1. Resume normal activities.
2. Interpret test results and monitor appropriately for adrenal insufficiency.
3. See Chapter 1 guidelines for safe, effective, informed *posttest* care.

GASTRIN

Normal Values

Adult male:	< 100 pg/ml, or 100 ng/L
Adult female:	< 75 pg/ml
Child:	10–125 pg/ml or ng/L

Background

Gastrin, a hormone secreted by the antral G cells in stomach mucosa, stimulates gastric acid production, affects antral motility, and affects the secretion of pepsin and intrinsic factor.

Explanation of Test

Measurement of serum gastrin is generally used to diagnose stomach disorders, such as gastrinoma and Zollinger–Ellison syndrome, in the presence of hyperacidity.

Procedure

Obtain a 5-ml fasting venous blood sample; serum is preferred. Observe universal precautions.

Interfering Factors

Values will be falsely increased in nonfasting patients or the elderly, diabetics taking insulin, after gastroscopy, or after administration of H_2 secretion blockers (cimetidine), steroids, or calcium.

Clinical Implications

1. *Increased gastrin levels* are found in
   a. Stomach carcinoma (reduction of gastric acid secretion)
   b. Gastric and duodenal ulcers
   c. Zollinger–Ellison syndrome (gastrinoma)
   d. Pernicious anemia (low secretion of hydrochloric acid results in elevated gastrin levels)
   e. End-stage renal disease (gastrin is metabolized by the kidneys)
   f. Antral G-cell hyperplasia
   g. Vagotomy without gastric resection
2. *Decreased gastrin levels* occur in
   a. Antrectomy with vagotomy
   b. Hypothyroidism

Patient Preparation

1. Explain test purpose and procedure.
2. Fasting is required for 12 hours preceding the test. Water is permitted.
3. See Chapter 1 guidelines for safe, effective, informed *pretest* care.

Patient Aftercare

1. Resume normal activities.
2. Interpret test results and monitor appropriately. Follow-up testing using gastric stimulation or gastrin suppression may be indicated.
3. See Chapter 1 guidelines for safe, effective, informed *posttest* care.

GROWTH HORMONE (hGH); SOMATOTROPIN ●

Normal Values

Adults:	< 5 ng/ml, or < 5 μg/L
Children:	0–10 ng/ml, or 0–10 μg/L
Newborn:	10–40 ng/ml, or 10–40 μg/L

NOTE: *Because of marked fluctuations of hGH, a random specimen has limited value. Stimulation or inhibitor tests give more information.*

Background

Growth hormone (somatotropin) is essential to the growth process and has an important role in the metabolism of adults. It is released by the pituitary gland secondary to exercise, deep sleep, hypoglycemia, and ingestion of protein. It also stimulates the production of ribonucleic acid (RNA), mobilizes fatty acids from fat deposits, and is intimately connected with insulinism. If the pituitary gland secretes too little or too much in the growth phase of life, dwarfism or giantism will result. An excess of growth hormone during adulthood leads to acromegaly.

Explanation of Test

The test confirms hypo- or hyperpituitarism so that therapy can be initiated as soon as possible. Challenge or stimulation tests are generally used to detect growth hormone deficiency.

Clinical Implications

1. Increased hGH levels are associated with giantism and acromegaly.
2. Decreased hGH levels are associated with dwarfism and hypopituitarism.
3. Following challenge testing to establish a pattern, the appropriate normal response is debatable. A response equal to or greater than 7 ng/ml is clearly normal. Also, the suppression of growth hormone levels of 0 to 3 ng/ml in 30 minutes to 2 hours following the ingestion of 100 g of glucose is considered a normal response in adults. In children, a rebound-stimulation effect may be seen from 2 to 5 hours following administration of glucose.

Interfering Factors

1. *Increased levels* are associated with the use of oral contraceptives, estrogens, arginine, glucagon, levodopa, low glucose, and insulin.

2. Levels will rise 15 times normal by the second day of starvation; also after deep sleep.
3. *Decreased levels* are associated with obesity and the use of corticosteroids.

Procedure

1. Obtain a 5-ml fasting venous blood sample. Observe universal precautions.
2. Check with your laboratory for specific challenge protocols for stimulation tests, such as insulin-induced hypoglycemia, arginine transfusion, glucagon infusion, L-dopa, and propranolol with exercise.

Patient Preparation

1. Explain test purpose and blood-drawing procedure.
2. Fasting from food for 8 to 10 hours is required; water is permitted. For accurate levels, the patient should be free of stress and at complete rest in a quiet environment for at least 30 minutes before specimen collection.
3. The physiologic state such as feeding, fasting, sleep, or activity should be noted in the healthcare record.
4. See Chapter 1 guidelines for safe, effective, informed *pretest* care.

Patient Aftercare

1. Resume normal activities.
2. Interpret test results and monitor appropriately. A glucose challenge test may be indicated for follow-up.
3. Follow Chapter 1 guidelines for safe, effective, informed *posttest* care.

PROLACTIN (hPRL) ●

Normal Values

Nonpregnant women:	0–17 ng/ml or μg/L
Pregnant women:	34–386 ng/ml or μg/L by third trimester
Adult males:	0–15 ng/ml or μg/L
Children:	3.2–20 ng/ml or μg/L

Background

Prolactin is a pituitary hormone essential for initiating and maintaining lactation. The sex difference in prolactin does not occur until puberty, when increased estrogen production results in higher prolactin levels in females. Circadian changes in prolactin concentration in adults are marked by episodic fluctuation and a sleep-induced peak in the early-morning hours.

Explanation of Test

This test may be helpful in the diagnosis, management, and follow-up of a prolactin-secreting tumor, accompanied by secondary amenorrhea or galactorrhea, hyperprolactinemia, and infertility. It is also useful in the management of hypothalamic disease and in monitoring the effectiveness of surgery, chemotherapy, and radiation treatment of prolactin-secreting tumors.

Procedure

Obtain a 12-hour fasting (at least 5-ml) venous blood (serum) sample. Procure specimens in the morning, 3 to 4 hours after awakening. Observe universal precautions.

Clinical Implications

1. *Increased prolactin values* are associated with
   - **a.** Galactorrhea or amenorrhea
   - **b.** Diseases of the hypothalamus and pituitary
   - **c.** Prolactin-secreting pituitary tumors
   - **d.** Acromegaly
   - **e.** Ectopic production of malignant tumors
   - **f.** Hypothyroidism, primary
   - **g.** Renal failure
   - **h.** Anorexia nervosa
   - **i.** Insulin-induced hypoglycemia
2. *Decreased prolactin values* are found in Sheehan's syndrome (pituitary apoplexy).

Interfering Factors

1. Increased values are associated with newborns, pregnancy, postpartum period, stress, exercise, sleep, nipple stimulation, and lactation.
2. Drugs may increase values (estrogens, methyldopa, tricyclic antidepressants, phenothiazines, antihypertensives).
3. Dopaminergic drugs inhibit prolactin secretion. Administration of L-dopa can normalize prolactin levels in galactorrhea, hyperprolactinemia, and pituitary tumor.

Clinical Alert

Levels over 200 ng/ml in a nonlactating female indicate a prolactin-secreting tumor. However, a normal prolactin level does not rule out pituitary tumor.

Patient Preparation

1. Explain test purpose. Fasting is required. Obtain blood-drawn specimen between 8:00 AM and 10:00 AM.
2. Avoid stress, excitement, stimulation (venipuncture itself can sometimes elevate prolactin).
3. Discontinue (if possible) prescribed medications that interfere with test.
4. See Chapter 1 guidelines for safe, effective, informed *pretest* care.

Patient Aftercare

1. Resume normal activities.
2. Interpret test outcome and counsel concerning repeat testing to monitor treatment. Magnetic resonance (MR) imaging may be indicated.
3. Follow Chapter 1 guidelines for safe, effective, informed *posttest* care.

PARATHYROID HORMONE ASSAY; PARATHYRIN; PARATHORMONE (PTH-C TERMINAL) ●

Normal Values

NH_2-terminal:	8–24 pg/ml (ng/L); COOH-terminal: 50–330 pg/ml (ng/L)
Intact molecule:	10–65 pg/ml (ng/L)
Calcium:	8.5–10.9 mg/dl

Background

Parathormone (PTH), a polypeptide hormone produced in the parathyroid gland, is one of the major factors in the regulation of calcium concentration in extracellular fluid. Three molecular forms of PTH exist: (1) intact, also called native or glandular hormone; (2) multiple NH_2-terminal fragments; and (3) COOH-terminal fragments.

Explanation of Test

This test studies altered calcium metabolism, establishes a diagnosis of hyperparathyroidism, and distinguishes nonparathyroid from parathyroid causes of hypercalcemia. A decrease in the level of ionized calcium is the primary stimulus for PTH secretions, whereas a rise in calcium inhibits secretions. This normal relationship is lost in hyperthyroidism, and PTH will be inappropriately high in relation to calcium. Acute changes of secretory activity are better reflected by the PTH, NH_2-terminal assay, which is usually decreased when hypercalcemia is due to neoplastic secretions (prostaglandins). The PTH, NH_2-terminal assay may be a more reliable indication of secondary hyperparathyroidism in patients with renal failure.

Creatinine is determined with all PTH assays to determine kidney function and for meaningful interpretation of results.

Procedure

1. Obtain a 10-hour fasting (at least 10-ml) venous blood sample in chilled vials and kept on ice. Observe universal precautions.
2. Immediately take specimen to the laboratory and centrifuge in a 4° centrifuge after blood has clotted.

Clinical Implications

1. *Increased PTH values* occur in primary hyperparathyroidism and in pseudohyperparathyroidism when there is a primary defect in renal tubular responsiveness to PTH (secondary hyperparathyroidism).

2. *Decreased PTH values* occur in
   a. Hypoparathyroidism (Graves' disease)
   b. Nonparathyroid hypercalcemia
   c. Secondary hypoparathyroidism (surgical)
   d. Magnesium deficiency
   e. Sarcoidosis
   f. Hyperthyroidism
   g. DiGeorge syndrome
3. *Increased PTH-N* values occur in primary hyperparathyroidism and secondary hyperparathyroidism.
4. *Decreased PTH* NH_2*-terminal values* occur in hypoparathyroidism, nonparathyroid hypercalcemia, aluminum-associated osteomalacia, and severely impaired bone mineralization.
5. *Increased COOH-terminal hormone (PTHC)* values are found in
   a. Primary hyperparathyroidism (very specific for)
   b. Some neoplasms with elevated calcium
   c. Renal failure (even if parathyroid disease is absent)
6. *Decreased COOH-terminal* (PTHC) values are found in hypoparathyroidism and nonparathyroid hypercalcemia.

Interfering Factors

1. Elevated blood lipids (interfere with test methods).
2. Milk ingestion (milk–alkali syndrome) may falsely lower PTH levels.
3. Recently administered radioisotopes.
4. Vitamin D deficiency will increase levels.
5. Many drugs: phosphates will raise levels up to 125%, and vitamin A and D overdoses will decrease levels.

Patient Preparation

1. Explain test purpose and procedure.
2. Fasting for at least 10 hours is required. Draw blood by 8:00 AM because of circadian rhythm changes.
3. See Chapter 1 guidelines for safe, effective, informed *pretest* care.

Patient Aftercare

1. Resume normal activities.
2. Interpret test results and monitor appropriately for calcium imbalance and hypo- or hyperparathyroidism.
3. Follow Chapter 1 guidelines for safe, effective, informed *posttest* care.

PROGESTERONE ●

Normal Values

Male: 0–0.4 ng/ml

Female:	Follicular	0.1–1.5 ng/ml
	Luteal	2.5–28.1 ng/ml
	1st trimester	9–47 ng/ml

2nd trimester	16.8–146 ng/ml
3rd trimester	55–255 ng/ml
> 60 yr	0–0.2 ng/ml
Prepubertal	0.1–0.3 ng/ml
Midluteal	5.7–28.1 ng/ml
Oral contraceptives	0.1–0.3 ng/ml

Background

Progesterone, a female sex hormone, is primarily involved in the preparation of the uterus for pregnancy and in its maintenance during pregnancy. The placenta begins producing progesterone at 12 weeks of gestation. Progesterone peaks in the midluteal phase of the menstrual cycle. In nonpregnant females, progesterone is produced by the corpus luteum. During the 12th week of gestation, the placenta begins producing progesterone.

Explanation of Test

This test is part of a fertility study to confirm ovulation, evaluate corpus luteum function, and assess risk for early miscarriage. Testing of several samples during the cycle is necessary. Ovarian production of progesterone is low during the follicular (first) phase of the menstrual cycle. After ovulation, progesterone levels rise for 4 to 5 days and then fall. During pregnancy, there is a gradual increase from the 9th to 32nd week, often to 100 times the level in the nonpregnant woman. Levels of progesterone in twin pregnancy will be higher than in a single pregnancy.

Procedure

1. Obtain a venous blood sample. Observe universal precautions. The test request should include sex, day of last menstrual period, and trimester of pregnancy.
2. Urine tests can also be done.

Clinical Implications

1. *Increased progesterone levels* are associated with
   - **a.** Congenital adrenal hyperplasia
   - **b.** Lipid ovarian tumor
   - **c.** Molar pregnancy
   - **d.** Chorionepithelioma of ovary
2. *Decreased progesterone levels* are associated with
   - **a.** Threatened abortion
   - **b.** Galactorrhea–amenorrhea syndrome

Interfering Factors

Recently administered radioisotopes.

Patient Preparation

1. Explain test purpose and procedure. Note date of last menstrual period.
2. No radioisotopes within 1 week of test.
3. See Chapter 1 guidelines for safe, effective, informed *pretest* care.

Patient Aftercare

1. Resume normal activities.
2. Interpret test results, counsel and monitor appropriately concerning fertility and pregnancy.
3. Follow Chapter 1 guidelines for safe, effective, informed *posttest* care.

SOMATOMEDIN-C, INSULINLIKE GROWTH HORMONE

Normal Values

Age in Years	*Male (U/ml)*	*Female (U/ml)*
0–2	0.8–1.10	0.11–2.20
3–5	0.12–1.60	0.18–2.40
6–10	0.22–2.80	0.41–4.50
11–12	0.28–3.70	0.99–6.80
13–14	0.90–5.60	1.20–5.90
15–17	0.91–3.10	0.71–4.10
>18	0.34–1.90	0.45–2.20

Background

Somatomedin-C, a polypeptide hormone produced by the liver and other tissues, affects growth hormone activity and glucose metabolism.

Explanation of Test

This test is used to monitor the growth of children, as well as to diagnose acromegaly and hypopituitarism. Normal somatomedin results rule out a deficiency of growth hormone.

Procedure

1. Obtain a fasting (preferred, 5-ml plasma) venous blood sample, using EDTA anticoagulant. Observe universal precautions.
2. Blood-drawing tubes must be chilled and placed on ice immediately after obtaining specimen.

Clinical Implications

1. *Increased somatomedin-C levels* are associated with acromegaly.
2. *Decreased somatomedin-C levels* are associated with
   - **a.** Dwarfism
   - **b.** Hypopituitarism
   - **c.** Hypothyroidism
   - **d.** Kwashiorkor
   - **e.** Laron dwarfism
   - **f.** Cirrhosis of liver and other hepatocellular diseases
   - **g.** Malnutrition
   - **h.** Anorexia
   - **i.** Emotional deprivation syndrome

Patient Preparation

1. Explain test purpose and procedure. Fasting is not required.
2. No radioisotopes within 1 week of testing.
3. See Chapter 1 guidelines for safe, effective, informed *pretest* care.

Patient Aftercare

1. Resume normal activities.
2. Interpret test results and monitor appropriately for abnormal growth and development.
3. Follow Chapter 1 guidelines for safe, effective, informed *posttest* care.

TESTOSTERONE (TOTAL); **TESTOSTERONE** (FREE) ●

Normal Value

Male:	Total, 300–1000 ng/dl or 10.4–34.7 mmol/L
Female:	20–75 ng/dl or 0.69–2.69 mmol/L
Pregnancy:	3–4 times higher
Postmenopause:	8–35 ng/dl or 0.28–1.22 mmol/L

TESTOSTERONE FREE

Age yr	*Male (pg/ml)*	*Female (pg/ml)*
20–29	19–41	0.9–3.2
30–39	18–39	0.8–3.0
40–49	16–33	0.6–2.5
50–59	13–31	0.3–2.7
> 60	9–26	0.2–2.2

Background

Testosterone hormone is responsible for the development of male secondary sexual characteristics. It is secreted by the adrenal glands and testes in men and by the adrenal glands and ovaries in women. Excessive production induces premature puberty in men and masculinity in women. Testosterone exists in serum both free and bound to albumin and to sex hormone-binding globulin (SHBG; testosterone-binding globulin). Unbound (free) testosterone is the active portion.

Explanation of Test

Testosterone measurements in men assess hypogonadism, pituitary gonadotropin function, impotency, and cryptorchidism; these measurements are also useful in the detection of ovarian tumors and viralizing conditions in women.

Procedure

1. Obtain a 5-ml venous blood sample; serum is preferred. Observe universal precautions.
2. Indicate age and sex on laboratory requisition.

Clinical Implications

1. Men: *decreased total testosterone levels* in
   a. Hypogonadism (pituitary failure) **b.** Klinefelter's syndrome

   c. Hypopituitarism (primary and secondary)
   d. Orchidectomy
   e. Hepatic cirrhosis
   f. Down syndrome
   g. Delayed puberty
2. Men: *decreased free testosterone levels* occur in hypogonadism and increase of sex hormone-binding globulin (TeBG), especially in elderly men.
3. Men: *increased total testosterone levels* occur in
   a. Hyperthyroidism
   b. Syndromes of androgen resistance
   c. Adrenal tumors or congenital adrenal hyperplasia
   d. Precocious puberty
   e. Idiopathic CNS lesion
4. Women: *increased total testosterone levels* are associated with
   a. Adrenal neoplasms
   b. Ovarian tumors, benign or malignant (virilizing)
   c. Trophoblastic disease during pregnancy
   d. Idiopathic hirsutism
   e. Hilar cell tumor
5. Women: *increased free testosterone levels* are associated with female hirsutism, polycystic ovaries, and virilization.

Clinical Alert

1. The testosterone level is normal in cryptorchidism, azoospermia, and oligospermia.
2. In general, there appears to be little advantage in doing urine testosterone measurements compared with (or in addition to) serum measurements, and the serum test is recommended.
3. Testosterone levels normally undergo large and rapid changes. Testosterone levels are highest in the morning. Male levels drop 30% to 50% and female levels drop 20% by midafternoon.

Interfering Factors

1. Alcoholism in males decreases levels.
2. Estrogen therapy in males increases levels.
3. Many drugs decrease levels, including androgens and steroids.

Patient Preparation

1. Explain test purpose and procedure. Draw blood at 7:00 AM for highest levels.
2. Multiple samples drawn at different times throughout the day and pooled may be necessary for more reliable results.
3. No radioisotopes within 1 week of test.
4. See Chapter 1 guidelines for safe, effective, informed *pretest* care.

Patient Aftercare

1. Resume normal activities.
2. Interpret test results and counsel appropriately concerning hormone dysfunction.
3. Follow Chapter 1 guidelines regarding safe, effective, informed *posttest* care.

● ENZYME TESTS

ACID PHOSPHATASE; PROSTATIC ACID PHOSPHATASE (PAP) ●

Normal Values

0–3.1 ng/ml

Background

Acid phosphatases are enzymes that are widely distributed in tissue, including the bone, liver, spleen, kidney, RBCs, and platelets. However, their greatest diagnostic importance is in the prostate gland, where acid phosphatase activity is 100 times higher than in other tissue.

Explanation of Test

This test diagnoses metastatic cancer of the prostate and monitors the effectiveness of treatment. Elevated levels of acid phosphatase are seen when prostate cancer has metastasized beyond the capsule to the other parts of the body, especially the bone. Once the carcinoma has spread, the prostate starts to release acid phosphatase, resulting in an increased blood level. The prostatic fraction procedure specifically measures the concentration of prostatic acid phosphatase secreted by cells of the prostate gland, in contrast with the total enzyme activity, which is an indirect measurement. Acid phosphatase is also present in high concentration in seminal fluid. Tests for presence of this enzyme may be used to investigate rape.

Procedure

Obtain a venous blood sample of 5 ml. Seminal fluid may also be tested. Observe universal precautions.

Clinical Implications

1. A significantly elevated acid phosphatase value is almost always indicative of metastatic cancer of the prostate. If the tumor is successfully treated, this enzyme level will drop within 3 to 4 days after surgery or 3 to 4 weeks after estrogen administration, also in benign prostatic hypertrophy.

2. Moderately elevated values also occur in the absence of prostate disease in
   a. Paget's disease
   b. Gaucher's disease
   c. Hyperparathyroidism
   d. Multiple myeloma
   e. Any cancer that has metastasized to the bone

Interfering Factors

1. Drugs may cause *increased* and *decreased* levels.
2. Palpation of prostatic gland and prostate biopsy before testing causes increases.

Patient Preparation

1. Explain test purpose and procedure.
2. No palpation of prostate gland 2 to 3 days before test and no rectal exams 2 to 3 days before test.
3. See Chapter 1 guidelines for safe, effective, informed *pretest* care.

Patient Aftercare

1. Resume normal activities.
2. Interpret test results and counsel appropriately concerning repeat testing. When elevated values are present, retesting and biopsy are considered.
3. Follow Chapter 1 guidelines for safe, effective, informed *posttest* care.

PROSTATE-SPECIFIC ANTIGEN (PSA) ●

Normal Values

Men: 0–4.0 ng/ml or μg/L

Background

Prostate specific antigen (PSA) is functionally and immunologically distinct from prostatic acid phosphatase. It is localized in both normal prostatic epithelial cells and prostatic carcinoma cells. It has proved to be the most prognostically reliable marker for monitoring recurrence of prostatic carcinoma.

Explanation of Test

Testing for both PSA and prostate acid phosphatase (PAP) increases detection of early-stage prostate cancer. PSA determines the effectiveness of therapy for prostate cancer and is used as an early indicator of prostate cancer recurrence. The greatest value of PSA is as a marker in the follow-up of patients at high risk for disease progression.

Procedure

Obtain a 2-ml venous blood sample. Observe universal precautions. Inform the laboratory of patient's age. Collect specimen before palpation of the prostate.

Clinical Implications

1. *PSA increases* occur in prostate cancer (80% of patients).
2. Patients with benign prostatic hypertrophy often demonstrate values between 4.0 and 8.0 μg/L. Results between 4.0 and 8.0 μg/L may represent benign prostatic hypertrophy or possible cancer of the prostate. Results above 8.0 μg/L are highly suggestive of prostatic cancer.
3. Increases above 4.0 ng/ml have been reported in about 8% of patients with no prostatic malignancies and no benign diseases.
4. If a prostate tumor is completely and successfully removed, *no* antigen will be detected.

Interfering Factors

Transient increases occur following prostate palpation or rectal examination.

Patient Preparation

1. Explain test purpose and procedure.
2. Do not schedule any prostatic exams, including rectal examination, prostate biopsy, or surgical transurethral resection of prostate (TURP) before the blood test.
3. See Chapter 1 guidelines for safe, effective, informed *pretest* care.

Patient Aftercare

1. Resume normal activities.
2. Interpret test results, monitor, and counsel as appropriate for response to treatment and progression or remission of prostate cancer.
3. Follow Chapter 1 guidelines for safe, effective, informed *posttest* care.

Clinical Alert

1. PSA is not a definitive diagnostic marker to screen for carcinoma of the prostate because it is also found in men with benign prostatic hypertrophy.
2. Digital rectal examination (DRE) is recommended by the American Cancer Society as the primary test for detection of prostatic tumor, recent studies indicate that serum PSA may offer additional information. PSA should be used in conjunction with DRE.

ALANINE TRANSAMINASE (AMINOTRANSFERASE; ALT); SERUM GLUTAMIC–PYRUVIC TRANSAMINASE (SGPT) ●

Normal Values

Adults:	7–56 U/L
Children:	10–35 U/L
Newborns:	6–50 U/L

Slightly higher in males and black persons. Normal values vary with method. Check with your laboratory.

Background

The enzyme ALT occurs in high concentration in the liver, and relatively low concentrations are found in the heart, muscle, and kidney.

Explanation of Test

This test is primarily used to diagnosis liver disease and to monitor the course of treatment for hepatitis, active postnecrotic cirrhosis, and the effects of later drug therapy. ALT also differentiates between hemolytic jaundice and jaundice caused by liver disease.

Procedure

1. Obtain a 5-ml venous blood sample. Observe universal precautions.
2. Avoid hemolysis during collection of the specimen.

Clinical Implications

1. *Increased ALT levels* are found in
   - **a.** Hepatocellular disease (moderate to high increase)
   - **b.** Active cirrhosis (mild increase)
   - **c.** Metastatic liver tumor (mild increase)
   - **d.** Obstructive jaundice or biliary obstruction (mild to moderate increase)
   - **e.** Viral, infectious, or toxic hepatitis (30–50 times normal)
   - **f.** Infectious mononucleosis
   - **g.** Pancreatitis (mild increase)
   - **h.** Myocardial infarction
   - **i.** Polymyositis
   - **j.** Severe burns
   - **k.** Trauma to striated muscle
   - **l.** Severe shock
2. Aspartate transaminase *(AST)/ALT comparison*: Although the AST level is *always* increased in acute myocardial infarction, the ALT level does not always increase proportionately. The ALT is *usually* increased more than the AST in acute extrahepatic biliary obstruction. ALT is less sensitive than AST to alcoholic liver disease.

Interfering Factors

1. Many drugs may cause falsely increased ALT levels.
2. Salicylates may cause decreased or increased ALT levels.

Clinical Alert

There is a correlation between the presence of elevated serum ALT and abnormal antibodies to the hepatitis B virus core antigen. Persons with elevated ALT levels should *not* donate blood.

Patient Preparation

1. Explain test purpose and blood-drawing procedure.
2. See Chapter 1 guidelines for safe, effective, informed *pretest* care.

Patient Aftercare

1. Resume normal activities.
2. Interpret test results and monitor as appropriate for liver disease.
3. Follow Chapter 1 guidelines regarding safe, effective, informed *posttest* care.

ALKALINE PHOSPHATASE (ALP) TOTAL; 5′-NUCLEOTIDASE ●

Normal Values

Age (yr)	*Males (U/L)*	*Both (U/L)*	*Females (U/L)*
0–4		145–320	
4–7		150–380	
7–10		175–420	
10–12		135–530	
12–14	200–495		105–420
14–16	130–525		70–230
16–20	65–260		50–130
Adult	17–142		17–142

Background

Alkaline phosphatase is an enzyme originating mainly in the bone, liver, and placenta, with some activity in the kidney and intestines. It is called *alkaline* because it functions best at a pH of 9. The ALP levels are age and sex dependent.

Explanation of Test

Alkaline phosphatase is used as a tumor marker and an index of liver and bone disease, when correlated with other clinical findings. In bone disease, the enzyme rises in proportion to new bone cell production resulting from osteoblastic activity and the deposit of calcium in the bones. In liver disease, the blood level rises when excretion of this enzyme is impaired as a result of obstruction in the biliary tract.

Procedure

1. Obtain a 5-ml venous blood (serum) sample. Anticoagulants may not be used. Observe universal precautions.
2. Refrigerate sample as soon as possible.
3. Note age and sex on requisition.

Clinical Implications

1. *Elevated levels of ALP and liver disease* (correlates with abnormal liver function tests) occur in

   a. Obstructive jaundice (gallstones obstructing major biliary ducts; accompanying elevated bilirubin)
   b. Space-occupying lesions of the liver, such as cancer (hepatic carcinoma) and malignancy with liver metastasis
   c. Hepatocellular cirrhosis
   d. Biliary cirrhosis
   e. Intrahepatic and extrahepatic cholestasis
   f. Hepatitis
   g. Infectious mononucleosis
2. Bone disease and *elevated ALP levels* occur in
   a. Paget's disease (osteitis deformans)
   b. Metastatic bone tumor
   c. Osteogenic sarcoma
   d. Osteomalacia (elevated levels help differentiate between osteomalacia and osteoporosis, in which there is no elevation
   e. Rickets
   f. Healing factors
   g. Celiac sprue
   h. Renal disorders
3. Other diseases and elevated levels
   a. Hyperparathyroidism (accompanied by hypercalcemia)
   b. Pulmonary and myocardial infarctions
   c. Hodgkin's disease
   d. Cancer of lung or pancreas
   e. Ulcerative colitis
   f. Sarcoidosis
   g. Perforation of bowel
   h. Amyloidosis
   i. Chronic renal failure
   j. Sepsis
4. *Decreased levels of ALP* are found in
   a. Hypophosphatasia
   b. Malnutrition
   c. Hypothyroidism
   d. Pernicious anemia and other severe anemias
   e. Scurvy

Interfering Factors

1. A variety of drugs produces mild to moderate elevations or decreased ALP levels.
2. Age: young children, those experiencing rapid growth, pregnant women, and all postmenopausal women have physiologically high levels of ALP; level is slightly increased in older persons.
3. After IV administration of albumin, there is sometimes a marked increase for several days.
4. The ALP increases at room temperature.
5. The ALP levels decrease if blood is anticoagulated.

Patient Preparation

1. Explain test purpose and blood-drawing procedure. Fasting is required.
2. See Chapter 1 guidelines for safe, effective, informed *pretest* care.

Patient Aftercare

1. Resume normal activities.
2. Interpret test results and monitor appropriately for liver or bone disease and evidence of tumor. Testing for 5′-nucleotidase provides supportive evidence in the diagnosis of liver disease. When ALP and 5′-nucleotidase test results are evaluated, they provide definitive diagnosis of Paget's disease and rickets, in which high levels of ALP accompanying normal (0–5 U/L) or marginally increased 5′-nucleotidase activity. 5′-Nucleotidase is increased in liver disease (eg, hepatic carcinoma, biliary cirrhosis, extrahepatic obstruction, and metastatic neoplasia of liver. 5′-Nucleotidase usually does not increase in skeletal disease.
3. Follow Chapter 1 guidelines for safe, effective, informed *posttest* care.

ALKALINE PHOSPHATASE ISOENZYMES (ISO) ●

Normal Values

AP-1, $alpha_2$: Values are reported as weak, moderate, or strong (liver).
AP-2, $beta_1$: Values are reported as weak, moderate, or strong (bone).
AP-3, $beta_2$: Values are reported as weak, moderate, or strong (intestines).
AP-4, placental.

Background

The isoenzymes of ALP are produced in various tissues. AP-1, $alpha_2$ in the liver and by proliferating blood vessels; AP-2, $beta_1$ by bone and placental tissue. The intestinal isoenzyme AP-3, $beta_2$ is present in small quantities, in group O and B individuals who are Lewis-positive secretors. Placental ALP is found in the last trimester of pregnancy.

Explanation of Test

Any patient with an elevation of serum total alkaline phosphatase is a candidate for ALP isoenzyme study. The ALP ISO is mainly used to distinguish between bone and liver elevations of alkaline phosphatase.

Procedure

Obtain a 5-ml venous blood sample. Add no anticoagulant. Observe universal precautions.

Clinical Implications

1. Liver (AP-1, $alpha_2$) isoenzymes are elevated in hepatic and biliary diseases:
   a. Cirrhosis (congestive)
   b. Hepatic carcinoma
   c. Biliary obstruction
2. Bone (AP-2, $beta_1$) isoenzymes are elevated in

   a. Paget's disease
   b. Rickets
   c. Bone cancer
   d. Osteomalacia
   e. Celiac disease
   f. Certain renal disorders
3. Intestinal (AP-3, beta$_2$) isoenzymes are elevated in
   a. Intestinal infarction
   b. Ulcerative lesions of stomach, small intestine and colon
   c. May be increased in cirrhosis of liver
   d. Patients undergoing hemodialysis
4. Placental AP-2–4 isoenzymes are increased in
   a. Pregnant women in third trimester
   b. Complications of pregnancy such as hypertension
   c. Placental-like isoenzymes in some cancers
      (1) Regan isoenzyme
      (2) Vagal isoenzyme

Interfering Factors

Same as for alkaline phosphatase.

Clinical Alert

1. This test should not be done if the total alkaline phosphatase level is normal.
2. For evaluation of the biliary tract, alternatives of GGT, leucine aminopeptidase (LAP), and 5′-nucleotidase are recommended, rather than alkaline phosphatase isoenzymes.
3. Alkaline phosphatase isoenzymes have little value in children and adolescence because bone and liver fractions will be elevated normally.

Patient Preparation and Patient Aftercare

See Total Alkaline Phosphatase Patient Preparation and Aftercare on pages 383–384. The same guidelines prevail for alkaline phosphatase isoenzymes.

ALDOLASE (ALD)

Normal Values

Adult:	1.5–8.1 U/L
1 mo–6 yr:	3.0–16 U/L
0–1 mo:	6.0–32.0 U/L

Background

Aldolase is an enzyme present in heart and skeletal muscle. It is important in the conversion of glycogen to lactic acid.

Explanation of Test

This test is helpful in complex diagnostic situations to evaluate muscle-wasting process, and skeletal muscle degeneration. As muscle mass diminishes, aldolase values decrease.

Procedure

Obtain a 5-ml fasting, venous blood (serum) sample. Observe universal precautions.

Clinical Implications

1. Highest aldolase levels are found in Duchenne's muscular dystrophy.
2. Lesser ALD elevations are found in
   a. Dermatomyositis
   b. Polymyositis
   c. Limb-girdle muscular dystrophy
   d. Acute hepatitis and other acute viral infections
   e. Portal cirrhosis, viral infections, obstructive jaundice
   f. Gangrene
   g. Some carcinomas with liver metastases
   h. Delirium tremens
   i. Burns
   j. Patients with acute psychosis or schizophrenia
   k. Granulocytic and megaloblastic anemias
   l. Myocardial infarction
3. Normal aldolase values are found in neurogenic atrophies, multiple sclerosis, and myasthenia gravis.

Patient Preparation

1. Explain test purpose and procedure. Fasting from midnight until the specimen is obtained is required. Water is permitted.
2. See Chapter 1 guidelines for safe, effective, informed *pretest* care.

Patient Aftercare

1. Resume normal activities.
2. Interpret test results and counsel appropriately. Aldolase is not specific for muscle disease. The assay of creatinine kinase (CK) has been the preferred test for muscle disease. The CK isoenzymes have a specific band for skeletal muscle.
3. Follow Chapter 1 guidelines for safe, effective, informed *posttest* care.

ANGIOTENSIN-CONVERTING ENZYME (ACE) ●

Normal Values

5–21 mmol/ml/min

Background

Angiotensin I is produced by the action of renin on angiotensinogen. Angiotensin I-converting enzyme (ACE) catalyzes the conversion of angiotensin I to the vasoactive peptide, angiotensin II. Angiotensin I is concentrated in the proximal tubules.

Explanation of Test

This test is used primarily to evaluate the severity and activity of sarcoidosis.

Procedure

Obtain a venous (at least 5-ml) blood sample; serum is used. Observe universal precautions.

Clinical Implications

1. *Increased levels* are associated with
   a. Sarcoidosis: ACE levels reflect the severity of the disease, with 68% positivity in stage 1 disease, 86% in stage 2, and 92% in stage 3.
   b. Gaucher's disease
   c. Leprosy
   d. Acute and chronic bronchitis
   e. Myeloma
   f. Amyloidosis
2. *Decreased levels* occur following prednisone treatment for sarcoidosis.

Interfering Factors

The test should not be done on persons under age 20 because they normally have a very high level of ACE. About 5% of the normal adult population have elevated levels.

Patient Preparation

1. Explain test purpose and blood-drawing procedure.
2. See Chapter 1 guidelines for safe, effective, informed *pretest* care.

Patient Aftercare

1. Interpret test results and monitor as appropriate for sarcoidosis and amyloid disease.
2. Follow Chapter 1 guidelines for safe, effective, informed *posttest* care.

AMYLASE AND LIPASE

Normal Values

Amyloid		*Lipase*	
Newborn:	6–65 U/L	Adults:	10–140 U/L
Adult:	25–125 U/L	Adults over 60 yr:	18–180 U/L
Elderly:	21–160 U/L		

Normal values vary widely depending on the method used. Check with your laboratory for reference ranges.

Background

Amylase, an enzyme that changes starch to sugar, is produced in the salivary glands, pancreas, liver, and fallopian tubes. If there is an inflammation of the pancreas or salivary glands, much amylase enters the blood. Amylase levels in the urine reflect blood changes by a time-lag of 6 to 10 hours (see *Amylase Excretion/Clearance,* Chap. 3). Lipase changes fats to fatty acids and glycerol. The pancreas is the major source of this enzyme. Lipase appears in the blood following pancreatic damage.

Explanation of Test

The amylase and lipase tests are used to diagnose and monitor treatment of acute pancreatitis and to differentiate pancreatitis from other acute abdominal disorders; 80% of patients with acute pancreatitis will have elevated amylase and lipase levels. The lipase test is useful in late diagnosis of pancreatitis when amylase levels may have returned to normal.

Procedure

Obtain a 5-ml venous blood (serum) sample. EDTA anticoagulant interferes with lipase testing. Observe universal precautions.

Clinical Implications

1. *Increased amylase levels* occur in
   a. Greatly increased levels in acute pancreatitis early in the course of the disease. The increase begins in 3 to 6 hours after the onset of pain.
   b. Amylase increases also occur in
      (1) Acute exacerbation of chronic pancreatitis
      (2) Partial gastrectomy
      (3) Obstruction of pancreatic duct
      (4) Perforated peptic ulcer
      (5) Alcohol poisoning
      (6) Mumps
      (7) Obstruction or inflammation of salivary duct or gland
      (8) Acute cholecystitis (common duct stone)
      (9) Intestinal obstruction with strangulation
      (10) Ruptured tubal pregnancy and ectopic pregnancy
      (11) Ruptured aortic aneurysm

2. *Decreased amylase levels* occur in
   a. Pancreatic insufficiency
   b. Hepatitis, severe liver disease
   c. Advanced cystic fibrosis
   d. Toxemia of pregnancy
   e. Severe burns
   f. Severe thyrotoxicosis

3. *Elevated lipase levels* occur in pancreatic disorders (eg, pancreatitis and pancreatic carcinoma). Elevations of lipase may not occur until 24 to 36 hours after onset of illness and remain elevated for up to 14 days. Lipase elevation occurs later and persists longer than blood amylase changes.

4. *Increased lipase values* are also associated with

a. Cholecystitis
b. Severe renal disease
c. Strangulated or impacted bowel
d. Peritonitis

Clinical Alert

Panic lipase level is greater than 600 IU/L.

Patient Preparation

1. Explain test purpose and procedure. Amylase and lipase testing are done together in the presence of abdominal pain, epigastric tenderness, nausea and vomiting. These findings characterize acute pancreatitis as well as other acute surgical emergencies.
2. If amylase/creatinine clearance is also being done, a single, random urine sample is collected at the same time the blood is drawn.
3. See Chapter 1 guidelines for safe, effective, informed *pretest* care.

Patient Aftercare

1. Resume normal activities.
2. Interpret test results and monitor as appropriate for pancreatitis or other acute abdominal conditions.
3. Follow Chapter 1 guidelines for safe, effective, informed *posttest* care.

ASPARTATE TRANSAMINASE (AMINOTRANSFERASE; AST) **OR SERUM GLUTAMIC–OXALOACETIC TRANSAMINASE** (SGOT)

Normal Values

Age	*U/L*
0–5 d	35–140
6 d–3 yr	20–60
3–6 yr	15–50
6–12 yr	10–50
12–18 yr	10–40
Adult	5–40

Background

Aspartate transaminase (AST) is an enzyme present in tissues of high metabolic activity, with decreasing concentration in the heart, liver, skeletal muscle, kidney, brain, pancreas, spleen, and lungs. The enzyme is released into the circulation following the injury or death of cells. Any disease that causes change in these highly metabolic tissues will result in a rise in AST. The amount of AST in the blood is directly related to the number of damaged cells and the amount of time that passes between injury to the tissue and the test. Following severe cell damage, the blood AST level will rise in 12 hours and remain elevated for about 5 days.

Explanation of Test

This test is used in the evaluation of liver and heart diseases.

Procedure

Obtain a 5-ml venous (serum) sample. Observe universal precautions. Hemolysis should be avoided.

Clinical Implications

1. *Increased AST levels* occur in myocardial infarction (MI):
   - **a.** In MI, the AST level may be increased four to ten times the normal values.
   - **b.** The AST level reaches a peak in 24 hours and returns to normal by the third or fourth day. Secondary rises in AST levels suggest extension or recurrence of MI.
   - **c.** The AST curve in MI parallels that of creatinine phosphokinase (CPK) (see page 392).
2. *Increases* in liver diseases (10–100 times normal):
   - **a.** Acute hepatitis and chronic hepatitis
   - **b.** Active cirrhosis
   - **c.** Infectious mononucleosis
   - **d.** Hepatic necrosis
   - **e.** Primary or metastatic carcinoma
   - **f.** Alcoholic hepatitis
   - **g.** Reye's syndrome
3. Other diseases associated with elevated AST levels include
   - **a.** Acute pancreatitis
   - **b.** Trauma or irradiation of skeletal muscle
   - **c.** Dermatomyositis
   - **d.** Polymyositis
   - **e.** Trichinosis
   - **f.** Cardiac catheterization and angiography
   - **g.** Recent brain trauma, with brain necrosis, cerebral infarction
   - **h.** Crushing and traumatic injuries
   - **i.** Progressive muscular dystrophy (Duchenne's)
   - **j.** Pulmonary emboli
   - **k.** Gangrene
   - **l.** Malignant hyperthermia, heat exhaustion
   - **m.** Mushroom poisoning
4. *Decreased AST levels* occur in azotemia and chronic renal dialysis.

Interfering Factors

1. Slight decreases occur during pregnancy when there is abnormal metabolism of pyridoxine.
2. Many drugs can cause elevated levels, salicylates may cause falsely decreased or increased AST levels, and alcohol ingestion affects it.

Patient Preparation

1. Explain test purpose and blood-drawing procedure. For diagnosis of MI, the AST levels should be done on 3 consecutive days because the peak is reached in 24 hours and levels are back to normal in 3 to 4 days.
2. See Chapter 1 guidelines for safe, effective, informed *pretest* care.

Patient Aftercare

1. Interpret test results and monitor appropriately for heart and liver diseases.
2. Levels are falsely decreased in diabetic ketoacidosis, beriberi, severe liver disease, and uremia.
3. Follow Chapter 1 guidelines for safe, effective, informed *posttest* care.

CREATINE PHOSPHOKINASE (CPK); CREATINE KINASE (CK), AND CPK, CK ISOENZYMES ●

Normal Values

Men:	
6–11 yr	56–185 U/L
12–18 yr	35–185 U/L
>19 yr	38–174 U/L
Women:	
6–7 yr	50–145 U/L
8–14 yr	35–145 U/L
15–18 yr	20–100 U/L
>19 yr	96–140 U/L
Newborn:	
68–580 U/L	
Isoenzymes:	
MM CK_3:	96%–100%
MB CK_2:	0%–4%
BB CK_1:	0%

Background

Creatine kinase (CPK/CK) is an enzyme found in higher concentrations in the heart and skeletal muscles and in much smaller concentrations in the brain tissue. Because CK exists in relatively few organs, this test is used as a specific index of injury to myocardium and muscle. CPK can be divided into three isoenzymes: MM or CK_3, BB or CK_1, and MB or CK_2. CK-MM is the isoenzyme that makes up almost all the circulatory enzymes in healthy persons. Skeletal muscle contains primarily MM; cardiac muscle, MM and MB; and brain tissue, GI and genitourinary tracts, BB. Normal CK levels are virtually 100% MM isoenzyme. A slight increase in total CPK is reflected from elevated BB from central nervous system injury. The isoenzyme studies help distinguish whether the CPK originated from the heart (MB) or the skeletal muscle (MM).

Explanation of Test

The CK (CPK) test is used in the diagnosis of myocardial infarction and as a reliable measure of skeletal and inflammatory muscle diseases. The CK levels can prove helpful in recognizing muscular dystrophy before clinical signs appear. Creatine kinase levels may rise significantly with central nervous system disorders, such as Reye's syndrome. The determination of CK isoenzymes may be helpful in a differential diagnosis. Elevation of MB, the cardiac isoenzyme, provides a more definitive indication of myocardial cell damage than total CK alone. MM isoenzyme is an indicator of skeletal muscle damage.

CK-BB may be a useful marker for monitoring therapy in cancer of the lung, breast, and prostate.

Procedure

Obtain a 5-ml venous blood sample. Observe universal precautions. If a patient has been receiving multiple injections intramuscularly, note this fact on the laboratory requisition. Avoid hemolysis.

Clinical Implications of Total CK Levels

1. With myocardial infarction (MI) the rise starts soon after an attack (about 4–6 hours) and reaches a peak of at least several times normal within 24 hour.
2. CK and CK-MB (CK_2 MB) peaks about 1 day following onset, as does AST.
3. Lactate dehydrogenase (LD) usually peaks at the second day when the LD_1–LD_2 inversion (flip) is found.
4. CK-MB, LD_1, LD_1/LD_2 ratio, total CK, and total LD classically increase with acute MI. CK-MB and LD_1 increase in percentage and absolutely (each isoenzyme percentage times the respective total enzyme), peak, then decrease.
5. AST (aspartate transaminase) with LD_1 and LD_2 isoenzymes is advocated when the patient reaches medical attention 48–72 hours after onset of a possible acute myocardial infarction.
6. Other diseases and procedures that cause increased CK/CPK levels include
   a. Acute cerebrovascular disease
   b. Progressive muscular dystrophy (levels may reach 300–400 times normal), Duchenne's muscular dystrophy, also familiar carriers of muscular dystrophy
   c. Dermatomyositis and polymyositis
   d. Delirium tremens and chronic alcoholism
   e. Electric shock, electromyography
   f. Cardiac surgery

g. Cardiac defibrillation
h. Convulsions, ischemia, or subarachnoid hemorrhage
i. Last weeks of pregnancy and during childbirth
j. Hypothyroidism
k. Acute psychosis
l. Central nervous system trauma, extensive brain infarction
m. Acromegaly

7. Normal values are found in myasthenia gravis and multiple sclerosis.
8. Decreased values have no diagnostic meaning: low muscle mass and bed rest (prolonged).

Clinical Implications of CK Isoenzymes

1. *Elevated MM (CK_3) isoenzyme levels* occur in MI (rises 4–6 hours after MI; not demonstrable after 24–36 hours—***peak*** with rapid fall):
   a. Myocardial ischemia, angina pectoris
   b. Duchenne's muscular dystrophy
   c. Polymyositis, dermatomyositis
   d. Significant myoglobinuria
   e. Reye's syndrome
   f. Muscle trauma, muscular exercise
   g. Following intramuscular injections
   h. Circulatory failure and shock
   i. Postoperatively in major surgical procedures
   j. Chronic renal failure
   k. Hypothymia, malignant hypothymia

2. BB (CK_1) elevations are seen in
   a. Reye's syndrome
   b. Some breast, small-cell, lung, and prostate cancers
   c. Severe shock syndrome
   d. Brain injury, neurosurgery
   e. Hypothermia
   f. Following coronary bypass surgery

Clinical Alert

1. After an MI, MB appears in the serum between 6 and 12 hours and remains for about 18 to 32 hours. The finding of MB in patient with chest pain is diagnostic of MI. In addition, if there is a negative CK-MB for 48 hours or more following a clearly defined episode, it is clear that the patient has not had an MI.
2. CK-MB, LD_1, LD_1/LD_2 ratio, total CK, and total LD classically increase with acute MI. CK-MB and LD_1, increase in percentage and absolutely (each isoenzyme percentage times the respective total enzyme), peak, then decrease.

Interfering Factors

1. Strenuous exercise, weight lifting, and surgical procedures that damage skeletal muscle may cause increased levels of CK.
2. High doses of salicylates may cause increased levels.
3. Athletes have a higher value because of greater muscle mass.

4. Multiple intramuscular injections may cause increased levels.
5. Drugs may cause increased levels.
6. Childbirth
7. Hemolysis of blood sample

Patient Preparation

1. Explain test purpose and need for three consecutive blood draws following episode.
2. Note on requisition when suspected cardiac episode had occurred.
3. No exercise before test.
4. See Chapter 1 guidelines for safe, effective, informed *pretest* care.

Patient Aftercare

1. Resume normal activities.
2. Interpret test results and monitor as appropriate for MI, muscular dystrophy, and other causes of abnormal test outcomes.
3. Follow Chapter 1 guidelines for safe, effective, informed *posttest* care.

GALACTOSE-1-PHOSPHATE URIDYLTRANSFERASE (GPT); GALACTOKINASE ●

Normal Values

Galactose-1-phosphate uridyltransferase: 18.5–28.5 U/g of hemoglobin
Galactokinase: 12.1–39.7 U/g of hemoglobin

Background

The enzyme galactose-1-phosphate uridyltransferase is needed in the use of galactose-1-phosphate so that it does not accumulate in the body. Its deficiency is a very rare genetic disorder resulting from an inborn (inherited or during intrauterine development) error of galactose metabolism.

Explanation of Test

This measurement is used to identify galactose defects that can result in widespread tissue damage and abnormalities, such as cataracts, liver disease, and renal disease. It also causes failure to thrive and mental retardation.

Procedure

Obtain (at least a 5-ml) venous blood sample, anticoagulated with heparin or EDTA. Observe universal precautions.

Clinical Implications

Decreased values are associated with galactosemia, a rare genetic disorder transmitted as an autosomal recessive gene. The resulting accumulation of galactitol or galactose-1-phosphate, or both, can result in juvenile cataracts, liver failure, failure to thrive, and mental retardation in galactose 1-phosphate uridyltransferase deficiency.

Patient Preparation

1. Explain test purpose and procedure. Genetic counseling may be necessary.
2. See Chapter 1 guidelines for safe, effective, informed *pretest* care.

Patient Aftercare

1. Interpret test results and counsel appropriately.
2. Parents of infants and children with positive test results should be instructed that the disease can be effectively treated by removing galactose-containing foods, especially milk, from the diet. With dietary galactose restriction, liver and lens changes are reversible.
3. Follow Chapter 1 guidelines for safe, effective, informed *posttest* care.

HEXOSAMINIDASE; TOTAL AND ISOENZYME A ●

Normal Values

Hexosaminidase A	*Total*
Noncarrier, 7.2–9.88 U/L	Noncarriers, 9.83–15.95 U/L
Heterozygous, 3.30–5.39 U/L	Heterozygous, 3.30–5.39 U/L
Tay–Sachs, 0 U/L	Homozygous Tay-Sachs, 17.1 U/L

Check with your laboratory because normal values are method dependent.

Background

Hexosaminidase A is a lysosomal isoenzyme, a deficiency of which characterizes patients with Tay–Sachs disease. In the brains of affected children, there is a 100 times increase of ganglioside owing to a deficiency to this enzyme.

Explanation of Test

Hexosaminidase A is used as a diagnostic test for Tay–Sachs disease and can be of help in identifying carriers among persons with no family history of this disease. This condition is due to an autosomal recessive trait, found predominantly, but not exclusively, in Ashkenazic Jewish people, and is characterized by the appearance during infancy of psychomotor deterioration, blindness, cherry red spot on the macula, and an exaggerated extension response to sound.

Procedure

Obtain a venous (at least 5-ml) blood sample. The test uses serum. If the test is not done immediately, serum must be frozen.

Clinical Implications

1. *Decreased hexosaminidase:* An almost total deficiency of the A component is diagnostic of Tay–Sachs disease or GM_2 gangliosidosis. The total hexosaminidase is of no value in Tay–Sachs.
2. In a variant of Tay–Sachs disease, Sandhoff's disease, both A and B-isoenzymes are defective, causing an absence of this enzyme. The total is also decreased in Sandhoff's disease.
3. *Increased hexosaminidase (total)* is found in
   a. Hepatic disease
   b. Gastric cancer
   c. Myeloma
   d. Myocardial infarction
   e. Vascular complications of diabetes mellitus

Interfering Factors

1. Total values are increased in pregnancy.
2. Oral contraceptives falsely increase values.

Clinical Alert

Critical values: Hexosaminidase A less than 50% of total activity = Tay–Sachs disease.

Patient Preparation

1. Explain test purpose and procedure.
2. Pregnancy or oral contraceptives are contraindications for testing.
3. See Chapter 1 guidelines for safe, effective, informed *pretest* care.

Patient Aftercare

1. Interpret test results and be prepared to do genetic counseling of patient and family.
2. Follow Chapter 1 guidelines for safe, effective, informed *posttest* care.

LACTIC ACID DEHYDROGENASE (LD, LDH)

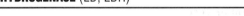

Normal Values

Reported values vary considerably. Check with your laboratory.

Age	*U/L*
0–5 yr	425–975
5–12 yr	370–840
12–14 yr	370–785
14–16 yr	370–645
Adult	313–618

Background

Lactic acid dehydrogenase is an intracellular enzyme that is widely distributed in the tissues of the body, particularly in the kidney, heart, skeletal muscle, brain, liver, and lungs. Increases in the reported value usually indicate cellular death and leakage of the enzyme from the cell.

Explanation of Test

Although elevated levels of LDH are nonspecific, this test is useful in confirming myocardial or pulmonary infarction when viewed in relation to other test findings. For example, LDH remains elevated longer than CK in myocardial infarction (MI). It is also helpful in the differential diagnosis of muscular dystrophy and pernicious anemia. More specific findings may be found by breaking down the LDH into its five isoenzymes. (When LDH values are reported or quoted, *total* LDH is meant.) LDH is also valuable as a tumor marker in seminoma or germ cell testis tumor, especially when AFP and hCG are not produced in the tumor.

Procedure

1. Obtain a 5-ml venous blood sample. Observe universal precautions.
2. Avoid hemolysis in obtaining blood sample

Clinical Implications

1. *LDH (LD) is increased* in MI: high levels occur within 36 to 55 hours after infarction and continue longer than AST (SGOT) or CPK (3–10 days). Differential diagnosis of acute MI may be accomplished with LDH isoenzymes.
2. In pulmonary infarction: increased LDH occurs within 24 hours of pain onset. The pattern of normal AST and elevated LDH that levels off 1 to 2 days after an episode of chest pain is indicative of pulmonary infarction.
3. *Elevated levels of LDH* are observed in various other conditions, such as
   a. Congestive heart failure
   b. Liver diseases (eg, cirrhosis, alcoholism, and acute viral hepatitis)
   c. Malignant neoplasms or cancer
   d. Hypothyroidism
   e. Lung diseases (pulmonary infarction)
   f. Skeletal muscle diseases (muscular dystrophy)
   g. Megaloblastic and pernicious anemia
   h. Sickle cell disease
4. Angina and pericarditis do *not* produce LDH elevations.
5. *Decreased LDH levels* are associated with a good response to cancer therapy.
6. *Elevated urine LDH* levels occur in
   a. Cancer of kidney or bladder
   b. Glomerulonephritis
   c. Malignant hypertension
   d. Lupus nephritis
   e. Acute tubular necrosis
   f. Renal transplantation and homograft rejection
   g. Pyelonephritis (sometimes)

Interfering Factors

1. Strenuous exercise and the muscular exertion involved in childbirth will cause increased levels.
2. Skin diseases can cause falsely increased levels.

3. Hemolysis of RBCs caused by freezing, heating, or shaking the blood sample will cause falsely increased levels.
4. Some drugs may cause increased and decreased levels.

Clinical Alert

LDH is found in nearly every tissue of the body. An elevated level, therefore, is of limited diagnostic value by itself. Differential diagnoses may be accomplished with LDH isoenzyme determination.

Patient Preparation

1. Explain test purpose and blood-drawing procedure.
2. See Chapter 1 guidelines for safe, effective, informed *pretest* care.

Patient Aftercare

1. Resume normal activities.
2. Interpret test results and monitor for myocardial and pulmonary infarction and other diseases related to abnormal results.
3. See Chapter 1 guidelines for safe, effective, informed *posttest* care.

LDH (LD) **ISOENZYMES** (ELECTROPHORESIS)

Normal Values

LDH Isoenzymes	*% of Total*
LDH_1	17–27
LDH_2	29–39
LDH_3	19–27
LDH_4	8–16
LDH_5	6–16

Background

Electrophoresis or separation of LDH identifies the five isoenzymes or fractions of LDH, each with its own physical characteristics and electrophoretic properties. Fractionation of the LDH activity sharpens its diagnostic value because LDH is found in many organs. The LDH isoenzymes are released into the bloodstream when tissue necrosis occurs. However, a complete knowledge of the clinical history is necessary to properly interpret the resulting patterns. The isoenzymes are elevated in terms of patterns established, not on the basis of the value of a single isoenzyme. The origins of the LDH isoenzymes are as follows: LD_1 and LD_2, cardiac, RBCs (brain, renal cortex);

LD_3, mainly lung, spleen, pancreas, also placenta; LD_4 and LD_5, skeletal muscle, liver, and skin.

Explanation of Test

The five isoenzyme fractions of LDH show different patterns in various disorders. Abnormalities in the pattern suggest which tissues have been damaged. This test is useful in the differential diagnosis of acute MI, megaloblastic anemia (folate deficiency, pernicious anemia); hemolytic anemia, and very occasionally, renal infarct. These entities are characterized by LD_1 increases, often with LD_1/LD_2 inversion (*flip*).

Procedure

Obtain a 5-ml venous blood sample; avoid hemolysis. Observe universal precautions.

Clinical Implications

1. Abnormal LD_1 and LD_2 patterns reflect damaged tissues.
   a. The appearance of an LD flip (when LD_1 is > LD_2) is extremely helpful in diagnosis of MI. The presence of an LD flip a day following or with the detection of CK-MB is essentially diagnostic of MI, if baseline cardiac enzymes/isoenzymes are normal and if rises and falls are as anticipated for the diagnosis of acute MI.
   b. Persistent LD_1/LD_2 flip following acute myocardial infarct may represent reinfarction. When acute myocardial infarction is complicated by shock, a normal pattern may be found. The LD_1/LD_2 inversion commonly appears subsequent to the isomorphic pattern in instances of acute myocardial infarction.
   c. The LDH pattern in hemolytic megaloblastic and sickle cell anemia cirrhosis, renal infarction, and testicular cancer will be essentially the same as in MI and other anemias. This is because red blood cells and the kidney have isoenzyme patterns similar to that of heart muscle. The time elapsed to peak values may help differentiate.
2. LD_3 increases occur in advanced cancer and malignant lymphoma; it should decrease following effective therapy. LD_3 occasionally is elevated in pulmonary infarction or pneumonia.
3. LD_5 is *increased* in
   a. Liver disease
   b. Congestive heart failure
   c. Striated muscle trauma
   d. LD_5 increase is more significant when the LD_5/LD_4 ratio is increased
4. In most cancers, one to three of the bands (LD_2, LD_3, and LD_4) are frequently increased. A notable exception is in seminomas and dysgerminomas when LD_1 is increased. Frequently, an increase in LD_3 may be the first indication of the presence of cancer.
5. All LDH isoenzymes are increased in systemic diseases (eg, carcinomatous collagen vascular, DIC, and sepsis.)

Clinical Alert

1. LDH isoenzyme testing should be reserved for diagnosis of complex cases. In 5% to 20% of patients with acute MI, the expected reversal of LD_1/LD_2 does not occur; in these patients there is often simply an increase in LD_1.
2. LDH isoenzymes should be interpreted in light of the clinical findings.

Patient Preparation

1. Explain test purpose and procedure. Repeat testing on 3 consecutive days is likely.
2. See Chapter 1 guidelines for safe, effective, informed *pretest* care.

Patient Aftercare

1. Resume normal activities.
2. Interpret test results and monitor appropriately for abnormal LDH patterns.
3. See Chapter 1 guidelines for safe, effective, informed *posttest* care.

RENIN (ANGIOTENSIN); **PLASMA RENIN ANGIOTENSIN** (PRA) ●

Normal Values

Adult normal sodium diet:

Supine:	0.1–3.1 ng/ml/hr
Standing:	1.6–7.4 ng/ml/hr

Adult low-sodium diet:

Supine:	2.1–4.3 ng/ml/hr
Standing:	5.0–13.6 ng/ml/hr

NOTE: *A restricted salt diet increases supine levels.*

Background

Renin is an enzyme that converts angiotensinogen to angiotensin I. Derived from the liver, angiotensinogen is an alpha$_2$-globulin in the serum. Angiotensin I is then converted in the lung to angiotensin II. Angiotensin II is a potent vasopressor agent, responsible for hypertension of renal origin, as well as a powerful releaser of aldosterone from the adrenal cortex. Both angiotensin II and aldosterone increase blood pressure. Renin levels increase when there is decreased renal perfusion pressure. The renin–aldosterone axis regulates sodium and potassium balance, blood volume, and blood pressure. Renal reabsorption of sodium affects plasma volume. Low plasma volume, low blood pressure, low sodium and increased potassium levels will induce renin release, thereby causing increased aldosterone production through stimulation of angiotensin. Potassium loss, acute blood pressure increases, and increased blood volumes suppress renin release.

Explanation of Test

This test is most useful in the differential diagnosis of hypertension, either essential, renal, or renovascular. In primary hyperaldosteronism, the findings will demonstrate that aldosterone secretion is exaggerated and secretion of renin is suppressed.

Procedure

1. Obtain a 5-ml fasting venous blood sample. Collect specimen with scrupulous attention to detail. Use EDTA as the anticoagulant, which aids in preservation of any angiotensin formed before examination. Observe universal precautions.
2. Draw blood in chilled tubes and place on ice immediately.
3. Record posture and dietary status of patient at time blood is drawn.

Clinical Implications

1. *Increased renin levels* occur in
   - **a.** Secondary aldosteronism (severe hypertension of renal origin)
   - **b.** Addison's disease
   - **c.** Low-sodium diet, diuretics, hemorrhage
   - **d.** Chronic renal failure
   - **e.** Salt-losing status owing to gastrointestinal disease
   - **f.** Renin-producing tumors of kidney
   - **g.** Few patients (15%) with essential hypertension
   - **h.** Bartter's syndrome (high renin hypertension)
2. *Decreased renin levels* are found in
   - **a.** Primary aldosteronism (98%)
   - **b.** Unilateral renal artery stenosis
   - **c.** Administration of salt-retaining steroids
   - **d.** Congenital adrenal hyperplasia, with 17-hydroxylase deficiency

Interfering Factors

1. Levels vary in healthy persons and increase under influences that tend to shrink the intravascular fluid volume.
2. Random specimens may be difficult to interpret unless dietary and salt intake of patient is regulated.
3. Values will be higher when the patient is in an upright position, early in the day, with low-salt diets, during pregnancy, and with drugs, such as diuretics, antihypertensives, estrogen, and oral contraceptives.
4. Recently administered radioisotopes interfere.

Patient Preparation

1. Explain test purpose and procedure.
2. A regular diet that contains 180 mEq of sodium and 100 mEq of potas-

sium must be maintained for 3 days before the specimen is obtained. A 24-hour urine sodium and potassium test should also be done to evaluate salt balance.

3. Instruct the patient that it is necessary to be in a supine position for at least 2 hours before obtaining the specimen. The specimen is drawn with patient in supine position.
4. Antihypertensive drugs, cyclic progestogens, estrogens, diuretics, or licorice should be terminated at least 2 weeks, and preferably 4 weeks, before a renin–aldosterone workup.
5. If a standing specimen is ordered, the patient must be standing for 2 hours before beginning, and blood is drawn in the sitting position.
6. No caffeine may be ingested the morning before or during the test.
7. See Chapter 1 guidelines for safe, effective, informed *pretest* care.

Patient Aftercare

1. Interpret test results and counsel appropriately concerning hypertension.
2. Resume normal activities.
3. Follow Chapter 1 guidelines for safe, effective, informed *posttest* care.

RENIN STIMULATION/CHALLENGE TEST ●

Challenge Test

A challenge test distinguishes primary from secondary hyperaldosteronism on the basis of renin levels, with the patient in both the recumbent and upright positions, and after the patient has been maintained on a low-salt diet. In normal persons and in those with essential hypertension, renin concentration will be increased by the reduction in volume caused by sodium restriction and the upright position. In primary aldosteronism, volume depletion does not occur and renin concentration remains low.

General Procedure for Renin Stimulation Test

1. The patient should be admitted to the hospital for this test. On admission, obtain weight and record.
2. A diet containing reduced sodium content, supplemented with potassium, is given for 3 days, along with diuretics (such as furosemide or chlorothiazide), as ordered.
3. Weigh again on the third day, record, and see that the patient remains upright for 4 hours participating in normal activities.
4. A venous heparinized blood sample for renin is obtained at 11 AM (when renin is usually at its maximum level). Place on ice and immediately send to the laboratory.

Interpretation of Renin Stimulation Test

In healthy persons and most hypertensive patients, the stimulation of a low-salt diet, a diuretic, and upright posture will raise renin activity to very high levels and result in weight loss. However, in primary aldosteronism, the plasma level is expanded and remains so. In these patients, there is little if any weight loss, and the renin level is very low or undetectable. A response within the normal range *can* occur in the presence of aldosterone.

Patient Preparation

1. Explain test purpose and procedure. The purpose of the preparation is to deplete the patient of sodium.
2. Check with the individual laboratory for specific practices.
3. See Chapter 1 guidelines for safe, effective, informed *pretest* care.

Patient Aftercare

1. Resume normal activities.
2. Interpret test results and counsel appropriately concerning hypertension.
3. Follow Chapter 1 guidelines for safe, effective, informed *posttest* care.

γ-GLUTAMYLTRANSFERASE (GGT); γ-GLUTAMYL TRANSPEPTIDASE (γGT); γ-GLUTAMYLTRANSFERASE (γGT) ●

Normal Values

Men:	5–85 U/L
Women:	5–55 U/L

Background

The enzyme γ-glutamyl transpeptidase is present mainly in the liver, kidney, prostate, and spleen. Despite the fact that the kidney has the highest level of the enzyme, the liver is considered the source of normal serum activity. Men will have higher normal levels because of the large amounts found in the prostate.

Explanation of Test

This test is used to determine liver cell dysfunction and to detect alcohol-induced liver disease. It also screens for the consequences of chronic alcoholism. Because GGT is very sensitive to the amount of alcohol consumed by chronic drinkers, it can be used to monitor the cessation or reduction of alcohol consumption. The γGT activity is elevated in all forms of liver disease. This test is much more sensitive than either the alkaline phosphatase test or the transaminase tests (AST, ALT) in detecting obstructive jaundice, cholangitis, and cholecystitis. It is also indicated in the differential diagnosis of liver disease in children and pregnant women who have elevated levels of LDH and alkaline phosphatase. γGT is also useful as a cancer marker because levels reflect remission and recurrence.

Procedure

Obtain a 5-ml venous blood (serum) sample. Observe universal precautions.

Clinical Implications

1. *Increased γGT levels* are associated with liver diseases
   a. Hepatitis
   b. Cirrhosis, obstructive and familial
   c. Liver metastasis and carcinoma
   d. Cholestasis (especially during or following pregnancy)
   e. Chronic alcoholic liver disease
   f. Infectious mononucleosis
2. It is also increased in pancreatitis and carcinoma of pancreas.
3. In MI, γGT is usually normal. However, if there is an increase, it occurs about the fourth day after an MI and probably implies liver damage secondary to cardiac insufficiency.
4. Hyperthyroidism.
5. *Decreased γGT levels* are found in hypothyroidism.
6. Values are normal in bone disorders, bone growth, pregnancy, skeletal muscle disease, strenuous exercise, and renal failure.

Interfering Factors

1. Various drugs
2. Alcohol (ethanol)
3. Oral contraceptives
4. Pregnancy

Patient Preparation

1. Explain test purpose blood-drawing procedure. No alcohol before test.
2. See Chapter 1 guidelines for safe, effective, informed *pretest* care.

Patient Aftercare

1. Resume normal activities.
2. Interpret test results and monitor as appropriate for liver, pancreatic, or thyroid disease, or for cancer recurrence.
3. Follow Chapter 1 guidelines for safe, effective, informed *posttest* care.

DRUG MONITORING

THERAPEUTIC DRUG MONITORING

Normal Values

See Tables 6-2 and 6-3 for maintenance levels.

Explanation of Test

Therapeutic drug monitoring is a reliable and practical approach to managing individual patient drug therapy. Determination of drug levels is especially important when the potential for drug toxicity is significant, or when

TABLE 6-2
Blood Plasma Concentration of Commonly Monitored Drugs

Drug	*Therapeutic* Maintenance*	*Toxic† (Panic or Critical)*
Acetaminophen (Tylenol)	1–30 μg/ml or 66–199 μmol/L	>200 μg/ml or >1324 μmol/L
Alcohol (Ethanol)	Driving while intoxicated: 100 mg/dl or 10.9–21.7 mmol/L	>400 mg/dl >86.8 mmol/L
Amitriptyline (Elavil)	120–250 mg/ml or 433–903 nmol/L	>500 mg/ml or >1805 nmol/L
Bromide	750–1500 μg/ml or 9.4–18.7 nmol/L	>1250 μg/ml or >15.6 nmol/L >15.6 nmol/L
Carbamazepine (Tegretol)	8–12 μg/ml or 34–51 μmol/L	>15 μg/ml or >63 mol/L
Chlordiazepoxide (Librium)	700–1000 ng/ml or 2.34–3.34 μmol/L	>5000 ng/ml or >16.70 μmol/L
Desopyramide (Norpace)	Variable	>7 μg/ml or >20.7 μmol/L
Diazepam (Valium)	100–1000 ng/ml or 0.35–3.51 μmol/L	>5000 ng/ml or >17.55 μmol/L
Digitoxin	20–35 ng/ml or 26–46 nmol/L	>45 ng/ml or >59 nmol/L
Digoxin	CHF: 0.8–1.5 ng/ml or 1.0–1.9 nmol/L Arrhythmias: 1.5–2.0 ng/ml or 1.9–2.6 nmol/L	>25 ng/ml or >3.2 nmol/L
Doxepin	30–150 ng/ml or 107–537 nmol/L	>500 ng/ml or >1790 nmol/L
Ethchlorvynol (Placidyl)	2–8 μg/ml or 14–55 μmol/L	>20 μg/ml or >138 μmol/L
Glutethimide (Doriden)	2–6 μg/ml or 9–28 μmol/L	>5 μg/ml or >23 μmol/L
Imipramine (Tofranil)	125–250 ng/ml or 446–893 nmol/L	>500 ng/ml or >1785 nmol/L
Lithium	0.6–1.2 mEq/L or 0.6–1.2 mmol/L	>2 mEq/L or >2 mmol/L
Lidocaine (Xylocaine)	1.5–6.0 μg/ml or 6.4–25.6 μmol/L	6–8 μg/ml or 25.6–34.2 μmol/L
Methotrexate	Variable	48 hr after high dose: 454 mg/ml or 1000 mmol/L
Methyprylon (Noludar)	8–10 μg/ml or 45–55 μmol/L	>50 μg/ml or >275 μmol/L

(continued)

TABLE 6-2 *(continued)*

Drug	Therapeutic* Maintenance	Toxic† (Panic or Critical)
Phenobarbital	15–40 g/ml or 65–172 mol/L	Varies 35–80 g/ml or 151–345 mol/L
Phenytoin (Dilantin)	10–20 g/ml or 40–79 mol/L	Varies with symptoms
Procainamide (Promestyl)	4–10 g/ml or 17–42 mol/L	10–12 g/ml or 42–51 mol/L
Primidone (Mysoline)	5–12 g/ml or 23–35 mol/L	15 g/ml or 69 mol/L
Propranolol (Inderal)	50–100 mg/ml or 193–386 nmol/L	Not defined
Quinidine	Varies considerably	
Salicylate	<100 µg/ml or <724 µmol/L	Quite variable: begins at 100 µg/ml or begins at 724 µmol/L
Theophylline	Bronchodilator: 8–20 µg/ml or 44–111 µmol/L Premature apnea: 6–13 µg/ml or 33–72 µmol/L	>20 µm/ml or >111 µmol/L
Valproic Acid (Depakene)	50–100 g/ml or 347–693 µmol/L	100 g/ml or 693 µmol/L

**Therapeutic value* refers to expected drug concentration associated with desirable clinical effects in majority of the patient population treated.
†*Toxic values* refer to the drug concentration associated with undesirable effects or, in certain cases, death.

inadequate or undesirable response follows the use of a standard dose. It provides an easier and more rapid estimation of dosage requirements than does observation of the drug effects themselves. For some drugs, monitoring is routinely useful (digoxin); for others, it can be helpful in certain situations (antibiotics). The plasma level of drugs needed to control the patient's symptoms is called the steady-state concentration, usually maintained by a combination of drug dosage and dosage interval. Monitoring at intervals minimizes the possibility of the development of dose-related side effects. If single-drug therapy is not effective, therapeutic monitoring allows the physician to select supplementary medication and monitor its effect on the primary drug.

Indications for Testing

1. To verify correct drug dosage and level. The drug source, dose, or regimen is changed.
2. If noncompliance (nonadherence) is suspected, and patient motivation to maintain medication is poor.

TABLE 6-3
Blood Plasma Concentration of Commonly Monitored Antibiotics

Antibiotic	*Peak**	*Trough*†
Amikacin	Therapeutic: 25–35 μg/ml or 43–600 μmol/L Toxic: >35 μg/ml or >6000 μmol/L	Less severe infections: 1–4 μg/ml Therapeutic: 1.71–6.84 μmol/L Toxic: >5 μg/ml or >17 μmol/L
Ethosuximide		Therapeutic: 40–100 μg/ml or 283–708 μmol/L Toxic: >150 μg/ml or >1062 μmol/L
Gentamicin	Less severe infection: Therapeutic: 5–8 μg/ml Toxic: >12 μg/ml	Less severe: Therapeutic: 1–4 μg/ml Toxic: >4 μg/ml
Kanamycin	Therapeutic: 8–25 μg/ml Toxic: >25 μg/ml	Therapeutic: 2–8 μg/ml Toxic: >8 μg/ml
Tobramycin	Less severe: Therapeutic: 5–9 μg/ml or 11–17 μmol/L Toxic: >12 μg/ml or 21–26 μmol/L	Less severe: 1–3 μg/ml Therapeutic: <2 μmol/L Toxic: >3 μg/ml or >4–9 μmol/L

**Peak drug level* refers to maximum drug concentration achieved following administration of a single dose. For a specific drug, both the concentration achieved and time interval between dosing and peak drug level required may vary considerably from patient to patient.
†*Trough drug level* refers to minimum drug concentration preceding administration of a single dose.

3. If the physiologic status is altered by factors such as weight, menstrual cycle, body water, stress, age, and thyroid function.
4. Coadministered (multiple) drugs may cause either synergistic or antagonistic drug reaction.
5. In pathology that influences drug absorption and elimination, such as
   a. Cardiovascular dysfunction
   b. Liver clearance
   c. Renal clearance (urinary output and pH)
   d. Gastrointestinal—poor absorption
   e. Altered plasma protein binding (or change in blood proteins that carry drug)
6. Some drugs have a very small safety range (therapeutic window or concentration). Factors that affect concentration include absorption, metabolism, excretion, tissue storage, and site of action.

Procedure

1. Obtain a venous sample of blood. Serum or plasma can be used, depending on the drug being tested and laboratory protocols.

2. Serum-separation tubes may not be used for drug monitoring because small amounts of the drug adhere to the separator testing gill.

Patient Preparation

1. Explain test purpose, procedure, and recommended regimen for drawing specimens for therapeutic drug testing.
2. See Chapter 1 guidelines for safe, effective, informed *pretest* care.

Patient Aftercare

1. Interpret test results, counsel and monitor appropriately. Assessment of changes in patient's condition and knowledge of drug interactions aid in the interpretation of test results. The importance of accurate sampling time in obtaining therapeutic drug-monitoring data cannot be overstated. Whatever sampling procedure is used, such as *peak* or *maximum* concentration or *trough* or *minimum* drug concentration, it is important that the same time interval between sampling and dose administration be used consistently when comparing results from serial samples on the same patient.
2. *Elimination half-life* refers to time required to eliminate drug from the body after the initial distribution phase is complete. Under certain conditions, elimination half-life dates are useful in estimating how long one should wait following initiation of therapy before sampling.

> **Clinical Alert**
>
> Factors influencing drug and chemical concentrations in living patients are frequently altered significantly after death.

BLOOD ALCOHOL CONTENT (BAC); **ETHANOL** (ETHYL ALCOHOL) ●

Normal Value

Negative: no alcohol detected

Background

Ethanol is absorbed rapidly from the GI tract, with peak blood levels usually occurring within 40 to 70 minutes on an empty stomach. (Food in the stomach depresses alcohol absorption.) Ethanol is metabolized by the liver to acetaldehyde. Once peak blood ethanol levels are reached, disappearance is linear; a 70-kg man metabolizes 7 to 10 g alcohol per hour (15 ±5 mg/dl/hr). Symptoms of intoxication in the presence of low alcohol levels could indicate a serious acute medical problem requiring immediate attention.

Explanation of Test

The test, done to detect the presence of alcohol, is an indication of overdose and alcohol-impaired driving.

Procedure

1. Obtain a 5-ml venous blood sample from the arm in living persons. From dead persons, take samples from the aorta. Observe universal precautions.
   a. Use nonalcohol solution for cleansing venipuncture site.
   b. Sodium fluoride or oxalate anticoagulant is recommended.
   c. Keep blood sample tightly stoppered.
2. A 20-ml sample of urine or gastric contents can be used.
3. Breath analyzer measures ethanol content at the end of expiration, following a deep inspiration.

Clinical Implications

1. At levels of 50 to 100 mg/dl, certain signs and symptoms are reported: flushing, slowing of reflexes, and impaired visual acuity.
2. At levels higher than 100 mg/dl, central nervous system depression is reported. This is the cut-off level for driving under the influence of alcohol.
3. At levels higher than 400 mg/dl, death is reported.
4. Properly collected urine samples will have an alcohol content 1.3 times that of blood. Saliva samples will have an alcohol content 1.2 times that of blood.

Intefering Factors

1. Increased blood ketones, as in diabetic ketoacidosis, can falsely elevate blood or breath test results.
2. Other alcohols, such as isopropanol or methanol, affect results.

Clinical Alert

A value of greater than 300 mg/dl is a critical or panic value. Report and initiate overdose treatment at once.

Patient Preparation

1. Explain test purpose and procedure. Proper collection, handling, and storage of the blood alcohol specimen are essential when the question of sobriety is raised.
2. Advise patient of legal rights in cases involving question of sobriety.
3. A witnessed signed consent form may have to be obtained.
4. See Chapter 1 guidelines for safe, effective, informed *pretest* care.

Patient Aftercare

1. Interpret test results and monitor as appropriate.
2. If alcohol levels are high, initiate treatment at once.
3. Follow Chapter 1 guidelines for safe, effective, informed *posttest* care.

● LIPOPROTEIN TESTS

Lipoprotein measurements are diagnostic indicators for hyper- and hypolipidemia. Hyperlipidemia is classified as I, IIa, IIb, III, IV, and V. Lipids are fatty substances made up of cholesterol, cholesterol esters (liquid compounds), triglycerides, nonesterized fatty acids, and phospholipids. Lipoproteins are unique plasma proteins that transport otherwise insoluble lipids. They are categorized as chylomicrons; beta-lipoproteins (low-density lipoproteins [LDL]); prebeta-lipoproteins (very low-density lipoproteins [VLDL]); and alpha-lipoproteins (very high-density lipoproteins [HDL]). Apolipoprotein A is composed mainly of HDL, chylomicrons, and VLDL. Apolipoprotein B is the main component of LDL. Lipids provide energy for metabolism, serve as precursors of steroid hormones (adrenals, ovaries, and testes) and bile acids, and play an important role in cell membrane development. A lipid profile usually includes cholesterol, triglycerides, LDL, and HDL.

CHOLESTEROL ●

Normal Values

Normal values vary with age, diet, and geographic or cultural region.

Adults: *Desirable level:* 140–199 mg/dl, or < 5.18 mmol/L
Borderline high: 200–239 mg/dl, or 5.18–6.19 mmol/L
High: 240 mg/dl or higher, or > 6.20 mmol/L

Children and adolescents (age 12–18):
Desirable level: < 170 mg/dl, or < 4.39 mmol/L
Borderline: 170–199 mg/dl, or 4.40–5.16 mmol/L
High: > 200 mg/dl, or > 5.18 mmol/L

Background

Cholesterol is a fat-soluble steroid alcohol found in animal fats and oils. It is widely distributed, especially in the blood, brain, liver, kidneys, and the nerve fibers' myelin sheaths, and is an essential component of cell membrane development and production of bile acids, adrenal steroids, and sex hormones.

Explanation of Test

Cholesterol testing detects disorders of blood lipids and indicates potential risk for atherosclerotic coronary artery disease. Elevated cholesterol levels are a major component in the hereditary hyperlipoproteinemias. Cholesterol studies are also frequently a part of thyroid and liver function studies.

Procedure

Obtain a fasting 5-ml venous blood sample; serum is preferred. Observe universal precautions.

Clinical Implications

1. Total blood cholesterol levels are the basis for classifying coronary heart disease (CHD) risk.
   - **a.** Levels greater than 240 mg/dl are considered high and should include follow-up lipoprotein analysis. Borderline-high levels (200–239 mg/dl), in the presence of CHD or two other CHD risk factors, should also include lipoprotein analysis or profiles.
   - **b.** The CHD risk factors include male sex, family history of premature CHD (myocardial infarction or sudden death before age 55 in a parent or sibling), smoking habit (more than 10 cigarettes per day), hypertension, low HDL-cholesterol levels (below 35 mg/dl, confirmed by repeat measurement), diabetes mellitus, history of definite cerebrovascular or occlusive peripheral vascular disease, and severe obesity (> 30% overweight).
   - **c.** In public-screening programs, all patients with cholesterol levels above 200 mg/dl should be referred to their physicians for further evaluation.

2. *Elevated cholesterol levels (hypercholesterolemia)* occur in
   - **a.** Type II familial hypercholesterolemia
   - **b.** Hyperlipoproteinemia (types I, IV, and V)
   - **c.** Hepatocellular disease, biliary cirrhosis
   - **d.** Cholestasis
   - **e.** Nephrotic syndrome, glomerulonephritis
   - **f.** Chronic renal failure
   - **g.** Pancreatic and prostatic malignant neoplasms
   - **h.** Hypothyroidism
   - **i.** Poorly controlled diabetes mellitus
   - **j.** Alcoholism
   - **k.** Glycogen storage disease (von Gierke's disease)
   - **l.** Werner's syndrome
   - **m.** Diet high in cholesterol and fats
   - **n.** Obesity

3. *Decreased cholesterol levels (hypocholesterolemia)* occur in
   - **a.** alpha-Hypoprotein deficiency (Tangier disease)
   - **b.** Hepatocellular disease
   - **c.** Malignant liver neoplasms
   - **d.** Hyperthyroidism
   - **e.** Malabsorption syndrome, malnutrition
   - **f.** Megaloblastic anemia or sideroblastic anemia
   - **g.** Severe burns
   - **h.** Conditions of acute illness
   - **i.** Chorionic obstructive lung disease

Interfering Factors

1. Estrogens decrease plasma cholesterol levels.
2. Certain drugs increase or decrease levels.
3. Seasonal variations in cholesterol levels have been observed—levels are higher in fall and winter and lower in spring and summer.

Patient Preparation

1. Explain test purpose and procedure. A 12-hour fast before testing is required, although water may be taken. Pretest, a normal diet should be consumed for 7 days. The patient should abstain from alcohol for 48 hours before testing.
2. Document drugs the patient is taking.
3. Encourage the patient to relax.
4. See Chapter 1 guidelines for safe, effective, informed *pretest* care.

Patient Aftercare

1. Interpret test results and counsel appropriately. Cholesterol levels are influenced by heredity, diet, body weight, and physical activity. Some lifestyle changes may be necessary to reduce elevated levels.
2. Cholesterol levels above 200 mg/dl should be retested and the results averaged. If the two results vastly differ, a third test should be done.
3. Once hyperlipidemia has been established, the diet should be low in animal fats and should replace saturated fats with polyunsaturated fats. Fruits and vegetables (especially greens) should be increased. Patients with diabetes, as well as others, should seek counsel from a dietitian concerning diet management if necessary. Therapy for hyperlipidemia should always begin with diet modification.
4. The American Heart Association and National Cholesterol Education Programs have excellent resources for diet and lifestyle management information.
5. At least 6 months of dietary therapy should be tried before initiating cholesterol-reducing drug therapy.
6. A comprehensive lipoprotein analysis should be done if cholesterol levels are not lowered within 6 months.

Clinical Alert

Cholesterol measurement should not be done immediately after myocardial infarction. A 3-month wait is suggested.

HIGH-DENSITY LIPOPROTEIN CHOLESTEROL (HDL-C) ●

Normal Values

Male:	37–70 mg/dl
Female:	40–85 mg/dl

Less than 25 mg/dl of HDL	CHD risk is at dangerous level
26–35 mg/dl of HDL	High CHD risk
36–44 mg/dl of HDL	Moderate CHD risk
45–59 mg/dl of HDL	Average CHD risk
60–74 mg/dl of HDL	Below average CHD risk
Greater than 75 mg/dl of HDL	Protection probable. Associated with longevity.

Background

The HDL-C is a class of lipoproteins produced by the liver and intestines. HDL is comprised of phospholipids and one or two apolipoproteins. It plays a role in the metabolism of the other lipoproteins and in cholesterol transport from peripheral tissues to the liver. LDL and HDL may combine to maintain cellular cholesterol balance through the mechanism of LDL moving cholesterol into the arteries and HDL removing it from the arteries. Decreased HDL levels are atherogenic, whereas elevated HDL levels protect against artherosclerosis by removing cholesterol from vessel walls and transporting it to the liver where it is removed from the body.

Explanation of Test

The HDL-C test assesses coronary artery disease risk and monitors persons with known low HDL levels. The HDL-C levels are inversely proportionial to coronary heart disease (CHD) risk.

Procedure

Obtain a 5-ml fasting venous blood sample. The HDL is precipitated out from the total cholesterol for analysis. A cholesterol/HDL-C ratio can be calculated from these values.

Clinical Implications

1. *Increased HDL-C values* occur in
   a. Familial hyperalphalipoproteinemia
   b. Chronic liver disease (cirrhosis, alcoholism, hepatitis)
   c. Long-term aerobic or vigorous exercise.
2. *Decreased HDL-C values* are associated with
   a. Increased risk for CHD and premature CHD
   b. Familial hypoalphalipoproteinemia (Tangier disease)
   c. Apo C-III deficiency
   d. Hypertriglyceridemia
   e. Poorly controlled diabetes mellitus
   f. Hepatocellular diseases
   g. Nephrotic syndrome
   h. Chronic renal failure
   i. 3% of males in the United States have low HDL (for unknown reasons), even though cholesterol and triglyceride values are normal

Interfering Factors

1. *Increased HDL* is associated with estrogen therapy, moderate alcohol intake, and other drugs, especially androgenic and related steroids.
2. Drugs such as β-adrenergic blockers and diuretics cause decreased HDLs.

Patient Preparation

1. Explain test purpose. A 12-hour fast is required, but water may be taken. Alcohol should not be consumed for at least 24 hours before the test.
2. If possible, all medication should be withheld for at least 24 hours before testing. Check with physician.
3. Encourage relaxation.
4. See Chapter 1 guidelines for safe, effective, informed *pretest* care.

Patient Aftercare

1. Interpret test results and counsel appropriately (see Cholesterol Patient Aftercare).
2. Low HDL levels can be raised by diet management, exercise, weight loss, and by smoking cessation. Many resources are available through the American Heart Association and other organizations.
3. Drug therapy may be necessary if other methods fail to raise HDL levels.
5. Follow Chapter 1 guidelines for safe, effective, informed *posttest* care.

Clinical Alert

Cholesterol and HDL-C levels should not be done immediately after myocardial infarction. A 3-month wait is suggested.

Clinical Alert

The cholesterol/HDL ratio gives more information than does either value alone. The higher the cholesterol/HDL ratio, the greater risk for developing atherosclerosis. This ratio should be reported with total cholesterol values.

Cholesterol/HDL-C Ratio	Total Cholesterol-HDL-C	
Risk Level for CHD	*Men*	*Women*
Low	3.43	3.27
Average	4.97	4.44
Moderate	9.55	7.05
High	23.99	11.04

VERY LOW-DENSITY LIPOPROTEINS (VLDL) **AND LOW-DENSITY LIPOPROTEINS** (LDL)

Desirable Values—LDL

Adults

< 130 mg/dl, or < 3.4 mmol/L: desirable LDL-cholesterol

140–159 mg/dl, or 3.4–4.1 mmol/L: borderline high-risk cholesterol
> 160 mg/dl, or > 4.1 mmol/L: high-risk LDL-cholesterol

Children and adolescents
< 110 mg/dl, or < 2.8 mmol/L: Desirable
110–129 mg/dl, or 2.8–3.4 mmol/L: Borderline high-risk
> 130 mg/dl, or > 3.4 mmol/L: High-risk

Background

Most serum cholesterol is present in the LDL. The LDLs are the cholesterol-rich remnants of the VLDL lipid transport vehicle. Because LDL has a longer half-life (3–4 days) then its precursor, VLDL, LDL is more prevalent in the blood. It is mainly catabolized in the liver and, possibly, also in nonhepatic cells. The very low-density lipoproteins (VLDL) are major carriers of triglycerides. Degradation of VLDL is a major source of LDL. Circulating fatty acids form triglycerides in the liver, and these are packaged with apoprotein and cholesterol to be exported into the blood as VLDLs. Therefore, LDH is the test of choice because of its longer half-life and because VLDLs are extremely hard to measure.

Explanation of Test

This test is specifically done to determine coronary heart disease risk. The LDLs are closely associated with increased incidence of atherosclerosis and CHD.

Procedure

LDL cholesterol levels are calculated by using the Friedwald formula:

$$\text{LDL cholesterol} = \text{total cholesterol} - \text{HDL cholesterol} - (\text{triglyceride}/5)$$

1. The formula is valid only if the triglyceride level is less than 400 mg/dl.
2. Lipoprotein analysis measures fasting levels of total cholesterol, total triglycerides, and HDL-cholesterol. The LDL-cholesterol is calculated from these values.

Clinical Implications

1. *Increased LDL levels* are caused by familial type II hyperlipidemia and familial hypercholesterolemia.
2. Secondary causes include
   - **a.** High-cholesterol and saturated fat diet
   - **b.** Hyperlipidemia secondary to hypothyroidism
   - **c.** Nephrotic syndrome
   - **d.** Multiple myeloma and other dysglobulinemias
   - **e.** Hepatic obstruction or disease
   - **f.** Anorexia nervosa
   - **g.** Diabetes mellitus
   - **h.** Chronic renal failure
   - **i.** Porphyria
   - **j.** Premature coronary heart disease
3. *Decreased LDL levels* occur with

a. Hypolipoproteinemia
b. Tangier disease
c. Type I hyperlipidemia
d. Apo-C-II deficiency
e. Hyperthyroidism
f. Chronic anemias
g. Severe hepatocellular disease
h. Reye's syndrome
i. Acute stress (burns, illness)
j. Inflammatory joint disease
k. Chronic pulmonary disease

Interfering Factors

1. *Increased LDLs* are associated with pregnancy, and certain drugs, such as estrogens, progestins, birth control pills, and androgens.
2. Disregard for pretest fasting.

Patient Preparation

Same as for HDL patient preparation.

Patient Aftercare

1. Interpret test results and counsel appropriately.
2. If patient has high LDH levels, repeat the test between 2 and 8 weeks later and average the values to establish an accurate baseline from which to devise a treatment plan.
3. The National Cholesterol Education Program offers excellent resource materials.

	Initiation Level	*Minimal Goal*
DIETARY TREATMENT		
Without CHD or two other risk factors*	>160 mg/dl	<160 mg/dl
With CHD or two other risk factors*	>130 mg/dl	<130 mg/dl
DRUG TREATMENT		
Without CHD or two other risk factors*	>190 mg/dl	<160 mg/dl
With CHD or two other risk factors*	>160 mg/dl	<130 mg/dl

NOTE: *Patients need a lower initiation level and goal if they are at high risk because of existing CHD or any two of the following risk factors: male sex, family history of premature CHD, smoking, hypertension, low HDL-cholesterol, diabetes mellitus, cerebrovascular or peripheral vascular disease, or severe obesity.*

4. A comprehensive history and physical, together with analysis of test results, determines whether high LDL-cholesterol is secondary to another disease or drug, or is of a familial lipid disorder. The patient's total coronary risk profile, clinical status, age, and sex are considered when prescribing a cholesterol-lowering treatment program.

Clinical Alert

Another method for assessing CAD/CHD risk is by calculating the LDH/HDL ratio (LDL − HDL-C).

LDL CHOL/HDL-C Ratio

Risk Level	*Men*	*Women*
Low	1.00	1.47
Average	3.55	3.22
Moderate	6.25	5.03
High	7.99	6.14

APOLIPOPROTEIN A AND B, APO A, APO B

Normal Values

	Male	*Female*
Apo A-I	96—166 mg/dl	106—179 mg/dl
Apo B	44—125 mg/dl	40—119 mg/dl
Apo A-I/Apo B (ratio)	> 1.32	

Background

Hypolipoproteins/apolipoproteins are surface proteins of lipoprotein particles and are important in the study of atherosclerosis. Apolipoprotein A is the main component of HDLs, chylomicrons, and VLDLs. Apolipoprotein B is the main component of LDL.

Explanation of Test

This test is used to diagnose coronary artery disease (CAD). Apo A_1 deficiencies are often associated with premature cardiovascular disease. Apo B plays an important role in LDL catabolism. The ratio of Apo A to Apo B correlates more closely with increased risk of CAD than cholesterol levels or LDL/HDL ratio.

Procedure

Obtain a 5-ml venous blood sample. Do not freeze. Observe universal precautions.

Clinical Implications

1. *Increased Apo-A-I* is associated with familial (inherited) hyperalphalipoproteinemia.
2. *Decreased Apo-A-I* is found with

a. β-Lipoproteinemia
b. Apo C-II deficiency
c. Apo A-I Melano disease
d. Apo A-I–C-III deficiency
e. Hypertriglyceremia
f. Poorly controlled diabetes
g. Premature coronary heart disease
h. Hepatocellular disease
i. Nephrotic syndrome and renal failure

3. *Increased Apo-B* is found with
   a. Hyperlipoproteinemia types IIa, IIb, and V
   b. Premature CHD
   c. Diabetes mellitus
   d. Hypothyroidism
   e. Nephrotic syndrome, renal failure
   f. Hepatic disease and obstruction
   g. Dysglobulinemia
   h. Porphyria
   i. Cushing's syndrome
   j. Wisnor's syndrome
4. *Decreased Apo-B* occurs with
   a. Tangier disease
   b. Hypo-β-lipoproteinemia
   c. Type I hyperlipidemia
   d. Apo C-II deficiency
   e. Hypothyroidism
   f. Malnutrition/malabsorption
   g. Chronic anemias
   h. Reye's syndrome
   i. Acute stress (burns, illness)
   j. Inflammatory joint disease

Interfering Factors

1. *Decreased Apo-A-I* is associated with diet high in polyunsaturated fats, smoking, and androgen or oral contraceptive use.
2. *Decreased Apo-B* is associated with diets high in polyunsaturated fats.
3. *Increased apolipoproteins* can be caused by various drugs.

Patient Preparation

1. Explain test purpose and procedure. A 12-hour fast is required, but water may be taken. Smoking is prohibited.
2. Encourage relaxation.
3. See Chapter 1 guidelines for safe, effective, informed *pretest* care.

Patient Aftercare

1. Resume normal activities.
2. Interpret test results and counsel appropriately concerning CAD risk and potential lifestyle changes.
3. Follow Chapter 1 guidelines for safe, effective, informed *posttest* care.

TRIGLYCERIDES ●

Normal Values

Age (yr)	*Male (mg/dl)*	*Female (mg/dl)*
0–9	30–100	35–110
9–14	32–125	37–131

Age (yr)	*Male (mg/dl)*	*Female (mg/dl)*
14–20	37–148	39–124
>20	40–160	35–135

Values are age and diet related.

Background

Triglycerides account for more than 90% of dietary intake and comprise 95% of fat stored in tissues. Because they are insoluble in water, they are the main plasma glycerol ester. Normally stored in adipose tissue as glycerol, fatty acids, and monoglycerides, the liver reconverts these metabolites to triglycerides.

Explanation of Test

This test evaluates suspected atherosclerosis and measures the body's ability to metabolize fat. Elevated triglycerides, together with elevated cholesterol, are atherosclerotic disease risk factors. Because cholesterol and triglycerides can vary independently of each other, measurement of both values is more meaningful.

Procedure

Obtain a fasting (at least 5-ml) venous blood sample. Observe universal precautions.

Clinical Implications

1. *Increased triglycerides* occur with
   - **a.** Types I, IIb, III, IV, and β-hyperlipoproteinemias
   - **b.** Liver disease and alcoholism
   - **c.** Nephrotic syndrome and renal disease
   - **d.** Hypothyroidism
   - **e.** Poorly controlled diabetes mellitus
   - **f.** Pancreatitis
   - **g.** Glycogen storage disease (von Gierke's disease)
   - **h.** Myocardial infarction (elevated levels may persist for several months)
   - **i.** Gout
2. *Decreased triglyceride* levels occur with congenital α–β-lipoproteinemia, malnutrition, and hyperthyroidism.

Interfering Factors

1. A transient increase will occur following a heavy meal or alcohol ingestion.
2. Increased values are associated with pregnancy and oral contraceptive use.

Patient Preparation

1. Explain test purpose and procedure. Fasting for at least 12 hours pretest is required, but water may be taken.

2. The patient should be on a normal diet for 1 week pretest. No alcohol is permitted for at least 24 to 48 hours before testing.
3. See Chapter 1 guidelines for safe, effective, informed *pretest* care.

Patient Aftercare

1. Interpret test results and counsel appropriately. Weight reduction, low-fat diet, and an exercise program can reduce high triglyceride levels.
2. Advise that triglycerides are not a strong predictor of CHD and, as such, are not an independent risk factor if under 250 mg/dl. However, increased levels may increase cardiovascular disease risk.
3. Follow Chapter 1 guidelines for safe, effective, informed *posttest* care.

Clinical Alert

1. Panic values of > 500 mg/dl indicate hypertriglyceridemia in the presence of diagnosed pancreatitis.
2. Values of > 1000 mg/dl present a substantial risk of pancreatitis.
3. Chylomicronemia, although associated with pancreatitis, is not accompanied by increased atherogenesis. Chylomicrons are not seen in normal fasting serum, but instead, are found as exogenous triglycerides in healthy persons after a fatty meal has been eaten.

LIPOPROTEIN ELECTROPHORESIS

Normal Values

For 12- to 14-hour fasting specimen:

Chylomicrons: 0%–2%	
β or LDL: 33%–52%	Mass fraction of total lipoprotein
Pre-β or VLDL: 7%–28%	Mass fraction of total lipoprotein
α or HDL: 10%–30%	Mass fraction of total lipoprotein
Plasma appearance: Clear	

Background

Lipoproteins comprise hydrophobic lipids, bound to protein, that produce a liquid-soluble complex. Chylomicrons primarily transport dietary triglycerides from the intestines. They are proteins derived from dietary sources and, if significantly increased, can extend into the pre-β area. In hyperchylomicronemia, chylomicrons represent dietary fat in transport. The standing plasma contains a cream layer over a clear layer in type I hyperlipidemia (in which chylomicrons are elevated), but not in type IV (in which both chylomicrons and triglycerides are elevated). Very low-density lipoproteins (VLDL) transport cholesterol and triglycerides that have been synthesized in the liver. Low-density lipoproteins (LDL) are the major cholesterol-transporting lipoproteins. Atherosclerotic plaque-cholesterol is derived from LDLs, and LDL elevations are associated with an increased coronary artery disease risk. On the other hand, high-density lipoproteins (HDL) provide protection against atherosclerosis, reversing cholesterol transport mechanisms. Levels of plasma HDL cholesterol are inversely proportional to the risk of heart disease.

Explanation of Test

Lipoprotein electrophoresis evaluates hyperlipidemia and determines abnormal serum lipoprotein distribution and concentration.

Procedure

Obtain a fasting, 5-ml sample of venous blood (serum). Do not freeze. Observe universal precautions.

Clinical Implications

1. Patients may be phenotyped using Frederickson's Classification System. Triglyceride, cholesterol, and lipoprotein levels are considered in this system.

Interfering Factors

1. Lipid phenotypes are affected by stress or dietary changes.
2. Phenotyping is invalid in the presence of secondary disorders such as diabetes mellitus, renal failure, or nephritis.
3. Certain drugs may alter the electrophoretic mobility of lipoproteins.
4. Heparinized blood is not acceptable; test results are not reliable during heparin therapy.

Patient Preparation

1. Explain test purpose and blood-drawing procedure. A 12-hour fast before the blood draw is required.
2. The patient should be on a normal diet for 2 weeks pretest.
3. See Chapter 1 guidelines for safe, effective, informed *pretest* care.

Patient Aftercare

1. Interpret test results and counsel appropriately concerning dietary and drug therapy. The National Cholesterol Education Program and other organizations have many resources available. (National Cholesterol Education Program, National Institutes of Health, 9000 Rockville Pike, Bethesda, MD 20184).
2. Follow Chapter 1 guidelines for safe, effective, informed *posttest* care.

FREE FATTY ACIDS AND FATTY ACID PROFILE ●

Normal Values

Adult: 8–25 mg/dl, or 0.30–0.90 mmol/L
Child: < 31 mg/dl, or < 1.10 mmol/L

Phytanic Acid Profile
Normal: > 0.3%
Borderline: 0.3%–0.5%
Refsum's disease: > 0.5%
Linolate: > 25% of total fatty acids
Arachnidate: 0%–6%
Oleic: 26%–35%
Palmitate: 23%–25%
Linoleic: 8%–16%
Steric: 10%–14%

Background

Free fatty acids are formed by lipoprotein and triglyceride breakdown. The amount of free fatty acids and triglycerides present in blood comes from dietary sources, fat deposits, or is synthesized by the body. Carbohydrates can be converted to fatty acids and then stored in fat cells as triglycerides.

Explanation of Test

This lipid fraction measurement is helpful in determining fat and carbohydrate metabolism. Fatty acid and carbohydrate metabolism is altered in fat breakdown process (eg, when fasting). Unusually high levels will be associated with untreated diabetes. It has been shown that the response of free fatty acids to treatment occurs more rapidly than the responses associated with blood sugar, plasma carbon dioxide, or ketone levels. Disorders identified with excess fatty acids are also usually associated with high VLDL levels.

Specific fatty acid measurement can be useful for monitoring nutritional status in the presence of malabsorption, starvation, and long-term parenteral nutrition. It is also valuable for the differential diagnosis of polyneuropathy when Refsum's disease is suspected. In this disease, the enzyme that degrades phytanic acid is lacking.

Procedure

Obtain a fasting, 5-ml blood sample. The blood serum should be separated from blood cells within 45 minutes of drawing and should be placed on ice. Observe universal precautions.

Clinical Implications

1. *Increased free fatty acid values* are associated with
   a. Poorly controlled diabetes mellitus
   b. Excessive release of lipoactive hormones, such as epinephrine, norepinephrine, glucagon, thyrotropin, and adrenocorticotropin
   c. Hyperthyroidism
   d. Huntington's chorea
   e. von Gierke's disease
   f. Alcoholism
   g. Acute myocardial infarction
   h. Reye's syndrome
2. *Decreased fatty acids* are found in

a. Cystic fibrosis
b. Malabsorption
c. Zinc deficiency (linoleate and arachidonate are low)
d. Refsum's disease (phytanate low)—a level of > 0.5% indicates Refsum's; repeat the test to confirm.

Interfering Factors

1. Values are elevated by exercise, anxiety, hypothermia, and certain drugs.
2. Values are decreased by food intake, long-term IV or parenteral nutrition therapy, and certain drugs.
3. Prolonged fasting or starvation (as much as three times normal) affects levels.

Patient Preparation

1. Explain test purpose and blood-drawing procedure. Fasting required, but water may be taken.
2. Patients receiving heparin therapy should not be tested.
3. Discontinue strenuous exercise before the test. Encourage relaxation.
4. See Chapter 1 guidelines for safe, effective, informed *pretest* care.

Patient Aftercare

1. Resume normal activities.
2. Interpret test results and monitor appropriately.
3. Follow Chapter 1 guidelines for safe, effective, informed *posttest* care.

● THYROID FUNCTION TESTS

Laboratory determinations of thyroid function are useful in distinguishing patients with euthyroidism (normal thyroid gland function) from those with hyperthyroidism (increased function) or hypothyroidism (decreased function).

PATIENT CARE FOR THYROID TESTING ●

Patient Preparation

1. Explain test purpose and blood specimen collection procedure. To understand the thyroid function tests, it is necessary to know these basic concepts: The thyroid gland takes iodine from the circulating blood, combines it with the amino acid tyrosine, and converts it to the thyroid hormones thyroxine (T_4) and triiodothyronine (T_3). Iodine constitutes about two-thirds of the weight of the thyroid hormones. The thyroid gland stores T_3 and T_4 until they are released into the bloodstream under the influence of thyrotropin (thyroid-stimulating hormone; TSH) from the pituitary gland. Only a small amount of these hormones is not bound to

protein; however, it is the free portion of the thyroid hormones that is the true determinant of the thyroid status of the patient.

2. Assess for signs and symptoms of thyroid disease and note thyroid and iodine medications. Fasting is required for some tests.
3. A typical thyroid panel includes the following tests:
   - **a.** T_3 uptake (TU)
   - **b.** Free T_4
   - **c.** Total T_4
   - **d.** Total T_3
   - **e.** FTI (T_7; free thyroxine index)
   - **f.** TSH
4. The most useful laboratory tests to confirm or exclude hyperthyroidism are total thyroxine (T_4), the free thyroxine index (FTI), and total triiodothyronine (T_3). The most useful tests to detect hypothyroidism are total T_4, the free thyroxine index (FTI), and thyrotropin (thyroid-stimulating hormone; TSH). A thyrotropin-releasing hormone (TRH) stimulation test can be valuable in establishing the thyroid status in some patients with equivocal signs of thyroid dysfunction and borderline laboratory values. It should be kept in mind that values obtained for the assessment of thyroid function can be influenced by factors other than disease, such as age, current illness, binding capacity of serum proteins, and some drugs.
5. See Chapter 1 guidelines for safe, effective, informed *pretest* care.

Patient Aftercare

1. Interpret test results, counsel and monitor appropriately for abnormal thyroid function and disease. Follow-up testing may be required.
2. Thyroid antibody testing also can be done for diagnosis of autoimmune thyroid testing.
3. Follow Chapter 1 guidelines for safe, effective, informed *posttest* care.

CALCITONIN ●

Normal Values

Male: <19 pg/ml or ng/L
Female: <14 pg/ml or ng/L

Calcium infusion (2.4 mg of calcium per kilogram)
Male: <190 pg/ml or ng/L
Female: <130 pg/ml or ng/L

Pentagastrin injection (0.5 µg/kg)
Male: <110 pg/ml or ng/L
Female: <35 pg/ml or ng/L

Background

Calcitonin, a hormone secreted by the C cells (parafollicular) of the thyroid gland, inhibits bone resorption by regulating the number and activity of osteoblasts. Calcitonin is secreted in direct response to high blood calcium levels and helps prevent abrupt changes in calcium levels and the excessive loss of calcium.

Explanation of Test

Measurement of calcitonin is used preoperatively to diagnose familiar medullary thyroid carcinoma and, postoperatively, to evaluate medullary thyroid carcinoma. This test is done to measure increases in immunoreactive calcitonin after stimulation with calcium or pentagastrin. Early detection of elevated calcitonin leads to diagnosis of tumor or abnormally secreting C cells before cancer spreads.

Procedure

Obtain a fasting, 5-ml venous blood specimen. The blood should be heparinized and chilled immediately. If testing is not done at once, blood should be frozen.

Clinical Implications

1. *Increased levels of calcitonin* are associated with
   - **a.** Medullary thyroid cancers
   - **b.** C-cell hyperplasia
   - **c.** Chronic renal failure
   - **d.** Pernicious anemia
   - **e.** Zollinger–Ellison syndrome
   - **f.** Cancer of lung, breast, pancreas (some patients)
   - **g.** Carcinoid syndrome
   - **h.** Alcoholic cirrhosis
   - **i.** Patients with pancreatitis and thyroiditis
2. In a small portion of patients who do have medullary cancer, the fasting level of calcitonin is normal. In these instances, a provocative test using calcium or pentagastrin should be done.
   - **a.** Very high levels > 1000 mg/L are evidence of medullary thyroid carcinoma.
   - **b.** These stimulation tests are not needed if the basal calcitonin test is diagnostically high.
   - **c.** In patients with elevated calcitonin levels who do not have medullary thyroid carcinoma, the response is not as vigorous.

Interfering Factors

Levels are normally *increased* in pregnancy at term and in newborns.

Clinical Alert

1. Screening with the calcitonin test of families of patients with proved medullary cancer of the thyroid is recommended because the tumor has both sporadic and familial incidence.
2. If the calcitonin test is normal in family members, it is advisable to repeat the calcium provocative test periodically (over a period of months or years).
3. Some patients who have medullary thyroid carcinoma do not respond to the stimulation test.

Patient Preparation

1. Explain test purpose and procedure.
2. Fasting from food overnight is required. Water is permitted.
3. If the provocative tests are to be done, the patient must also be fasting.
   a. Blood samples are drawn before the injection for baseline value of calcitonin. A blood sample is drawn 1.5, 2, and 5 minutes after the injection.
   b. Calcium, 2.0 mg/kg, is injected after baseline is drawn. A blood sample is drawn 5 and 10 minutes after injection.
4. See Chapter 1 guidelines for safe, effective, informed *pretest* care.

Patient Aftercare

1. Interpret test outcome and monitor appropriately.
2. The patient may experience transient nausea or fatigue after injection and may experience chest pain for a short time.
3. Resume normal activities when symptoms abate.
4. Follow Chapter 1 guidelines for safe, effective, informed *posttest* care.

FREE THYROXINE T_4 (FT_4) ●

Normal Values

0.8–2.4 ng/dl or 10.3–31.0 pmol/L

For patients taking levothyroxine (Synthroid), up to 5.0 ng/dl

Background

Free thyroxine (T_4) constitutes a small fraction of the total thyroxine. The free T_4 is available to the tissues and is the metabolically active form of this hormone. This fraction (about 5% of the circulatory thyroxine T_4) exists in a free state, unbound to protein.

Explanation of Test

This test determines thyroid status, rules out hypo- and hyperthyroidism, and evaluates thyroid replacement therapy. The FT_4 has diagnostic value in situations in which total hormone levels do not correlate with the thyrometabolic state, and there is not suspected abnormality in binding protein levels. It is, however, a useful test when there are definite or probably abnormalities in binding levels; it provides a more accurate picture of the thyroid status in persons with abnormal thyroxine-binding globulin levels in pregnancy, and in those who are receiving estrogens, androgens, phenytoin, and salicylates.

Procedure

Obtain a venous blood (at least 5-ml) sample. Accurate results can be obtained in as little as 0.5 ml for pediatric cases. Serum is needed for this test. Observe universal procedures.

Clinical Implications

1. *Increased FT_4 levels* are associated with Graves' disease and thyrotoxicosis caused by overproduction of T_4.
2. *Decreased FT_4 levels* are associated with
   a. Primary hypothyroidism
   b. Secondary hypothyroidism (pituitary)
   c. Tertiary hypothyroidism (hypothalamic)
   d. Thyrotoxicosis caused by overproduction of T_3

Interfering Factors

1. Values are increased in infants at birth. This value rises even higher after 2 to 3 days of life.
2. Free T_4 levels are decreased in adolescents, compared with adults.
3. Heparin will cause falsely elevated values.
4. Levels can fluctuate in patients with severe or chronic illness.
5. Radioisotopes will interfere with the test.

Patient Preparation and Aftercare

See Patient Care for thyroid testing. The same protocols prevail.

FREE TRIIODOTHYRONINE T_3 (FT_3) ●

Normal Values

Adult: 260–480 pg/dl or 4.0–7.4 pmol/L

Explanation of Test

This is one of the determinations used to evaluate thyroid function and measure that fraction of the circulatory T_3 that exists in the free state in the blood, unbound to protein. It is done to rule out T_3 toxicosis, hypothyroidism, and hyperthyroidism; to determine thyroid status; and to evaluate thyroid replacement therapy.

Procedure

Obtain a venous blood (at least 5-ml) sample. Observe universal precautions.

Interfering Factors

Recently administered radioisotopes and high altitude affect results.

Clinical Implications

1. *Increased FT_3 values* are associated with
   a. Hyperthyroidism
   b. T_3 toxicosis
   c. Peripheral resistance syndrome

2. *Decreased FT_3 values* are associated with hypothyroidism (primary and secondary) and in the third trimester of pregnancy.

Patient Preparation and Aftercare

See Patient Care for thyroid testing. The same protocols prevail.

FREE THYROXINE INDEX (FTI) (T_7)

Normal Values

Adult: 1.5–4.5 index (These are arbitrary units.)

Explanation of Test

This index is a mathematical calculation used to correct the estimated total thyroxine (T_4) for the amount of thyroxine-binding globulin (TBG) present. To perform this calculation, two results are needed: the T_4 value and the T_3 uptake ratio. The product of these two members is the free thyroxine index (FTI). The FTI is useful in the diagnosis of hyper- and hypothyroidism, especially in patients with known or suspected abnormalities in thyroxine-binding protein levels. In such patients, blood levels and clinical signs may seem contradictory unless both T_4 and TBG are considered as interrelated parameters of thyroid status. Measurement of the free T_4 also gives a more accurate picture of the thyroid status when the TBG is abnormal in pregnant women or in those persons who are being treated with estrogen, androgens, phenytoin, or salicylates.

Procedure

A calculation is made, based on results of T_3 uptake and T_4 total.

$$FTI = T_4 \text{ total} \times T_3 \text{ uptake } (\%)/100.$$

The free thyroxine index permits meaningful interpretation by balancing out most nonthyroidal factors.

Clinical Implications

Application of the equation of the FTI includes the following:

This is a mathematical calcuation that does not involve the patient.

Status	*TBG*	*T_3 Uptake*	×	*T_4*	=	*FTI*
Euthyroid (normal thyroid function)	Normal	35%		9.0		3.1
Euthyroid	Low	52%		4.0		2.1
Euthyroid	High	13%		16.0		2.8
Hypothyroid	High	24%		4.0		0.9
Hyperthyroid	Low	46%		13.0		6.0

NEONATAL THYROTROPIN-RELEASING HORMONE (TRH) ●

Normal Values

Newborn screen: < 20 μU/ml

TRH surges at birth, peaking at 30 minutes at 25–160 μU/ml. It declines and reaches adult levels by the first week of life.

Background

Neonatal primary hypothyroidism is characterized not only by low T_4 levels in blood serum, but also by elevated thyrotropin-releasing hormone (TRH) levels (so as to differentiate from TSH test).

Explanation of Test

This measurement is used as a confirmatory test for infants with positive T_4 screens or low blood serum T_4 levels. Although TRH measurement has been suggested as the primary screening test for neonatal hypothyroidism, infants with secondary (hypothalamic or hypopituitary) hypothyroidism, which constitutes about 10% of all neonatal hypothyroid cases, would be missed in such a screening system.

Procedure

1. Cleanse the skin with an antiseptic and puncture the infant's heel with a sterile disposable lancet. Collect 3 to 7 days after birth.
2. If bleeding is slow, it helps to hold the leg dependent for a short time before spotting the blood on the filter paper.
3. The circles on the filter paper must be completely filled. This can best be done by placing one side of the filter paper against the infant's heel and watching for the blood to appear on the front side of the paper and completely fill the circle.
4. Air-dry for 1 hour, fill in all information, and send to the laboratory immediately. Do not expose to extreme heat or light.

Clinical Implications

An elevated TRP test is associated with neonatal hypothyroidism.

Patient Preparation

1. Inform the parents or mother about test purpose and method of specimen collection.
2. See Patient Care for thyroid testing.

Patient Aftercare

Be prepared to counsel parents or mother on steps to take if TRP test is abnormal.

NEONATAL THYROXINE (T_4); NEONATAL SCREEN FOR HYPOTHYROIDISM

Normal Values

1–5 days:	> 7.5 μg/dl
6–8 days:	> 6.5 μg/dl

Background

Normal brain growth and development cannot take place without adequate thyroid hormone. Congenital hypothyroidism (cretinism) is characterized by low levels of T_4 and elevated levels of TSH.

Explanation of Test

This is a screening test of thyroxine (T_4) activity to detect neonatal hypothyroidism. Specimens should be obtained after the first 24 hours of protein feeding, or within the first week. Thyroxine is obtained from whole blood spotted on paper using a radioimmune assay technique.

Procedure

1. Cleanse the skin with an antiseptic and puncture the infant's heel with a sterile disposable lancet.
2. If bleeding is slow, it helps to hold the leg dependent for a short time before spotting the blood on the filter paper.
3. The circles on the filter paper must be completely filled. This can best be done by placing one side of the filter paper against the infant's heel and watching for the blood to appear on the front side of the paper and completely fill the circle.
4. Air-dry for 1 hour, fill in all requested information, and send to the laboratory immediately. Protect from extreme heat and light.

Clinical Implications

1. Low values are associated with hypothyroidism.
2. Several nonthyroid conditions can result in depressed T_4 levels (eg, low birth weight, prematurity, twinning, fetal distress, and deficient TBG levels).

Patient Preparation and Aftercare

Refer to Neonatal TRH Testing for care. The same protocols prevail.

Clinical Alert

1. Do not interpret this test in terms of the blood serum T_4 values. This is an entirely different procedure, using a different type of specimen.
2. Notify the attending physician and the parents of positive results within 24 hours.
3. If T_4 results are abnormal, a TRP test should be done.

THYROGLOBULIN (Tg)

Normal Values

3–42 ng/ml or µg/L
Newborn at 48 hr: 36–48 ng/ml

Background

Thyroglobulin is normally present in the blood and is composed of glycoprotein and the iodinated secretions of epithelial cells of the thyroid. These iodinated secretions contain both the precursors of T_4 and T_3, and these hormones themselves.

Explanation of Test

This test is helpful in the diagnosis of hyperthyroidism and to monitor the course of differentiated or metastatic thyroid cancer. It is not useful in the diagnosis of thyroid cancer. Levels will decrease following successful initial treatment, and in recurrence of metastasis, the level will again rise. A lack of sensitivity and specificity limits the value of the test.

Procedure

Obtain a 5-ml venous blood sample.

Clinical Implications

1. *Increased thyroglobulin levels* are associated with
    - **a.** Untreated and metastatic differentiated thyroid cancers (not medullary carcinoma)
    - **b.** Hyperthyroidism (not good correlation with elevated T_4)
    - **c.** Subacute thyroiditis
    - **d.** Benign adenoma (some cases)
    - **e.** Levels rise when metastases develop after initial treatment.
2. *Decreased thyroglobulin levels* found in thyrotoxicosis factitia.

Interfering Factors

1. Newborns have very high levels that drop to adult levels by 2 years of age.
2. Autoantibodies to thyroglobulin cause decreased values. Thyroglobulin antibody test may have to be done to confirm decreased levels.

Patient Preparation

1. See Patient Care for thyroid testing on page 424.
2. Patient should be off of thyroid medication for 6 weeks before specimen collection.
3. Determination of thyroglobulin levels may be substituted for ^{131}I scans in patients with low risk for thyroid cancer.

Patient Aftercare

1. Resume thyroid medication and normal activities.
2. Monitor as appropriate for metastatic thyroid cancer.

3. The Patient Aftercare for thyroid testing on pages 424–425 is to be as followed.

THYROID-STIMULATING HORMONE (THYROTROPIN; TSH)

Normal Values

Adult: 0.2–5.4 μU/ml
Neonate: 3–20 μU/ml by day 3 of life

Background

The thyroid is unique among the endocrine glands because it has a large store of hormone and a slow rate of normal turnover. Stimulation of the thyroid gland by the TSH, which is produced by the anterior pituitary gland, will cause the release and distribution of stored thyroid hormones. Thyrotropin stimulates secretion of T_4 (thyroxine) and T_3. The TSH secretion is physiologically regulated by T_3 and T_4 (feedback inhibition) and is stimulated by TRH (thyrotropin-releasing hormone) from the hypothalamus. The TSH is the single most sensitive test for primary hypothyroidism. If there is clear evidence for hypothyroidism and the TSH is not elevated, than an implication of possible hypopituitarism exists.

Explanation of Test

This measurement is used in the diagnosis of primary hypothyroidism when there is thyroid gland failure owing to intrinsic disease, and it is used to differentiate primary from secondary hypothyroidism by determining the actual circulatory level of TSH: TSH is high in primary hypothyroidism; low TSH levels occur in hyperthyroidism. This is the single most sensitive test for primary hypothyroidism.

Procedure

Obtain a 5-ml venous sample. Observe universal precautions.

Clinical Implications

1. *Increased TSH levels* are seen in
   a. Adults and neonates with primary hypothyroidism
   b. Thyrotropin-producing tumor
   c. Thyrotoxicosis
2. *Decreased levels* are associated with
   a. Hyperthyroidism
   b. Secondary and tertiary hypothyroidism

Interfering Factors

1. Values are normally high in neonatal cord blood. There is hypersecretion of TSH in newborns, up to two to three times normal. The TSH level returns to normal by 14 days of life.

2. Values are suppressed during treatment with T_3, aspirin, corticosteroids, and heparin.
3. Values are abnormally increased during drug therapy with lithium, potassium iodide, and TSH injection.
4. Radioisotopes administered within the last week before test.

Patient Preparation

1. Explain test purpose and procedure.
2. See Chapter 1 guidelines for safe, effective, informed *pretest* care.

Patient Aftercare

1. Resume normal activities.
2. Interpret test results and counsel as appropriate for hypo- or hyperthyroidism.
3. Follow Chapter 1 guidelines for safe, effective, informed *posttest* care.

THYROTROPIN-RELEASING HORMONE (TRH) STIMULATION TEST; THYROID-STIMULATING HORMONE (THYROTROPIN; TSH) STIMULATION TEST ●

Normal Values

Thyrotropin baseline: 0.2–5.4 μIU/L 30 minutes. After stimulation, TSH should increase approximately two times baseline and is usually greater in women than in men.

Background

Thyrotropin, or thyroid-stimulating hormone (TSH), is a tripeptide secreted by the anterior lobe of the pituitary that stimulates the pituitary gland. It also releases prolactin from the pituitary.

Explanation of Test

This test assesses the responsiveness of the anterior lobe of the pituitary gland and differentiates between the three types of hypothyroidism: primary, secondary, and tertiary. When TRH is injected, a rise in TSH indicates that the pituitary gland is functioning.

Procedure

1. Obtain a baseline 5-ml, fasting blood sample.
2. A bolus of TRH is given intravenously (protirelin [Thypinone] or thyrotropin [Thytropar]).
3. Thirty minutes after injection, obtain another blood sample.
4. Both samples are tested for TSH levels.

Clinical Implications

1. The TSH level shows a very slight increase or no response in hyperthyroidism after injection.

2. In hypothyroidism, differing responses will be seen in the various types of hypothyroidism:
   a. In primary (thyroid gland failure), there is an increase of two or more times the normal response with an elevated base.
   b. In secondary (anterior pituitary failure), there is no response.
   c. In tertiary (hypothalamic failure), the TSH rises after a delay. Multiple injections of TRH may be necessary to induce the appropriate TSH response.

Patient Preparation

1. Explain test purpose and procedure.
2. The patient must fast from midnight. No water is permitted.
3. After baseline TSH is drawn, the patient receives the IV injection of Thypinone.
4. 30 minutes later, a postinjection TSH blood test is drawn.
5. See Chapter 1 guidelines for safe, effective, informed *pretest* care.

Patient Aftercare

1. Resume normal activities.
2. See Patient Care for thyroid testing.
3. Follow Chapter 1 guidelines for safe, effective, informed *posttest* care.

THYROXINE-BINDING GLOBULIN (TBG) ●

Normal Values

Male Adult:	15–30 μg/dl	
Female:	Nonpregnant,	11.5–32.2 μg/dl
	Pregnant 1st trimester,	19.8–64.7 μg/dl
	2nd trimester,	41.4–63.9 μg/dl
	3rd trimester,	31.0–73.6 μg/dl
	Oral contraceptives,	23.1–47.9 μg/dl

Background

Almost all of the thyroid hormones in the blood are protein-bound: albumin, thyroid-binding prealbumin and, most important, thyroxine-binding globulin (TBG). Variations in TBG levels have a major effect on bound and free (metabolically active) forms of T_4 and T_3.

Explanation of Test

This measurement is useful to distinguish between hyperthyroidism causing high T_4 and euthyroid individuals, with increased binding by TBG, who have increased T_4 and normal levels of free hormones; to identify hereditary deficiency or increase of TBG; or for workup of thyroid disease in hypothyroid populations, when the mean TBG concentration is significantly higher than the mean level in normal thyroid populations. In hyperthyroid populations, the mean TBG concentration level is lower than the mean level in normal thyroid populations.

Procedure

Obtain a 2-ml venous blood specimen. Observe universal precautions.

Clinical Implications

1. The TBG test is *increased* in
   a. Genetically determined high TBG
   b. Hypothyroidism (some cases)
   c. Infectious hepatitis and other liver diseases
   d. Acute intermittent porphyria
   e. Estrogen-producing tumors
2. The TBG test is *decreased* in
   a. Genetic deficiency of TBG
   b. Nephrotic syndrome
   c. Major illness or surgical stress
   d. Acromegaly
   e. Severe acidosis
   f. Testosterone-producing tumors
   g. Hepatic disease
   h. Marked hypoproteinemia, malnutrition

Interfering Factors

1. Many drugs increase (estrogens, oral contraceptives) or decrease (androgens, steroids) values.
2. Neonates have higher values.
3. Recently administered radioisotopes affect the value.

Patient Preparation and Aftercare

See Patient Care for thyroid testing on pages 424–425.

THYROXINE; TOTAL T_4 ●

Normal Values

Adult:	5.4–11.5 μg/dl, or 57–148 nmol/L
Child:	6.4–13.3 μg/dl, or 83–172 nmol/L

If testing is done by immunoassay, it is reported out as T_4 RIA.

Background

Thyroxine is the thyroid hormone with four atoms of iodine; hence, called T_4. The combination of the serum T_4 and T_3 uptake as an assessment of thyroxine-binding globulin (TBG), helps determine whether an abnormal T_4 value is due to alterations in serum thyroxine-binding globulin or to changes of thyroid hormone levels. Deviations of both tests in the same direction usually indicate that an abnormal T_4 level is due to abnormalities in thyroid hormone. Deviations of the two tests in opposite directions provide evidence that an abnormal T_4 level may relate to alterations in TBG.

Explanation of Test

Thyroxine, one of the thyroid function panel tests, is a direct measurement of the concentration of T_4 in the blood serum. The total T_4 level is a good index of thyroid function when the TBG is normal: the increase in thyroxine-binding globulin (TBG) levels normally seen in pregnancy and with estrogen therapy will increase the total T_4 levels; the decrease of TBG levels in persons receiving anabolic steroids, in chronic liver disease, and in nephroses will decrease the total T_4 value. This test is commonly done to rule out hyperthyroidism and hypothyroidism. The T_4 test also can be used as a guide in establishing maintenance doses of thyroid in the treatment of hypothyroidism. In addition, it also can be used in hyperthyroidism to follow the results of antithyroid drugs.

Procedure

Obtain a 5-ml venous blood sample. If the patient is already receiving thyroid treatment, it must be stopped 1 month before the test. Observe universal precautions.

Interfering Factors

1. Total thyroxine levels increase during the second or third month or pregnancy as a result of increased estrogen production.
2. Values also are increased with the use of drugs such as estrogens, anticonvulsants, heroin, and methadone.
3. Contrast radiopaque substance used for x-rays and other diagnostic procedures will affect results.
4. Values are decreased with salicylates and anticoagulant drugs.

Clinical Implications

1. *Increased T_4 values* are found in
   - **a.** Hyperthyroidism
   - **b.** Clinical status that increases TBG
   - **c.** Thyrotoxicosis factitia
   - **d.** Acute thyroiditis
   - **e.** Hepatitis, liver disease
   - **f.** Neonates
   - **g.** D-Thyroxine therapy
2. *Decreased T_4 values* are found in
   - **a.** Hypothyroidism
   - **b.** Disorders of decreased TBG
   - **c.** Hypoproteinemia
   - **d.** Treatment with triiodothyronine

Patient Preparation

1. Explain test purpose and procedure. T_4 is usually the first test used in the diagnosis of hypo- or hyperthyroidism.
2. Avoid strenuous exercise.
3. No radiopaque contrast administered for 1 week before testing.
4. If patient is receiving thyroid therapy, stop treatment for 1 month for baseline values.
5. See Chapter 1 guidelines for safe, effective, informed *pretest* care.

Patient Aftercare

1. Resume normal activities.
2. See Patient Care for thyroid testing.

> **Clinical Alert**
>
> T_4 values are higher in neonates owing to elevated TBG. Values rise abruptly in the first few hours after birth and decline gradually until the age of 5.

TRIIODOTHYRONINE T_3, TOTAL; RADIOIMMUNOASSAY (T_3-RIA)

Normal Values

> 24 yr: 80–200 ng/dl
15–23 yr: 100–220 ng/dl
1–14 yr: 125–250 ng/dl

If the radioimmunoassay is used, the result is reported as T_3 RIA.

Background

T_3 has three atoms of iodine, compared with four atoms in T_4. T_3 is more active metabolically than T_4, but its effect is shorter. There is much less T_3 than T_4 in the serum, and it is bound less firmly to thyroid-binding globulin.

Explanation of Test

This measurement is a quantitative determination of the total T_3 concentration in the blood and is the test of choice in the diagnosis of T_3 thyrotoxicosis. *It is not the same as the T_3-uptake test that measures the unsaturated TBC in serum.* It can also be very useful in the diagnosis of hyperthyroidism. T_3 thyrotoxicosis refers to a variant of hyperthyroidism in which a thyrotoxic patient will have elevated T_3 values and normal T_4 values. It is of limited value in diagnosing hypothyroidism.

Procedure

Obtain a venous, 5-ml blood sample. Observe universal precautions.

Clinical Implications

1. *Increased T_3 values* are associated with
   - **a.** Hyperthyroidism
   - **b.** T_3 thyrotoxicosis
   - **c.** Daily dosage of 25 μg or more of T_3
   - **d.** Acute thyroiditis
   - **e.** TBG elevation from any cause
   - **f.** Daily dosage of 300 μg or more of T_4
2. *Decreased T_3 levels* are associated with
   - **a.** Hypothyroidism (however, some clinically hypothyroid patients will have normal levels)

b. Starvation and state of nutrition, acute illness
c. TBG decrease from any cause

Interfering Factors

1. Values are increased in pregnancy and with the use of drugs such as estrogens and antiovulatory compounds, methadone, and heroin.
2. Values are decreased with the use of drugs such as anabolic steroids, androgens, large doses of salicylates, and phenytoin.
3. Fasting cause T_3 to decrease.

Clinical Alert

Panic values of < 50 ng/dl or > 300 ng/dl.

Patient Preparation and Aftercare

Care is the same as for T_4 testing on page 427.

TRIIODOTHYRONINE UPTAKE (T_3Up; T_3U)

Normal Values

0.8–1.30, which is a ratio between patient specimen and the standard control.

25%–35% uptake (These are arbitrary units.)

Explanation of Test

This test is a indirect measurement of the unsaturated thyroxine-binding globulin (UTBG) in the blood. This determination, expressed in arbitrary terms, is inversely proportional to the TBG. For this reason, low T_3Up levels are indicative of situations that result in elevated levels of UTBG. For example, in hypothyroidism, when insufficient T_4 is available to produce saturation of TBG, UTBG is elevated and the T_3Up values are low. Similarly, in pregnant patients or those receiving estrogen, TBG levels are increased proportionately more than are T_4 levels, resulting in high levels of UTBG, which are reflected in low T_3Up results. This test should not be ordered alone. It is useful only when T_4 is done. It is also used to calculate the T_7 or free thyroxine index (FTI).

Clinical Implications

1. See Explanation of Test.
2. *Decreased T_3Up levels* occur in normal pregnancy, with estrogens, antiovulatory drugs, methadone, and heparin.
3. *Increased T_3Up levels* occur with drugs such as dicumarol, heparin, androgens, anabolic steroids, phenytoin, and large doses of salicylates.

Patient Preparation and Aftercare

See Patient Care for thyroid testing on pages 424–425. Pre- and posttest care is the same as for T_4 testing on page 427.

Clinical Alert

1. This test has nothing to do with the actual T_3 blood level, in spite of its name, which is sometimes confusingly abbreviated to the T_3 test. It is emphasized that the T_3Up and the true T_3 are entirely different tests. The T_3Up gives only an indirect measurement of overall binding.
2. It should be used only in conjunction with the T_4 test to calculate the free thyroxine index (FTI).
3. Some methods of T_3Up assessment have a direct relation with T_4. Check reference values of your laboratory.

BIBLIOGRAPHY

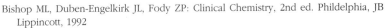

Bishop ML, Duben-Engelkirk JL, Fody ZP: Clinical Chemistry, 2nd ed. Phildelphia, JB Lippincott, 1992

Burritt ME et al: Pediatric reference intervals for 19 biologic variables in healthy children. Mayo Clinic Proceedings 65:329, 1990

Cohen MC, Muller JE: Chromobiology of acute myocardial infarction. Laboratory Medicine 25(8):494–499, August 1994

Demers LM: The influence of nonthyroidal factors on thyroid function. 24(8):495–499, August 1993

Detmer WM et al: Pocket Guide to Diagnostic Tests. A Lange Medical Book. Norwalk, CT, Appleton & Lange, 1992

Expert Panel 2nd Report: Detection, evaluation and treatment of high blood cholesterol in adults. Bethesda, MD, National Institution of Health, 1993

Fish H, Lipshultz LI: Diagnosing male factors in infertility. Archives Pathology and Laboratory Medicine 116:398–405, 1992

Garnick M: Prostate cancer: Screening, diagnosis and management. Annals of Internal Medicine 118(10):804–818, May 15, 1993

Greenspan FS (ed): Basic and Clinical Endocrinology, 3rd ed. Norwalk, CT, Appleton & Lange, 1991

Harr R: Measurement of adrenal corticosteroids by high performance liquid chromatography. Clinical Laboratory Science 7(1):50–56, Jan/Feb 1994

Katan MB, Mensim RP: Omega fatty acids and serum lipoproteins. Nutrition Reviews 50, 1992

LeGrys VA: Trends and methodology in sweat testing for cystic fibrosis. Laboratory Medicine 21(3):155–158, March 1990

Little RR, Goldstein DE: Long-term glucose monitoring with glycosylated proteins. Laboratory Medicine 23(8):533–530, August 1992

Mehta JB et al: Effects of antituberculosis therapy on angiotensin-converting enzyme levels in tuberculosis patients. Laboratory Medicine 21(4):223–228, April 1990

Mikkelson SL et al: Comparison of therapeutic drug-monitoring assays. Laboratory Medicine 24(1):729–738, November 1993

Miller S: Saliva testing—a non-traditional diagnostic tool. Clincial Laboratory Science 7(1):39–43, Jan/Feb 1994

Sowell A: Simple, rapid method for assessments of serum vitamin A concentration. Clinical Laboratory Practice 7(3), May/June 1994

Speicher CE: The Right Test: A Physician's Guide to Laboratory Medicine, 2nd ed. Philadelphia, WB Saunders 1993

Steffes MW: The clinical laboratory and diabetes mellitus in the future. Medicine 21(8):489–496, August 1990

Tietz NW: Clinical Guide to Laboratory Tests, 3rd ed. Phildelphia, WB Saunders, 1995

Wallace J: Interpretation of Diagnostic Tests: A Synopsis of Laboratory Medicine, 5th ed. Boston, Little, Brown & Co, 1992

Yoder PE, Burroughs RG, Domonice P: Lead still poisoning our children. RN 28-30, February 1993

7

Microbiologic Studies

● OVERVIEW OF MICROBIOLOGIC STUDIES

Diagnostic Testing and Microbes

Microorganisms, as referred to in diagnostic testing, are termed **pathogens.** The word **pathogenic** is usually defined as "causing infectious disease"; however, organisms that are pathogenic under one set of conditions may, under other conditions, reside within or on the surface of the body without causing disease. When these organisms are present, but do not cause harm to the host, they are considered **commensals.** But, once they begin to multiply and to cause tissue damage, they are considered pathogens, with the potential for causing or increasing a pathogenic process (Table 7-1). Many

TABLE 7-1
Pathogens Detectable in Body Tissue and Fluid by Diagnostic Methods

NASOPHARYNX
- β-Hemolytic streptococci
- *Bordetella pertussis*
- *Candida albicans*
- *Corynebacterium diphtheriae*
- *Haemophilus influenzae* (large counts)
- Meningococci
- Pneumococci (large counts)
- *Staphylococcus aureus*
- *Klebsiella* spp.
- *Capnocytophaga* spp.

URINE
- β-Hemolytic streptococci, groups B and D
- Coliform bacilli (100,000 count or more) including *Escherichia coli, Klebsiella, Enterobacter–Serratea*
- Enterococci: *Streptococcus faecalis*
- Gonococci: *Neisseria gonorrhoeae*
- *Mycobacterium tuberculosis*
- *Pseudomonas aeruginosa*
- *Staphylococcus aureus*
- *Staphylococcus saprophyticus*
- *Salmonella* and *Shigella* spp.
- *Trichomonas vaginalis*
- *Candida albicans* and other yeasts
- *Staphylococcus epidermidis*

CEREBROSPINAL FLUID
- *Bacteroides* spp.
- *Brucella abortus*
- Coliform bacilli
- *Cryptococcus neoformans*
- *Haemophilus influenzae*
- *Leptospira* spp.
- *Mycobacterium tuberculosis*
- *Neisseria meningitidis*
- Pneumococci: *Streptococcus pneumoniae*
- *Pseudomonas*
- Staphylococci
- Streptococci
- *Toxoplasma gondii*
- Viruses and fungi
- *Listeria monocytogenes*
- *Enterobacteriaceae*

BLOOD
- *Streptococcus* spp.
- *Staphylococcus aureus*
- *Listeria monocytogenes*
- *Corynebacterium* JK group
- *Haemophilus influenzae*
- *Enterobacteriaceae*
- *Salmonella typhi*
- *Pseudomonas aeruginosa*
- *Bacteroides fragilis* and anaerobic bacteria
- *Candida albicans* and other yeasts
- *Mycobacterium* spp.

SPUTUM
- *Blastomyces dermatitidis*
- *Bordetella pertussis*

(continued)

TABLE 7-1 *(Continued)*

SPUTUM

- *Candida albicans*
- *Coccidiodes immitis*
- Hemolytic streptococci
- *Histoplasma capsulatum*
- *Klebsiella* spp.
- *Mycobacterium tuberculosis*
- *Yersinia pestis*
- *Francisella tularensis*
- Pneumococci
- *Staphylococcus aureus*
- *Mycoplasma* spp.
- *Eikenella corrodens*
- *Legionella* spp.

SKIN

- *Bacteroides* spp.
- *Clostridium*
- Coliform bacilli
- Fungi
- *Proteus*
- *Pseudomonas*
- *Staphylococcus aureus*
- *Streptococcus pyogenes*

VAGINAL DISCHARGE

- β-Hemolytic streptococci
- *Candida albicans*
- Coliform bacilli
- Enterococci
- *Gardnerella vaginalis*
- *Listeria monocytogenes*
- *Mycoplasma* spp.
- *Neisseria gonorrhoeae*
- *Treponema pallidum*
- *Haemophilus ducreyi*
- *Chlamydia trachomatis*
- Herpes simplex virus
- *Trichomonas vaginalis*
- *Ureaplasma urealyticum*
- *Mobiluncus* spp. and other anaerobes

FECES

- *Candida albicans*
- *Campylobacter jejuni*
- *Clostridium botulinum*
- *Entamoeba histolytica*
- *Escherichia coli* (toxogenic strains)
- *Mycobacterium tuberculosis*
- *Pseudomonas* (large counts)
- *Salmonella*
- *Shigella*
- Staphylococci
- *Vibrio cholerae*
- *Vibrio comma*
- *Vibrio parahaemolyticus*
- *Yersina enterocolitica*
- *Clostridium difficile*

EAR

- *Aspergillus fumigatus*
- *Candida albicans* and other fungi
- Coliform bacilli
- Hemolytic streptococci
- *Proteus* sp.
- Pneumococci (*Streptococcus pneumoniae*)
- *Pseudomonas aeruginosa*
- *Staphylococcus aureus*
- *Haemophilus influenzae*
- *Moraxella catarrhalis*
- *Mycoplasma pneumoniae*
- *Peptostreptococcus* spp.
- *Bacteroides fragilis*
- *Fusobacterium nucleatum*

URETHRAL DISCHARGE

- *Chlamydia trachomatis*
- Coliform bacilli
- Cytomegalovirus
- *Haemophilus ducreyi*
- Herpes simplex virus
- *Neisseria gonorrhoeae*
- *Treponema pallidum*
- *Trichomonas vaginalis*
- *Mycoplasma* spp.

newly discovered organisms exhibit clinical relevance. Some of these organisms, formerly considered as insignificant contaminants or *commensals,* have taken on roles as causative agents for opportunistic diseases in patients with human immunodeficiency virus (HIV) infection and other immunodeficiency syndromes, as well as other diseases associated with a compromised health state. Consequently, virtually any organism recovered in pure culture from a body site must be considered a *potential pathogen.*

Basics of Infectious Disease

Infectious diseases cause pathologic conditions. Infectious processes demonstrate observable physiologic and other human responses to the invasion and multiplication of the offending microorganisms. Once an infectious disease is suspected, appropriate cultures should be done or nonculture techniques, such as serologic testing for antigens and antibodies, monoclonal antibodies, and DNA probes, should be used. Proper specimen collection and appropriate blood and skin tests are necessary to detect and diagnose the presence of the microorganism.

Opportunity for infection depends on host resistance; organism volumes; ability of the organisms to find a portal of entry; and ability to overcome host defenses, invade tissues, and produce toxins. Organisms may become seated in susceptible persons through inhalation, ingestion, direct contact, inoculation, break in natural skin or mucous membrane barriers, changes in organism volumes, alterations in normal flora balances, or changes in other host defense mechanisms.

Host Factors

The following factors influence development of an infectious disease: patient's general health, normal defense mechanisms, previous contact with the offending organism, past clinical history, and type and location of infected tissue. Mechanisms of host resistance are detailed in the following lists:

Primary Host Defenses

1. Anatomic barriers
   - **a.** Intact skin surfaces
   - **b.** Nose hairs
   - **c.** Respiratory tract cilia
   - **d.** Coughing and flow of respiratory tract fluids and mucus
   - **e.** Swallowing and GI tract peristalsis
2. Physiologic barriers
   - **a.** High or low pH and oxygen tension (prevents proliferation of organisms)
   - **b.** Chemical inhibitors to bacterial growth, such as proteases
   - **c.** Bile acids
   - **d.** Active lysozymes in saliva and tears
   - **e.** Fatty acids on skin surfaces

CHART 7-1
Reportable Diseases, Conditions, and Outbreaks*

Acquired immunodeficiency syndrome (AIDS) and symptomatic immunodeficiency virus infection
Amebiasis
Animal bites
Anthrax
Botulism
Brucellosis
Chancroid
Cholera
Diphtheria
Encephalitis
Gonococcal Infection
Haemophilus infuenzae type B invasive disease
Hepatitis, viral (A, B, C, D, and E undetermined)
Kawasaki syndrome
Legionellosis
Leprosy
Leptospirosis
Lyme disease
Malaria
Measles (rubeola)
Meningitis (viral, bacterial, parasitic, and fungal)
Meningococcal diseases
Mumps (infectious parotitis)
Mycobacteriosis other than tuberculosis and leprosy
Pertussis
Pertussis vaccine, adverse reaction
Plague
Poliomyelitis
Psittacosis
Rabies
Rocky Mountain spotted fever
Rubella (German measles) and congenital rubella syndrome
Salmonellosis
Septicemia in newborns
Shigellosis
Syphilis
Tetanus
Trichinosis
Tuberculosis
Tularemia
Typhoid fever (case of carrier, or both of *Salmonella typhi)*

*Based on 1993 data from State of Maryland Communicable Disease Regulations.

Secondary Host Defenses

1. Physiologic barriers
   a. Responses of complement, lysozymes, opsonins, and secretions
   b. Phagocytosis
   c. IgA, IgG, and IgM antibody formation
   d. Cell-mediated immune responses

Decreased Host Resistance Factors

1. Age: The very young and very old are more susceptible
2. Presence of chronic diseases such as cancer, cardiovascular diseases, or diabetes
3. Use or history of select therapeutic modalities such as radiation, chemotherapy, corticosteroids, antibiotics, or immunosuppressants
4. Toxins, including alcohol, street drugs, legitimate therapeutic drugs,

venom or toxic secretions from reptile, insect, or other nonhuman bites or punctures

5. Others, including excessive physical or emotional stress states and presence of foreign material at site

COLLECTION OF SPECIMENS

General Principles

The healthcare professional is responsible for collecting specimens for diagnostic examinations. Because procedures vary, check institutional protocols for specimen retrieval, delivery, preservation, and reporting of test results.

Precautions

Without routine precautions for collecting and handling specimens, the patient's condition may be incorrectly diagnosed, laboratory time may be wasted, effective treatment may be delayed, or pathogenic organisms may be transmitted to healthcare workers and other patients.

Sources of Specimens

Microbiologic specimens may be collected from many sources, such as blood, pus or wound exudates or drainage, urine, sputum, feces, genital discharges or secretions, cerebrospinal fluid, and eye or ear drainage. During specimen collection, these general procedures should be followed:

1. Generally, label specimens properly with the following information (institutional requirements may vary):
   - **a.** Patient's name, age, sex, address, hospital ID numbers, and physician's full name
   - **b.** Specimen source (eg, throat, conjunctiva)
   - **c.** Time of collection–time completed
   - **d.** Specific studies ordered
   - **e.** Clinical diagnosis; suspected microorganisms
   - **f.** Patient history
   - **g.** Patient's immune state
   - **h.** Previous and current infections
   - **i.** Previous or current antibiotic therapy
   - **j.** Isolation status—state type of isolation (eg, respiratory, wound)
   - **k.** Body weight and height
   - **l.** Other requested information pertinent to testing
2. Avoid contaminating the specimen. Maintain aseptic or sterile technique as required:
   - **a.** Special supplies may be required:
     - **(1)** For anaerobes, sterile syringe aspiration of pus or other body fluid
     - **(2)** Carbon dioxide–containing transport medium for select tissue specimens
   - **b.** Sterile specimen containers
   - **c.** Precautions to take during specimen collection include

(1) Care to maintain clean outside container surfaces
(2) Use of appropriate-fitting covers or plugs for specimen tubes and bottles
(3) Replacing sterile plugs and caps that have become contaminated
(4) Observing universal precautions

3. Preserving specimens: prompt delivery to the laboratory is desirable; however, many specimens may be refrigerated (not frozen) for a few hours without any adverse effects. Note the following exceptions:
  a. Urine culture samples must be *refrigerated.*
  b. Cerebrospinal fluid specimens should be transported to the lab as soon as possible. If this is problematic, the culture should be *incubated* (a suspected meningococcus will not withstand refrigeration).

4. Transporting specimens: specimen material should be quickly transported to the lab to prevent the specimen from drying out and death of the microorganisms.
  a. For anaerobic microbe cultures, no more than 10 minutes should elapse between time of collection and culture. Anaerobic specimens should be placed into a butyl rubber-stoppered gased-out glass tube.
  b. Urine specimens should be *refrigerated* until tested.
  c. Feces suspected of harboring *Salmonella* or *Shigella* organisms should be placed in a special transport medium, such as buffered glycerol–saline, if culturing of the specimens will be delayed.

5. Specimen quantity: with few exceptions, the quantity of the specimen should be as large as possible. When only a small quantity is available, swabs should be moistened with sterile saline just before collection, especially for nasopharyngeal cultures.

6. Specimen collection
  a. Whenever possible, specimens should be collected before antibiotic regimens are instituted. For example, complete all blood culture sampling before starting antibiotic therapy.
  b. Collection must be geared to the rise in symptoms such as fever. (The practitioner should be familiar with the clinical course of the suspected disease.)

DIAGNOSIS OF BACTERIAL DISEASE: GENERAL OBSERVATIONS

Bacteriologic studies try to trace the specific organism causing an infection (Table 7-2). This organism may be specific to one disease, such as *Mycobacterium tuberculosis,* for tuberculosis, or may cause a variety of infections, such as those associated with *Staphylococcus* species. Antibiotic sensitivity studies then determine the response of a specific organism to different classes and types of antibiotics. Obviously, an antibiotic that inhibits bacterial growth would be the logical choice for treating the infection.

Some questions that need to be asked when searching for bacteria as the cause of a disease process include the following: (1) Are bacteria responsi-

TABLE 7-2
Bacterial Diseases and Their Laboratory Diagnosis

Disease	*Causative Organism*	*Source of Specimen*	*Diagnostic Tests*
Anthrax	*Bacillus anthracis*	Blood, sputum, sore	Blood, sputum, skin smear and culture; specific serologic test; biopsy
Brucellosis (undulant fever)	*Brucella melitensis, B. abortus, B. suis*	Blood, bone marrow, CSF, tissue	Culture, skin test; specific serologic test
Bubonic plague	*Yersina pestis*	Buboes (enlarged and inflamed lymph nodes) blood, sputum	Skin, blood and sputum smear; culture; agglutination test
Chancre	*Haemophilus ducreyi*	Genital lesion	Lesion smear and culture; biopsy; serologic test
Cholera	*Vibrio cholerae*	Feces	Stool smear and culture; skin biopsy
Chlamydia, once considered virus because of small size	*Chlamydia psittaci* (psittocosis)	Blood, sputum, lung	Culture, smears, serologic tests (immunofluorescent and enzyme immunoassay)
Diphtheria	*Corynebacterium diphtheriae*	Nasopharynx	Nasopharyngeal smear and culture
Erysipeloid	*Erysipelothrix rhusiopathiae*	Lesion, blood	Culture
Gonorrhea	*Neisseria gonorrhoeae*	Vagina, urethra, CSF, blood joint fluid, throat	Smear, culture and fluorescent antibody test
Granuloma inguinale	*Calymmatobacterium granulomatis*	Groin lesion	Smears and culture from lesion

Leprosy (Hansen's disease)	*Mycobacterium leprae*	Skin scrapings	Skin smear, biopsy, serologic test
Lymphogranuloma venereum	*Chlamydia trachomatis*	Genital swab, conjunctiva swab	Culture and smear, immuno-fluorescent test
Listerosis	*Listeria monocytogenes*	Stool, blood, CSF amniotic fluid, placenta, vagina	Smears and culture, serologic test
Pertussis (whooping cough)	*Bordetella pertussis*	Trachea, bronchi, naospharynx	Cultures of swabs of trachea and nasopharynx and bronchi; serologic test (CRP)
Pneumonia	*Haemophilus influenzae, Klebsiella pneumoniae, Staphylococcus aureus, Streptococcus pneumoniae*	Bronchoscopy secretions, sputum, blood, lung aspirate or biopsy	Smear and culture
Strep throat, scarlet fever, impetigo	*Streptococcus pyogenes*	Throat, lesion	Culture, serology
Tetanus	*Clostridium tetani*	Wound	Wound smear and culture
Toxic shock syndrome	*Staphylococcus aureus*	Tissue	Culture
Tuberculosis	*Mycobacterium tuberculosis*	Sputum, gastric washings, urine, CSF	Smear and culture of sputum; gastric washings, urine and CSF; skin test
Tularemia	*Francisella tularensis*	Skin, lymph node, ulcer tissue biopsy, sputum, bone marrow	Foshay skin test; serologic test
Typhoid	*Salmonella typhi*	Blood (after first week of infection); feces (after second week of infection)	Culture and serologic test
Whooping cough	*Bordetella pertussis*	Nasopharyngeal swab	Culture, fluorescent antibody test

ble for this disease? (2) Is antimicrobial therapy indicated? Most bacterial-related diseases produce a febrile course. From a practical standpoint during evaluation of the febrile patient, the sooner a diagnosis can be reached and the sooner a decision can be made concerning antimicrobial therapy, the less protracted the period of recovery.

Anaerobic bacterial infections are commonly associated with localized necrotic abscesses: these may yield several different strains of bacteria. Because of this, the term *polymicrobic disease* is sometimes used to refer to anaerobic bacterial diseases. These are in sharp contrast with the "one organism–one disease" concept that characterizes other infections, such as typhoid fever, cholera, or diphtheria. Isolation and identification of the different strains of anaerobic bacteria through sensitivity studies are desirable so that appropriate therapy may be given.

SENSITIVITY (SUSCEPTIBILITY) STUDIES OF BACTERIA TO ANTIMICROBIAL AGENTS ●

A sensitivity (susceptibility) test detects the type and the amount of antibiotic or chemotherapeutic agent required to inhibit bacteria growth. Often, culture and sensitivity tests are ordered together. Sensitivity studies also may be indicated when altering an established regimen of treatment.

The most common and useful test for evaluating antibiotic sensitivity is the disk method. A basic set of antibiotic-impregnated disks on agar is inoculated with a culture derived from the specific bacteria being tested. After a suitable period of incubation, the degree of bacterial growth within the different antibiotic zones on the disks is determined by microscopic observation and measurement. Growth zone diameters, measured in millimeters, are compared against set standards to determine if the organism is truly sensitive to the antibiotic, or if it falls into the intermediate category. The drug zone showing the least amount of bacterial growth is considered to be the drug of choice during treatment.

Clinical Implications

1. The terms *sensitive* or *susceptible* imply that an infection caused by the bacterial strain tested will respond favorably in the presence of the indicated antimicrobial.
2. The terms *intermediate, partially resistant,* or *moderately susceptible* mean that the bacterial strain tested is not completely inhibited by therapeutic concentrations of a test drug.
3. *Indeterminant* means that the bacterial organism may either be susceptible or resistant to the antibiotic test sample. Usually these organisms will be susceptible to high blood levels of select antibiotics.
4. The organism is not inhibited by antibiotics.
5. Physicians tend to rely more on published reports of the antibiotic's effectiveness, rather than on the sensitivity report. Sensitivity is an *in vitro* (in glass) test, whereas the antibiotic will be working *in vivo* (in the body).

DIAGNOSIS OF MYCOBACTERIAL INFECTIONS

The genus *Mycobacterium* contains several species of bacteria pathogenic to humans (Table 7-3). For example, *Mycobacterium tuberculosis* is spread from person to person through inhalation of airborne respiratory secretions containing mycobacteria expelled during coughing, sneezing, or talking. In patients with acquired immunodeficiency syndrome (AIDS), *M avium–intracellulare* (MAI) is acquired through the gastrointestinal tract, often through ingestion of contaminated water or food.

The disease progression of mycobacteriosis, particularly in patients with AIDS, is quite rapid, measured in a time span of a few weeks. This decreased time span has led to new methods for rapidly recovering and identifying mycobacteria so that antibiotic therapy can be promptly instituted. These newer techniques involve the use of certain radiometric instruments that shorten the growth period for mycobacteria to 1 to 2 weeks. Isotopic nucleic acid probes are available for culture identification of *M. tuberculosis, M. avium–intracellulare* (MAI complex), *M. kansasii,* and *M. gordonae.* Polymerase chain reaction (PCR), using DNA technology to directly detect mycobacteria in clinical specimens is also available to clinical laboratories.

Collection of Specimens

1. Sputum and bronchial aspirates and lavages produce the best samples for diagnosis of pulmonary infection. Purulent sputum (5 to 10 ml) from the

TABLE 7-3
Mycobacterial Infections and Their Laboratory Diagnosis

Causative Organism	*Source of Specimen*	*Diagnostic Tests*
Mycobacterium tuberculosis	Sputum, urine, CSF, tissue, bone marrow	Culture and smear; skin test
M. avium–intracellulare	Sputum, stool, CSF, tissue, blood, semen, lymph nodes	Culture and smear
M. kansasii	Skin, joint, lymph nodes, sputum, tissue	Culture and smear
M. leprae	Cerebrospinal fluid, skin, bone marrow, lymph nodes	Histopathologic examination of lesion
M. marinum	Joint lesion	Culture and smear
M. xenopi	Sputum	Culture and smear
M. fortuitum	Surgical wound, bone, joint, tissue, sputum	Culture and smear
M. chelonei	Surgical wound, sputum, tissue	Culture and smear

first productive cough of the morning should be expectorated into a sterile container. If the specimen is not processed immediately, it should be refrigerated. Pooled specimens collected over several hours are not acceptable. For best results, three to five specimens should be collected over several days.

2. If the patient is unable to produce sputum, an early-morning gastric sample may need to be aspirated and cultured. This specimen must be hand-delivered to the laboratory to be processed or neutralized immediately.
3. Suspected renal disease patients should provide early-morning urine specimens collected for 3 to 5 days in a row. Pooled 24-hour urine collections are not recommended. Unless processed immediately, the specimen should be refrigerated.
4. If tuberculosis meningitis is suspected, at least 10 ml of cerebrospinal fluid (CSF) should be obtained.
5. Sterile body fluids, tissue biopsies, and aspirated material from skin lesions are acceptable specimens for mycobacterial cultures. The least desirable specimen is one obtained on a swab.
6. Feces are commonly the first specimen to be positive for *M. avium–intracellulare*. An acid-fast stain is usually performed on the local smear. Culture is performed only if the smear tests positive.

DIAGNOSIS OF RICKETTSIAL DISEASE: GENERAL OBSERVATIONS

Rickettsiae are small, gram-negative coccobacilli that structurally resemble bacteria but are one-tenth to one-half as large. Polychromatic stains (Giemsa stain) are better than simple stains or the Gram stain for demonstrating rickettsiae in cells.

Rickettsiosis is the general name given to any disease caused by rickettsiae (Table 7-4). These organisms are considered to be *obligate intracellular parasites;* that is, they cannot exist anywhere except inside the bodies of living organisms. Diseases caused by rickettsiae are transmitted by *arthropod vectors,* such as lice, fleas, ticks, or mites (Table 7-5). Generally rickettsial diseases are divided into the following groups:

1. Typhuslike fevers
2. Spotted fever
3. Scrub typhus
4. Q fever
5. Other miscellaneous groups

Q fever, caused by *Coxiella burnetii,* is characterized by an acute febrile illness, severe headache, rigors, and possibly pneumonia or hepatitis. It may cause encephalitis in children and has been isolated in breast milk and the placentas of infected mothers, making it possible for a fetus to be infected in utero. Both complement fixation and fluorescent antibody tests can detect antibodies to the organism. *Coxiella burnetii* displays an antigenic variation during an infection. Phase I antibodies are preponderant during the chronic phase, whereas phase II antibodies are preponderant during the acute

TABLE 7-4
Rickettsial Diseases and Their Laboratory Diagnosis

Disease		**Geographic Distribution**	*Natural Cycle*		**Transmission to Humans**	**Serologic Diagnosis**
Group and Type	*Agent*		*Antropod*	*Mammal*		
Typhus epidemic	*Rickettsia prowazekii*	Worldwide	Body louse	Human	Infected louse feces into broken skin	Positive group- and type-specific agglutination IgG antibody
Brill's disease	*R. prowazekii*	N. America, Europe	*			
Endemic	*R. typhi*	Worldwide	Flea	Rodents	As above	Specific immunofluorescent pattern
Spotted fever; Rocky Mountain spotted fever	*R. rickettsii*	Western Hemisphere	Ticks	Wild rodents, dogs	Tick bite	Immunofluorescent latex agglutination
North Asian tick-borne rickettsiosis	*R. sibirica*	Siberia, Mongolia	Ticks	Wild rodents	Tick bite	Complement fixation
Boutonneuse fever	*R. conorii*	Africa, Europe, Mideast, India	Ticks	Wild rodents, dogs	Tick bite	Positive group- and type-specific

(continued)

TABLE 7-4 *(Continued)*

Disease		Geographic Distribution	Natural Cycle		Transmission to Humans	Serologic Diagnosis
Group and Type	*Agent*		*Antropod*	*Mammal*		
Queensland tick typhus	*R. australis*	Australia	Ticks	Marsupials, wild rodents	Tick bite	Complement fixation
Rickettsial pox	*R. akari*	N. America, Europe	Blood-sucking mite	House mouse, other rodents	Mite bite	Microimmunofluorescence
Scrub typhus	*R. tsutsugamushi*	Asia, Australia, Pacific Islands	Tromiculid mite	Wild rodents	Mite bite	Specific complement fixation positive in about 50% pts and indirect immunofluorescence
Q fever	*Coxiella burnetti*	Worldwide	Ticks	Small mammals, cattle, sheep, and goats	Inhalation of dried, infected material, milk, products of conception	Positive for complement fixation phase I and II
Trench fever	*Rochalimaea quintana*	Europe, Africa, N. America	Body louse	Human	Infected louse feces into broken skin	Specific complement fixation reaction
Oroya fever	*Bartonella bacilliformis*	Peru, Ecuador, Columbia, Brazil	Sand fly	Human	Bite of sand fly	Specific complement fixation reaction

*Recurrence years after original attack of epidemic typhus.

TABLE 7-5
Modes of Transmission of the Major Rickettsial Diseases

Disease in Man	Etiologic Agent	Chain of Transmission
Epidemic typhus	*R. prowazekii*	Man → louse → man → louse
Endemic typhus	*R. typhi*	Rat → rat flea → rat → rat flea → rat → man
Rocky Mountain spotted fever (boutonneuse fever, other spotted fevers)	*R. rickettsii*	Tick → tick → tick → tick → dog → man Tick → man
Scrub typhus (tsutsugamushi fever)	*R. tsutsugamushi*	Mite → field mouse → mite → field mouse → man
Rickettsialpox	*R. akari*	Mite → house mouse → mite → house mouse→ man
Q fever	*Coxiella burnetii*	Tick → small mammal → tick → cattle .→ (airborne) → man

phase. A diagnosis is made when a phase I titer in a convalescent serum specimen is four times greater than that in an acute serum specimen.

Signs and Symptoms

1. Fever
2. Skin rashes
3. Parasitism of blood vessels
4. Prostration
5. Stupor and coma
6. Headache
7. Ringing in the ears
8. Dizziness

> **NOTE:** *Rickettsial diseases are often characterized by an incubation period of 10 to 14 days, followed by an abrupt onset of the preceding signs and symptoms. This follows a history of arthropod bites. Cultures of rickettsia are performed only in reference laboratories. Rickettsial infections are usually diagnosed by serologic methods, by using acute and convalescent serum specimens. A fourfold rise in serum antibody titer is preferable, but a single titer of greater than 1:64 is highly suggestive of infection (see Chap. 8).*

DIAGNOSIS OF PARASITIC DISEASE: GENERAL OBSERVATIONS

Many parasitic infections are either asymptomatic or produce only mild symptoms. Routine blood and stool examinations will uncover many unsuspected infections (Table 7-6).

Approximately 70 species of animal parasites commonly infect the human

TABLE 7-6
Parasitic Diseases and Their Laboratory Diagnosis

Disease	*Causative Organism*	*Source of Specimen*	*Diagnostic Tests*
1. Amebiasis	1. *Entamoeba histolytica*	1. Stool	1. Stool smear, rectal biopsy and serologic test
2. Ascariasis	2. *Ascaris lumbricoides*	2. Stool, sputum	2. Stool and sputum smear; serologic test
3. Cestodiasis of intestine (tapeworm disease)	3. *Taenia saginata* *T. solium* *Diphyllobothrium* *Hymenolepis nana* *H. diminuta*	3. Stool	3. Stool smear and Scotch tape test
4. Chagas disease	4. *Trypanosoma cruzi*	4. Blood, spinal fluid	4. Blood and spinal fluid smear; animal inoculation
5. Cryptosporidiosis	5. *Cryptosporidium parvum*	5. Stool, lung, gallbladder	5. Stool, lung and gallbladder smear
6. Cysticercosis	6. *Taenia solium* larvae	6. Muscle and brain	6. Muscle and brain cyst biopsy
7. Echinococcosis	7. *Echinococcus granulosus*	7. Sputum and urine	7. Sputum and urine smear; serologic test; Casoni skin test; liver and bone biopsy
8. Enterobiasis (pinworm disease)	8. *Enterobius vermicularis*	8. Stool	8. Scotch tape smear
9. Filariasis	9. *Wucheria bancrofti* *Brugia malayi* *Loaloa*	9. Blood	9. Blood smear; lymph node biopsy; serologic test

10. Giardiasis	10. *Giardia lamblia*	10. Stool, duodenal aspirate or biopsy	10. Stool smear; Enterotest, immunologic test
11. Hookworm disease	11. *Ancylostoma duodenale* *Necator americanus*	11. Stool	11. Stool smear
12. Isospora	12. *Isospora belli*	12. Stool	12. Stool smear
13. Kala-azar	13. *Leishmania donovani*	13. Liver, bone marrow, blood	13. Liver, bone marrow and blood smear and culture; lymph node and spleen biopsy
14. Malaria	14. *Plasmodium falciparum* *Plasmodium malariae* *Plasmodium vivax* *Plasmodium ovale*	14. Blood, bone marrow	14. Blood and bone marrow smear, serologic test
15. Acanthamoebiasis	15. *Acanthomoeba culbertsoni*	15. CSF, corneal biopsy or scraping	15. Smear and tissue culture
16. Naegleriosis	16. *Naegleria fowleri*	16. CSF	16. Smear
17. Sarcocystosis	17. *Sarcocystis hominis* or *S. suishiominis*	17. Stool	17. Smear
18. Blastocytosis	18. *Blastocystis hominis*	18. Stool	18. Smear
19. Pneumocystosis	19. *Pneumocystis carinii*	19. Lung biopsy, bronchoalveolar lavage	19. Smear; serologic test
20. Onchocerciasis	20. *Onchocerca volvulus*	20. Skin	20. Skin biopsy
21. Paragonimiasis	21. *Paragonimus westermani*	21. Sputum, stool	21. Sputum and stool smear; serologic test; skin test

(continued)

TABLE 7-6 *(Continued)*

Disease	*Causative Organism*	*Source of Specimen*	*Diagnotic Tests*
22. Scabies	22. *Sarcoptes scabiei*	22. Skin	22. Skin smear, serologic test, skin test
23. Schistosomiasis of intestine and bladder	23. *Schistosoma mansoni* *S. japonicum* *S. haemotobium*	23. Stool, urine	23. Urine and stool smear; serologic test; skin test; rectal, bladder, and liver biopsy
24. Strongyloidiasis	24. *Strongyloides stercoralis*	24. Stool, duodenal aspirate	24. Stool and gastric smear; serologic test
25. Toxoplasmosis	25. *Toxoplasma gondii*	25. Blood, tissue	25. Serologic test; skin test; tissue smear
26. Trichinosis	26. *Trichinella spiralis*	26. Muscle	26. Serologic test; skin test, muscle biopsy
27. Trichomoniasis	27. *Trichomonas vaginalis*	27. Vagina, bladder, urethra	27. Vaginal and urethral smear and culture
28. Trichuriasis	28. *Trichuris trichiura*	28. Stool	28. Stool smear
29. Trypanosomiasis	29. *Trypanosoma rhodesiense, T. gambiense*	29. Blood, spinal fluid, lymph node	29. Blood, spinal fluid and lymph node smear; serologic test
30. Visceral larva migrans	30. *Toxocara canis, T. cati*	30. Liver	30. Serologic test; skin test; liver biopsy
31. Trematodes	31. *Fasciola hepatica* *Clonorchis sinensis* *Fasciolopsis buskii*	31. Stool	31. Stool smear

body. More than half of these can be detected by examining stool specimens because the parasites inhabit the GI tract and its environs. Of the parasites that can be diagnosed by stool examinations, approximately one-third are single-celled protozoa and two-thirds are multicellular worms. Only six or seven types of intestinal protozoa are clinically important, but almost all of the worm classes are potentially pathogenic.

Diagnosis for parasites begins with ova and parasite examination. Other diagnostic options include sigmoidoscopy smears, biopsies, barium radiologic studies, and serologic tests. For ova and parasite examination, ideally, one specimen should be collected every other day for a total of three specimens. At the most, these specimens should be gathered within 10 days.

For detection of *Giardia,* other diagnostic tests, such as the Entero-test capsule (string test) and duodenal aspiration or biopsy may be necessary.

Cryptosporidium parvum has long been recognized as an animal parasite but is also capable of infecting humans, especially physically compromised patients. Organisms have been recovered from the gallbladder, the lungs, and the stool.

Another protozoan infecting humans is *Pneumocystis carinii.* This organism causes pneumonia in the physically compromised patient, especially in the presence of HIV infection. An open-lung biopsy or a specimen from bronchoalveolar lavage presents the specimens of choice. For extraintestinal diagnosis of amebiasis, tests include hepatic scans, ultrasound studies, and needle aspiration.

Collection of Specimens

1. Generally, it is not possible to accurately identify a parasite from a single specimen.
2. Most parasites found in humans are identified in blood or feces but may also be evident in urine, sputum, tissue fluids, or biopsy tissues.

Clinical Alert

The number of worms harbored is the most important factor in the diagnosis of parasitic worms.

Clinical Considerations

1. General
   a. *Eosinophilia* is considered a definite indicator for parasitic infection. Protozoa also may produce associated eosinophilia.
   b. Protozoa and helminths, particularly larvae, may be found in organs, tissues, and blood.
2. Specimen-related
   a. *Hepatic puncture* can reveal visceral leishmaniasis. Liver biopsy may yield toxocara larvae and schistosomal worms and eggs.

b. *Bone marrow* may be positive for trypanosomiasis and malaria when blood samples produce negative results. Bone marrow specimens are obtained through puncture of the sternum, iliac crest, vertebral processes, trochanter, or tibia.

c. Puncture or biopsy samples from a *lymph node* may be examined for the presence of trypanosomiasis, leishmaniasis, toxoplasmosis, and filariasis.

d. *Mucous membrane* lesion or *skin samples* may be obtained through scraping, needle aspiration, or biopsy.

e. *Cerebrospinal fluid* may contain trypanosomes and toxoplasma.

f. *Sputum* may reveal *Paragonimus westermani* (lung fluke) eggs. Occasionally, the larvae and hookworm of *Strongyloides stercoralis* and *Ascaris lumbricoides* may be expectorated during pulmonary migration. In pulmonary *echinococcosis* (hydatid disease), hydatid cyst contents may be found in sputum.

DIAGNOSIS OF FUNGAL DISEASE: GENERAL OBSERVATIONS

Fungal diseases, also known as mycoses, are believed to be more common now than in the past because of increased antibacterial and immunosuppressive drug use (Table 7-7). Fungi prefer the debilitated host, the individual with impaired immunity or presence of chronic disease, or one who has been receiving prolonged antibiotic therapy.

Of more than 50,000 species of fungi, approximately 50 of these species are generally recognized as being pathogenic for humans. Fungi live in soil enriched by decaying nitrogenous matter and are capable of maintaining a separate existence through a parasitic cycle in humans or animals. The systemic mycoses are not communicable in the usual sense of human-to-human or animal-to-animal transfer. Humans become accidental hosts through inhalation of spores, or by spore introduction into tissues through trauma. Altered susceptibility may result in fungal lesions, as in patients having a debilitating disease, diabetes, or impaired immunologic responses from steroid or antimetabolite therapy. Prolonged administration of antibiotics can result in a fungal superinfection.

Fungal diseases can be classified according to the type of tissues involved.

1. *Dermatophytoses* include superficial and cutaneous mycoses, such as athlete's foot, ringworm, and "jock itch." Species of *Microsporum, Epidermophyton,* and *Trichophyton* are the causative organisms of the dermatophytoses.
2. *Subcutaneous mycoses* involve the subcutaneous tissues and muscles.
3. *Systemic mycoses* involve the deep tissues and organs and are the most serious of all three groups.

TABLE 7-7
Fungal Diseases and Their Laboratory Diagnosis

Disease	*Causative Organism*	*Source of Specimen*	*Diagnostic Tests*
Actinomycosis	*Actinomyces israelii*	Skin, subcutaneous tissue, sputum	Skin, subcutaneous tissue, sputum culture, smear*
Aspergillosis	*Aspergillus fumigatus* *A. flavus* *A. niger* *A. terreus*	Sputum, tissue, ear	Culture, smear, serologic test
Blastomycosis	*Blastomyces dermatidis*	Skin, sputum, bone, joint	Skin and sputum smear and culture; serologic skin†
Candidiasis	*Candida albicans*	Mucous membrane, sputum	Mucous membrane and sputum‡
Coccidioidomycosis	*Coccidioides immitis*	Sputum, bone, skin, joint	Smear culture, serologic§
Cryptococcosis	*Cryptococcus neoformans*	CSF, sputum, urine	Serology, culture, smear
Histoplasmosis	*Histoplasma capsulatum*	Sputum, urine, blood, bone marrow	Smear, culture, test, skin test and biopsy
Mucormycosis	Members of order *Mucorales* (*Absidia, Rhizopus, Mucor*)	Nose, pharynx, stool, CSF, sputum	Nose, pharynx, stool and CSF sputum culture
Nocardiosis	*Nocardia asteroides* *N. brasiliensis*	Sputum, spinal fluid	Sputum, spinal fluid culture, smear; biopsy

(continued)

TABLE 7-7 *(Continued)*

Disease	Causative Organism	Source of Specimen	Diagnostic Tests
Paracoccidioidomycosis	*P. brasiliensis*	Lung tissue, sputum	Culture, serology
Sporotrichosis	*Sporothrix schenckii*	Skin	Skin culture, biopsy; serologic test
Tinea pedis (athlete's foot)	*Epidermophyton* spp. and *Candida albicans* *Trichophyton mentagrophytes* *T. rubrum*	Skin	Hair, skin, nail scrapings for culture
Tinea capitis (ringworm of scalp)	*Microsporum* (any species) and *Trichophyton* (all except *T. concentricum*)	Skin	Hair/skin scrapings for culture As above
Tinea barbae (ringworm of beard, barber's itch)	*Trichophyton* and *Microsporum* spp.	Skin	As above
Tinea cruris (jock itch)	*Epidermophyton* spp. and *Candida albicans*	Skin	As above
Tinea corporis (ringworm of the body)	*Trichophyton rubrum, T. ton surans*	Skin	Skin scrapings for culture

*Skin, subcutaneous tissue, and sputum culture and smear; biopsy
†Skin and sputum smear and culture; serologic test; skin test
‡Mucous membrane and sputum smear and culture
§Smear, culture, serologic test, skin test, biopsy

Collection of Hair and Skin Specimens

1. Cleanse the suspected area with 70% alcohol to remove bacteria.
2. Scrape the peripheral erythematous margin of "ringworm" lesions with a sterile scalpel or wooden spatula and place the scrapings in a covered sterile container.
3. Clip samples of the infected scalp or beard hair and place in a covered sterile container.
4. Pluck hair stubs out with a tweezer because the fungus is usually found at the base of the hair shaft. The use of a Wood's light in a darkened room will help identify the infected hairs.
5. Samples from infected nails should be procured from beneath the nail plate to obtain softened material from the nail bed. If unable to do so, collect shavings from the deeper portions of the nail and place in a covered sterile container.

Common Diagnostic Methods

1. Direct microscopic examination of tissue samples placed on a slide to determine whether a fungus is actually present.
2. Use of a Wood's light to determine presence of a fungus. A Wood's light is a lamp using 3660 Angstrom units of ultraviolet rays. When used in a darkened room, infected hairs fluoresce a bright yellow-green.
3. The potassium hydroxide (KOH) test to determine the presence of mycelial fragments, arthrospores, spherules, or budding yeast cells involves mixing the specimen with KOH on a glass slide, covering the slide, and exposing it to gentle heat. The slide is then microscopically examined for fungal elements.
4. Cultures are done to identify the specific type of fungus. Fungi are slow-growing and subject to overgrowth by contaminating and more rapidly growing organisms. Fungemia (fungus in the blood) is an opportunistic infection, and often a blood culture reveals the earliest suggestion of the causative organism. The use of the DuPont Isolator System, a lysis-centrifugation system, not only shortens the time necessary for detection, but also improves the rate of detection.
5. A fluorescent brightener, Calcofluor white, fluoresces when exposed to ultraviolet light. This reagent stains the fungi, causing them to exhibit a fluorescence that can be microscopically detected. It can be used on tissue and has the same sensitivity as potassium hydroxide. Moreover, it allows for easier and faster detection of fungal elements. Calcofluor white-stained specimens can also be examined under bright-field or phase-contrast microscopy.
6. For fungal serology tests, single titers of > 1:32 usually indicate the presence of disease. A fourfold or greater rise in titer of samples drawn 3 weeks apart is significant. However, serologic diagnosis for *Candida* and *Aspergillus* species can be disappointing. The latex serology test for *cryptococcal* antigen detects 95% of *cryptococcal meningitis* cases. Complement fixation tests for *histoplasmosis* and *coccidioidomycosis* can

aid diagnosis of these diseases. The immunodiffusion test is helpful for diagnosis of *blastomycosis*.

Types of Specimens

1. Skin
2. Nails
3. Hair
4. Ulcer scrapings
5. Pus
6. Cerebrospinal fluid
7. Urine
8. Blood
9. Bone marrow
10. Stool
11. Bronchial washings
12. Tissue biopsies
13. Prostatic secretions
14. Sputum

DIAGNOSIS OF SPIROCHETAL DISEASE: GENERAL OBSERVATIONS

Spirochetes present as spiral and curved bacteria. The four genera of spiral and curved bacteria—*Borrelia, Treponema, Leptospira,* and *Spirillum* (Table 7-8)—include several human pathogens.

Clinical Considerations

BORRELIA

1. Borrelia appear in the blood at the onset of various forms of relapsing fever. Louse-borne relapsing fever is caused by *B. recurrentis,* tick-borne relapsing fever by several other *Borrelia* species, and Lyme disease by *B. burgdorferi.*
2. *Treponema (Borrelia) vincentii* is the species responsible for ulcerative gingivitis (trench mouth).

TREPONEMA

1. *Treponema pallidum* is the species responsible for venereal syphilis in humans.
2. *Treponema pallidum* subsp. *pertenue* is the causative agent of yaws.
3. *Treponema carateum* causes pinta (carate).
4. *Treponema pallidum* subsp. *endemicum* is the cause of endemic non-venereal syphilis or bejel.

LEPTOSPIRA

1. *Leptospira* is the genus of microorganism responsible for Weil's disease (infectious jaundice), swamp fever, swineherd's disease, and canicola fever.
2. The organism is widely distributed in the infected person and appears in the blood early in the disease process.
3. After 10 to 14 days the organisms appear in considerable numbers in the urine.
4. Patients with Weil's disease show striking antibody responses; serologic testing is useful for diagnosis of this disease.

TABLE 7-8
Spirochetal Diseases and Their Laboratory Diagnosis

Disease	*Causative Organism*	*Source of Specimen*	*Diagnostic Tests*
Pinta	*Treponema carateum*	Skin	Skin smear, serologic test
Rat-bite fever	*Spirillum minor, Streptobacillus moniliformis*	Blood, joint fluid, abscess	Skin, blood, joint fluid
Relapsing fever	*Borrelia recurrentis*	Blood	Blood smear
Syphilis	*Treponema pallidum*	Skin	Skin smear, TPI and FTA-Ab test
Weil's disease (leptospiral jaundice)	*Leptospira ictero haemorrhagiae*	Urine, blood, CSF	Urine, blood and CSF smear
Yaws	*Treponema pertenue*	Skin	Culture, serologic test
Lyme disease	*Borrelia burgdorferi*	Skin	Skin, smear and serologic test
Nonveneral syphilis	*Treponema endemicum*	Skin, blood	Serologic test, characteristic erythema, chronicum migrans lesion

SPIRILLUM

Streptobacillus moniliformis as well as *Spirillum minor* are the species responsible for rat-bite fever. Although this condition occurs worldwide and is common in Japan and Asia, it is uncommon in North and South America and most European countries. Cases in the United States have been tied to bites by laboratory rats.

DIAGNOSIS OF VIRAL AND MYCOPLASMAL DISEASE: GENERAL OBSERVATIONS

Viral diseases are the most common of all human infections. Once thought to be confined to the childhood years, viral infections in adults have increasingly been recognized and implicated as the cause for many cases of morbidity and death. Viruses can be responsible for such infectious diseases as hepatitis, AIDS, and other sexually transmitted diseases; they are being considered as possible etiologic agents in cancer. They also affect immunosuppressed patients and the elderly.

Viruses are submicroscopic, filterable, infectious organisms that exist as intracellular parasites. They are divided into two groups according to the type of nucleic acid they contain: ribonucleic acid (RNA) or deoxyribonucleic acid (DNA). The *mycoplasmas* are scotobacteria without cell walls and are surrounded by a single triple-layered membrane. They are also known as *pleuropneumonia-like* organisms (PPLO).

Viruses and mycoplasmas are infectious agents small enough to pass through bacteria-retaining filters. Although small size is the only property they have in common, viruses and mycoplasmas cause illnesses that are often indistinguishable from each other as they relate to clinical signs and symptoms; both frequently occur together as a double infection. Thus, the serologic (antigen–antibody) procedures commonly used for diagnosing viral disease are also used for diagnosing mycoplasmal infections (Table 7-9).

Physiologically, mycoplasmas are generally considered as an intermediate-stage disease between bacteria and rickettsiae. One species, *Mycoplasma pneumoniae,* is recognized as the causative agent of primary atypical pneumonia and bronchitis. Other species are suspected as possible causal agents for urethritis, infertility, early-term spontaneous abortion, rheumatoid arthritis, myringitis, and erythema multiforme.

Approach to Diagnosis

1. Isolation of the virus in tissue culture remains the "gold standard" for detecting many common viruses. Diagnostic modalities include the following:
   - **a.** Tissue culture
   - **b.** Use of special culture media
   - **c.** Typing, such as for herpes simplex
   - **d.** Use of identification reagents, immunofluorescence and immunoperoxidase, latex agglutination, or enzyme-linked immunosorbent assay (ELISA)
   - **e.** Visualization through an electron microscope
   - **f.** Direct nucleic acid probe and polymerase chain reaction (PCR)-DNA technology
2. Serologic studies for antigen–antibody detection.
3. Available cell cultures vary greatly in their sensitivity to different viruses. It must be understood that one cell type or species may be more sensitive than another for detecting the virus in low titers. For example, primary human or monkey kidney (1 MK) can be used for adenovirus, enterovirus, herpes simplex, measles, influenza and parainfluenza, and rubella; however, human embryonic kidney (HEK) cannot be used for cytomegalovirus or myxovirus.
4. The critical first step in successful viral diagnosis is the timely and proper collection of specimens. The choice of which specimen to collect depends on typical signs and symptoms and the suspected virus. Improper

TABLE 7-9
Virus Study Procedures

Disease or Syndrome	*Clinical Specimens*	*Suspected Viral Agents*
Nervous system Aseptic meningitis Encephalitis Poliomyelitis	Stool Throat swab CSF (Acute and convalescent sera)	Enteroviruses (Coxsackie, echo, polio) Mumps Cytomegalovirus
Respiratory/upper respiratory infections Croup Bronchiolitis Influenza Viral pneumonia Infectious mononucleosis	Throat washing or swab, stool Nasopharyngeal swab (Acute and convalescent sera) Serology Serology	Adenovirus, rhinovirus, enterovirus, respiratory, syncytial, influenza A Parainfluenza 1–3 Adenovirus, influenza, rhinovirus, respiratory syncytial, coxsackievirus, coronavirus Epstein–Barr
Exanthema and rashes Chickenpox Zoster (shingles) Herpes simplex Herpangina Measles Rubella	Vesicle swab Throat swab Stool Urine (Acute and convalescent sera)	Varicella zoster Herpes simplex Coxsackievirus A Measles Rubella
Perinatal infections Cytomegalic inclusion disease Rubella syndrome Herpes simplex	Urine Throat swab CSF (Acute and convalescent sera)	Cytomegalovirus Rubella Herpes simplex
Gastrointestinal diarrhea	Stool (for ELISA or EM) 10–20 g as soon after onset as possible	Rotavirus, Enterovirus, Adenovirus, Norwalk agent
Myocarditis, pericarditis Pleurodynia Epidemic myalgia Myopericarditis Lymphadenopathy	Stool Throat swab Pericardial or pleural fluid (Acute and convalescent sera)	Coxsackievirus B and A Echovirus Other etiology
Eye infections	Conjunctival swab or scraping	Herpes simplex, varicella zoster, adenovirus
Hepatitis	Serology	B, A, and non-A, non-B(C)

specimen choice and collection is one of the biggest factors in diagnostic delays.

Specimen Collection

1. Collect specimens for viruses as early as possible during the course of the illness, preferably within the first 4 days after symptom onset. If specimen collection is delayed for 7 or more days after symptoms appear, diagnosis will be compromised.

2. Sampling procedure

a. For localized infection:

(1) Direct sampling of affected site (eg, throat swab or skin scraping).

(2) Indirect sampling. For example, if cerebrospinal fluid (CSF) is the target sample in a central nervous system (CNS) infection, the indirect approach would involve obtaining throat swabs or stool specimens for culture.

(3) Sampling from more than one site (eg, in disseminated disease or nonspecific clinical findings).

(4) The type of applicators used to obtain specimens may affect accurate results. Do not use wooden applicators or cotton swabs because they are toxic to viruses.

(5) When transporting specimens:

(a) Keep in mind that viral specimens are unstable and rapidly lose infectivity outside of living cells. Prompt delivery to the laboratory is essential. Samples must be refrigerated or placed on ice or cold packs in transit.

(b) Freezing and thawing of specimens diminishes the quantity of available viable virus.

Clinical Considerations

1. Herpes simplex virus is the most frequently isolated virus diagnosed in the laboratory.

2. Acute viral titers are the most common serologic tests requested.

3. Viral culture results are normally available within 3 to 5 days, although rapid test results (24 hours) are accurate and available for certain viruses, such as cytomegalovirus (CMV).

4. Significance of viral cultures

a. Positive viral culture results from the following sources are diagnostically accurate:

(1) Autopsy specimens

(2) Blood

(3) Biopsy

(4) Cerebrospinal fluid (CSF)

(5) Other body fluids

(6) Cervix

(7) Eye

(8) Skin lesions

b. *Probably diagnostically accurate* (diagnostic if confirmed by serology):

(1) Throat

(2) Urine

c. *Possibly diagnostically accurate:* Stool
d. Viruses do not compromise normal bacterial flora in the body. However, bacterial or fungal contamination of specimens can occur.

DIAGNOSIS OF SEXUALLY TRANSMITTED DISEASES: GENERAL OBSERVATIONS

Sexually transmitted diseases present a serious increasing public health problem. They are caused by a variety of etiologic agents (Table 7-10). Some conditions, such as chlamydia and nongonococcal urethritis (NGU), have reached epidemic proportions. Although NGU is a nonreportable disease in the United States, it is estimated that more than 2 million new cases occur each year. Manifestations of these infections range from being an asymptomatic carrier, to diseases with obvious symptoms, such as cervicitis, conjunctivitis, endometritis, epididymitis, infertility, pharyngitis, proctitis, lymphogranuloma venereum, salpingitis, trachoma, urethritis and, in the neonate, conjunctivitis and pneumonia. The causative agent of *lymphogranuloma venereum* (LGV) is *Chlamydia trachomatis.* The primary lesion associated with LGV appears as a small, painless vesicle. Other signs and symptoms include manifestations of pelvic inflammatory disease, inguinal lymphadenopathy, fever, chills, and malaise. Occasionally, a genitoanorectal syndrome that exhibits signs of a bloody, mucopurulent rectal discharge, occurs within this disease. Diagnosis is usually made by isolating the causative organism; complement fixation (CF) and macroimmunofluorescence tests also can be helpful.

Suggested Specimens

1. Urine
2. Semen
3. Urethral, vaginal, cervical or oral swabs
4. Prostatic secretion
5. Tissue biopsy
6. Blood
7. Stool

Common Diagnostic Methods

1. Viral isolation in tissue cell cultures
2. Specific serologic antibody assays and syphilis detection tests
3. Cytologic techniques, such as Papanicolaou (PAP) and Tzanck smears to demonstrate giant cells associated with herpes virus infection.
4. Gram stain
5. ELISA and immunoperoxidase assay to detect causative agent
6. Fluorescein or enzyme-tagged monoclonal antibodies to detect and identify etiologic agents.

Clinical Considerations

1. Patients presenting with one sexually transmitted disease are frequently infected with other types of sexually transmitted pathogens.

TABLE 7-10
Sexually Transmitted Diseases and Their Laboratory Diagnoses

*Disease**	*Causative Agents†*	*Diagnosis*
Chancroid	*Haemophilus*	Culture of lesion or aspirate. Differential diagnosis should include syphilis, herpes, and LAV monoclonal antibody test, DNA probes.
Gonorrhea	*Neisseria gonorrhoeae*	Gram stain of male urethra, culture of male urethra or female cervix, rectum, or pharynx. When indicated, urogenital swab tested for direct antigen.
Granuloma inguinale (donovanosis)	*Calymmatobacterium granulomatis* (formerly *Donovania granulomatis*)	Wright's Giemsa stain of lesion, tissue biopsy.
Hepatitis B	Hepatitis B virus (HBV)	Serologic testing HB, AG—most infectious state of disease. HB,AG: presence and persistence of infectivity and chronicity usually appear before symptoms.
Genital herpes	Herpes simplex virus (HSV) types 1 and 2	Culture from unroofed blister, scrapings examined by fluorescent microscopy or cytologic stains
Lymphogranuloma venereum (LGV)	*Chlamydia trachomatis* serotypes L_1, L_2, and L_3	Culture of aspirate of bubo, serologic tests of blood (immunofluorescence and enzyme immunoassay).
Molluscum contagiosum	Molluscum contagiosum virus	Clinical appearance of lesions (pearly white, painless, umbilicated papules), microscopic exam of scrapings.

Chlamydia	*Chlamydia trachomatis* serotypes D–K	Cell culture, urogenital swabs for direct antigen test, or fluorescent microscopy.
Candidosis (monilia)	*Candida albicans*	Culture, KOH wet mount, Gram stain.
Pelvic inflammatory disease (PID)	*Neisseria gonorrhoeae, Chlamydia trachomatis*	Clinical symptoms, cervical culture, laparoscopy or culdocentesis.
Pediculosis pubis	*Phthirus pubis* (pubic or crab louse)	Adult lice or nits appear on body hairs.
Scabies	*Sarcoptes scabiei*	Characteristic lesions, scrapings for microscopy.
Syphilis	*Treponema pallidum*	Darkfield microscopic exam of primary and secondary lesions for *T. pallidum*. Nontreponemal reagin tests (VDRL, RPR) and specific tests (FTA–ABS, MHA–TP) are used to identify active and latent syphilis.
Trichomoniasis	*Trichomonas vaginalis*	Vaginal, urethral, prostatic secretion examined microscopically in a drop of saline for motile trichomonas; culture; speculum exam reveals foamy, greenish discharge and presence of bright red dots in vaginal wall and cervix.
Nonspecific urethritis (non gonococcal urethritis—NGU)	*Chlamydia trachomatis* (50% of cases), *Ureaplasma urealyticum,* a human T-strain mycoplasma (*Mycoplasma hominis*), *Trichomonas vaginalis, Candida , albicans* herpes simplex virus	Failure to demonstrate *N. gonorrhoeae* in cell culture; culture of genital specimen, tissue, urine.
Nonspecific vaginitis	*Gardnerella vaginalis* *Mobiluncus cortisii* *M. mulieris*	Wet mount for "clue" cells or PAP smear; fishy smell is released when specimen fluid is mixed with 10% KOH. Culture or enzyme immunoassay to RD gonorrhea.

(continued)

TABLE 7-10 *(Continued)*

Disease*	***Causative Agents***[†]	***Diagnosis***
Condylomata acuminata (venereal warts)	Human papilloma DNA virus	Typical clinical lesion; cauliflower-like, soft, pink growths around vulva, anus, labia, vagina, glans penis, urethra and perineum; rule out syphilis.
Acquired immunodeficiency syndrome (AIDS)	HIV virus	Serology
Gastrointestinal (giardiasis) amebiasis, shigellosis, campylobacteriosis, and anorectal infections	Enteric infections:	Stool-polyvinyl alcohol fixative or formalin ethyl acetate sedimentation (FES); same as above.
	Giardia lamblia, Entamoeba histolytica, Cryptosporidum spp.	Stool stain
	Shigella spp.,	Rectal stool swab culture
	Campylobacter fetus,	Rectal stool swab culture
	Strongyloids spp. (worms)	Stool (FES)
	Anorectal:	
	Neisseria gonorrhoeae	Anal canal swab specimen, culture
	Chlamydia trachomatis	Anal swab or rectal biopsy culture
	Treponema pallidum	Dark-field microscopy plus serology, lesion swab, culture
	Herpes simplex virus	Signs and symptoms, tissue culture
	Human papillomavirus	Signs and symptoms, tissue culture

*The major diseases are syphilis and gonorrhea.

†The pathogens causing sexually transmitted diseases span the full range of medical microbiology. The only common characteristic of these pathogens is that they may cause genital disease or may be transmitted by genital contact.

2. Asymptomatic carriers are more common than generally realized.
3. Tracing sexual partners is a very important part of diagnosis and treatment.
4. The disease may recur because the patient becomes reinfected by the nontreated sexual partner.

● DIAGNOSTIC PROCEDURES

Six different categories of laboratory tests are used for the diagnosis of infectious diseases. These include smears and stains, cultures, animal inoculation, tissue biopsy, serologic testing, and skin testing. Cultures and skin testing are described in detail in this chapter. Serologic testing is described in Chapter 8. A brief description of each of these procedures follows.

The Smear

A smear specimen for microscopic study is prepared by spreading a small quantity of the specimen material across a glass slide. If the material is also to be stained, it is generally fixed to the slide by quickly passing the slide through the flame of a Bunsen burner. Smears also can be fixed in a methanol solution.

The Stain

Smears are most often observed after they have been stained. Stains are salts composed of a positive and negative ion, one of which is colored. Structures present in the specimen pick up the stains, and make the organism visible under the light microscope. One staining procedure, called the *negative stain,* colors the background but leaves the organisms themselves uncolored. The gross structure of the organisms can then be studied.

TYPES OF STAINS

Bacterial stains are of two major types: *simple* and *differential.* A *simple stain* consists of a coloring agent such as gentian violet, crystal violet, carbol-fuchsin, methylene blue, or safranine. A thin smear of sampled organisms is stained and then observed under an oil-immersion lens. A *differential stain* is one in which two chemically different stains are applied to the same smear. Organisms that are physiologically different will pick up different stains.

The *Gram stain* is the most important of all bacteriologic differential stains. It divides bacteria into two physiologic groups: gram-positive and gram-negative. The staining procedure consists of four major steps: (1) staining the smear with gentian or crystal violet; (2) washing off the violet stain and flooding the smear with an iodine solution; (3) washing off the iodine solution and flooding the smear with 95% alcohol; and (4) counterstaining the smear with safranine, a red dye.

In addition to permitting morphologic study of the bacteria under question, the Gram stain, as mentioned before, divides all bacteria into two physiologic groups according to their ability or inability to pick up one or both of the two stains. The two categories of bacteria (gram-positive and gram-negative) exhibit different properties, which helps to identify and differentiate them.

Stains other than the Gram stain are used for examining bacteriologic smears. Some, such as the *acid-fast stain,* can identify organisms of the genus *Mycobacterium.* Other stains differentiate certain structures, such as capsules, endospores, and flagella.

Cultures

Preparing a culture involves growth of microorganisms or living tissue cells on a special medium that will support the growth of a given material. Cultures may be maintained in test tubes, petri dishes, dilution bottles, or other suitable containers. The container holds a food (called the *culture medium*) that is either solid, semisolid, or liquid. Each organism has its own special requirements for growth (proper combination of nutritive ingredients, temperature, and presence or absence of oxygen). The culture is prepared in accordance with its food needs. Later, it is either refrigerated or incubated, according to the temperature requirements for supporting growth.

Animal Inoculation

Animal inoculation is used to isolate bacteria when other means have failed. For example, when tuberculosis is suspected, but smears fail to confirm the disease, guinea pig inoculation is used. The organisms responsible for plague (*Yersinia pestis*) and tularemia (*Francisella tularensis*) may be isolated by animal inoculation. When viruses, certain spirochetes, certain fungi, and some parasites must be identified, animal inoculation is often used.

Tissue Biopsy

At times, microorganisms are isolated from small quantities of body tissue that have been surgically removed. Such tissue is removed using full aseptic technique and is transferred to a sterile container to be rapidly transported to the laboratory for analysis. Generally, the specimens are finely ground in a sterile homogenizer and then plated out.

Serologic Testing

Serologic testing is a method for analyzing blood specimens for antigen–antibody reactions. This form of testing is diagnostically valuable later in the disease course. Specimens should be collected at onset of the disease and again in 3 to 4 weeks.

Skin Testing

Skin testing determines hypersensitivity to the toxic products formed in the body by pathogens. Three types of skin tests are generally performed: scratch tests, patch tests, and intradermal tests.

BLOOD CULTURES

Normal Value

Negative for pathogens.

Explanation of Test

Blood for culture is probably the single most important specimen submitted to the microbiologic laboratory for examination. Blood cultures are collected whenever there is reason to suspect bacteremia or septicemia. Although mild transitory bacteremia is a frequent finding in many infectious diseases, a persistent, continuous, or recurrent bacteremia indicates a more serious condition that may require immediate treatment.

Indications for Blood Culture

1. Bacteremia
2. Septicemia
3. Unexplained postoperative shock
4. Postoperative shock following genitourinary tract manipulation or surgery
5. Unexplained fever of several days' duration
6. Chills and fever in patients with
   - **a.** Infected burns
   - **b.** Urinary tract infections
   - **c.** Rapidly progressing tissue infections
   - **d.** Postoperative wound sepsis
   - **e.** Indwelling venous or arterial catheters
7. Debilitated patients receiving
   - **a.** Antibiotics
   - **b.** Corticosteroids
   - **c.** Immunosuppressives
   - **d.** Antimetabolites
   - **e.** Parenteral hyperalimentation

NOTE

1. *During an acute febrile illness, immediately draw two separate blood samples from opposite arms and promptly begin antibiotic therapy.*
2. *For fever of unknown origin, two blood cultures can initially be drawn 45 to 60 minutes apart. If necessary, two more sets of samples can be drawn 24 to 48 hours later.*
3. *In cases of acute endocarditis, three separate samples should be drawn during the first 1 to 2 hours of evaluation. Then therapy should begin. In cases of suspected endocarditis, on the first day, obtain three samples at least 30 minutes apart. If results are negative, two more sets on subsequent days may be obtained.*

Procedure for Obtaining Blood Culture

Clinical Alert

During venipuncture, because the potential for infecting the patient is quite high, aseptic technique must be used. Keypoints are listed as follows:

1. Observe universal precautions. The proposed puncture site should be scrubbed with an antiseptic such as povidone–iodine or 70% alcohol. Allow to dry for 1 to 2 minutes.
2. The rubber stoppers of culture bottles should be cleansed with iodine and allowed to air dry. They should then be cleansed with 70% alcohol.
3. Venipuncture should be performed using a sterile syringe and needle; avoid contamination of the cleansed puncture site.
4. Approximately 10 to 20 ml of blood should be withdrawn into a 20-ml syringe or directly into the culture tubes. Because of the danger of accidental needle sticks, the practice of changing needles to transfer the specimen into blood culture bottles has been replaced by direct injection with the original phlebotomy needle.
5. If two culture bottles are to be inoculated (one anaerobic and one aerobic), the anaerobic bottle should be inoculated before the aerobic bottle.
6. Both bottles should be mixed gently. To vent the aerobic bottle, use a cotton-plugged needle especially designed for that purpose.
7. Properly label the specimens and immediately transfer them to the laboratory.

Clinical Alert

1. Handle all blood specimens according to universal precautions.
2. After disinfection, *do not palpate* the venipuncture site unless sterile gloves are worn or the finger has been disinfected. Palpation is the greatest potential cause of blood culture contamination.
3. The attending physician should be notified immediately about positive cultures so that appropriate treatment may be started.
4. Specimens can be drawn from two or three different sites to exclude a skin-contaminating organism. Taking more than three blood cultures in a 24-hour period does not produce significantly increased positive results.

Clinical Implications

1. *Negative cultures*
   If all cultures, subcultures, and Gram-stained smears are negative, the blood culture may be reported as *no growth, aerobic* or *anaerobic, after a 3-day incubation. . . . Final report: No growth after 7 to 14 days of incubation.*
2. *Positive cultures.*
   Pathogens most commonly found in blood cultures include
   - **a.** *Bacteroides* species
   - **b.** *Brucella* species
   - **c.** Coliform bacilli
   - **d.** *Pseudomonas aeruginosa*
   - **e.** *Haemophilus influenzae*
   - **f.** *Listeria monocytogenes*
   - **g.** *Streptococcus pneumoniae*
   - **h.** Enterococci
   - **i.** *Staphylococcus aureus, S. epidermidis*
   - **j.** *Streptococcus pyogenes*
   - **k.** *Salmonella* species
   - **l.** *Candida albicans*
   - **m.** *Clostridium perfringens*

Interfering Factors

1. Blood cultures are subject to contamination, especially by skin bacteria. These skin organisms should be identified if possible.
2. Nonfilterable blood contains abnormal proteins.

Special Situation

In those patients who have already received antibacterial therapy, certain enzymes may be incorporated into the growth medium to eliminate the activity of the antibacterial agent on the blood sample.

Patient Preparation

1. Explain purpose and culture procedure.
   See Chapter 1 guidelines for safe, effective, informed *pretest* care.

Patient Aftercare

1. Interpret test results, monitor for bacteremia, septicemia, and other febrile illness, and counsel appropriately.
2. Follow Chapter 1 guidelines for safe, effective, informed *posttest* care.

URINE CULTURES ●

Normal Values

Negative: fewer than 10,000 organisms per milliliter. Bacteria found are either skin contaminants or pathogens.

Clinical Alert

1. A bacterial count of fewer than 10,000/ml does not indicate infection; the findings may be due to contamination. A count of 100,000 or more bacteria per milliliter indicates infection.
2. Urine cultures showing *Escherichia coli* are significant if they show more than 100,000 organisms per milliliter.

Explanation of Test

Urine cultures are most commonly used to diagnose bacterial urinary tract infection (kidneys, ureter, bladder, and urethra). Urine is an excellent culture and growth medium for most organisms that infect the urinary tract. The combination of pyuria (pus in the urine) and significant bacteriuria strongly suggests the presence of a urinary tract infection.

Collection of Specimens for Culture: General Principles

1. Whenever possible, early-morning specimens should be obtained because bacterial counts are highest at that time.
2. A clean-voided urine specimen of at least 3 to 5 ml should be collected into a sterile container. Catheterization or suprapubic or indwelling catheter aspiration are alternative methods for procuring urine specimens.
3. Urine specimens for culture must never be retrieved from a urine collection bag that is part of an indwelling catheter drainage system.

Clinical Alert

Catheterization heightens the risk of introducing a urinary tract infection. If possible, avoid collecting urine by this method. **Do not** catheterize when only a bacteriologic specimen is needed.

4. Ideally, urine should be taken to the laboratory and examined as soon as possible. When this is not possible, the urine can be refrigerated for up to 2 hours before being cultured. If the specimen is collected for diagnosis of cytomegalovirus, it should be kept at room temperature. *If refrigerated, the cytomegalovirus will be destroyed.*
5. Two successive clean-voided or midstream urine specimens should be collected to establish that true bacteriuria is present.
6. Whenever possible, specimens should be obtained before antibiotic or antimicrobial therapy begins.
7. Professional health personnel should instruct the patient concerning proper specimen collection technique. Failure to isolate a causative organism is frequently the result of faulty cleansing or collection techniques

that can come from misinformation about the proper collection procedure.

8. Provide proper supplies and privacy for cleansing and urine collection. Instruct patients in proper cleansing techniques. The patient who is unable to comply with instructions should be assisted by healthcare personnel.
9. The urine specimen should be properly covered and labeled. Pertinent information includes
   a. Patient's identification information
   b. Physician's name
   c. Suspected clinical diagnosis
   d. Method of collection
   e. Precise time obtained
   f. Whether forced fluids or IVs have been administered
   g. Specific chemotherapeutic agents being administered

Procedure for Collection of Clean-Catch Urine Specimen or Midstream Specimen

Clinical Alert

Urine is an excellent culture medium. At room temperature it promotes growth of many organisms. Specimen collection should be as aseptic as possible. Samples should be transported to the laboratory and examined as soon as possible. The specimen must be refrigerated (2 hours maximum) if there is a delay in examination.

1. For females:
   a. Remove lower undergarments and clothing.
   b. Thoroughly wash and dry hands.
   c. Remove the cap from the sterile container and place it so that the outer surface touches whatever it is placed on.
   d. Cleanse the area around the urinary meatus from front to back with an antiseptic sponge.
   e. With one hand, spread and keep the labia apart. Hold the sterile container in the other hand, using care not to contaminate the inside surface.
   f. Void the first 25 ml into the toilet, then catch the rest of the urine directly into the sterile container without stopping the urine stream until sufficient quantity is collected. Hold the collection cup in such a way that it avoids contact with the legs, vulva, or clothing. Keep fingers away from the rim and inner surface of the container.
   g. Recap the specimen container using care not to contaminate the inside surface of the cap.
   h. Wash and dry hands thoroughly.

   i. Healthcare personnel should observe universal precautions when handling specimens.

2. For males:

   a. Thoroughly wash and dry hands. Prepare the container as cited in c for females.

   b. Completely retract the foreskin to expose the glans.

   c. Cleanse the area around the meatus with antiseptic sponges.

   d. Void the first 25 ml of urine directly into the toilet and then void a sufficient amount of urine into the sterile specimen container. Do not collect the last few drops of urine.

   e. Follow instructions g, h, i, as listed for females.

3. For infants and young children:

   a. For infants and young children, urine may be collected in a suitable plastic collection apparatus. Because the collection bag touches skin surfaces and picks up commensals, the specimen must be analyzed as soon as possible.

   b. Before applying collection bag, thoroughly cleanse and dry urethral area.

   c. Cover collection bag with a diaper or undergarment to prevent dislodging.

Clinical Implications

1. A count of 100,000 or more bacteria per milliliter indicates infection. A bacterial count of fewer than 10,000 bacteria per milliliter does not necessarily indicate infection, but possible contamination.

2. The following organisms, when present in the urine in sufficient titers, may be considered pathogenic:

   a. *Escherichia coli*

   b. Enterococci

   c. *Neisseria gonorrhoeae*

   d. *Klebsiella–Enterobacter–Serratia* species

   e. *Mycobacterium tuberculosis*

   f. *Proteus* species

   g. *Pseudomonas aeruginosa*

   h. Staphylococci: coagulase-positive and coagulase-negative

   i. Streptococci: β-hemolytic, usually group B

   j. *Trichomonas vaginalis*

   k. *Candida albicans* and other yeasts

Interfering Factors

1. Patients who are receiving forced fluids may sufficiently dilute the urine to reduce colony counts below 105/ml.

2. Bacterial contamination comes from sources such as

   a. Perineal hair

   b. Bacteria beneath the prepuce in males

   c. Bacteria from vaginal secretions, from the vulva, or from the distal urethra in females

   d. Bacteria from the hands, skin, or clothing

Patient Preparation

1. Explain the purpose and procedure of the test.
2. The cleansing procedure must be done correctly to remove contaminating organisms from the vulva, urethral meatus, and perineal area so that any bacteria found in the urine can be assumed to have come only from the bladder and urethra.
3. See Chapter 1 guidelines for safe, effective, informed pretest care.

Patient Aftercare

1. Interpret test outcomes, monitor for urinary tract infection, and counsel appropriately.
2. Follow Chapter 1 guidelines for safe, effective, informed *posttest* care.

Clinical Alert

The urine culture sample should *not* be taken from a urinal or bedpan and should *not* be brought from home. The urine needs to be collected directly into the sterile container that will be used for culture.

Special Situation

In the case of suspected urinary tuberculosis, three consecutive early-morning specimens should be collected. Special care should be taken when cleaning the external genitalia to reduce the risk of contamination with commensal acid-fast *Mycoplasma smegmatis.*

RESPIRATORY TRACT CULTURES

Normal Values

The following organisms may be present in the nasopharynx of apparently healthy individuals:

1. *Candida albicans*
2. Diphtheroid bacilli
3. *Haemophilus hemolyticus*
4. *Haemophilus influenzae*
5. *Branhamella catarrhalis*
6. *Staphylococcus aureus* (occasionally)
7. Staphylococci (coagulase-negative)
8. Streptococci (α-hemolytic)
9. Streptococci (nonhemolytic)
10. Micrococci

Explanation of Test

Four major types of cultures may be used to diagnose infectious respiratory tract diseases: (1) sputum, (2) throat swabs, (3) nasal swabs, and (4) nasopharyngeal swabs. At times, the purposes for which certain tests are ordered will overlap.

Clinical Alert

1. Twenty percent of normal adults carry *Staphylococcus aureus;* 10% are carriers of group A hemolytic streptococci.
2. A new 10-minute strep test gives results after 10 minutes, instead of 24 to 48 hours. It shows a false-negative rate of 5% to 10%, about the same as traditional methods. It permits rapid diagnosis and treatment.
3. Both throat and urine cultures are done to detect Epstein–Barr virus (EBV) and cytomegalovirus (CMV).

SPUTUM CULTURES

Normal Value

Negative for infection.

Explanation of Test

Sputum is *not* material from the postnasal region and is *not* spittle or saliva. A sputum specimen comes from deep within the bronchi. Effective coughing usually enables the patient to produce a satisfactory sputum specimen.

Indications for Collection

Sputum cultures are important for diagnosis of the following conditions:

1. Bacterial pneumonia
2. Pulmonary tuberculosis
3. Chronic bronchitis
4. Bronchiectasis
5. Suspected pulmonary mycotic infections
6. Mycoplasmal pneumonia
7. Suspected viral pneumonia

Procedure

1. Sputum must be coughed up from the bronchi.
2. Collect the specimen in a sterile container and cap the container with a sterile lid. If possible, procure an early-morning specimen.
3. Expectorated material of 1 to 3 ml is sufficient for most examinations, except tuberculosis testing.
4. Ascertain that the specimen is truly sputum and not saliva before sending it to the laboratory. Culturing saliva can result in misleading results because the actual infecting agent may not be observed.

Maintenance and Delivery of Specimen

1. Do not refrigerate specimens.
2. Deliver specimens to the laboratory promptly, so that organisms remain viable.
3. Label specimens properly. Note the suspected disease.

Patient Preparation

1. Instruct the patient that this test requires tracheobronchial sputum from deep in lungs. Instruct the patient to take two or three deep breaths, then to take another deep breath and forcefully cough with exhalation.
2. When the cough is not productive, inhalation of superheated hypertonic aerosols may assist sputum production. Document use of this modality.
3. See Chapter 1 guidelines for safe, effective, informed *pretest* care.

Patient Aftercare

1. Interpret test outcomes, counsel, and monitor for respiratory tract infections.
2. Follow Chapter 1 guidelines for safe, effective, informed *posttest* care.

Clinical Alert

A laryngeal swab may be taken from children or adults who cannot produce sputum specimens.

THROAT CULTURES (SWAB OR WASHINGS)

Normal Value

Negative: No growth.

Explanation of Test

1. Throat cultures are important for diagnosis of the following conditions:
   - **a.** Streptococcal sore throat
   - **b.** Diphtheria—throat and nasopharyngeal cultures should be obtained.
   - **c.** Thrush (candidal infection)
   - **d.** Viral infection
   - **e.** Tonsillar infection
   - **f.** Gonococcal pharyngitis
   - **g.** *Bordetella pertussis* and recovery of viruses
2. Throat cultures can establish the focus of infection in
   - **a.** Scarlet fever
   - **b.** Rheumatic fever
   - **c.** Acute hemorrhagic glomerulonephritis
3. Throat cultures can be used to detect the carrier state of individuals harboring such organisms as
   - **a.** β-Hemolytic streptococcus
   - **b.** *Neisseria meningitidis*
   - **c.** *Corynebacterium diphtheriae*
   - **d.** *Staphylococcus aureus*

Clinical Implications

Positive findings are associated with infections in the presence of

1. Group A β-hemolytic streptococci
2. *Neisseria gonorrhoeae*
3. *Corynebacterium diphtheriae*
4. *Bordella pertussis*
5. *Capnocytophaga* species

Procedure

1. Place the patient's mouth in good visual light.
2. Use a sterile throat culture kit, with a polyester-tipped applicator or swab, and a sterile container or tube of culture medium.
3. Depress the patient's tongue with a tongue blade and visualize the throat as well as possible. Rotate the swab firmly and gently over the back of the throat, around both tonsils or fossae, and on areas of inflammation, exudation, or ulceration.
   a. Avoid touching the tongue or lips with the swab.
   b. Because most patients will gag or cough, the collector should wear a face mask for protection.
4. Replace the swab into the designated receptacle so that it comes in contact with the culture medium. Immediately send the specimen to the laboratory.
5. A throat culture can be refrigerated if examination is delayed.

Procedure for Pediatric Patients

1. Seat the patient in the adult's lap.
2. Have the adult encircle the child's arms and chest to prevent the child from moving.
3. The collector should place one hand on the child's forehead to stabilize the head and to prevent movement.
4. Proceed with the technique used for collection of the throat and nose culture as cited under *Throat Culture* and *Nasal Culture*.

For throat washings, the patient should gargle with 5 to 10 ml of sterile saline solution and should then expectorate it into a sterile cup. This method provides more specimen than a throat swab and is more definitive for viral isolation.

Patient Preparation

1. Explain purpose and procedure to patient or parents.
2. See Chapter 1 guidelines for safe, effective, informed *pretest* care.

Patient Aftercare

1. Interpret test outcomes, monitor for throat infection, and counsel appropriately.
2. Follow Chapter 1 guidelines for safe, effective, informed *posttest* care.

NASAL CULTURES (SWAB) ●

Indications for Collection

1. Acute leukemia patients
2. Transplant recipients

3. Intermittent dialysis patients
4. Tracing and tracking epidemics

Procedure

Swab both external nares and the deeper, more moist recesses of the nose. Both nose and throat specimens are preferred for diagnosis of paramyxoviruses.

WOUND CULTURES ●

Normal Values

Clinical specimens taken from wounds can harbor any of the following microorganisms. Pathogenicity is dependent on the quantity of organisms present.

1. *Actinomyces* species
2. *Bacteroides* species
3. *Clostridium perfringens* and other species
4. *Escherichia coli*
5. Other gram-negative enteric bacilli
6. *Mycobacterium marinum*
7. *Nocardia* species
8. *Pseudomonas* species
9. *Staphylococcus aureus*
10. Coyneform JK bacillus
11. *Streptococcus faecalis*
12. *Streptococcus:* β-hemolytic

Explanation of Test

Material from infected wounds will reveal a variety of aerobic and anaerobic microorganisms. Because anaerobic microorganisms are the preponderant microflora in humans and are consistently present in the upper respiratory, gastrointestinal, and genitourinary tracts, they are also likely to invade other parts of the body to cause severe, and sometimes fatal, infections.

Clinical Implications

Clinically significant pathogens are likely to be present in the following specimens:

1. Pus from deep wounds or abscesses, especially if associated with a foul odor
2. Necrotic tissue or debrided material from suspected gas gangrene infection
3. Samples from infections bordering mucous membranes
4. Postoperative wound drainage
5. Ascitic fluid

Procedure for Wound Culture

1. Observe universal precautions.
2. Most wounds need some form of preparation to reduce the risk of introducing extraneous organisms into the collected specimen. In the presence of moderate to heavy pus or drainage, irrigate the wound with ster-

ile saline until all visible debris has been washed away. When culturing chronically present wounds (pressure sores), debride the wound surface of any loose necrotic, sloughed material before culturing.

3. Next, apply sterile gauze pads to absorb excess saline and to expose the culture site. Always culture highly vascular areas of granulation tissue. Wearing sterile gloves, separate margins of deep wounds with thumb and forefinger to permit insertion of the swab deep into the wound cavity. Press and rotate the swab several times over the clean wound surfaces to extract tissue fluid containing the potential pathogen. Avoid touching the swab to intact skin at the wound edges.
4. The swab should then be immediately placed into the appropriate transport container.

Procedure for Anaerobic Collection of Aspirated Material

1. The culture site should first be decontaminated with surgical soap and 70% ethyl or isopropyl alcohol.
2. Aspirate at least 1 ml of fluid using a sterile 3-ml syringe with an appropriately gauged needle. Immediately transfer the aspirate to an anaerobic transport medium.
3. Aspiration cultures are commonly done for closed wounds, such as soft-tissue abscesses, cellulitis, or infected skin flaps. On the other hand, tissue biopsies are more often performed during surgery when infected tissue is more easily accessible.

INFORMATION FOR THE MICROBIOLOGY LABORATORY

Properly label the specimen with the patient's ID information and physician's name. Include the following:

1. Date and time the specimen was collected
2. Anatomic site or specific source of the specimen
3. Type of specimen (granulation tissue, abscess fluid, postsurgical wound)
4. Examination requested
5. Patient's diagnosis
6. Current antibiotic therapy

Clinical Alert

A microscopic examination of pus and wound exudates can be very helpful in diagnosing a pathogenic organism. Consider the following:

1. Pus from streptococcal lesions is thin and serous.
2. Pus from staphylococcal infections is gelatinous.
3. Pus from *Pseudomonas aeruginosa* infections is blue-green.
4. Actinomycosis infections show "sulfur" granules.

Patient Preparation

1. Explain purpose and wound culture procedure.
2. See Chapter 1 guidelines for safe, effective, informed *pretest* care.

Patient Aftercare

1. Interpret test outcomes, monitor site of infection, and counsel appropriately.
2. Follow Chapter 1 guidelines for safe, effective, informed *posttest* care.

SKIN CULTURES ●

Normal Values

The following organisms may be present on the skin of a healthy person. When present in low numbers, some of these organisms may be considered normal commensals; at other times, when they multiply to excess these same organisms may become pathogens.

1. *Clostridium* species
2. Coliform bacilli
3. Diphtheroids
4. Enterococci
5. Mycobacteria
6. *Proteus* species
7. Staphylococci
8. Streptococci
9. Yeasts and fungi

Explanation of Test

The most common bacteria implicated in skin infections include staphylococci, streptococci (group A), and *Arcanobacterium (Corynebacterium) haemolyticum*. The common abnormal skin conditions include

1. Pyoderma
   a. Staphylococcal impetigo characterized by bullous lesions with thin, amber, varnishlike crusts
   b. Streptococcal impetigo characterized by thick crusts
2. Erysipelas
3. Folliculitis
4. Furuncles
5. Carbuncles
6. Secondary invasion of burns, scabies, and other skin lesions
7. Dermatophytes, especially athlete's foot, scalp and body ringworm, and "jock itch"

Procedure for Obtaining Vesicular Lesions or Skin Scrapings

1. Observe universal precautions.
2. Clean the affected site with sterile saline, wipe gently with alcohol, and allow it to air-dry.
3. Aspirate fluid sample from fresh, intact vesicles with a 25-gauge needle

attached to a tuberculin syringe and transfer the specimen to the transport medium by ejecting it from the syringe.

4. If fluid cannot be aspirated, open the vesicles and use a cotton-, rayon-, or Dacron-tipped applicator to swab the base of the lesion to collect infected cells. Place the swab directly into transport medium.
5. To make smears for stains, use a scalpel blade to scrape the base of the lesion, using care not to macerate the cells. Spread scraped material in a thin layer on a slide.
6. Immediately transport the specimen to the laboratory for viral cultures.

Clinical Alert

The most useful and common specimens for analysis include skin scrapings, nail scrapings, and hairs (see *Fungal Diseases*).

Clinical Implications

1. When present on the skin in significant quantities, the following organisms may be considered pathogenic and indicative of an abnormal condition:
   - **a.** *Bacteroides* species
   - **b.** *Clostridium* species
   - **c.** Coliform bacilli
   - **d.** Fungi (*Sporotrichum, Actinomyces, Nocardia, Candida albicans, Trichophyton, Microsporum, Epidermophyton*)
   - **e.** *Staphylococcus aureus* (coagulase-positive)
   - **f.** *Streptococcus pyogenes*
   - **g.** *Pseudomonas aeruginosa*
   - **h.** Varicella–zoster virus
   - **i.** Herpes simplex virus

STOOL AND ANAL CULTURES AND SMEARS

Normal Values

1. The following organisms may be present in the stool of apparently healthy people:
   - **a.** *Candida albicans*
   - **b.** Clostridia
   - **c.** Enterococci
   - **d.** *Escherichia coli*
   - **e.** *Proteus* species
   - **f.** *Pseudomonas aeruginosa*
   - **g.** *Anaerobic streptococci*
   - **h.** Staphylococci
2. Several "new" gastrointestinal pathogens include
   - **a.** *Helicobacter (Campylobacter) cinaedi* and *Helicobacter (Campylobacter) fennelliae*
   - **b.** *Aeromonas* spp.
   - **c.** *Blastocystis hominis*
   - **d.** Adenovirus

Explanation of Test

Stool cultures are commonly done to identify parasites, enteric disease organisms, and viruses in the intestinal tract. Of all specimens collected, feces are the most likely to contain the greatest number and greatest variety of organisms. For a routine stool culture, the stool is examined to detect and to rule out *Salmonella, Shigella, Campylobacter, Yersinia,* enteropathogenic *E. coli* and pure cultures of *Staphylococcus.*

A single negative stool culture should not be considered the endpoint in testing. At least three stool cultures are recommended if the patient's clinical picture suggests bacterial involvement, in spite of previous negative cultures. Moreover, once a positive diagnosis has been made, the patient's personal contact people should also be tested to prevent a potential spread of infection.

Procedure for Collection

1. Observe universal precautions.
2. Feces should be collected into a dry container or clean, dry bedpan. Do not mix stool with urine.
3. A freshly passed stool is best. The entire stool volume should be collected.
4. Only a small amount of stool is needed. A stool the size of a walnut is usually adequate; however, the entire passed stool should be sent for examination.
5. Diarrheal stool usually gives acceptable results.
6. Stool must not be retrieved from the toilet for specimen use.
7. Do not place toilet tissue with the specimen. It may contain bismuth, which interferes with laboratory tests.
8. Transfer stool specimens from bedpan to the container with tongue blades.
9. Properly label the sealed specimen container and immediately send it to the laboratory.

Procedure for Obtaining a Rectal Swab

1. Observe universal precautions.
2. Gently insert the swab into the rectum (to a depth of at least 3 cm) and rotate it to retrieve a visible amount of fecal material (Fig. 7-1).
3. Place the swab into the transport medium receptacle.
4. Properly label the specimen and send it to the laboratory as soon as possible.

Clinical Alert

Fecal specimens are far superior to rectal swab specimens. Often rectal swabs reach only the anal canal and provide material of limited diagnostic significance.

Culture Maintenance

1. Specimens processed within 1 hour of collection do not require added preservatives.

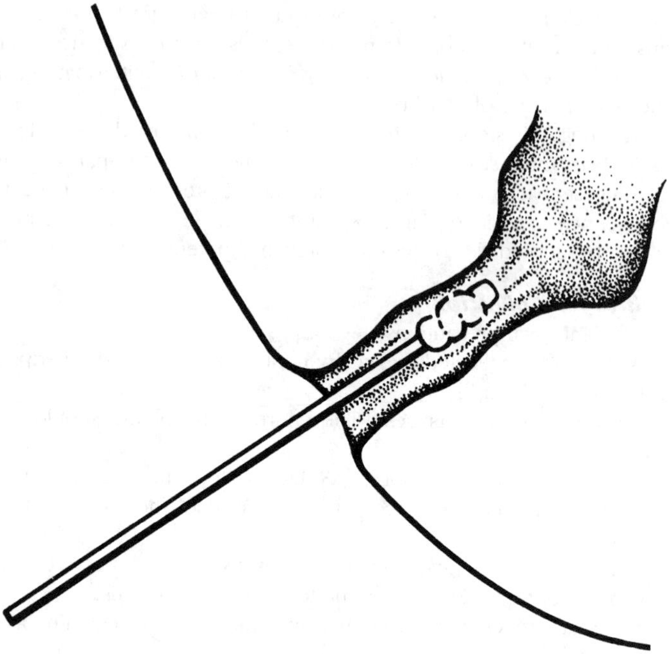

FIGURE 7-1
Method for obtaining the rectal culture.

2. If a delay longer than 2 hours is likely, the specimen should be placed into a transport medium such as Cary–Blair medium.
3. The culture medium should be immediately inoculated by the rectal swabs or otherwise placed into a suitable transport medium to prevent drying out of the specimen.

Procedure for Performing Cellophane Tape Test

1. Observe universal precautions.
2. The tape test is indicated in cases of suspected enterobiasis (pinworms).
3. Apply a strip of clear cellophane tape (not micropore or adhesive type tape) to the perineal region. Remove and spread the tape on a slide for microscopic examination.
4. A paraffin-coated swab can be used in place of the cellophane tape test. If used, place the swab within a stoppered test tube.
5. It may be necessary to repeat examinations on consecutive days.
6. Test for pinworm eggs in the morning before the patient has defecated or bathed.

7. Testing children: In about one-third of the cases involving infected children, pinworm eggs can be obtained from beneath the fingernails. Follow instructions on the testing kit.

Clinical Implications

1. *Candida albicans, Staphylococcus aureus,* and *Pseudomonas aeruginosa,* found in large numbers in the stool, are considered pathogenic in the presence of previous antibiotic therapy. Alterations of normal flora by antibiotics often change the "environment" so that normally harmless organisms become pathogens.
2. *Cryptosporidiosis* is a cause of severe, protracted diarrhea in immunosuppressed patients.
3. The organism, *Helicobacter pylori,* has been associated with gastritis and peptic ulcer disease. *Helicobaction pylori* is found only on the mucus-secreting epithelial cells of the stomach. Detection of *H. pylori* in gastric specimens necessitates collecting the specimens in sterile containers. Smears and cultures should be examined for the presence of this organism. Initial culture incubation requires 7 days. Therefore, results of gastric specimen cultures may take 8 to 10 days to obtain.
4. *Clostridium difficile:* Whenever normal flora are reduced by antibiotic therapy or other host factors, the syndrome known as "pseudomembranous colitis (PMC)" occurs. This condition is often caused by the anaerobic organism known as *C. difficile.* It may be present in small numbers in the normal person, or it may occur in the hospital environment. When normal flora are reduced, *C. difficile* can multiply and produce its toxins.

   The definitive diagnosis of *C. difficile*–associated diarrhea is based on clinical criteria. Endoscopic visualization of a characteristic pseudomembrane or plaque, together with a history of prior antibiotic therapy is diagnostic for *C. difficile.* Three laboratory tests are also available. These include stool culture for *C. difficile* (nonspecific; requires at least 48 hours for result); tissue culture for detection of cytotoxin (requires 48 hours for result); and rapid tests that include enzyme immunoassay and latex agglutination, both of which are sensitive and specific for *C. difficile.*

Interfering Factors

Feces from patients receiving barium, bismuth, oil, or antibiotics are not satisfactory specimens for identifying protozoa.

Patient Preparation for Stool Specimen Collection

1. Explain purpose and procedure. Instruct the patient to defecate into a clean, dry bedpan or large-mouthed container.
2. Do not defecate into the toilet bowl or urinate into the bedpan or collecting container because urine has an adverse effect on protozoa.

3. Do not place toilet paper into the bedpan or collection container because it may contain bismuth, which can interfere with testing.
4. See Chapter 1 guidelines for safe, effective, informed *pretest* care.

Patient Aftercare

1. Interpret test outcomes, monitor for intestinal infection, and counsel appropriately.
2. Follow Chapter 1 guidelines for safe, effective, informed *posttest* care.

Clinical Alert

1. In the institutional setting, patients with diarrhea should remain in isolation until the cause for the diarrhea is determined.
2. When pathogens are found in the diarrheic stool, the patient usually remains isolated until the stool becomes formed and antibiotic therapy is completed.

CEREBROSPINAL FLUID (CSF) CULTURES AND SMEARS

Normal Values

Flora are not normally present in cerebrospinal fluid. However, the specimen may be contaminated by normal skin flora during the process of CSF procurement.

Indications for Collection

1. Viral meningitis
2. Pyogenic meningitis
3. Tuberculosis meningitis
4. Chronic meningitis (caused by *Cryptococcus neoformans*)

Explanation of Test

Bacteriologic examination of cerebrospinal fluid (CSF) is an essential step in the diagnosis of any case of suspected meningitis. Acute bacterial meningitis is an infection of the meninges (the membrane covering the brain and spinal cord) and is a rapidly progressive, fatal disease if untreated or if treated inadequately. Death can occur within hours of symptom onset. Prompt identification of the causative agent is necessary for appropriate antibiotic therapy and aggressive treatment. Meningitis is caused by a variety of gram-positive and gram-negative microorganisms. Bacterial meningitis also can be secondary to infections in other areas of the body.

A smear and culture should be done on all CSF specimens obtained from persons with suspected meningitis, whether the CSF fluid is clear or cloudy. (Normal CSF is clear.)

In bacterial meningitis, which is caused by a variety of bacteria, the CSF shows the following characteristics:

1. Purulent (usually)
2. Increased numbers of white blood cells
3. Preponderance of polymorphonuclear cells
4. Decreased CSF glucose levels
5. Elevated CSF protein levels

In meningitis caused by the tubercle bacillus, viruses, fungi, or protozoa, the CSF shows the following characteristics:

1. Nonpurulent (usually)
2. Decreased mononuclear white cell counts; increased lymphocytes
3. Normal or decreased CSF glucose levels

In those persons with suspected meningitis, the CSF fluid is generally submitted for chemical and cytologic examinations as well as for culture.

Procedure

1. The specimen must be collected under sterile conditions, must be sealed immediately to prevent leakage or contamination, and must be sent to the laboratory without delay.

> **Clinical Alert**
>
> In cases of suspected meningitis, a culture needs to be done and a diagnosis made as quickly as possible. This is important because some causative organisms cannot tolerate temperature changes.
>
> If a viral cause is suspected, a portion of the CSF fluid should be stored at refrigerated temperatures (0–4°C). It is not recommended to freeze specimens unless inoculation into tissue culture will take longer than 5 days.

2. Label the specimen properly. Alert laboratory staff so that the specimen can be examined immediately.

> **Clinical Alert**
>
> Alert the laboratory that the CSF sample will be delivered and will need to be evaluated immediately. Time is of the essence; cells disintegrate if the sample is kept at room temperature for longer than 1 hour.

3. Notify the attending physician as soon as results are obtained so that appropriate treatment can be started in a timely fashion.

Clinical Implications

1. Pathogens found in CSF include
   a. Coliform bacilli
   b. *Cryptococcus* and other fungi
   c. *Haemophilus influenzae* (especially in infants and children)
   d. *Leptospira* species
   e. *Naegleria* or *Acanthamoeba* species
   f. Viruses (usually enteroviruses)
   g. *Angiostrongylus cantonensis*
   h. *Toxoplasma gondii*
   i. *Listeria monocytogenes*
   j. *Mycobacterium tuberculosis*
   k. *Neisseria meningitidis*
   l. Streptococcal pneumococci
   m. Staphylococci
   n. *Streptococcus agalactiae* (group B)
   o. *Treponema pallidum*
2. Positive CSF cultures occur in
   a. Meningitis
   b. Trauma
   c. Abscess of brain or ependyma of spine
   d. Septic thrombophlebitis of venous sinuses

Maintenance of Culture

1. If the CSF specimen cannot be delivered to the laboratory immediately, the container should be stored at a temperature of 37°C (98.6°F).
2. No more than 4 hours should elapse before laboratory analysis takes place because of the low survival rates of the organisms causing meningitis (especially *H. influenzae* and the meningococcus).

Patient Preparation

1. Explain purpose and lumbar puncture procedure (see Chapter 4).
2. See Chapter 1 guidelines for safe, effective, informed *pretest* care.

Patient Aftercare

1. Interpret test outcomes, monitor for meningitis, and counsel appropriately (see Chap. 4).
2. Follow Chapter 1 guidelines for safe, effective, informed *posttest* care.

CERVICAL, URETHRAL, ANAL, AND OROPHARYNGEAL CULTURES AND SMEARS FOR GONORRHEA AND OTHER SEXUALLY TRANSMITTED DISEASES ●

Normal Value

Negative cultures for sexually transmitted diseases.

Explanation of Test

These tests are done for persons with positive genital ulcers, vaginal lymphadenopathy, lesions affecting epithelial surfaces, signs and symptoms of bacterial sexually transmitted diseases (STDs), pelvic inflammatory disease, urethritis, or abnormal discharges and itching.

Procedure for Obtaining Cultures

FEMALE PATIENTS

CERVICAL CULTURE The cervix is the best site from which to obtain a culture specimen (Fig. 7-2). Observe universal precautions.

1. Moisten the vaginal speculum with warm water; do *not* use a lubricant.
2. Remove cervical mucus, preferably with a cotton ball held in a ring forceps.
3. Insert a sterile, cotton-tipped swab into the endocervical canal; move the swab from side to side; allow several seconds for absorption of organisms by the swab.

Because *Trichomonas vaginalis* may be present in urethral or vaginal discharge, material for culture should be collected as stated previously; however, the swab should be placed in a tube containing 0.5 ml of sterile saline and should be delivered to the laboratory immediately.

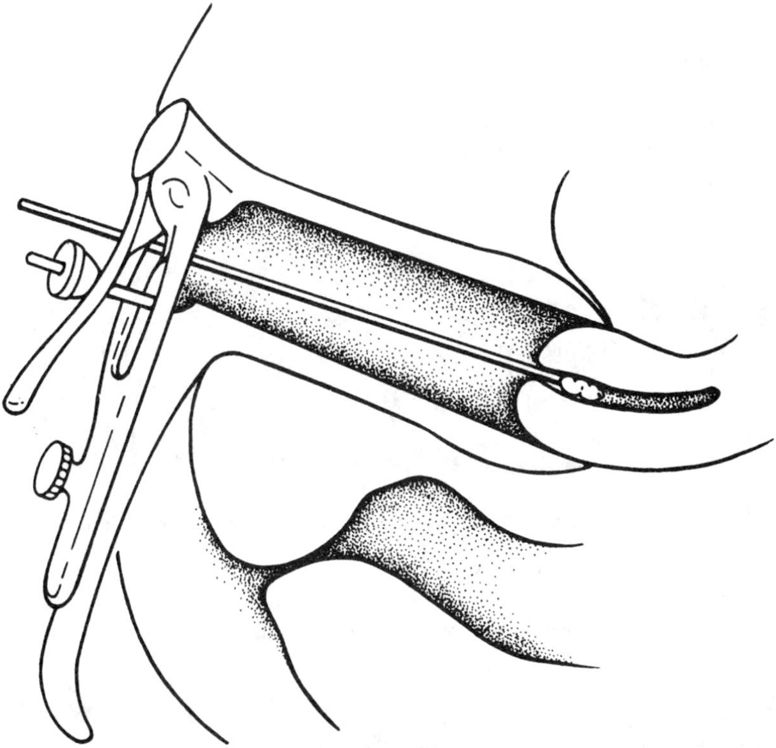

FIGURE 7-2
Method for obtaining the endocervical culture.

Swabs for culture should be transported to the laboratory in Stuart's transport medium and should be held at room temperature until processed. If specimens are not processed within several hours, they should be refrigerated. Recovery of a pathologic organism may be more difficult because of delay in processing.

ANAL CANAL CULTURE This site is most likely to be positive when a cervical culture is negative.

> **NOTE:** *The anal canal specimen can be obtained after the cervical specimen without changing the patient's position and without using the anoscope. Observe universal precautions.*

1. Insert a sterile, cotton-tipped swab approximately 1 in. into the anal canal. (If the swab is inadvertently pushed into feces, use another swab to obtain the specimen.)
2. Move the swab from side to side in the anal canal to sample the crypts; allow several seconds for absorption of organisms by the swab.

URETHRAL CULTURE (MALE PATIENTS)

1. Use a sterile swab to obtain the specimen from the anterior urethra by gently scraping the urethral mucosa (Fig. 7-3).
2. For chlamydia, the swab should be rotated 360° to dislodge some of the epithelial cells. *Neisseria gonorrhoeae* organisms inhabit the exudate, whereas *Chlamydia trachomatis* organisms are intracellular within the epithelial cells.

Clinical Alert

If the male urethral culture is negative, but gonorrhea is still suspected, prostatic massage may produce an increased number of organisms in the urethral discharge. The first morning specimen before urination may be the best.

ANAL CANAL CULTURE Follow the same procedure as for female patients.

BOTH MALE AND FEMALE PATIENTS

See oropharyngeal culture: Culture specimens should also be obtained from the oropharynx in those persons who engage in oral sex.

Clinical Alert

The finding of repeated negative cultures for gonococci does not always exclude a diagnosis of gonorrhea.

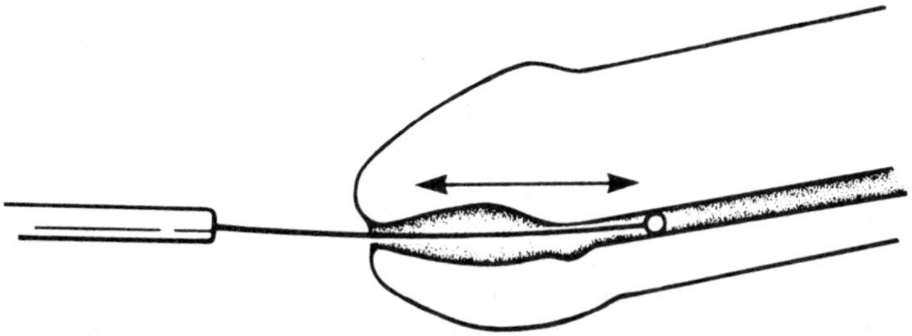

FIGURE 7-3
Method for obtaining the urethral culture.

Patient Preparation

1. Explain culture purpose and collection procedure.
2. Place the patient in the dorsal lithotomy position and appropriately drape for genital procedures. Provide as much privacy as possible.
3. Follow universal precautions.
4. See Chapter 1 guidelines for safe, effective, informed *pretest* care.

Patient Aftercare

1. Interpret test outcomes and counsel appropriately.
2. Explain need for possible follow-up testing and treatment.

● SKIN TESTS

Normal Values (for skin tests)

Positive reactions indicate

1. Lack of immunity to specific disease such as tuberculosis-producing agent
2. Sensitivity to a specific allergen (such as mold)

Explanation of Test

Skin testing is done for three major reasons: (1) to detect sensitivity to allergens, such as dust and pollen; (2) to determine sensitivity to microorganisms believed to cause disease; and (3) to determine whether cell-mediated, immune functions are normal. The test that detects sensitivity to allergens will be mentioned only briefly in this chapter. Most of this discussion will focus on skin tests used to determine sensitivity to pathogens.

In general, the following three types of skin tests are used:

SCRATCH TESTS

Scratches approximately 1 cm long and 2.5 cm apart are made in rows on the patient's back or forearms. Extremely small quantities of allergens are introduced into these scratches. Positive reaction: shows swelling or redness at the site within 30 minutes.

PATCH TESTS

A small square of gauze is impregnated with the suspected allergen and is applied to the skin of the forearm. A positive reaction shows swollen or reddened skin at the patch site within a given time period.

INTRADERMAL TESTS

The substance being tested is injected into the layers of skin with a tuberculin syringe fitted with a short-bevel, 26- or 27-gauge needle. A positive reaction shows red, inflamed area at the site of the injection within a given time period (eg, 72 hours for the Mantoux test for tuberculosis).

Skin tests that show a hypersensitivity to a toxin from a disease-producing agent may also signal immunity to the disease. Positive reactions may also indicate an active or inactive phase of the disease under study. The following categorizes skin tests according to their nature and purpose:

1. Tests to determine possible susceptibility (or resistance) to infection; for example, Schick test (positive reaction = lack of immunity to diphtheria). Dick test (positive reaction = lack of immunity to scarlet fever).
2. Tests to indicate a present or past exposure to the infectious agent; for example, tuberculin test (positive reaction = presence of active or inactive tuberculosis).
3. Tests to show sensitivity to materials toward which a person may react in an exaggerated manner; for example, allergenic extracts such as house dust and pollen (positive reaction = sensitivity to allergen extracts).
4. Tests to detect impaired cellular immunity. Intradermal skin testing with several common antigenic microbial substances can determine whether immune function is normal (eg, PPD tuberculin skin tests, mumps virus, *Candida albicans,* skin fungi, and streptokinase–streptodornase). This would be important in treating leukemia and cancer with chemotherapy. (Negative reaction to any intradermal antigen is indicative of impaired immunity owing to autoimmune function.)

Procedure for Skin Tests

1. Most diagnostic skin tests are prepackaged as sterile kits. Follow the manufacturer's instructions carefully.
2. Generally, 0.1 ml of the test material is injected intradermally on the volar aspect of the forearm.
3. Positive reaction = redness or swelling of more than 1 cm in diameter at the injection site. A central area of necrosis is a highly significant finding.

Clinical Alert

Material for diagnostic skin tests may be inadvertently injected into subcutaneous tissue, rather than intradermal tissue. A subcutaneous injection will yield a false-negative result.

Procedure for Patch Tests

1. Cleanse and dry the skin.
2. Firmly apply the patch to the forearm or the interscapular region of the back secondary to package instructions.

Procedure for Scratch Tests

The scratch method is especially recommended for patients who give a history of extreme sensitivity. Use universal precautions.

1. Cleanse the skin with alcohol (or acetone if allergic to alcohol); allow site to dry. Use forearm or interscapular sites on the back. Avoid elbow and wrist areas because they are less reactive.
2. Stretch the skin taut, using the thumb and index finger.
3. Use a sterile lancet to puncture the epidermis and make a scratch approximately 1 to 4 mm long. This is done to raise the skin. Do not draw blood. If blood appears, do not use that site.
4. Apply 1 drop of the testing material to the scratch site; take care not to touch the skin with the dropper.
5. Control tests should be done for baseline comparison.

TUBERCULIN SKIN TEST
(FOR DETECTION OF TUBERCULOSIS) ●

Normal Values

Negative or not significant.

Explanation of Test

The intradermal tuberculin (TB) skin test detects tuberculosis infection; it does not distinguish active TB from dormant TB. Tuberculin is a protein fraction of the tubercle bacilli; when it is introduced into the skin of a person with active or dormant tuberculosis infection, it causes a localized skin erythema and induration at the injection site because of accumulated small, sensitized lymphocytes.

The Mantoux test is the test of choice. The tuberculin is injected into the intradermal skin layer with a syringe and fine-gauge needle.

The multiple puncture test (tine test) is used for screening purposes for asymptomatic persons. However, the Mantoux test is the far more accurate of the two.

Indications for Testing

1. Persons who exhibit signs (x-ray film abnormality) or symptoms (cough, hemoptysis, weight loss, or other) suggestive of tuberculosis.
2. Recent close contacts with persons known to have or suspected of having tuberculosis.
3. Persons who show abnormal chest roentgenograms compatible with past tuberculosis exposure.
4. Persons with medical conditions that increase the risk of contradicting tu-

berculosis (silicosis, gastrectomy, diabetes, immunosuppressive therapy, lymphomas, AIDS).

5. Groups at high risk for sustaining infection with *M. tuberculosis,* such as immigrants from Asia, Africa, Latin America, and Oceania; poverty-prone and "skid row" populations; personnel and long-term residents in health-care facilities and institutions, such as nursing homes, mental institutions, and prisons.

Procedure

INTRADERMAL SKIN TEST (MANTOUX)

1. Observe universal precautions. Draw up PPD-t into a tuberculin syringe (follow manufacturer's directions carefully) with a 1/2-in. 26- or 27-gauge needle. Use 0.1 ml of 5 tuberculin units for each test.
2. Cleanse the skin on the volar or dorsal aspect of the forearm with alcohol and allow to dry.
3. Stretch the skin taut.
4. Hold the tuberculin syringe close to the skin so that the hub of the needle touches the skin as the needle is introduced under the skin. A discrete pale elevation of the skin—a wheal—6 to 10 mm in diameter should be produced when the prescribed amount of purified protein derivative (PPD)-t (0.1 ml) is injected into the intradermal skin layer.

Clinical Implications

1. The test should be "read" at 48 to 72 hours after injection. The larger the area size of the skin reaction, the more likely it is to represent tuberculosis infection. Positive test will show reddened area of 5 to 15 mm in size. However, a significant reaction to the skin test does not necessarily signify the presence of tuberculosis.
2. A significant reaction does not distinguish between active and dormant TB infection; the stage of infection can be determined from the results of clinical bacteriologic sputum tests and chest roentgenograms.
3. A significant reaction in the clinically ill patient means that a case of active tuberculosis should be considered as a possible cause for illness.
4. A significant reaction in a healthy person usually signifies either a healed tuberculosis or an infection caused by a different mycobacteria. Chest roentgenograms can confirm absence of an active disease process.

Clinical Alert

1. Tuberculin test material should never be transferred from one container to another.
2. Intradermal skin tests should be given immediately after the tuberculin is drawn up.

(continued)

(Clinical Alert continued)

3. The greatest value of tuberculin skin testing is in the negative results; a negative test result in the presence of signs and symptoms of lung disease is strong evidence against active tuberculosis in most cases.
4. A presumptive diagnosis of tuberculosis must be bacteriologically confirmed.
5. Incidence of tuberculosis is higher among older persons, men, nonwhites, and the foreign-born.
6. Typical new case scenario: Born in 1930s, infected in 1940s, developed TB in 1980s.
7. Sixteen percent of tuberculosis cases are extrapulmonary.
8. Tuberculosis is acquired through close, frequent, and prolonged exposure to the disease.
9. A diagnosed case of tuberculosis averages nine contacts, of which 21% are infected.
10. Persons who received BCG vaccine prophylactically as well as for bladder cancer treatment will always test positive for TB.
11. Periodic chest x-ray films are valuable adjuncts to following patients who test positive because there is no foolproof way of predicting who will develop active TB.
12. Bacille Camette-Guerin (BCG) is a freeze-dried preparation of a live, attenuated bovine strain of mycobacteria. It is used for TB immunization in children (eg, negative TB test = infant who lives in a household with untreated or ineffectively treated cases of TB).

Interfering Factors

False-negative results may occur even in the presence of active tuberculosis or whenever sensitized T lymphocytes are temporarily depleted in the body.

Reading the Test Results

1. The test should be read 48 to 72 hours after injection.
2. Examine the injection site in good light.
3. The patient should flex the forearm at the elbow.
4. Inspect the skin for induration (hardening or thickening).
5. Rub a finger lightly from the normal skin area to the indurated zone (if present).
6. Circle the zone of induration with a pencil and measure the diameter in millimeters. Disregard erythema; it is clinically insignificant.
7. Large reactions may still be evident 7 days after the test.

Interpreting the Test Results

1. The test interpretation is based on the presence or absence of induration.
2. Negative/no significant reaction: zone of induration smaller than 5 mm in diameter. Positive/significant reaction: zone of induration 10 mm or larger in diameter.
3. For those in *good* health with no risk factors, an induration of 15 mm is usually considered positive. However, because those at increased risk (poor health) for TB will have decreased hypersensitivity, a 5-mm induration may be considered positive. Retest within 3 weeks of the previous test.

Potential Causes of False Nonsignificant Tuberculin Test

Reactions can be categorized according to the following factors:

FACTORS RELATED TO PERSON BEING TESTED

Presence of infections
  Viral (measles, mumps, chickenpox)
  Bacterial (typhoid fever, brucellosis, typhus, leprosy, pertussis, overwhelming tuberculosis, tuberculous pleurisy)
  Fungal (South American blastomycosis)
Live virus vaccinations (measles, mumps, polio)
Metabolic derangements (chronic renal failure)
Nutritional factors (severe protein depletion)
Diseases affecting lymphoid organs (Hodgkin's disease, lymphoma, chronic lymphocytic leukemia, sarcoidosis)
Drugs (corticosteroids and other immunosuppressive agents)
Age (newborns, elderly patients with "waned" sensitivity)
Recent or overwhelming *M. tuberculosis* infection
Stress (surgical procedure, burns, mental illness, graft-versus-host reactions)

FACTORS RELATED TO TUBERCULIN INJECTED

Improper storage (exposure to light, heat)
Improper dilution
Chemical denaturation
Contamination
Adsorption (partially controlled by adding Tween 80)

OUTDATED FACTORS RELATED TO METHOD OF ADMINISTRATION

Injection of too little or too much antigen
Delayed administration after drawing up dose
Injection too deep or too shallow

FACTORS RELATED TO TEST INTERPRETATION AND RECORDING OF RESULTS

Test not read within prescribed time frame
Inexperienced reader

Conscious or unconscious bias
Recording error
Measurement error

Patient Preparation

1. Explain TB skin test purpose and procedure.
2. See Chapter 1 guidelines for safe, effective, informed *pretest* care.

Patient Aftercare

1. Interpret test outcomes at the prescribed time; monitor, and counsel appropriately for follow-up testing. Institute exposure control plan.
2. Follow Chapter 1 guidelines for safe, effective, informed *posttest* care.

SCHICK TEST ●

Normal Values

See "Clinical Implications."

Background

Diphtheria is a respiratory disease caused by the bacterium *Corynebacterium diphtheriae.* A person immune to diphtheria will produce significant quantities of antitoxins that will circulate in the blood to act on the intradermal injected toxin. A person susceptible to diphtheria will lack (or have very low levels of) antitoxins and, therefore, will not be able to neutralize the diphtheria toxin injected intradermally during the Schick test.

Explanation of Test

The Schick test determines the presence or absence of a significant quantity of diphtheria antitoxins in the blood. It also gives a rough estimate of the quantity of antitoxins circulating in the blood. The presence of these antitoxins indicates immunity to diphtheria.

1. If the skin test causes erythema and skin flaking at the injection site, the person tested is susceptible to diphtheria. This is considered a positive reaction.
2. A negative reaction, indicated by the absence of flaking or erythema, means that under normal exposure, the person will not contract diphtheria.

Procedure

1. Observe universal precautions. One-tenth milliliter of purified diphtheria *toxin* (0.02 of the amount necessary to kill a guinea pig) dissolved in human serum albumin is injected intradermally on the volar surface of the forearm. A 0.1-ml quantity of inactivated diphtheria *toxoid* is injected into the other arm as a control to rule out sensitivity to culture proteins. Note which arm receives which injection.

2. These areas are examined in 24 hours, 48 hours, and between the third and fourth days after injection.

Interpreting Test Results

1. Positive test: Site of *toxin* injection begins to redden in 24 hours, increases, and reaches maximum size in about 1 week, when it will be swollen, tender, and as large as 3 cm in diameter. Usually a small, dark red central zone that gradually turns brown and leaves a pigmented area is present. The area of *toxoid* injection shows no reaction.
2. Negative test: No reaction at either site.
3. Document test results in patient's record.

Clinical Implications

1. If the allergic response at the toxoid control site parallels that of the toxin site in size and duration of reaction, the test is recorded as a negative Schick.
2. If, however, the reaction to the unheated toxin is at least 50% larger and persists longer than the reaction to the control, the individual is both susceptible to the toxin and allergic to the contaminating substances that are not destroyed by heating; a positive Schick is recorded.
3. If a reaction occurs (ie, a positive test), the person does not have enough antibodies to neutralize the toxin and, therefore, is susceptible to diphtheria. In other words, the person is not immune to diphtheria.
4. Persons who have been well immunized with four injections of diphtheria toxoid show uniformly negative reactions to the Schick test.
5. If the test is positive in a well-immunized person, this presents strong evidence of the person's inability to produce sufficient antibodies against diphtheria.
6. A negative test means that the person has immunity to diphtheria.
7. The Schick test has limited use in the United States.

Clinical Alert

The major categories of persons who are significant reservoirs of diphtheria include formerly immunized persons, particularly the elderly, whose immunity has waned, and nonimmunized children.

Patient Preparation

1. Explain skin test purpose and procedure.
2. See Chapter 1 guidelines for safe, effective, informed *pretest* care.

Patient Aftercare

1. Interpret test outcomes and counsel about immune status.
2. Follow Chapter 1 guidelines for safe, effective, informed *posttest* care.

DICK TEST

Normal Values

See "Clinical Implications."

Background

Scarlet fever, also called *scarlatina,* is a communicable, hemolytic streptococcal infection caused by *Streptococcus pyogenes*. This disease causes generalized toxemia, a typical rash, and scaling of skin during the recovery period.

The occurrence of scarlet fever has decreased in recent years. Scarlatinal or erythrogenic toxin is responsible for the rash that occurs with scarlet fever.

Explanation of Test

The Dick test is a diagnostic skin test that measures susceptibility to scarlet fever. It also indicates the degree of immunity to the disease. A solution of dilute scarlatinal toxin is injected intradermally to detect antibodies and to determine immunity to scarlet fever.

Procedure

1. Observe universal precautions. Inject a 0.1-ml dilute solution of scarlet fever (Dick) toxin intradermally on the volar surface of the forearm.
2. Examine the test area within 24 hours.

Interpreting Test Results

1. Read the test within 18 to 24 hours after injection.
2. Positive reaction: injection site is very red and markedly swollen (3 to 5 cm in diameter). The swollen area has sharply raised edges. A positive test indicates damage done by the injected toxin that has not been neutralized by antibodies.
3. Negative reaction: no more than a faint pink streak along the course of the needle injection site.
4. Slightly positive reaction: faint red area measuring less than 1 cm in diameter; no swelling.
5. Document findings in patient's record.

Clinical Implications

1. A positive reaction signifies insufficient amounts of circulating antitoxins to neutralize the Dick toxin. This person is susceptible to scarlet fever. A positive test reverts to a negative reaction following infection by *Streptococcus pyogenes.*
2. A negative reaction signifies relative immunity to scarlet fever.

Clinical Alert

There are three immunologically rare, but distinct, toxins that may account for second attacks of scarlet fever.

Patient Preparation

1. Explain skin test purpose and procedure.
2. See Chapter 1 guidelines for safe, effective, informed *pretest* care.

Patient Aftercare

1. Interpret test outcomes and counsel about immune status.
2. Follow Chapter 1 guidelines for safe, effective, informed *posttest* care.

MUMPS TEST

Normal Values

See "Clinical Implications."

Background

Mumps, the common disease causing swelling and tenderness of the parotid glands, is caused by a myxovirus.

Explanation of Test

An antigen made from infected monkeys or chickens is injected intradermally. A control material made from noninfected monkeys or chickens also is injected intradermally at the same time. A positive mumps skin test may indicate either prior or existing infection and, therefore, is not very effective as a diagnostic tool. The test is primarily used as part of a battery of skin tests to determine immunocompetence.

Procedure

1. Observe universal precautions. Before injecting antigen, assess for allergy to eggs. Persons who are allergic would be at risk for an anaphylactic reaction to mumps antigen.
2. Inject mumps antigen intradermally.
3. Inject control material intradermally.
4. Note which area is injected with the antigen and with the control.

Clinical Implications

1. A positive reaction indicates resistance to the mumps virus.
2. A negative reaction indicates susceptibility to mumps virus.
3. Before injecting antigen into the patient, determine allergic reactions to eggs. An allergic patient would be at risk for an anaphylactic reaction to the mumps antigen.

Interpreting Test Results

1. Read the test 48 hours from the time of injection.
2. Positive reaction: erythema and a lesion larger than 10 mm in diameter
3. Negative reaction: No erythema and a lesion smaller than 10 mm in diameter

Patient Preparation

1. Explain skin test purpose and procedure.
2. See Chapter 1 guidelines for safe, effective, informed *pretest* care.

Patient Aftercare

1. Interpret test outcomes about immunocompetence.
2. Follow Chapter 1 guidelines for safe, effective, informed *posttest* care.

CANDIDA AND TETANUS TOXOID TESTS ●

Candida and tetanus toxoid are additional skin tests that can be done to detect delayed-type hypersensitivity (DTH). The candida/antigen is a mixture of trichophytin and oidium. Both antigens are administered in a manner similar to the tuberculin skin test.

To interpret skin tests for anergy, the following Centers for Disease Control and Prevention guidelines are recommended. For high-risk patients (HIV-positive, IV drug abusers, immunocompromised patients) an induration area of 5 mm or larger is positive. For moderate risk patients (institutionalized patients, healthcare workers), a 10-mm or larger induration area is significant. In patients with no significant risk factors, an indurated area of 15 mm or larger is considered positive.

These additional skin tests are helpful in evaluating a negative PPD test in an immunosuppressed individual. No reactions with mumps, tetanus, or candida testing may indicate a false-negative PPD test. However, an induration larger than 2 mm with the mumps, candida, or tetanus antigen confirm the negative PPD result.

BLASTOMYCOSIS (GILCHRIST'S DISEASE) **TEST** ●

Normal Value

Negative reaction.

Background

Blastomycosis, a condition characterized by cutaneous, pulmonary, and systemic lesions, is caused by organisms of the genus *Blastomyces*.

Explanation of Test

Blastomycin, an antigen, is injected intradermally. The test is reasonably specific for blastomycosis, but in practice, this skin-test antigen is usually injected simultaneously with histoplasmin, coccidioidin, and tuberculin.

Blastomycosis is also diagnosed by recovery of the organism from pus, sputum, or tissue specimens.

Procedure

Observe universal precautions. Inject the blastomycin intradermally.

Interpreting Test Results

1. Read the test 48 hours from time of injection.
2. Positive reaction is an area of erythema and induration 5 by 5 mm or larger.
3. Doubtful reaction is an area of induration smaller than 5 mm in diameter; only erythema present.
4. Negative reaction is no induration; erythema smaller than 5 mm in diameter

Clinical Implications

A positive reaction may indicate

1. Past infections
2. Mild, chronic, or subacute infection
3. Improvement in cases of serious symptomatic blastomycosis that previously had been blastomycin-negative

Patient Preparation

1. Explain purpose and skin test procedure.
2. See Chapter 1 guidelines for safe, effective, informed *pretest* care.

Patient Aftercare

1. Interpret test outcomes at proper time and counsel about skin reaction.
2. Follow Chapter 1 guidelines for safe, effective, informed *posttest* care.

COCCIDIOIDOMYCOSIS TEST ●

Normal Value

Negative reaction.

Background

Coccidioidomycosis, an infectious fungus disease that occurs in both an acute form and a progressive form, is caused by *Coccidioides immitis*.

Explanation of Test

Coccidioidin, an antigen prepared from culture, is injected intradermally. Coccidioidomycosis also can be diagnosed by recovery of the causative organism from pus, sputum, or tissue specimens.

Procedure

1. Observe universal precautions.
2. Inject the antigen intradermally.

Interpreting Test Results

1. The test must be read in 24 to 72 hours. If an immediate reaction occurs, it is nonspecific for coccidioidomycosis and is ignored.
2. Positive reaction is an area of erythema and induration 5 mm or larger in diameter. The reaction disappears within 24 to 72 hours.

Clinical Implications

1. The skin test becomes positive in more than 80% of the cases of coccidioidomycosis during the first week of clinical symptoms and in almost 100% of patients after the first week of symptoms.
2. A positive reaction to coccidioidomycosis persists for many years; however, this does not imply that an active infection is present (only exposure). If a positive reaction occurs during the course of infection, but an earlier test was negative, it can indicate a currently active infectious process.
3. Conversion to positive in a person who has been in an endemic area is virtually diagnostic for coccidioidal infection.

Patient Preparation

1. Explain purpose and skin test procedure.
2. See Chapter 1 guidelines for safe, effective, informed *pretest* care.

Patient Aftercare

1. Interpret test outcomes at correct time and counsel about skin reaction.
2. Follow Chapter 1 guidelines for safe, effective, informed *posttest* care.

HISTOPLASMOSIS TEST

Normal Values

See "Clinical Implications."

Background

Histoplasmosis, a systemic fungus infection of the reticuloendothelial system, is caused by the organism *Histoplasma capsulatum*.

Explanation of Test

Histoplasmin, an antigen prepared from culture, is injected intradermally. Skin reactions to histoplasmin are of relatively little diagnostic value because anergy may provide false-negative results. Histoplasmosis is also diagnosed by identification of the causative agent in pus, sputum, or tissue specimens.

Procedure

1. Observe universal precautions.
2. Inject the antigen intradermally.
3. Note site of injection.

Interpreting Test Results

1. The test should be read in 24 to 48 hours. If an immediate reaction occurs, it is nonspecific for histoplasmosis and should be ignored.
2. Positive reaction is an area of erythema and induration 5 mm or larger in diameter
3. Negative reaction is no induration; erythema smaller than 5 mm in diameter
4. Document findings in patient record.

Clinical Implications

1. A positive test indicates past or present infection.
2. Acutely ill patients may not have a positive reaction.

Clinical Alert

The skin test for histoplasmosis should be given after specimens for complement-fixation tests have been collected. The skin test reagent may induce or increase the titer of complement-fixing antibodies, even in the absence of active histoplasmosis.

Patient Preparation

1. Explain skin test purpose and procedure.
2. See Chapter 1 guidelines for safe, effective, informed *pretest* care.

Patient Aftercare

1. Interpret test outcomes at proper time and counsel about skin reaction.
2. Follow Chapter 1 guidelines for safe, effective, informed *posttest* care.

BIBLIOGRAPHY

Avey M: TB skin testing: How to do it right. American Journal of Nursing September: 42–44, 1993

Balows A et al (eds): Manual of Clinical Microbiology, 5th ed. Washington DC, American Society for Microbiology, 1991

Carpenter D, Zielinski D: How do you treat—and control—*C. difficile* infection? American Journal of Nursing September: 22–24, 1992

Cates W Jr, Hinman AR: Sexually transmitted diseases in the 90's. New England Journal of Medicine 325:1368, 1991

Cuzzell J: The right way to culture a wound. American Journal of Nursing May: 48–50, 1993

Davis BD et al: Microbiology, 4th ed. Philadelphia, JB Lippincott, 1990

Feld R: Q fever. Diagnostic and Clinical Testing 28:30–32, Mar 1990

Finegold S, Baron E: Bailey and Scott's Diagnostic Microbiology, 8th ed. St. Louis, CV Mosby, 1990

Garcia LS: Parasitology update. Teleconference Network of Texas, April 10, 1990

Hong R: Recurrent infections. Pediatrics in Review II:180–183, 1990

Koneman EW et al (eds): Color Atlas and Textbook of Microbiology, 4th ed. Philadelphia, JB Lippincott, 1992

Lavin J: Anergy testing—a vital weapon. RN September: 31–32, 1993

Pauker SG: HIV screening: Nosocomial epidemiologic risks and decision analysis. Law Med Health Care 18(1/2):33–40, Spring-Summer 1990

Sacher RA, McPherson RA: Widmann's Clinical Interpretation of Laboratory Tests, 10th ed. Philadelphia, FA Davis, 1991

Sodeman T, Colmer J: Contemporary pathogens of the gastrointestinal system. Laboratory Medicine 22(3):173–178, March 1991

Sodeman T, Colmer J: Contemporary pathogens of the upper respiratory tract. Laboratory Medicine 22(5):313–317, May 1991

Spelcher CE: The Right Test—A Physician's Guide To Laboratory Medicine, 2nd ed. Philadelphia, WB Saunders, 1993

8

Immunodiagnostic Studies

Frances Fischbach: A MANUAL OF LABORATORY & DIAGNOSTIC TESTS, Fifth Edition.

OVERVIEW OF IMMUNODIAGNOSTIC STUDIES ●

Overview of Tests

Immunodiagnostic or serodiagnostic testing studies antigen–antibody reactions for diagnosis of infectious disease, autoimmune disorders, immune allergies, and neoplastic disease. These modalities also test for blood grouping and typing, tissue and graft transplant matching, and cellular immunology. The blood serum is tested for antibodies against a particular antigen.

Antigens are substances that stimulate and subsequently react with the products of immune response. They may be bacterial, viral, parasitic, fungal, or enzymatic. *Antibodies* are proteins produced by the body's immune system in response to an antigen. The antigen–antibody response is the body's natural defense against invading organisms.

Pathologically, *autoimmune disorders* are produced by autoantibodies, that is, antibodies against *self,* such as in rheumatoid disease or lupus erythematosus.

Immunodeficiency diseases exhibit a lack of one or more basic components of the immune system, which includes B lymphocytes, T lymphocytes, phagocytic cells, and the complement system. These diseases are classified as primary (congenital) and secondary (acquired).

Hypersensitivity reactions are defined as abnormally increased immune responses to some allergens (eg, allergic reaction to bee stings or pollens).

Types of Tests

Many methods of varying sophistication can detect antibodies. Results demonstrate that antigen–antibody reactions have taken place (see the table entitled Some Tests That Determine Antigen–Antibody Reactions).

Collection of Serum for Immunologic Tests

1. *Procure two samples.* One sample should be obtained at illness onset (acute phase) and the other sample drawn 3 to 4 weeks later (convalescent phase). In general, serologic test usefulness depends on a titer increase in the time interval between the acute and the convalescent phase.

   For a few serologic tests, *one* serum sample may be adequate because the antibody presence indicates an abnormal condition, or the antibody titer is unusually high. The following tests require a single sample:

   a. Antinuclear antibody
   b. Heterophilic antibody titer
   c. Histoplasmosis CF
   d. Toxoplasmosis (IFA)
   e. Rubella titer
   f. VDRL test
2. *Perform the serologic test before doing skin testing.* Skin testing often induces antibody production and could interfere with serologic test results.
3. *Label the sample properly and submit requested information.*
4. *Send samples to the laboratory promptly. Hemolyzed samples cannot yield accurate results.* Hemoglobin in the serum sample can interfere with complement-fixing antibody values.

Interpreting Results of Immunologic Tests

The following factors will affect test results:

1. History of previous infection by the same organism.
2. Previous vaccination (determine time frame).
3. Anamnestic reactions caused by heterologous antigens. (An *anamnestic reaction* is the appearance of antibodies in the blood after administration of an antigen to which the patient has previously developed a primary immune response.)
4. Cross-reactivity: Antibodies produced by one species of an organism reacting with an entirely different species (eg, Tularemia antibodies may agglutinate *Brucella* and vice versa or rickettsial infections may produce antibodies reactive with *Proteus* ϕX19).
5. Presence of other serious illness states (eg, lack of immunologic response in agammaglobulinemia or cancer treatment with immunosuppressant drugs).

Serologic Versus Microbiologic Methods

Serologic testing or microbial immunology evaluates antigens of bacteria, viruses, fungi, and parasites. The best means of establishing infectious dis-

Some Tests That Determine Antigen–Antibody Reactions

Name of Test	*Reaction*	*Visible Observable Change*	*Tests For*
1. Agglutination, hemagglutination (HA), immune hemagglutination assay (IHA)	Particulate antigen reacts with corresponding antibody. Antigen may be in form of RBCs (hemagglutination, latex or charcoal coated with antigen)	Clumping	Rubella, thyroid cold agglutin antibodies
2. Precipitation (eg, immunodiffusion [ID] and counterimmunoelectrophoresis [CIE])	Soluble antigen reacts with corresponding antibody by immunodiffusion (ID) or count	Precipitates	Fungal antibodies; food poisoning
3. Complement fixation (CF)	Competition between two antigen–antibody systems—test and indicator systems	Complement activation, hemolysis	Viral antibodies
4. Immunofluorescence (eg, Indirect fluorescent antibody [IFA])	Fluorescent-tagged antibody, reacts with antigen–antibody complex in the presence of ultraviolet light	Visible microscopic fluorescence	Antinuclear antibodies (ANAs) and antimitochondrial antibodies (AMAs)
5. Enzyme immunoassay (EIA)	Enzymes are used to label induced antigen–antibody reactions	Chromogenic fluorescent or luminescent change in substrate	Extractable nuclear antigens (ENAs); antiribonucleoproteins (RNPs)
6. Enzyme-linked immunosorbent assay (ELISA)	Indirect EIA for quantification of an antigen or antibody enzyme, and substrate	Color change indicates enzyme substrate reaction	Amyloid beta-protein in Alzheimer's
7. Immunoblot (eg, Western blot [WB])	Electrophoretic separation of antigen subspecies	Detection of antibodies of specific mobility	Confirms HIV-I

(continued)

Some Tests That Determine Antigen–Antibody Reactions *(Continued)*

Name of Test	*Reaction*	*Visible Observable Change*	*Tests For*
8. Polymerase chain reaction (PCR); *state of the art procedure*	Amplifies low levels of specific DNA sequences. Each cycle doubles the amount of specific DNA sequence	Exponential accumulation of DNA fragment being amplified	Even slightest trace of infection can be detected with this technique; more accurate than traditional tests for chlamydia
9. Rate nephelometry	Measures either antigen or antibody in solution through the scattering of a light beam; antibody reagent used to detect antigen IgA, IgG, IgM; concurrent controls are run to establish amount of background scatter in reagents and test samples.	Light-scatter proportionately increases as numbered size of immune complexes increase.	Quantitative immunoglobulins IgA, IgG, IgM recorded in mg/dl or IU/ml.
10. Flow cytometry	Blood cell types are identified with monoclonal antibodies (mABs) specific for cell markers by means of a flow cytometer with an argon laser beam. As the cells pass the beam, they scatter the light. Light energy is converted into electrical energy cells and stained with green (fluorescence) or orange (phycoerythrin) (Fig. 8-1).	Light scatter identifies cell size and granularity of lymphocytes, monocytes, and granulocytes. Color fluorochromes tagged to monoclonal antibodies bend to specific surface antigens for simultaneous detection of lymphocyte subsets.	Lymphocyte immunophenocytology differentiates B cells from T cells and T-helper cells from T-suppressor cells.

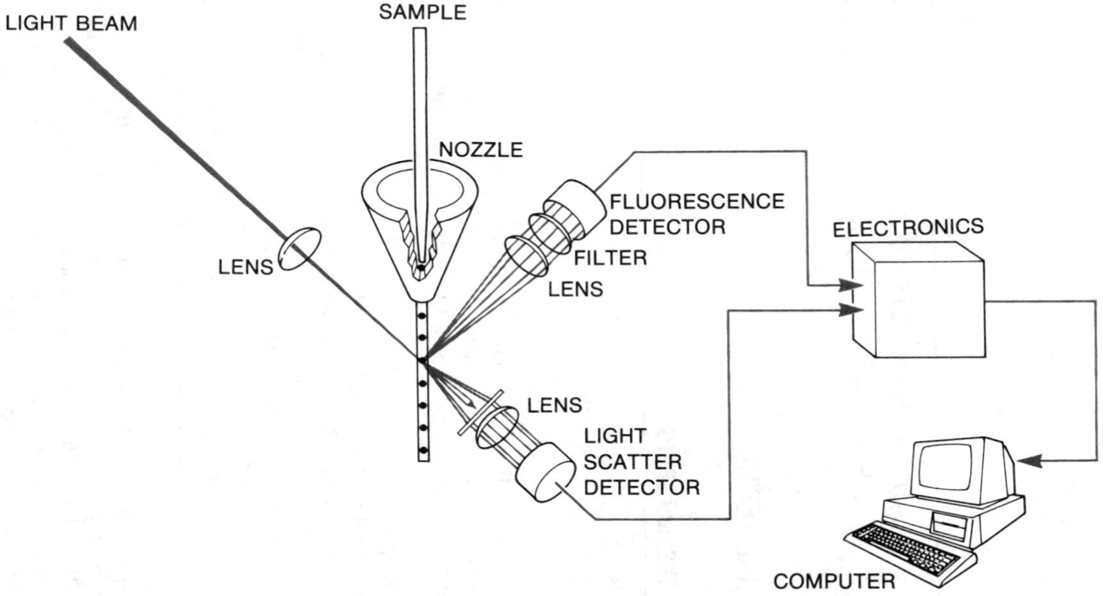

FIGURE 8-1
Schematic diagram of a flow cytometer.

ease etiology is by isolation and confirmation of the involved pathogen. Serologic methods can assist or confirm microbiologic analysis under the following circumstances: the patient is tested late in the disease course; antimicrobial therapy has suppressed organism growth; culture methods cannot verify a causative agent.

Serologic Tests of Bacterial, Viral, Fungal, and Parasitic Diseases

BACTERIAL TESTS

SYPHILIS DETECTION TESTS

Normal Value

Nonreactive: negative for syphilis

Background

Syphilis is a venereal disease caused by *Treponema pallidum,* a spirochete with closely wound coils, approximately 8 to 15 μm long. Untreated, the disease progresses through three stages that may extend over many years.

Explanation of Tests

Antibodies to syphilis begin to appear in the blood 4 to 6 weeks after infection (Table 8-1). Nontreponemal (nonspecific) tests determine the presence of reagin, which is a nontreponemal autoantibody directed against cardiolipin antigens. These tests include RPR (agglutination test) and VDRL (flocculation test). The Centers for Disease Control and Prevention (CDC) recommend these tests for *syphilis screening*. However, they may show negative results in some cases of late syphilis. Biological false-positive results can also occur (Table 8-2).

On the other hand, treponemal (specific) tests detect antibodies to *T. pallidum.* These tests include the microhemagglutination *Treponema pallidum* test (MHA-TP) and the fluorescent treponemal antibody test (FTA-ABS). These tests confirm syphilis when a positive nontreponemal test result is obtained. Because these tests are more complex, they are not used for screening.

Procedure

A 5-ml venous blood serum sample is used. Observe universal precautions. Fasting is usually *not* required.

TABLE 8-1
Serologic Tests for Syphilis (STS)

Name of Test	*Type/Description*	*Comments*
FTA-ABS (fluorescent treponemal antibody absorption)	Fluorescent antibody absorbs out antibody to nonpathogenic treponemes	Detects treponemal antibodies; differentiates biologic false-positives from true syphilis-positives and diagnoses syphilis when definite clinical signs of syphilis are present, but other tests are negative.
RPR (rapid plasma reagin)	Agglutination	Reagin reacts with lipid antigens; used as screening test; shows presence of reagin; more sensitive than VDRL. Patients treated for syphilis should have baseline RPR.
VDRL	Flocculation	Used as a screening test; developed in the Venereal and Research Laboratories of the U. S. Public Health Service; shows presence of reagin.
MHA-TP (microhemagglutination assay for *Treponema pallidum* antibodies)	Hemagglutination	Shows presence of treponemal antibody; even more specific than an FTA-ABS.

Clinical Implications

1. Diagnosis of syphilis requires correlation of patient history, physical findings, and results of syphilis antibody tests. *Treponema pallidum* infection is diagnosed when *both* the screening and the confirmatory tests are reactive.
2. Treatment of syphilis may alter both the clinical course and the serologic pattern of the disease. Treatment related to tests that measure *reagin* (RPR and VDRL) includes the following:
   a. If the patient is treated at the seronegative primary stage (eg, after the

TABLE 8-2
Nonsyphylitic Conditions Giving Biological False Positives (BFPs) Using VDRL and RPR Tests

Disease	*Percentage (Approximate) BFPs*
Malaria	100
Leprosy	60
Relapsing fever	30
Active immunization in children	20
Infectious mononucleosis	20
Lupus erythematosus	20
Lymphogranuloma venereum	20
Pneumonia, atypical	20
Rat-bite fever	20
Typhus fever	20
Vaccinia	20
Infectious hepatitis	10
Leptospirosis (Weil's disease)	10
Periarteritis nodosa	10
Trypanosomiasis	10
Chancroid	5
Chickenpox	5
Measles	5
Rheumatoid arthritis	5–7
Rheumatic fever	5–6
Scarlet fever	5
Subacute bacterial endocarditis	5
Pneumonia, pneumococcal	3–5
Tuberculosis, advanced pulmonary	3–5
Blood loss, repeated	? (low)
Common cold	? (low)
Pregnancy	? (low)

appearance of the syphilitic chancre but before appearance of reaction or reagin), the VDRL will remain nonreactive.

b. If the patient is treated in the seropositive primary stage (eg, after the appearance of a reaction) the VDRL usually becomes nonreactive within 6 months of treatment.

c. If the patient is treated during the secondary stage, the VDRL usually becomes nonreactive within 12 to 18 months.

d. If treated 10 or more years after disease onset, the VDRL usually remains unchanged.

3. A negative serologic test may indicate that

a. The patient does not have syphilis

b. The infection is too recent for antibodies to be produced. Repeat tests should be performed at 1-week, 1-month, and 3-month intervals to establish presence or absence of disease.

c. The syphilis is in a latent or inactive phase.
d. The patient has a faulty immunodefense mechanism.
e. Laboratory techniques were faulty.

FALSE-POSITIVE AND FALSE-NEGATIVE REACTIONS

A positive reaction is not conclusive for syphilis. Several conditions will produce biologic false-positive results for syphilis. Biologic false-positive reactions are by no means "false." They may reveal the presence of other serious diseases. It is theorized that reagin (reaction) is an antibody against tissue lipids. Lipids are presumed to be liberated from body tissue in the normal course of activity. These liberated lipids may then induce antibody formation. Nontreponemal biologic false-positive (BFP) reactions can occur in the presence of drug abuse, lupus erythematosus, mononucleosis, malaria, leprosy, viral pneumonia, the recently immunized, or, on rare occasions, during pregnancy. False-negative reactions may occur early in the disease course or during inactive or later stages.

Interfering Factors

1. Excess chyle in the blood interferes with test results.

Clinical Alert

Avoid drawing the blood sample immediately after a meal.

2. Alcohol decreases reaction intensity in tests that detect reagin; therefore, alcohol ingestion should be avoided for at least 24 hours before blood is drawn.

Patient Preparation

1. Explain test purpose and procedure. Assess for interfering factors. Instruct the patient to abstain from alcohol for at least 24 hours before the blood sample is drawn.
2. See Chapter 1 guidelines for safe, effective, informed *pretest* care.

Patient Aftercare

1. Interpret test results and counsel appropriately. Explain biologic false-positive or false-negative reactions. Repeat testing may be necessary.
2. Follow Chapter 1 guidelines for safe, effective, informed *posttest* care.

Clinical Alert

1. Sexual partners of syphilitic patients should be evaluated for the disease.
2. After treatment, patients with early-stage syphilis should be tested at 3-month intervals for 1 year to monitor for declining reactivity.

LYME DISEASE TEST

Normal Values

Indirect fluorescent antibody titer: < 1:256

Enzyme-linked immunosorbent assay (ELISA): nonreactive or negative for Lyme disease.

Explanation of Test

This test diagnoses Lyme disease, a multisystem disorder caused by the spirochete, *Borrelia burgdorferi*. It is transmitted by the bite of very tiny deer ticks residing on deer and other wild animals. Lyme disease is present worldwide, but certain geographic areas show higher incidences. Transmission to humans is highest during the spring, summer, and early fall months. Tests for antibodies include indirect fluorescent antibody (IFA), ELISA, Western blot assay (confirmatory), and polymerase chain reaction (PCR). The tick bite usually produces a characteristic rash, termed erythema chronicum migrans. If untreated, sequelae lead to serious joint, cardiac, and central nervous system symptoms. Antibody formation takes place in the following manner: IgM is detected 3 to 4 weeks after Lyme disease onset, peaks at 6 to 8 weeks, then gradually disappears. IgG is detected 2 to 3 months after infection and may remain elevated for years.

Procedure

Obtain a 5-ml venous blood sample. Observe universal precautions. Cerebrospinal fluid also may be used for the test.

Interfering Factors

1. False-positive results may occur with high levels of rheumatoid factors or in the presence of other spirochete infections, such as syphilis (cross-reactivity).
2. Asymptomatic individuals who spend time in endemic areas may have already produced antibodies to *B. burgdorferi*.

Clinical Implications

1. Serologic tests sometimes lack the degree of sensitivity, specificity, and standardization necessary for diagnosis in the absence of clinical history. The antigen capture–detection assay for bacterial proteins is a promising new test for this organism.
2. In patients presenting with a clinical picture of Lyme disease, negative serologic tests are inconclusive during the first month of infection.
3. Repeat paired testing should be performed if borderline values are reported.
4. The CDC laboratory criteria for diagnosis of Lyme disease include:
   - **a.** Isolation of *B. burgdorferi* from a clinical specimen
   - **b.** IgM and IgG antibodies in blood or CSF.

c. Paired, acute and convalescent blood samples show significant antibody response to *B. burgdorferi.*

Patient Preparation

1. Assess patient's clinical history, exposure risk, and knowledge about the test. Explain test purpose and procedure, as well as possible follow-up testing.
2. See Chapter 1 guidelines for safe, effective, informed *pretest* care.

Patient Aftercare

1. Interpret test outcomes for a positive test. Advise that follow-up testing may be required to monitor response to antibiotic therapy.
2. Patients with a negative test result and clinical findings suggestive of Lyme disease should also receive antibiotic treatment. They may require repeat testing because patients in early stages may test negative.
3. Follow Chapter 1 guidelines for safe, effective, informed *posttest* care.

LEGIONNAIRES' DISEASE ANTIBODY TEST ●

Normal Values

Negative for legionnaires' disease by indirect fluorescent antibody (IFA) test or enzyme-linked immunosorbent assay (ELISA).

Explanation of Test

This test diagnoses legionnaires' disease, a respiratory condition caused by *Legionella pneumophila.* It is best diagnosed by organism culture; however, the organism is difficult to grow. Detection of *L. pneumophila* in respiratory specimens by means of direct fluorescent antibody (DFA) technique is useful for rapid diagnosis but lacks sensitivity when only small numbers of organisms are available. Serologic tests should be used only if specimens for culture are not available, or if culture and DFA produce negative results.

Procedure

1. Obtain 5-ml blood serum sample. Observe universal precautions.
2. Follow-up testing is usually requested 3 to 6 weeks after initial symptom appearance.

Clinical Implications

1. A dramatic rise of titer to levels > 1:128 in the interval between acute- and convalescent-phase specimens occurs with recent infections.
2. Serologic tests are not the method of choice because they indicate retrospective values weeks after the acute phase.
3. Serologic testing is valuable because it provides a confirmatory diagnosis of *L. pneumophila* infection when other tests have failed. IFA is the serologic test of choice because it can detect all classes of antibodies.

Patient Preparation

1. Assess clinical history and knowledge about the test. Explain purpose and blood test procedure.
2. See Chapter 1 guidelines for safe, effective, informed *pretest* care.

Patient Aftercare

1. Interpret test outcomes and significance. Advise that negative results do not rule out *L. pneumophila*. Follow-up testing is usually needed.
2. Follow Chapter 1 guidelines for safe, effective, informed *posttest* care.

CHLAMYDIA ANTIBODY IgG TEST ●

Normal Values

Negative for chlamydia antibody by complement-fixation (CF), indirect fluorescent antibody (IFA), and polymerase chain reaction (PCR) tests.

Explanation of Test

This test diagnoses the presence of chlamydia infection (*Chlamydia* spp. are bacteria that require living cells for growth; they are classified as obligate cell parasites). Recognized species include *C. psittaci* and *C. trachomatis: C. psittaci* causes psittacosis in birds and humans; *C. trachomatis* is grouped into three serotype groups. One group causes lymphogranuloma venereum (LGV), a venereal disease. Another group causes trachoma, an eye disease. The third group causes genital tract infections different from LGV. Culture of the organism is definitive for the presence of chlamydiae. Because these organisms are difficult to culture and grow, serologic testing aids in diagnosis of such an infection.

Procedure

Obtain a 5-ml venous blood sample. Observe universal precautions.

Clinical Implications

1. Presence of antibody titer indicates chlamydial infection in the past. A fourfold or greater rise in antibody titer between acute and convalescent specimens indicates recent infection. Serologic tests cannot differentiate between the species of *Chlamydia*.
2. Infection with psittacosis shows an increase in antibody titer. History will reveal contact with infected birds as pets or as poultry.
3. In males, LGV is characterized by swollen and tender inguinal lymph nodes. For females, swelling occurs in the intra-abdominal, perirectal, and pelvic lymph nodes. Chlamydia causes urethritis in males. It can infect the female urethra and endocervix, and it is also a cause of pelvic inflammatory disease in females. Eye disease caused by chlamydia is endemic in parts of Africa, the Middle East, and Southeast Asia, although its

presence is established worldwide. Culture and stained smear identification of the organism is diagnostic.

Interfering Factors

Depending on geographic location, nonspecific titers can be found in the general healthy population.

Patient Preparation

1. Assess patient knowledge concerning the test and explain purpose and procedure. Elicit history of possible exposure to the organism.
2. See Chapter 1 guidelines for safe, effective, informed *pretest* care.

Patient Aftercare

1. Interpret test outcomes and significance of test results.
2. Follow Chapter 1 guidelines for safe, effective, informed *posttest* care.

STREPTOCOCCAL ANTIBODY TESTS: ANTISTREPTOLYSIN O TITER (ASO), STREPTOZYME, ANTI-DNASE B (ADB; STREPTODORNASE) ●

Normal Values

ASO titer: less than 166 Todd units

Anti-DNase B (ADB): birth to 4 years < 170 units
5 to 19 years < 480 units
20 years and older < 340 units

Streptozyme: negative for streptococcal antibodies

Explanation of Test

These tests diagnose streptococcal infections or illnesses associated with streptococcal infections. Group A β-hemolytic streptococci produce several enzymes that include streptolysin O, hyaluronidase, and DNase B. Serologic tests that detect these enzyme antibodies include (1) antistreptolysin O titer (ASO), which detects streptolysin O; (2) streptozyme—a screening test that detects antibodies to multiple enzymes; and (3) anti-DNase B (ADB) test, which detects DNase B. Serologic detection of streptococcal antibodies helps establish *prior* infection, but the tests are of no value for diagnosing *acute* streptococcal infections. Acute infections should be diagnosed by direct streptococcal cultures, or by the presence of streptococcal antigens.

The ASO test aids in the diagnosis of several conditions associated with streptococcal infections, such as rheumatic fever, glomerulonephritis, endocarditis, and scarlet fever. Serial rising titers over several weeks are more significant than is a single result. Anti-DNase B antibodies may appear earlier than ASO in streptococcal pharyngitis, and this test is more sensitive for streptococcal pyoderma.

Procedure

1. Obtain a 5-ml venous blood serum sample. Observe universal precautions.
2. Repeat testing 10 days after the first test is recommended.

Clinical Implications

1. In general, a titer higher than 166 Todd units is considered a definite elevation.
2. The ASO or the ADB test alone will be positive in 80% to 85% of streptococcal A infections (eg, streptococcal pharyngitis, rheumatic fever, pyoderma, glomerulonephritis).
3. When ASO and ADB are run concurrently, 95% of streptococcal infections can be detected.
4. A repeated low titer is good evidence for the absence of active rheumatic fever. Conversely, a high titer does not necessarily mean that rheumatic fever or glomerulonephritis is present; however, it does indicate the presence of a streptococcal infection.
5. ASO production is especially high in rheumatic fever and glomerulonephritis. These conditions show marked ASO titer increases during the symptomless period preceding an attack. Also, ADB titers are particularly high in pyoderma.

Interfering Factors

1. An increased titer can occur in healthy carriers.
2. Antibiotic therapy will suppress streptococcal antibody response.
3. Increased β-lipoprotein levels inhibit streptolysin O and produce falsely high ASO titers.

> **Clinical Alert**
>
> The ASO test is impractical in patients who have recently received antibiotics or who are scheduled for antibiotic therapy; the treatment suppresses the antibody response.

Patient Preparation

1. Assess patient's clinical history and test knowledge. Explain test purpose and procedure.
2. See Chapter 1 guidelines for safe, effective, informed *pretest* care.

Patient Aftercare

1. Interpret test outcomes (see page 514 for interpretation of immunologic test results) and explain test results. Inform that repeat testing is frequently required.
2. Advise patient that prior antibiotic therapy may suppress antibody forma-

tion. If antibiotics have been prescribed, the entire amount should be taken before retesting.

3. Follow Chapter 1 guidelines for safe, effective, informed *posttest* care.

● VIRAL TESTS

INFECTIOUS MONONUCLEOSIS TESTS: ROUTINE; HETEROPHIL ANTIBODY TITER TEST; EPSTEIN–BARR VIRUS (EBV) ANTIBODY TESTS ●

Normal Values

Negative for infectious mononucleosis and Epstein–Barr antibodies.

Background

The Epstein–Barr virus (EBV) is a herpes virus found throughout the world. The most common symptomatic manifestation of EBV infection is a disease known as infectious mononucleosis (IM). This disease induces formation of increased numbers of abnormal lymphocytes in the lymph nodes and stimulates increased heterophil antibody formation. IM occurs most often in young adults not previously infected. Symptoms include fever, pharyngitis, and lymphadenopathy. EBV is also thought to play a role in the etiology of Burkitt's lymphoma, nasopharyngeal carcinoma, and chronic fatigue syndrome.

Explanation of Test

The most common test for Epstein–Barr virus (EBV) is the rapid slide test (monotest) for heterophil antibody agglutination. Heterophil antibody agglutination is not specific for EBV and, therefore, is not useful for evaluating chronic disease. If the heterophil test is negative in the presence of acute IM symptoms, specific EBV antibodies should be determined. These include antibodies to viral capsid antigen (anti-VCA) and antibodies to EBV nuclear antigen (EBNA).

Diagnosis of infectious mononucleosis is based on the following criteria: clinical features compatible with IM, hematologic picture of relative and absolute lymphocytosis, and presence of heterophil antibodies. Tests for IM antibodies include heterophil antibodies, antibody agglutination, and specific EBV antibodies with IFA and ELISA tests.

Procedure

Obtain a 5-ml venous blood sample. Observe universal precautions.

Clinical Implications

1. The presence of heterophil antibodies (monospot test), along with clinical signs and other hematologic findings, is diagnostic for infectious mononucleosis.

2. Heterophil antibodies remain elevated for 8 to 12 weeks after the symptom appearance.

Patient Preparation

1. Assess patient's clinical history, symptoms, and test knowledge. Explain test purpose and procedure. If preliminary tests are negative, follow-up tests may be necessary.
2. See Chapter 1 guidelines for safe, effective, informed *pretest* care.

Patient Aftercare

1. Interpret test outcomes. Explain treatment. Note that recurrence of infectious mononucleosis is rare.
2. Resolution of infectious mononucleosis usually follows a predictable course: pharyngitis disappears within 14 days after onset, fever subsides within 21 days, and fatigue, lymphadenopathy, and liver and spleen enlargement regress by 21 to 28 days.
3. Follow Chapter 1 guidelines for safe, effective, informed *posttest* care.

RUBELLA ANTIBODY TESTS ●

Normal Values

HAI titer: < 1:10 = susceptible to rubella virus
HAI titer: > 1:10 = immune to rubella virus
ELISA: negative = not immune; positive = immune
Latex agglutination: negative = not immune; positive = immune

Background

Rubella virus causes German measles, a contagious disease characterized by fever and rash. Rubella acquired by a pregnant female during the first trimester of pregnancy is associated with congenital fetal abnormalities, miscarriage, and stillbirth.

Explanation

These tests determine susceptibility and immunity to rubella. Women of childbearing age and others, such as healthcare workers, should be tested to identify rubella immune status or carrier status. Testing for the IgM antibody is also indicated with any low-birth-weight newborn who also has symptoms of congenital rubella. Rubella infection will induce IgM and IgG antibody formation. Therefore, presence of an IgM antibody titer in an infant is diagnostic for congenital rubella infection (rubella antibodies do not cross the placenta.) Tests for the rubella virus include hemagglutination inhibition (HAI), ELISA, and latex agglutination.

Procedure

1. Obtain a 5-ml blood serum sample. See collection of serum for immunologic tests. Observe universal precautions.
2. Follow-up testing may be requested.

Clinical Implications

1. A fourfold rise in titer values between the acute and convalescent samples, together with clinical symptoms, is diagnostic of recent rubella infection. IgM is not detectable until 8 weeks after infection.
2. After infection, titer remains high for many years. Repeat infections are rare.
3. Rubella vaccine immunization produces formation of rubella antibodies.
4. Negative titers indicate ***no*** previous rubella infection and, therefore, ***no*** immunity to disease. Positive titers indicate past rubella infection and immunity to the disease.
5. Passively acquired rubella antibody levels in the infant will decrease markedly within 2 to 3 months after mother's infection.

Patient Preparation

1. Assess patient's test knowledge. Explain test purpose and procedure. Advise pregnant women that rubella acquired in the first trimester of pregnancy is associated with an increased incidence of miscarriage, stillbirth, and congenital abnormalities.
2. See Chapter 1 guidelines for safe, effective, informed *pretest* care.

Patient Aftercare

1. Interpret test outcome and counsel appropriately. Advise women of childbearing age, who test negative, to be immunized before becoming pregnant. Immunization is contraindicated during pregnancy. Advise patients who test positive that they are normally immune to further rubella infection.
2. Follow Chapter 1 guidelines for safe, effective, informed *posttest* care.

HEPATITIS TESTS ●

Normal Values

Radioimmune assay (RIA) and enzyme-linked immunosorbent assay (ELISA) are negative for hepatitis A, B, C, and D.

Background

Hepatitis can be caused by viruses, bacteria, drugs, toxins, and alcohol ingestion. Five major viral hepatitis types have been identified: hepatitis A, B, C, D, and E (Table 8-3). Diagnosing the specific virus is difficult because the symptoms each viral type presents are similar. Additionally, some individuals may be asymptomatic or have very mild symptoms that are ascribed to the "flu." Serologic tests for specific hepatitis virus markers have made it easier to define the specific type.

Hepatitis A virus (HAV), acquired through enteric transmission, infects the gastrointestinal tract and is eliminated through the feces. Serologically, presence of the IgM antibody to hepatitis A virus (IgM anti-HAV) and the total antibody to hepatitis A virus (total anti-HAV) identifies the disease.

TABLE 8-3
Summary of the Clinical and Epidemiological Features of Viral Hepatitis Agents

Features	*Hepatitis A*	*Hepatitis B*	*Hepatitis C*	*Hepatitis D*	*Hepatitis E*
Incubation period	2–6 weeks	8–24 weeks	2–52 weeks	3–13 weeks	3–6 weeks
Onset	Abrupt	Insidious	Insidious	Abrubt	Abrupt
SYMPTOMS					
Jaundice	Children: 10% Adults: 70%–80%	25%	25%	Varies	Unknown
Asymptomatic patients	Most Children	Most Children Adults: 50%	About 75%	Rare	Rare
ROUTES OF TRANSMISSION					
Fecal/oral	Yes	No	No	No	Yes
Parenteral	Rare	Yes	Yes	Yes	No
Sexual	No	Yes	Possible	Yes	No
Perinatal	No	Yes	Possible	Possible	No
Water/food	Yes	No	No	No	Yes
Chronic state	No	Adults: 6%–10% Children: 25%–50% Infants: 70%–90%	50%	10%–15%	No
Case fatality rate	0.6%	1%–4%	1%–2%	30%	1%–2% Pregnant women: 20%

Hepatitis B virus (HBV) demonstrates a central core containing the core antigen and a surrounding envelope containing the surface antigen. Detection of core antigen (HBcAg), envelope antigen (HBeAg), and surface antigen (HBsAg), or their corresponding antibodies, constitutes hepatitis B serologic assessment. Viral transmission occurs by exposure to contaminated blood or blood products through an open wound (eg, needlesticks, lacerations).

Hepatitis C virus (HCV), formerly non-A, non-B hepatitis, is also transmitted parenterally. Hepatitis C infection is confirmed serologically by presence of antibodies to hepatitis C (anti-HCV).

Hepatitis D virus (HDV) is encapsulated by the hepatitis B surface antigen. Without the HBsAg coating, HDV cannot survive. Because HDV can cause infection only in the presence of active HBV infection, it is usually found in areas where a high incidence of HBV occurs. Transmission is parenteral. Serologic HDV determination is made by detection of the hepatitis D antigen (HDAg) early in the course of the infection and by detection of anti-HDV antibody (anti-HDV) in the latter disease stages.

Hepatitis E virus (HEV) is serologically distinct. Enteric transmission is associated with poor hygienic practices and unsafe water supplies, especially in developing countries. [It is quite rare in the United States.]

Explanation of Test

These measurements are used for differential diagnosis of viral hepatitis. Serodiagnosis of viral hepatitis is complex because of the number of serum markers necessary to determine the stage of illness. Testing methods include radioimmunoassay (RIA) and enzyme-linked immunosorbent assay (ELISA).

Types of Hepatitis Virus

Disease Stages	*HVA*	*HVB*	*HVC*	*HVD*
Acute disease	IgM anti-HAV	IgM anti-HBc, HBsAg	Anti-HCV	HDAg
Chronic disease	None	HBsAg	Anti-HCV	Total anti-HDV
Infectivity	None	HBeAg, HBsAg, HBV-DNA	Anti-HCV	Total anti-HDV
Recovery	None	Anti-HBe, Anti-HBs	None	None
Carrier state	None	HBsAg	None	HDAg, anti-HD
Screening immunity	Total anti-HAV	Anti-HBs, total anti-HBc	None	None

Procedure

Obtain a 5-ml blood serum sample. Observe universal precautions.

Clinical Implications

1. Individuals with hepatitis may have generalized symptoms resembling the flu and may dismiss their illness as such.
2. A specific type of hepatitis cannot be differentiated by clinical observations alone. Testing is the only sure method to define the category.
3. Rapid diagnosis of acute hepatitis is essential both for the patient, so that treatment can be instituted, and for those who have close patient contact, so that protective measures can be taken to prevent disease spread.
4. Persons at higher risk for acquiring hepatitis A include patients and staff in healthcare and custodial institutions, people in daycare centers, IV drug abusers, and those who travel to undeveloped countries or those regions where food and water supplies may be contaminated.
5. Persons at higher risk for hepatitis B include those with a history of sexually transmitted diseases, IV drug abusers, infants born to infected mothers, hemodialysis patients, and healthcare workers.

Hepatitis Markers Following Infection

Serological Marker	*Time Marker Appears After Infection*	*Clinical Implications*
HEPATITIS A VIRUS		
HAV-Ab/IgM	4–6 wk	Positive for acute stage of hepatitis A; develops early in disease course
HAV-Ab/IgG	8–12 wk	Indicates previous exposure and immunity to hepatitis A
HEPATITIS B VIRUS		
HBsAg: hepatitis B surface antigen	4–12 wk	Positive in acute stage of hepatitis B; earliest indicator of acute infection; also indicates chronic infection
HBeAg	4–12 wk	Positive in acute active stage with viral replication (infectivity factor; "highly infectious")

(continued)

Hepatitis Markers Following Infection *(Continued)*

Serological Marker	Time Marker Appears After Infection	Clinical Implications
HEPATITIS B VIRUS		
HBcAb: hepatitis B core antibody	6–14 wk	This marker may remain in serum for a longer time; together with HBsAB represents convalescent stage; indicates past infection
ABcAbIgM	6–14 wk	Indicates acute infection
HBeAb antibody	8–16 wk	Indicates acute infection resolution
HbsAb antibody	4–10 mo	Indicates previous exposure, clinical recovery, immunity to hepatitis B; not necessarily to other types of hepatitis; the marker for permanent immunity to hepatitis B.

6. Healthcare workers should be periodically tested for hepatitis exposure and should always observe universal precautions when caring for patients.

Patient Preparation

1. Assess patient's social and clinical history and knowledge of test. Explain test purpose and procedure.
2. See Chapter 1 guidelines for safe, effective, informed *pretest* care.

Patient Aftercare

1. Explain significance of test results and counsel appropriately concerning presence of infection, recovery, and immunity. Counsel healthcare workers and family about protective and preventive measures necessary. Instruct patient to alert healthcare workers and others about hepatitis history in future situations during which exposure to body fluids and wastes may occur.
2. Pregnant women may need special counseling.
3. Follow Chapter 1 guidelines for safe, effective, informed *posttest* care.

Clinical Alert

1. Observe enteric and universal precautions (continue for 7 days after onset of symptoms or jaundice) in hepatitis A. Hepatitis A is most contagious before symptoms or jaundice appear.
2. Use universal blood and body fluid precautions for type B hepatitis and hepatitis B antigen carriers. Precautions apply until the patient is HBsAg-negative and the anti-HBs appear. Avoid sharp (needles, scalpel blades) injuries. Should accidental injury occur, encourage some bleeding and wash area well with a germicidal soap. Report injury to proper department and follow-up with necessary interventions. Put on gown when blood splattering is anticipated. A private hospital room and bathroom may be indicated.
3. *If* one has had a blood transfusion, he or she should not donate blood for 6 months. Transfusion-acquired hepatitis may not show up for 6 months posttransfusion. Persons who test positive for HBsAg should *never* donate blood or plasma.
4. Persons who have sexual contact with hepatitis B—infected individuals run a greater risk of acquiring that same infection. HBsAg appears in most body fluids, such as saliva, semen, and cervical secretions.
5. Universal precautions must be observed in all cases of suspected hepatitis until the diagnosis and hepatitis type are confirmed.
6. Immunization of persons exposed to the infection should be done as soon as possible. In the case of contact with hepatitis B, both HBIg [or, immunoglobulin (Ig)] and HBV vaccine should be administered within 24 hours of skin break and within 14 days of last sexual contact. For hepatitis A, Ig should be given within 2 weeks. In daycare centers, Ig should be given to all contacts, both children and personnel.

VIRAL ANTIBODY TESTS

Normal Values

Negative titer for viral disease: < 1:8 for complement fixation tests.

Explanation of Test

The antibody studies establish the presence of various viral diseases. Viral diseases are classified according to site as respiratory, gastrointestinal, central nervous system (CNS), and exanthem (skin eruption).

Procedure

1. Obtain a 5-ml blood serum sample. Observe universal precautions.
2. A follow-up, convalescent stage serum test is required. Spinal fluid can be tested for CNS viral determinates.

Clinical Implications
A fourfold increase in antibody titer values from acute stage to convalescent stage serum specimens indicates presence of viral infection.

Patient Preparation
1. Assess patient's clinical history and knowledge about test. Explain test purpose and procedure.
2. See Chapter 1 guidelines for safe, effective, informed *pretest* care.

Patient Aftercare
1. Interpret test outcome. Explain significance of results to patient and necessity for repeat testing.
2. Follow Chapter 1 guidelines for safe, effective, informed *posttest* care.

RABIES ANTIBODY TESTS

Normal Values
Indirect fluorescent antibody (IFA) < 1:16 or direct fluorescent examination of the animal brain for presence of the virus.

Explanation of Test
Serologic testing is diagnostic for the presence of rabies in animals. It also indicates the degree of antibody responses to rabies immunization (eg, for persons who routinely work with animals).

Procedure for Humans
Obtain a 5-ml blood serum sample. Observe universal precautions.

Procedure for Animals
1. If the suspect animal exhibits abnormal behavior, standard procedure is to sacrifice it and examine its brain for negative body inclusions in the nerves.
2. Rabies testing is usually performed in a public health laboratory.

Clinical Implications
An elevated titer in humans indicates an adequate response after immunization. A rabies titer of 1:16 or higher is considered protective.

Clinical Alert

1. Prevention: Preexposure vaccine (HDCV, human diploid cell rabies vaccine) should be given to persons at high risk, such as veterinarians, wildlife personnel, zoo workers, quarantine kennel workers, and those employed in laboratories that use animals.

(continued)

(Clinical Alert continued)

2. Postbite: Administer rabies immunoglobulin (RIg) as soon as possible after the bite, regardless of time interval, to neutralize the virus in the wound. Human diploid cell rabies vaccine in five, 1-ml intramuscular doses should be given in the deltoid muscle. The first HDCV dose is given concurrently with the RIg and then 3, 7, 14, and 28 days after the first dose.
3. The animal brain should be tested as soon as possible. Holding the animal for observation is not recommended.

Patient Preparation

1. Explain test purpose and procedure.
2. See Chapter 1 guidelines for safe, effective, informed *pretest* care.

Patient Aftercare

1. Interpret test results after immunization.
2. Follow Chapter 1 guidelines for safe, effective, informed *posttest* care.

ANTIBODY TO HUMAN IMMUNODEFICIENCY VIRUS (HIV-1/2); **ACQUIRED IMMUNODEFICIENCY SYNDROME** (AIDS) **TEST** ●

Normal Values

Negative: Nonreactive for HIV types 1 and 2 by ELISA, Western blot (WB), and indirect fluorescent antibody (IFA).

Explanation of Test

These tests detect human immunodeficiency viruses, types 1 and 2 (HIV-1/2), that cause acquired human immunodeficiency syndrome (AIDS). Infection with HIV-1 is most prevalent in the United States and Western Europe. Most cases associated with HIV-2 are reported in West Africa. Tests to detect the presence of HIV-1 antibody screen blood and blood products that will be used for transfusion. Persons at high risk for developing AIDS (homosexual men, intravenous [IV] drug users) also use the test. The diagnosis of AIDS must be clinically established. Tests used to determine the presence of antibodies to HIV-1 include ELISA, WB, and IFA.

A single reactive ELISA test by itself cannot be used to diagnose AIDS. It should always be repeated in duplicate with the same blood sample. If repeatedly reactive, follow-up tests using WB or IFA should be done. A positive WB or IFA is considered confirmatory for HIV. Recently, it has been recommended that the combination HIV-1/2 test replace the HIV-1 test when screening blood and blood products for transfusion. It is used for testing potential organ transplant donors.

Procedure

Obtain a 5-ml blood serum sample. Observe universal precautions.

Clinical Implications

1. A positive ELISA that fails to be confirmed by WB or IFA should not be considered negative, especially in the presence of symptoms or signs of AIDS. Repeat testing in 3 to 6 months is suggested.
2. A positive result may occur in noninfected persons because of unknown factors.
3. Negative tests tend to rule out AIDS in high-risk patients who do not have the characteristic opportunistic infections or tumors.
4. An HIV infection is described as a continuum of different stages that range from the acute, transient, mononucleosis-like syndrome associated with seroconversion, to asymptomatic HIV infection, to symptomatic HIV infection and, finally, to AIDS. AIDS is end-stage HIV infection.
5. Treatments are more effective and less toxic when begun early in the course of HIV infection.

Interfering Factors

1. Nonreactive HIV test results occur during the acute stage when the virus is present, but antibodies are not sufficiently developed to be detected. This may take up to 6 months. During this stage, the test for the HIV antigen may confirm an HIV infection.
2. Test kits for HIV are extremely sensitive. As a result, nonspecific reactions may occur if the tested person has been previously exposed to HIV human cells or the growth medium.

Clinical Alert

1. Issues of confidentiality surround HIV testing. Access to test results should be given judiciously on a need-to-know basis, unless the patient specifically expresses otherwise. Interventions to block general computer access to this information are necessary. Each healthcare facility must determine how best to accomplish this.
2. On the other hand, healthcare workers directly involved with the care of the HIV–AIDS patient have a right to know the diagnosis so that they may protect themselves from exposure.
3. All results, both positive and negative, must be somehow entered in the patient's healthcare records while maintaining confidentiality. People are more likely to test voluntarily when they trust that inappropriate disclosure of HIV-testing information will not occur. Long-term implications include potential loss of jobs, housing, insurance coverage, and relationship estrangements.

(continued)

(Clinical Alert continued)

4. The physician must sign a legal form stating that the patient has been informed about test risks.
5. A person who exhibits HIV antibodies is presumed to be HIV-infected; appropriate counseling, medical evaluation, and health-care interventions should be discussed and instituted.
6. Positive test results must be reported to the state public health authorities according to prescribed state regulations and protocols.
7. Anonymous testing and reporting are available.

Patient Preparation

1. An informed, witnessed consent form must be properly signed by any person being tested for HIV–AIDS. This consent form must accompany the patient and the specimen.
2. It is essential that counseling precede and follow the HIV antibody test. This test should not be performed without the subject's informed consent, and persons who need to legitimately access results must be mentioned. Discussion of the clinical and behavioral implications derived from the test results should address the accuracy of the test and should encourage behavioral modifications (eg, sexual contact, shared needles, or blood transfusions).
3. Infection control measures mandate use of universal precautions (see Appendix).
4. See Chapter 1 guidelines for safe, effective, informed *pretest* care.

Patient Aftercare

1. Interpret test outcomes. Explain significance of test results. Advise patient that screening tests must be confirmed before they are reported as HIV reactive. Provide options for immediate counseling if necessary.
2. See Chapter 1 guidelines for safe, effective, informed *posttest* care.

HERPES SIMPLEX VIRUS (HSV) ANTIBODIES: HSV-1 AND HSV-2 TEST ●

Normal Values

Some level of antibodies can be found in the normal population. Negative for HSV-1 and -2, IFA, EIA, and IHA tests.

Background

Two types of herpes simplex virus exist. Herpes simplex virus type 1 (HSV-1) causes orofacial herpes; type 2 (HSV-2) causes genital and neonatal herpes. Serologic differentiation is difficult. Therefore, type-specific antibody tests are required.

Explanation of Test

These tests identify the herpes simplex infections. Human HSV infections are found worldwide. The clinical course is variable, and symptoms may be mild enough to go unrecognized. Major signs and symptoms include oral and skin eruptions, genital tract infections and lesions, and neonatal herpes. Herpes simplex is also common in those individuals with immune system deficiencies (cancers, HIV–AIDS, chemotherapy treatment). Testing for HSV antibody is also widely used for bone marrow recipients and donors.

Procedure

1. Obtain a 5-ml blood serum sample. Observe universal precautions.
2. Follow-up testing is usually required.

Clinical Implications

1. Most persons in the general population have been infected with HSV by the age of 20. After the primary infection, antibody levels fall and stabilize until a subsequent infection occurs.
2. Diagnosis of current infection is related to determining a significant increase in antibody titers between the acute stage and the convalescent stage blood samples.
3. Serologic tests cannot indicate the presence of active genital tract infections. Instead, direct examination with procurement of lesion cultures should be done.
4. Newborn infections are acquired during delivery through the birth canal and may present as localized skin lesions or more generalized organ systems involvement.

Patient Preparation

1. Assess patient's knowledge about the test. Explain test purpose and procedure.
2. See Chapter 1 guidelines for safe, effective, informed *pretest* care.

Patient Aftercare

1. Interpret test outcomes. Refer to page 514 for interpreting results of immunologic tests. Advise pregnant women that the newborn may be infected during birth by presence of active genital area infection. Explain need for repeat testing.
2. Follow Chapter 1 guidelines for safe, effective, informed *posttest* care.

CYTOMEGALOVIRUS (CMV) **ANTIBODY TEST** ●

Normal Values

Negative for CMV antibodies by immunofluorescent assay–enzyme-linked immunoadsorbent assay and latex agglutination.

Background

Cytomegalovirus (CMV) is a ubiquitous human viral pathogen that belongs to the herpesvirus family. Infection with CMV is usually asymptomatic and can persist, in the host, as a chronic or latent infection. Cytomegalovirus has been linked with sexually transmitted infections. Blood banks routinely screen for CMV antibodies and report these as CMV-negative or CMV-positive.

Explanation of Test

This test determines the presence of CMV antibodies (eg, congenitally infected newborns, immunocompromised patients, and sexually active persons who present with mononucleosis-like symptoms). Antibody titers must be evaluated in the context of the patient's current clinical symptoms and viral culture results.

Procedure

1. Obtain a 5-ml blood serum sample. Observe universal precautions.
2. Posttransplant (organ) titers are recommended to be monitored at weekly intervals (particularly following bone marrow transplant).

Clinical Implications

1. Infants who acquire CMV during a primary infection of the mother are prone to develop severe cytomegalic inclusion disease (CID). This disease may be fatal or may cause neurologic sequelae, such as mental retardation, deafness, microcephaly, or motor dysfunction.
2. Transfusion of CMV-infected blood products or transplantation of CMV-infected donor organs may produce interstitial pneumonitis in an immunocompromised recipient.
3. Seroconversion or a significant rise in titer may indicate presence of a recent infection; however, it cannot differentiate between a primary or a recurrent antibody response.

Patient Preparation

1. Explain test purpose and procedure.
2. See Chapter 1 guidelines for safe, effective, informed *pretest* care.

Patient Aftercare

1. Interpret test results (see page 514 for interpreting results of immunologic tests) and counsel appropriately.
2. Follow Chapter 1 guidelines for safe, effective, informed *posttest* care.

HUMAN T-CELL LYMPHOTROPIC VIRUS-1 (HTLV-1) ANTIBODY TEST ●

Normal Value

Negative for human T-cell lymphotropic virus-1 (HTLV-1) antibodies.

Explanation of Test
This test detects antibodies to human T-cell lymphotropic virus 1, a retrovirus associated with adult T-cell leukemia (ATL) and demyelinating neurologic disorders. The presence of HTLV-1 antibodies in an asymptomatic person excludes that person from donating blood. (However, this finding does not mean that a leukemia or a neurologic disorder exists or will develop.)

Procedure
Obtain a 5-ml blood serum sample. Observe universal precautions.

Clinical Implications
1. Positive results (antibodies to HTLV-1) occur in the presence of HTLV-1 infection. Infection transmitted to recipients of HTLV-1–infected blood is well documented.
2. The presence of antibodies to HTLV-1 bears no relation to the presence of antibodies to HIV-1; it does not put one at risk of HIV–AIDS.
3. HTLV-1 is endemic to the Caribbean, Southeastern Japan, and some areas of Africa.
4. In the United States, HTLV-1 has been detected in persons with adult T-cell leukemia (ATL), intravenous drug users, healthy persons, and from donated blood products. Transmission can also take place through ingestion of breast milk, sexual contact, and sharing of contaminated intravenous drug paraphernalia.

Patient Preparation
1. Assess patient's knowledge about test. Explain test purpose and procedure.
2. See Chapter 1 guidelines for safe, effective, informed *pretest* care.

Patient Aftercare
1. Interpret test outcome. Inform that a positive outcome excludes person from donating blood. Assess for transmission exposure.
2. Follow Chapter 1 guidelines for safe, effective, informed *posttest* care.

PARVOVIRUS B-19 ANTIBODY TEST ●

Normal Value
Negative for parvovirus B-19-specific IgM and IgG antibodies by ELISA and IFA.

Explanation of Test
These tests detect parvovirus B-19, the only parvovirus known to cause human disease. The B-19 virus destroys red blood cell precursors and interferes with normal red blood cell production. In young children, it is associated with erythema infectiosum, a self-limiting mild disease, characterized by

a low-grade fever and rash. Recently, it has been associated with aplastic crisis in patients with chronic hemolytic anemia and those immunodeficient patients who have bone marrow failure.

Procedure

Obtain a 5-ml blood serum sample. Observe universal precautions.

Clinical Implications

Parvovirus B-19 infection has been implicated in aplastic anemia associated with organ transplants. Therefore, it is recommended that this test be included in the serologic assessment of prospective organ donors.

Patient Preparation

1. Assess patient's knowledge about test. Explain purpose and blood test procedure. Advise any prospective organ donor that this test is part of a panel of tests performed before organ donation to protect the organ recipient from potential infection.
2. See Chapter 1 guidelines for safe, effective, informed *pretest* care.

Patient Aftercare

1. Interpret test outcome (see page 514 for interpreting immunologic test results). Explain significance of test results.
2. Follow Chapter 1 guidelines for safe, effective, informed *posttest* care.

> **Clinical Alert**
>
> Repeat positive tests need to be confirmed by Western blot assay.

FUNGAL TESTS

FUNGAL ANTIBODY TESTS (HISTOPLASMOSIS, BLASTOMYCOSIS, COCCIDIOIDOMYCOSIS)

Normal Values

Negative for fungal antibodies; complement-fixation (CF) titer = < 1:8; immunodiffusion = negative

Background

Certain fungal species are associated with human respiratory diseases acquired by inhaling spores from sources such as dust, soil, and bird droppings. Serologic tests may be used for diagnosis. Fungal diseases are categorized as either "superficial" or "deep." For the most part, the superficial mycoses are limited to the skin, mucous membranes, nails, and hair. The deep mycoses involve the deeper tissues and internal organs. Histoplasmosis, coccidioidomycosis, and blastomycosis result from the deep mycoses.

Explanation of Test

These tests detect serum precipitin antibodies and complement-fixing antibodies present in the fungal diseases of coccidioidomycosis, blastomycosis, and histoplasmosis. Coccidioidomycosis (desert fever, San Joaquin fever, valley fever) is contracted through inhalation of *Coccidioides immitis* spores found in dust or soil. Blastomycosis is caused by the genus *Blastomyces*. Histoplasmosis is a granulomatous infection caused by *Histoplasma capsulatum*.

Procedure

Obtain a 7-ml blood serum sample. Observe universal precautions.

Clinical Implications

Antibodies to coccidioidomycosis, blastomycosis, and histoplasmosis appear early in the course of the disease (weeks 1–4) and then disappear.

Interfering Factors

1. Antibodies against fungi may be found in blood samples from apparently healthy people.
2. When testing for blastomycosis, cross-reactions with histoplasmosis may occur.

Patient Preparation

1. Explain test purpose and procedure. Assess for history of exposure.
2. See Chapter 1 guidelines for safe, effective, informed *pretest* care.

Patient Aftercare

1. Interpret test results (see page 514 for interpreting immunologic test results) and counsel appropriately.
2. Follow Chapter 1 guidelines for safe, effective, informed *posttest* care.

CANDIDA ANTIBODY TEST ●

Normal Values

Negative for candidal antibodies. Precipitins are occasionally found in the normal population.

Background

Candidiasis is usually caused by *Candida albicans* and affects the mucous membranes, skin, and nails. Compromised individuals with depressed T-cell function are most likely to have invasive disease.

Explanation of Test

Identifying the candidal antibody can be helpful when the diagnosis of systemic candidiasis cannot be shown by culture or tissue sample. Clinical symptomology must be present for the test to be meaningful. Tests include counterimmunoelectrophoresis (CIE), particularly valuable on CSF and urine, and latex agglutination (LA).

Procedure

Obtain a 7-ml venous blood sample. Observe universal precautions.

Clinical Implications

1. A titer higher than 1:8 by latex agglutination indicates systemic infection.
2. A fourfold rise in titers of paired blood samples 10 to 14 days apart indicates acute infection.
3. Patients receiving long-term intravenous therapy with broad-spectrum antibiotics and those who are diabetics, commonly have disseminated infections caused by *C. albicans*. Disease also occurs in bottle-fed newborns or in urinary bladder of catheterized patients.
4. Vulvovaginal candidiasis, common in late pregnancy, can transmit candidiasis to the infant through the birth canal.

Interfering Factors

1. Approximately 25% of the normal population tests positive for candida.
2. Cross-reaction can occur with LA testing in those cases who also have cryptococcosis and tuberculosis as clinical entities.
3. Positive results can occur in the presence of mucocutaneous candidiasis or severe vaginitis.

Patient Preparation

1. Explain test purpose and procedure.
2. See Chapter 1 guidelines for safe, effective, informed *pretest* care.

Patient Aftercare

1. Interpret test results (see page 514 for interpreting results of immunologic tests) and counsel appropriately. Repeat testing is usually indicated.
2. Follow Chapter 1 guidelines for safe, effective, informed *posttest* care.

ASPERGILLUS ANTIBODY TEST ●

Normal Value

Negative for aspergillus antibody by immunodiffusion.

Background

The aspergilli, especially *Aspergillus fumigatus, A. flavus,* and *A. niger,* are associated with pulmonary infections and invasive fatal disease sequelae in immunosuppressed patients. Manifestations of aspergillus infections include allergic bronchopulmonary disease, lung mycetoma, endophthalmitis, and disseminated brain, kidney, heart, and bone disease.

Explanation of Test

This test detects antibodies present in aspergillosis infections.

Procedure

1. Obtain 2-ml blood serum sample. Cerebrospinal fluid also can be tested. Observe universal precautions.

Clinical Implications

1. Positive tests are associated with pulmonary infections in compromised patients and aspergillus infections of prosthetic heart valves.
2. If blood serum exhibits one to four bands, aspergillosis is strongly suspected. Weak bands suggest an early disease process or hypersensitivity pneumonitis.

Patient Preparation

1. Explain test purpose and procedure.
2. See Chapter 1 guidelines for safe, effective, informed *pretest* care.

Patient Aftercare

1. Interpret test outcome (see page 514 for interpretation of results of immunologic tests) and counsel appropriately.
2. Follow Chapter 1 guidelines for safe, effective, informed *posttest* care.

CRYPTOCOCCUS ANTIBODY TEST ●

Normal Value

Negative for cryptococcus antibody.

Background

Cryptococcus neoformans, a yeastlike fungus, causes a lung infection thought to be acquired by inhalation. The organism has been isolated from several natural environments, especially those where weathered pigeon droppings accumulate. Symptoms include fever, headache, dizziness, ataxia, somnolence, and occasionally, cough.

Explanation of Test

This test detects antibodies present in cryptococcal infections. About 50% of patients who present with antibodies have a predisposing condition, such as lymphoma or sarcoidosis or are being treated with steroid therapy. Infection with *C. neoformans* has long been associated with Hodgkin's disease and other malignant lymphomas. In fact *C. neoformans,* in conjunction with malignancy, occurs to such a degree that some researchers have raised the question about the possible etiologic relation between the two diseases. Tests ordered for this disease include latex agglutination testing for antigens or antibodies.

Procedure

Obtain a 1-ml venous blood sample or a 2-ml spinal fluid sample. Observe universal precautions.

Clinical Implications

Positive *C. neoformans* tests are associated with infections of the lower respiratory tract by inhalation of aerosols containing *C. neoformans* cells disseminated by the fecal droppings of pigeons.

Patient Preparation

1. Explain test purpose and procedure. Obtain clinical history and assess for exposure.
2. See Chapter 1 guidelines for safe, effective, informed *pretest* care.

Patient Aftercare

1. Interpret test results (see page 514 for interpretation of results of immunologic tests) and counsel appropriately.
2. Follow Chapter 1 guidelines for safe, effective, informed *posttest* care.

● PARASITIC TESTS

TOXOPLASMOSIS (TPM) ANTIBODY TESTS ●

Normal Values

Normal

Titer < 1:16: no previous infection (*except* for ocular infection) by indirect fluorescent antibody (IFA) tests.

Titer 1:16 to 1:256: prevalent in general population

Background

Toxoplasmosis is caused by the sporozoan parasite *Toxoplasma gondii,* a severe, generalized, granulomatous central nervous system disease. It may be either congenital or postnatal and is found in humans, domestic animals (cats), and wild animals. Humans may acquire the infection through ingestion of inadequately cooked meat or other contaminated material. Congenital toxoplasmosis may cause fetal death. Symptoms of subacute infection may appear shortly after birth or much later. Complications of congenital toxoplasmosis include hydrocephaly, microcephaly, convulsions, and chronic retinitis. It is believed that one-quarter to one-half of the adult population is asymptomatically infected with toxoplasmosis. The Centers for Disease Control and Prevention (CDC) recommend serologic testing during pregnancy.

Explanation of Test

The IFA test helps differentiate toxoplasmosis from infectious mononucleosis. Toxoplasmosis antibodies appear within 1 to 2 weeks and peak at 6 to 8 months. IFA is also a valuable screening test for latent toxoplasmosis.

Procedure

Obtain a 5-ml blood serum sample. Observe universal precautions.

Clinical Implications

The IFA test is considered positive under any of the following conditions:

1. Titer of 1:256 or higher indicates recent exposure or current infection; rising titer is of greatest significance.
2. Any titer value in a newborn infant
3. Titer of 1:1024 or higher is significant for active disease.
4. Titer of 1:16 or lower occurs with ocular toxoplasmosis.

Patient Preparation

1. Explain test purpose and procedure. Obtain clinical history and assess for ingestion of contaminated material.
2. See Chapter 1 guidelines for safe, effective, informed *pretest* care.

Patient Aftercare

1. Interpret test results (see page 514 for interpretation of results of immunologic tests) and counsel appropriately.
2. Follow Chapter 1 guidelines for safe, effective, informed *posttest* care.

AMEBIASIS (*ENTAMOEBA HISTOLYTICA*) ANTIBODY TEST ●

Normal Values

Negative for amebiasis antibodies by indirect hemagglutination, latex agglutination, and counterimmunoelectrophoresis (CIE).

Explanation of Test

Entamoeba histolytica, the causative agent of amebiasis, is a pathogenic intestinal parasite. The *E. histolytica* test determines the presence or absence of specific serum antibodies to this parasite. Stool examination is considered the definitive diagnostic tool. However, the absence of detectable stool organisms does not necessarily rule out the disease; antibiotic therapy, oil enemas, and barium may alter the ability to isolate this organism in the stool.

Procedure

Obtain a 5-ml blood serum sample. Observe universal precautions.

Clinical Implications

1. Positive test of 1:128 and higher indicates active or recent infection.

   NOTE: *A positive test may only reflect past but not current infections.*

2. Amebic liver abscess and amebic dysentery produce positive results.
3. In persons currently infected, titers range from 1:256 to 1:2048 in the presence of current active amebiasis.
4. Titers of 1:32 or lower generally exclude amebiasis.

Patient Preparation

1. Explain test purpose and procedure.
2. See Chapter 1 guidelines for safe, effective, informed *pretest* care.

Patient Aftercare

1. Interpret test results (see page 514 for interpretation of immunologic test results) and counsel appropriately for infection.
2. Follow Chapter 1 guidelines for safe, effective, informed *posttest* care.

● MIXED TESTS

TORCH TEST ●

Normal Values

Negative for toxoplasma, rubella, cytomegalovirus, and herpes simplex antibodies.

Background

TORCH is an acronym that stands for *Toxoplasma,* rubella, cytomegalovirus, and herpes simplex virus. These pathogens are frequently implicated in congenital or neonatal infections that are not clinically apparent, but that may result in serious central nervous system impairment.

Explanation of Test

Both mother and newborn are tested for exposure to these agents. The test differentiates those of acute, congenital, and intrapartum infections caused by *Toxoplasma gondii,* rubella virus, cytomegalovirus, and herpes virus disorders. The presence of IgA- or IgM-associated antibodies in newborns reflects actual fetal antibody production. High levels of IgM at birth indicate fetal in utero response to an antigen. In this instance, an intrauterine infection should be considered. TORCH is more useful in excluding, rather than establishing, etiology.

Procedure

Obtain a 3-ml venous blood sample. Observe universal precautions.

Clinical Implications

1. Persistent rubella antibodies in an infant older than 6 months highly suggest congenital infection. Congenital rubella is characterized by neurosensory deafness, heart anomalies, cataracts, growth retardation, and encephalitic symptoms.
2. A diagnosis of toxoplasmosis is established through sequential testing, rather than by a single positive result. Sequential examination reveals rising antibody titers, changing titers, and the conversion of serologic tests from negative to positive. A titer of 1:256 suggests recent infection. About one-third of infants who acquire infection in utero will show signs of cerebral calcifications and chorioretinitis at birth. The rest who are infected will be born without symptoms.
3. A marked and persistent rise in complement-fixing antibody titer over time is consistent with a diagnosis of rubella in infants younger than 6 months.
4. Presence of herpes antibodies in CSF, together with signs of herpetic encephalitis and persistent herpes virus type 2 or 1 antibody levels in a newborn, who shows no obvious external lesions, is consistent with a diagnosis of herpes simplex.

Patient Preparation

1. Explain test purpose and procedure.
2. See Chapter 1 guidelines for safe, effective, informed *pretest* care.

Patient Aftercare

1. Interpret test results (see page 514 for interpretation of immunologic test results), monitor, and counsel appropriately for intrauterine and congenital infections.
2. Follow Chapter 1 guidelines for safe, effective, informed *posttest* care.

COLD AGGLUTININS (ACUTE AND CONVALESCENT STUDIES) ●

Normal Values

Normal: ≤ 1:16 by red cell agglutination at 4°C.

Background

Cold agglutinins are usually IgM autoantibodies that cause agglutination of the patient's own red blood cells at temperatures in the range of 0 to 10°C.

These antibodies, with maximum activity at temperatures below 37°C, are termed *cold* and are found in small amounts in the blood of normal persons.

Explanation of Test

This test most commonly diagnoses primary atypical viral pneumonia caused by *Mycoplasma pneumoniae* as well as certain hemolytic anemias (cold agglutination disease). The diagnosis depends on demonstrating a fourfold or higher increase in antibody titers between an early acute-phase blood serum sample and a blood serum sample taken in the convalescence phase, 7 to 10 days after the first sample. Positive reaction frequency and titer elevation both appear to be directly related to infection severity.

Procedure

Obtain a 10-ml venous blood sample. Observe universal precautions. The sample should be prewarmed to 37°C for at least 15 minutes before the serum is separated from the cells. This allows the cold agglutinating antibodies to be collected from the red cell membranes so they can be detected in the agglutination procedure using blood group O-negative indicator cells (pooled, group O donors).

Clinical Implications

1. In viral pneumonia, the titer rises 8 to 10 days after onset, peaks in 12 to 25 days, and decreases 30 days after onset. Up to 90% of persons with severe illness will exhibit positive titers.
2. Chronic increased titer levels are associated with
   - **a.** Cold antibody hemolytic anemia
   - **b.** Chronic cold agglutinin disease
   - **c.** Paroxysmal cold hemoglobinuria
   - **d.** Severe Raynaud's phenomenon (may lead to gangrene)
   - **e.** B-cell chronic lymphocytic leukemia
3. More important than any single high value is the rise in titer during the course of illness. The titer will usually decrease by the 4th to 6th week after onset of illness.
4. Transient increases in titers are associated with primary atypical viral pneumonia, infectious mononucleosis, congenital syphilis, hepatic cirrhosis, and trypanosomiasis.

Interfering Factors

1. A high cold agglutinin titer interferes with blood typing and crossmatching.
2. High titers are sometimes spontaneous in older persons and may persist for years.
3. Antibiotic therapy may interfere with cold agglutinin development.

Patient Preparation

1. Explain test purpose and procedure. Obtain clinical history and assess for interfering factors.
2. See Chapter 1 guidelines for safe, effective, informed *pretest* care.

Patient Aftercare

1. Interpret test results (see page 514 for interpretation of immunologic test results) and counsel appropriately. Cold agglutinin titers rise during the 2nd or 3rd week of illness before rapidly returning to baseline levels. The test should be repeated at appropriate intervals.
2. Follow Chapter 1 guidelines for safe, effective, informed *posttest* care.

C-REACTIVE PROTEIN (CRP) **TEST** ●

Normal Values

<0.8 mg/dl by rate nephelometry

Background

During any inflammatory process, a specific abnormal protein, named C-reactive protein (CRP) appears in the blood. This protein is virtually absent from the blood serum of healthy persons. CRP appears rapidly in blood and body fluids in response to injurious stimuli. It is thought to be mainly synthesized in the liver. Large amounts appear in peritoneal, pleural, pericardial, and synovial body fluids. CRP is the classic and most dramatic acute-phase reactant, with levels that increase up to 1000-fold, then decline rapidly when the inflammatory process regresses.

Explanation of Test

The CRP test is nonspecific for evaluating inflammatory disease course and severity in those conditions in which there is tissue necrosis, such as in myocardial infarction, malignancy, or rheumatoid arthritis. Blood serum CRP can be detected within 18 to 24 hours after the onset of tissue damage. CRP is useful for following the progress of rheumatic fever therapy and for interpreting the sedimentation rate. It has its place in monitoring the wound-healing process, especially with internal incisions, burns, and organ transplantation.

Procedure

Obtain a 10-ml blood serum sample. Observe universal precautions.

Clinical Implications

1. CRP is positive in the following conditions:
   - **a.** Rheumatic fever
   - **b.** Rheumatoid arthritis

   c. Myocardial infarction
   d. Malignancy (active, widespread)
   e. Bacterial and viral infections (acute)
   f. Postoperatively (no complications); will decline after fourth postoperative day.
2. The presence of CRP has added significance over and above elevated erythrocyte sedimentation rates (ESR), which may be influenced by altered physiologic states.
3. The CRP level tends to increase before rises in antibody titers and ESR levels occur. CRP levels also tend to decrease sooner than ESR levels.

Patient Preparation

1. Explain test purpose and procedure. Instruct the patient to fast for 8 to 12 hours before test (if required). Water may be taken.
2. See Chapter 1 guidelines for safe, effective, informed *pretest* care.

Patient Aftercare

1. Interpret test results, counsel, and monitor appropriately. Repeat testing is often necessary. A positive test indicates active inflammation but not its cause. It is an excellent tool for monitoring disease activity.
2. In rheumatoid arthritis, the test becomes negative with successful treatment and indicates that the inflammatory reaction has subsided, even though the sedimentation rate may be abnormal.
3. Follow Chapter 1 guidelines for safe, effective, informed *posttest* care.

Immunologic Tests for Immune Dysfunction, Autoimmune Diseases, and Related Disorders of the Immune System

PROTEIN TOTAL, PROTEIN ELECTROPHORESIS (BLOOD AND URINE); **SERUM PROTEIN ELECTROPHORESIS** (SPEP); **URINE PROTEIN ELECTROPHORESIS** (UPEP); **ALBUMIN, ALPHA, BETA, GAMMA GLOBULINS**

Normal Values: Serum Protein

Total protein g/dl		*Albumin g/dl*	
Adult	6.0–8.0	Adult	3.8-5.0
<5 d	5.4–7.0	Newborn	2.6–3.6
		1–3 y	3.4–4.2

Total protein g/dl		*Albumin g/dl*	
1–3 y	5.9–7.0	4–6 y	3.5–5.2
4–6 y	5.9–7.8	7–9 y	3.7–5.6
7–9 y	6.2–8.1	10–19 y	3.7–5.6
10–19 y	6.3–8.6		

$alpha_1$ Globulin:	0.1–0.3 g/dl	beta Globulin:	0.7–1.4 g/dl
$alpha_2$ Globulin:	0.6–1.0 g/dl	gamma Globulin:	0.7–1.6 g/dl

Normal Values: Urine Protein Electrophoresis (UPE):
A descriptive report is prepared by the pathologist.

Background

Serum proteins represent a diverse microenvironment. They are a source of nutrition and a buffer system. Immunoglobulins and related proteins function as immunologic agents. Carrier proteins (eg, haptoglobin, prealbumin, and transferrin) transport certain ions and molecules to their destinations. Antiproteases (eg, $alpha_1$-antitrypsin and $alpha_2$-macroglobulin) regulate the activity of various proteolytic enzymes and other classes of proteins that regulate oncotic pressure, genetic component pressures (chromosomal), and metabolic substances (hormones). Blood serum and urine are commonly screened for the monoclonal immunoglobulin component by means of serum protein electrophoresis (SPEP). Immunoglobulins are the major component of the serum gamma globulin fraction. In health, the immunoglobulins are polyclonal instead of monoclonal. When a monoclonal band is observed, it frequently signals a neoplastic process, such as multiple myeloma or Waldenstrom's macroglobulinemia. SPEP enhances follow-up procedures, such as specific protein quantification of immunoglobulins (IgA, IgG, IgM) and immunofixation. It provides one of the best tools for general screening of the human health state.

Explanation of Test

These tests can diagnose some inflammatory and neoplastic states, nephrotic syndromes, liver disease, and immune dysfunctions and can evaluate nutritional states and osmotic pressures in edematous and malnourished patients. Serum protein electrophoresis produces electrophoretic separation of the five major protein fractions (albumin and globulins: $alpha_1$, $alpha_2$, beta, and gamma) in serum and urine specimens so that a more definitive diagnosis can be made. Major components present in each protein fraction or zone exhibit characteristic and unique electrophoretic patterns. Zones are defined as the **albumin zone** (albumin) **$alpha_1$ zone**, $alpha_2$-lipoproteins (HDL, $alpha_1$-antitrypsin); **$alpha_2$ zone** ($alpha_2$-macroglobulin, haptoglobin, β-lipoprotein); **beta zone,** transferrin and C3 (complement); **gamma zone,** fibrinogen, IgA, IgM, and IgG.

Procedure

1. Obtain a 5-ml venous blood sample. Observe universal precautions. Avoid venous stasis during venipuncture.

2. First-voided morning urine specimen, or 24-hour timed specimen, is preferred. A 100-ml sample from a 24-hour urine collection is submitted for a urine protein electrophoresis.
3. To quantify the amount of protein in each fraction, separate proteins are scanned and separated according to net molecular charge by means of a densitometer and are expressed as grams per deciliter (g/dl).

Clinical Implications

1. The most frequent protein abnormalities in protein quantification and SPEP include
   - **a.** Total serum protein (the sum of circulating serum proteins) *increases* (hyperproteinemia) in dehydration and hemoconcentration states owing to fluid loss (eg, vomiting, diarrhea, poor kidney function); also found in
     - **(1)** Liver disease
     - **(2)** Multiple myeloma and other gammopaths
     - **(3)** Waldenstrom's microglobulinemia
     - **(4)** Tropical disease
     - **(5)** Sarcoidosis and other granulomatous diseases
     - **(6)** Collagen disorders, such as systemic lupus erythematosus (SLE) and rheumatoid arthritis (RA)
     - **(7)** Chronic inflammatory states
     - **(8)** Chronic infections
   - **b.** Total serum protein *decreases* (hypoproteinemia) with
     - **(1)** Insufficient nutritional intake (starvation or malabsorption)
     - **(2)** Severe liver disease and alcoholism
     - **(3)** Renal disease, nephrotic syndrome
     - **(4)** Diarrhea (Crohn's disease, ulcerative colitis)
     - **(5)** Severe skin diseases and burns
     - **(6)** Severe hemorrhage (when plasma volume is replaced more rapidly than protein)
     - **(7)** Heart failure
     - **(8)** Hypothyroidism
     - **(9)** Prolonged immobilization (eg, trauma, orthopedic surgery)
   - **c.** Serum albumin *increases* with intravenous infusions, dehydration (elevated hemoglobin and hematocrit indicate higher albumin levels).
   - **d.** Serum albumin *decreases* in
     - **(1)** Decreased synthesis states, such as liver diseases, alcoholism, malabsorption syndromes, Crohn's disease, other protein-losing enteropathies, starvation states, congenital analbuminemia
     - **(2)** *Increased* albumin loss (eg, nephrotic syndrome, third-degree burns)
     - **(3)** Poor nutrition states, inadequate iron intake
     - **(4)** Low albumin/globulin (A/G) ratio (eg, collagen disease, chronic inflammation, liver diseases, macroglobulinemia, severe infections, cachexia, burns, ulcerative colitis)

e. alpha$_1$-Globulin increases with infections (acute and chronic) and febrile reactions

f. alpha$_1$-Globulin decreases with nephrosis and alpha-antitrypsin deficiency.

g. alpha$_2$-Globulin increases in

- **(1)** Biliary cirrhosis
- **(2)** Obstructive jaundice
- **(3)** Nephrosis
- **(4)** Multiple myeloma (rare)
- **(5)** Ulcerative colitis

h. alpha$_2$-Globulin decreases in acute hemolytic anemia.

i. beta Globulin increases in biliary cirrhosis, obstructive jaundice, multiple myeloma (occasional).

j. beta Globulin decreases in nephrosis.

k. gamma Globulin increases in

- **(1)** Chronic infections
- **(2)** Hepatic diseases
- **(3)** Autoimmune diseases
- **(4)** Collagen diseases
- **(5)** Multiple myeloma
- **(6)** Waldenstrom's macroglobulinemia
- **(7)** Leukemia and other cancers

l. gamma Globulin decreases in agammaglobulinemia, hypogammaglobulinemia, and nephrotic syndrome.

Interfering Factors

1. Decreased albumin can be seen with rapid IV fluid infusions and hydration and during all trimesters of pregnancy.
2. Excessive hemolysis will decrease albumin 0.5 g/ml when patients are in the supine position. Conversely, hemolysis and dehydration will elevate the total serum protein.
3. Prolonged bed rest and the last trimester of pregnancy lowers total protein.

Patient Preparation

1. Explain test purpose and specimen collection procedure.
2. If a 24-hour urine is to be collected, the patient will need specific instructions, an appropriate container, and a receptacle for catching the voided urine (see Chap. 3, Urine Studies).
3. Follow guidelines in Chapter 1 for safe, effective, informed *pretest* care.

Patient Aftercare

1. Interpret test outcome and monitor appropriately. Very low levels of protein and albumin are associated with edema and hypocalcemia. Assess the patient for signs and symptoms related to these. Report and document same. Rarely is any one type of electrophoretic analysis used to diagnose a gammopathy. Follow-up testing may include immunofixation electrophoresis (IFE), quantitative immunoglobulins, or bone marrow studies.
2. Follow guidelines in Chapter 1 for safe, effective, informed *posttest* care.

Clinical Alert

Normally, very little protein is excreted in the urine. However, relatively large amounts may escape in certain disease states. In the presence of lipoid nephrosis, selective proteinuria produces excess albumin excretion. With nonselective proteinuria (eg, glomerulonephritis), all types of serum proteins usually appear in the urine. Urine protein electrophoresis can identify Bence Jones proteins, which migrate in the beta and gamma globulin regions. See Chapter 3 for complete explanation of urine protein and albumin.

QUANTITATIVE IMMUNOGLOBULINS: IgA, IgG, IgM

Normal Values

IMMUNOGLOBULINS

IgG: 700–1500 mg/dl for men and women ≥ 18 years of age
IgA: 60–400 mg/dl for men and women ≥ 18 years of age
IgM: 60–300 mg/dl for men and women ≥ 18 years of age

These values are derived from rate nephelometry.

PEDIATRIC NORMALS

(Results reported in mg/dl; ranges ±250)

IgA (males and females)	
0–4 mo	5–64
5–8 mo	10–87
9–14 mo	17–94
15–23 mo	22–178
2–3 y	24–192
4–6 y	26–232
7–9 y	33–258
10–12 y	45–285
13–15 y	47–317
16–17 y	55–377

IgG (males and females)	
0–4 mo	141–930
5–8 mo	250–1190
9–11 mo	320–1250
1–3 y	400–1250
4–6 y	560–1307
7–9 y	598-1379
10–12 y	638-1453
13–15 y	680–1531
16–17 y	724–1611

IgM (males)	
0–4 mo	14–142
5–8 mo	24–167
9–23 mo	35–200
2–3 y	41–200
4–17 y	47–200

IgM (females)	
0–4 mo	14–142
5–8 mo	24–167
9–23 mo	35–242
2–3 y	41–242
4–17 y	56–242

Background

Five classes of immunoglobulins (antibodies)—IgA, IgG (with four subclasses $IgG_{1,2,3,4}$, IgM, IgD, and IgE—have been isolated. Immunoglobulins function to neutralize toxic substances, support phagocytosis, and destroy microorganism functions. For example, IgA takes two forms: serum and secretory. Serum IgA is present in blood serum; secretory IgA is found in saliva, tears, colostrum, and bronchial, GI, and GU secretions where it can protect against microorganism invasion.

IgG, the only immunoglobulin that can cross the placenta, is responsible for protection of the newborn during the first months of life. IgM possesses antibody activity against gram-negative organisms and rheumatoid factors and forms the natural antibodies, such as the ABO blood group. IgM does not cross the placenta and, therefore, is usually absent in the newborn. It is observed approximately 5 days after birth.

Explanation of Test

Quantitative immunoglobulin measurements can monitor the course of a disease and its treatment. If there is a monoclonal protein or M component present on serum protein electrophoresis (SPEP), a quantitative measurement of IgA, IgG, and IgM, can identify the specific immunoglobulin. IgD and IgE are present in trace amounts.

Procedure

Obtain a 10-ml venous blood sample. Observe universal precautions.

Clinical Implications

1. IgA (accounts for 10%–15% of total immunoglobulin) *increases* occur in
- **a.** Chronic, nonalcoholic liver diseases, especially primary biliary cirrhosis (PBC).
- **b.** Obstructive jaundice
- **c.** Exercise
- **d.** Alcoholism
- **e.** Subacute and chronic infections

2. IgA *decreases* occur in
- **a.** Ataxia-telangiectasia
- **b.** Chronic sinopulmonary disease
- **c.** Congenital deficit
- **d.** Late pregnancy
- **e.** Prolonged exposure to benzene
- **f.** Abstinence from alcohol after a period of 1 year
- **g.** Drug and dextrin immunosuppressive therapy
- **h.** Protein-losing gastroenteropathies

Clinical Alert (for IgA)

Persons with IgA deficiency are predisposed to autoimmune disorders and can develop antibody to IgA, with possible anaphylaxis occurring if transfused with IgA blood.

3. IgG (75%–80% of total immunoglobulins) *increases* occur in
   a. Chronic granulomatous infections
   b. Hyperimmunization
   c. Liver disease
   d. Malnutrition (severe)
   e. Dysproteinemia
   f. Disease associated with hypersensitivity granulomas, dermatologic disorders, and IgG myeloma
   g. Rheumatoid arthritis
4. IgG *decreases* occur in
   a. Agammaglobulinemia
   b. Lymphoid aplasia
   c. Selective IgG, or IgA deficiency
   d. IgA myeloma
   e. Bence Jones proteinemia
   f. Chronic lymphoblastic leukemia
5. IgM (5%–10% of total antibody) *increases* (in adults) occur in
   a. Waldenstrom's macroglobulinemia
   b. Trypanosomiasis
   c. Malaria
   d. Infectious mononucleosis
   e. Lupus erythematosus
   f. Rheumatoid arthritis
   g. Dysgammaglobulinemia (certain cases)

Clinical Alert

In the newborn, a level of IgM above 20 mg/dl indicates in utero stimulation of the immune system (eg, rubella virus, cytomegalovirus, syphilis, or toxoplasmosis).

6. IgM *decreases* occur in
   a. Agammaglobulinemia
   b. Lymphoproliferative disorders (certain cases)
   c. Lymphoid aplasia
   d. IgG and IgA myeloma
   e. Dysgammaglobulinemia
   f. Chronic lymphoblastic leukemia

Patient Preparation

1. Explain test purpose and specimen collection procedure. Assess for relevant clinical history.
2. See guidelines in Chapter 1 for safe, effective, informed *pretest* care.

Patient Aftercare

1. See posttest care for protein electrophoresis. The same guidelines prevail.
2. Interpret test outcome. Follow-up immunoglobulin testing may be necessary, along with serum viscosity to monitor a patient with monoclonal gammopathy.
3. Follow Chapter 1 guidelines for safe, effective, informed *posttest* care.

IMMUNOFIXATION ELECTROPHORESIS (IFE OR IEP): URINE AND BLOOD

Normal Values

No abnormality present.

Background

Monoclonal immunoglobulins consist of heavy and light chains. Immunofixation electrophoresis (IFE) identifies the presence or absence of a monoclonal protein and determines its heavy-chain and light-chain types.

Explanation of Test

This test measures immune status and competence by identifying monoclonal and particle protein band immunoglobulins involved in the immune response. IFE is a follow-up test when a monoclonal spike is observed on SPEP, or if a monoclonal gammopathy is suggested on the basis of the patient's immunoglobulin concentrations.

Procedure

1. Obtain a fasting 15-ml venous blood sample or 24-hour urine specimen, or both. Observe universal precautions. Submit 25 ml from a 24-hour urine collection if a urine IFE is to be run simultaneously.
2. In IFE, high-resolution electrophoresis produces stained bands. By comparing the location of the stained immunofixed band with a band in the same location in the SPEP reference pattern, a particular protein band can be identified.

Clinical Implications

1. *Monoclonal* protein in the serum or urine suggests a neoplastic process; a *polyclonal* increase in immunoglobulins is seen in chronic liver disease, connective tissue disease, and infection.
2. In multiple myeloma, 99% of patients will have a monoclonal protein in the serum or urine. Waldenstrom's macroglobulinemia is always characterized by the presence of a serum monoclonal IgM protein.
3. A monoclonal light chain (kappa or Bence Jones protein) is found in the urine of approximately 75% of patients with multiple myeloma. Approximately 75% of patients with Waldenstrom's macroglobulinemia will have a monoclonal light chain in the urine. Heavy-chain fragments as well as free light chains may be seen in the urine of patients with multiple myeloma or amyloidosis.

Patient Preparation

1. Explain test purpose and specimen collection procedure.
2. If a blood sample is needed, fasting is required. Note patient's age (this procedure is seldom indicated in patients younger than 30, as monoclonal proteins are rarely identified in this age group).
3. A 24-hour urine specimen is preferred. Provide instructions and a 24-hour collection container (see Chap. 3 Urine Studies for protocols).
4. See Chapter 1 guidelines for safe, effective, informed *pretest* care.

Patient Aftercare

1. Interpret test outcomes and monitor appropriately for neoplasms, infection, liver, and connective tissue disease.
2. Follow Chapter 1 guidelines for safe, effective, informed *posttest* care.

TOTAL HEMOLYTIC COMPLEMENT (CH50)

Normal Values

25–110 units/ml by hemolytic tube titration

Background

Complement (C) is a complex sequential cascade system in which inactive proteins become active and interact very much like the clotting system. The complement system is very important as part of the body's defense mechanism against infection. Activation of complement results in cell lysis, release of histamine from mast cells and platelets, increased vascular permeability, contraction of smooth muscle, and chemotaxis of leukocytes. These inactive proteins make up about 10% of the globulins in normal blood serum. The complement system is also interrelated with the coagulation, fibrinolytic, and kinin systems. The action of complement, however, is not always beneficial. The potent reactions mediated by this complex system cannot always be contained. In the presence of gram-negative bacteremia, the complement can escape its built-in control mechanisms, causing severe damage to the body in the process. It is not clear how this happens, but it is known that complement abnormalities develop before shock occurs.

Explanation of Test

This test screens for certain autoimmune diseases, estimates the extent of immune complex formation, and detects all inherited and most acquired complement deficiencies. Serial measurements monitor disease course and treatment in systemic lupus erythematosus, rheumatoid arthritis, and glomerulonephritis. It is a useful adjunct for rheumatoid factor (RF) and systemic lupus erythematosus (SLE) testing when immune complexes appear to be the primary mediators of tissue injury.

Procedure

Obtain a 10-ml venous blood sample. Observe universal precautions. A joint fluid specimen (at least 1 ml) also can be collected in a tube without additives.

Clinical Alert

Complement deteriorates at room temperature and serum or fluid samples should be brought to the laboratory as soon as possible. Separate serum from clot and freeze at −70°C until test is performed. Both blood and fluid must be processed and frozen within 2 hours after the time of specimen collection. Failure to process in this manner may lead to falsely decreased functional activity levels.

Clinical Implications

1. *Increased total complement values* are associated with most inflammatory responses; these acquired elevations are usually transient and concentrations return to normal when the situation is resolved.
2. *Decreased total complement values* are associated with hereditary defects of a specific complement's components. In C2 deficiency, autoimmune disorders, such as lupus erythematosus and C1q deficiency, may cause agammaglobulinemia. Lack of one of the complement system inhibitors such as complement esterase inhibitor occurs in hereditary angioedema. Complement consumption by activation of the alternative pathway, an amplification of the classical pathway not requiring an "immunologic" stimulus, can be seen in
   - **a.** Gram-negative septicemia
   - **b.** Subacute bacterial endocarditis
   - **c.** Acute poststreptococcal glomerulonephritis (APSGN)
   - **d.** Membranoproliferative glomerulonephritis (MPGN)
3. Complement consumption owing to activation of the classic pathway by immune complex formation is seen in
   - **a.** Systemic lupus erythematosus
   - **b.** Serum sickness
   - **c.** Acute vasculitis
   - **d.** Severe rheumatoid arthritis
   - **e.** Hepatitis
   - **f.** Cryoglobulinemia

Patient Preparation and Patient Aftercare

See special section on collagen, rheumatic, and connective tissue disease diagnosis.

C3 COMPLEMENT COMPONENT ●

Normal Values

70–150 mg/dl by rate nephelometry

Background

C3 composes 70% of the total protein in the complement system and is essential to the activation of both the classical and alternative pathways. Along with the other components of the complement system, C3 may be used up in reactions that occur in some antigen–antibody reactions. C3 is synthesized in liver, macrophages, fibroblasts, lymphoid cells, and skin.

Explanation of Test

This test is done when it is suspected that individual complement component concentrations are abnormally reduced. This test and C1q and C4 are the most frequently ordered complement measurements. There is a correlation between most forms of nephritis, the degree of nephritis severity, and C3 levels.

Procedure
Obtain a 2-ml or greater venous blood sample. Observe universal precautions.

Clinical Implications
1. *Decreased C3 levels* are associated with most active diseases with immune complex formation.
   - **a.** Severe recurrent bacterial infections owing to C3 homozygous deficiency
   - **b.** Absence of C3b inactivator factor
   - **c.** Acute poststreptococcal glomerulonephritis (APSGN)
   - **d.** Immune complex disease
   - **e.** Active systemic lupus erythematosus
   - **f.** Membranoproliferative glomerulonephritis (MPGN)
   - **g.** Autoimmune hemolytic anemia
   - **h.** Nephritis
   - **i.** Rheumatoid arthritis
   - **j.** Disseminated intravascular coagulation (DIC) disorder
   - **k.** Liver disease
2. *Increased levels* are found in numerous inflammatory states.

Patient Preparation and Patient Aftercare
See special section on collagen, rheumatic, and connective tissue disease diagnosis.

> **Clinical Alert**
>
> Patients with low C3 levels are in danger of shock, leading to death.

C4 COMPLEMENT COMPONENT

Normal Values
10–30 mg/dl by rate nephelometry

Background
C4 is another of the components of the complement system, as synthesized in bone and lung tissue. C4 may be bypassed in the alternative complement pathway when immune complexes are not involved, or it may be used up in the very complicated series of reactions that follow many antigen–antibody reactions.

Explanation of Test
This is a follow-up test done when total complement levels are abnormally decreased.

Procedure
Obtain a 2-ml or larger venous blood sample. Observe universal precautions.

Clinical Implications

1. *Decreased C4 levels* are associated with
   - **a.** Acute systemic lupus erythematosus
   - **b.** Early glomerulonephritis
   - **c.** Immune complex disease
   - **d.** Cryoglobulinemia
   - **e.** Inborn C4 deficiency
   - **f.** Hereditary angioneurotic edema
2. *Increased C4 levels* are associated with malignancies.

Patient Preparation and Patient Aftercare

See special section on collagen, rheumatic, and connective tissue disease diagnosis.

C′1 ESTERASE INHIBITOR (C′1 INH)

Normal Values by Radial Immunodiffusion (RID)

Functional (reported as functional or nonfunctional).

Background

C′1 esterase inhibitor is a glycoprotein. It acts as a regulatory brake on the complement activation process. Decreased production of this glycoprotein results in hereditary angioedema (HAE).

Explanation of Test

This determination is an important tool for diagnosing HAE, a disorder caused by low concentration of C′1 esterase inhibitor or by an abnormal structure of the protein. Affected persons are apparently heterozygous for the condition. It is also used in the differential diagnosis of the more prevalent, less serious, allergic and nonfamilial angioedema.

Procedure

Obtain at least a 1-ml venous blood sample. Observe universal precautions.

Clinical Implications

Decreased values are associated with HAE, a genetic disease characterized by acute edema of subcutaneous tissue, GI tract, or upper respiratory tract. During acute attacks of the disease, C4 and C2 components can be markedly reduced.

Patient Preparation and Patient Aftercare

See special section on collagen, rheumatic, and connective tissue disease diagnosis.

Clinical Alert

Prednisolone and transfusions of fresh frozen plasma have been successfully used to treat HAE.

SOLUBLE AMYLOID BETA-PROTEIN PRECURSOR (sBPP) ●

Normal Value

Greater than 450 units/L (age-matched controls of 55 years) based on ELISA.

Background

A hallmark of Alzheimer's disease is deposition of the amyloid beta protein in senile plaques within the brain. In some studies, sBPP has been neuroprotective, whereas in others, amyloid beta protein has demonstrated neurotoxic effects. The sBPP is normally found in *cerebrospinal fluid* (CSF) of healthy individuals.

Explanation of Test

This test is used in the diagnosis of Alzheimer's disease. sBPP in the CSF of some, but not all, elderly patients suffering from dementia is lower than that in the CSF of normal, elderly control subjects.

Procedure

A CSF sample is collected by lumbar puncture, and a small portion is tested by ELISA. The exact amount of CSF fluid needed should be confirmed with the laboratory performing the assay.

Clinical Implications

1. Low CSF levels of sBPP suggest alteration in amyloid beta protein precursor processing and amyloid beta protein formation.
2. Correspondingly low sBPP levels correlate with clinically diagnosed and autopsy-confirmed Alzheimer's disease.

Patient Preparation

1. Explain spinal tap purpose and procedure. See Chapter 4 for protocols.
2. Follow guidelines in Chapter 1 for safe, effective, informed *pretest* care.

Patient Aftercare

1. Interpret test outcomes and counsel appropriately. As a result of performing this laboratory test, the diagnosis and understanding of Alzheimer's disease may become clearer, and appropriate counseling and support to the patient and family may be provided with a higher degree of confidence. Recently, the drug, tacrine (Cognex), has been approved for treatment of Alzheimer's disease. Measuring sBPP helps in selecting patients for clinical trials and in identifying patients who may benefit from therapy.
2. Follow Chapter 1 guidelines for safe, effective, informed *posttest* care.

LYMPHOCYTE IMMUNOPHENOTYPING: T AND B CELLS

Normal Values of Adult Peripheral Blood by Flow Cytometry

T AND B SURFACE MARKERS

Cells	*Percentage (%)*
Total T cells (CD3)	53–88
T-helper cells ($CD3^+$ $CD4^+$)	32–61
T-suppressor cells ($CD3^+$ $CD8^+$)	18-42
B-cells (CD19)	5–20
Natural killer cells (CD16)	4–32

ABSOLUTE COUNTS (BASED ON PATHOLOGIST'S INTERPRETATION)

Cells	*Number of Cells (μl)*
Lymphocytes	0.66–4.60 thousand
Total T cells (CD3)	812–2318
T-helper cells ($CD3^+$ $CD4^+$)	589–1505
T-suppressor cells ($CD3^+$ $CD8^+$)	325–997
B-cells (CD19)	92–426
Natural killer cells (CD16)	78-602

LYMPHOCYTE RATIO

T-helper/T-suppressor > 1.0

Background

Lymphocytes are divided into two categories, T and B cells, according to their primary function within the immune system. In the body, T and B cells work together to help provide protection against infectious and oncogenic agents and foreign tissue; they also play a vital role in regulating self-destruction or autoimmunity.

The majority of circulating lymphocytes are T cells, with a lifespan of months to years. The B cells constitute 10% to 30% of the lymphocytes, and lifespan measured in days. The *B cells* (*antibody*) are considered "bursa- or bone marrow-dependent," and are responsible for humoral immunity (in which antibodies are present in the serum). The *T cells (cellular)* are thymus-derived and responsible for cellular immunity. The T cells are further divided into T-helper ($CD3^+$ $CD4^+$) cells and T-suppressor ($CD3^+$ $CD8^+$) cells.

Explanation of Test

Evaluation of lymphocytes in the clinical laboratory is performed by quantitation of the lymphocytes and their subpopulations and by assessment of their functional activity. These laboratory analyses have become an essential component of the clinical assessment of two major disease states: 1)

Lymphoproliferative—characterization of the malignant cell in terms of lineage and stage of differentiation has provided valuable information to the oncologist treating a patient with leukemia or lymphoma, ie, prognosis, appropriate therapy and 2) Immunodeficient—evaluations in alterations in the immune system secondary to infection, ie, HIV-positive patients and monitoring organ transplant patients.

The method of lymphocyte quantitation and characterization is based on the detection of cell surface makers by very specific monoclonal antibodies. For cell surface immunophenotyping, flow cytometry rapidly has become the method of choice. Cell surface phenotyping is accomplished by reacting cells from an appropriate specimen with one or more labeled monoclonal antibodies and passing them though a flow cytometer, which counts the proportion of labeled cells.

Procedure

A venous blood sample is obtained. The sample must not be refrigerated or frozen. It should remain at room temperature until testing can be performed. A separate venous blood sample for hematology should be collected at the same time. Because the interpretation of data is based on absolute values, it is imperative that a WBC and Diff be perrformed so the appropriate data can be obtained.

Clinical Implications

1. Standard immunosuppressive drug therapy usually *decreases* lymphocyte totals.
2. Patients with an absolute T-helper ($CD3^+$ $CD4^+$) cell count of fewer than $200/mm^3$ are at greatest risk for developing clinical AIDS.
3. *Decreased* T cells occur in congenital immunodeficiency diseases (eg, DiGeorge syndrome, thymic hypoplasia).
4. *Decreased* T cells occur in kidney and heart transplant patients receiving OKT-3, an immunomodulatory drug to prevent rejection.
5. A marked *increase* in B cells occurs in lymphoproliferative disorders (eg, chronic lymphocytic leukemia [CLL]). The typical case of CLL would be positive for either kappa or lambda light chains (indicating monoclonality) and express CD19 (a B-cell antigen).

Patient Preparation

1. Explain purpose and specimen collection procedure. A recent viral cold can cause a decrease in total T cells, as can medications such as corticosteroids. Nicotine and strenuous exercise also decrease lymphocyte counts.
2. Follow guidelines in Chapter 1 for safe, effective, informed *pretest* care.

Patient Aftercare

1. Interpret test outcomes and possible need for repeat testing. Lymphocyte immunophenotyping is performed to monitor patients who are HIV-positive and have begun medication treatment. Transplant patients are

also retested at regular intervals to assess threat of organ rejection or host infection.

2. See guidelines in Chapter 1 for safe, effective, informed *posttest* care.

THYROID ANTIBODY GROUP (ANTITHYROGLOBULIN AND ANTIMICROSOMAL) ●

Normal Values by Gelatin Particle Agglutination

< 1:100 by gelatin

Background

Antibodies to thyroid gland components occur in various thyroid disorders. Several autoantibodies are involved, including one reaction against thyroglobulin and another against the microsomal component of thyroid epithelial cells. In certain destructive thyroid diseases, intact thyroglobulin may be released from the thyroid gland, stimulating antibody formation. These antibodies may be responsible for further destruction of this gland.

Explanation of Test

These studies detect elevated thyroid antibodies in certain thyroid diseases, such as Hashimoto's disease. When tests for both thyroglobulin antibodies and thyroid microsomal antibodies are done in combination, the specificity for detection of thyroid autoimmune antibodies is greatly increased and is more sensitive than a single test used for detection. Patients with low thyroid antibody titers should be tested periodically because the presence of the antibody may be an early sign of autoimmune disease.

Procedure

Obtain a 10-ml venous blood sample. Observe universal precautions.

Clinical Implications

1. High titers of both antibodies are found in Hashimoto's disease (hypothyroid), idiopathic myxedema, Grave's disease, nontoxic goiter, thyroid cancer, pernicious anemia.
2. Patients with Hashimoto's thyroiditis have a higher frequency of other autoimmune disorders (eg, Sjogren's syndrome and SLE). About 30% of the patients also have antiparietal cell antibodies.

Interfering Factors

About 10% of the population may have low titers of thyroid antibodies, with no symptoms of disease. Prevalence is higher in women and increases with age.

Patient Preparation

1. Explain test purpose. Thyroid antibody group testing is done to confirm diagnosis and monitor the course of disease activity.
2. See Chapter 1 guidelines for safe, effective, informed *pretest* care.

Patient Aftercare

1. Interpret test outcomes and need for possible follow-up testing. Diagnosis of autoimmune thyroiditis is made on the basis of clinical observations, thyroid function tests, and the presence of circulating autoantibodies (eg, antithyroglobulin and antimicrosomal).
2. Follow Chapter 1 guidelines for safe, effective, informed *posttest* care.

ANTI–SMOOTH-MUSCLE ANTIBODY (ASMA) TEST ●

Normal Values

Negative by indirect immunofluorescence.
If possible, serum will be titered.

Background

The ASMA is associated with liver and bile duct autoimmune diseases. The immune response itself is believed responsible for disease process.

Explanation of Test

This measurement differentiates chronic active hepatitis and primary biliary cirrhosis from other liver diseases in which anti–smooth-muscle antibodies (ASMAs) are seldom present (eg, systemic lupus erythematosus).

Procedure

Obtain a 10-ml venous blood sample. Observe universal precautions.

Clinical Implications

1. ASMAs are found in chronic active hepatitis, a progressive disease of unknown etiology found predominantly in young women; it has factors characteristic of both acute and chronic hepatitis (80% of patients). If this disease is associated with a positive antinuclear antibody test, the disease is often called *lupoid hepatitis*. ASMAs are also found in biliary cirrhosis.
2. ASMA antibodies are seldom present in
   a. Extrahepatic biliary obstruction
   b. Drug-induced liver disease
   c. Acute alcoholic hepatitis
   d. Hepatoma
3. More than 20% of patients with intrinsic asthma have ASMAs. (See Table 8-4 on the prevalence of autoantibodies in liver disease.)

Patient Preparation

1. Explain test purpose and procedure.
2. See guidelines in Chapter 1 for safe, effective, informed *pretest* care.

Patient Aftercare

1. Interpret test outcomes and monitor appropriately. Detection of ASMA by immunofluorescence will assist in determining the presence of chronic

TABLE 8-4
Prevalence of Autoantibodies in Liver Disease

Disease	*Anti–Smooth Muscle (%)*	*Antimitochondrial (%)*	*ANA*
Chronic active hepatitis	70–90	30–60	60
Chronic persistent hepatitis	45	15–20	15–30
Acute viral hepatitis	10–30	5–20	20
Acute alcoholic hepatitis	0	0	0
Biliary cirrhosis	30	60–70	5
Cryptogenic cirrhosis	15	30	0
Alcoholic (Laennee's) cirrhosis	0	0	0
Extrahepatic biliary obstruction	5–10	5–10	5

active hepatitis (CAH) and the need for therapy when used in conjunction with other laboratory tests, such as those used to evaluate liver enzymes, antinuclear antibodies, and IgG levels. All of these are elevated in most patients with CAH.

2. Follow guidelines in Chapter 1 for safe, effective, informed *posttest* care.

ANTIMITOCHONDRIAL ANTIBODY (AMA) TEST ●

Normal Values

Negative by indirect immunofluorescence.
If positive, serum will be titered.

Background

Antimitochondrial antibody (AMA) is non–organ- and non–species-specific and is directed against a lipoprotein in the inner mitochondrial membrane. The AMAs are preponderantly of the IgG class; however, they have not been proved to directly cause liver cell or bile duct destruction.

Explanation of Test

This measurement aids in the diagnosis of primary biliary cirrhosis (PBC). This is a progressive disease most commonly seen in women in the second half of their reproductive period. These antibodies are also associated with autoantibodies and autoimmune disease.

Procedure

Obtain a 10-ml venous blood sample. Observe universal precautions.

Clinical Implications

1. A titer of 1:160 or higher is present in 79% to 94% of patients with primary biliary cirrhosis.
2. High titers are also associated with long-standing hepatic obstruction, chronic hepatitis, and cryptogenic cirrhosis.
3. They are occasionally present in patients with:
   - **a.** Systemic lupus erythematosus
   - **b.** Rheumatoid arthritis
   - **c.** Thyroid disease
   - **d.** Pernicious anemia
   - **e.** Idiopathic Addison's disease

Patient Preparation

1. Explain test purpose and procedure.
2. Follow guidelines in Chapter 1 for safe, effective, informed *pretest* care.

Patient Aftercare

1. Interpret test outcomes and monitor appropriately. Immunofluorescence testing, along with quantitation of IgM and liver enzymes, both of which tend to be elevated in PBC, are reliable follow-up protocols.
2. See Chapter 1 guidelines for safe, effective, informed *posttest* care.

ANTIPARIETAL CELL ANTIBODY (APCA) TEST ●

Normal Values

Negative for APCA by indirect immunofluorescence.
If positive, serum will be titered

Background

The disruption of normal intrinsic factor production or function by autoimmune processes can lead to pernicious anemia. Antibodies to two antigens of the gastric parietal cell, antiparietal cell antibodies (APCAs) and intrinsic factor antibodies, are found in pernicious anemia.

Explanation of Test

This measurement is helpful in diagnosing chronic gastric disease and differentiating autoimmune pernicious anemia from other megaloblastic anemias. Persons with other anemias will not have detectable APCAs.

Procedure

Obtain a 10-ml venous blood sample. Observe universal precautions.

Clinical Implications

1. The APCAs occur in 80% to 90% of patients with autoimmune pernicious anemia; 50% will have antibodies to intrinsic factor.
2. Occasionally, APCAs are present in

a. Gastric ulcer
b. Gastric cancer
c. Atrophic gastritis
d. Thyroid disease
e. Diabetes mellitus

Interfering Factors

In normal children, there is a 2% incidence of APCAs and up to a 10% to 20% prevalence in the elderly.

Patient Preparation

1. Explain test purpose and procedure.
2. Follow guidelines in Chapter 1 for safe, effective, informed *pretest* care.

Patient Aftercare

1. Interpret test outcomes and monitor appropriately. Detection of AMA by immunofluorescence along with quantitation of IgM and liver enzymes, both of which tend to be elevated in primary biliary cirrhosis (PBC), constitute reliable follow-up treatment protocols.
2. See Chapter 1 guidelines for safe, effective, informed *posttest* care.

ANTIGLOMERULAR BASEMENT MEMBRANE (AGBM) ANTIBODY TEST ●

Normal Values

Negative:	< 20 units by EIA (enzyme immunoassay)
Borderline:	20–99 units
Positive:	> 100 units

Background

Antibodies specific for renal structural components, such as the glomerular basement membrane of the kidney, can bind to respective tissue-fixed antigens to produce an immune response.

Explanation of Test

This test is primarily used in the differential diagnosis of glomerular nephritis (induced by antiglomerular basement membrane antibodies [AGBMs]) from other types of glomerular nephritis. The AGBMs cause about 5% of glomerular nephritis; about two-thirds of these patients may also develop pulmonary hemorrhage (Goodpasture's syndrome).

Procedure

Obtain a 5-ml venous blood sample. Observe universal precautions.

Clinical Implications

The AGBM antibodies are detected in

1. Anti-GBM glomerular nephritis
2. Tubulointerstitial nephritis
3. Anti-GM Goodpasture's syndrome
4. Some patients with systemic lupus erythematosus (SLE)

Patient Preparation

1. Explain test purpose and procedure.
2. Follow Chapter 1 guidelines for safe, effective, informed *pretest* care.

Patient Aftercare

1. Interpret test outcomes and need for follow-up testing and treatments that involve immunosuppressants and plasmapheresis (effective if treatment is started before renal failure is well advanced).
2. See Chapter 1 guidelines for safe, effective, informed *posttest* care.

ACETYLCHOLINE RECEPTOR (AChR)-BINDING ANTIBODY TEST ●

Normal Values

Negative for AChR or ≤ 0.02 nmol/L by radioimmunoassay (RIA).

Background

Acetylcholine receptor antibodies (AChRs) appear in myasthenia gravis (MG). It is believed that this disease involves destruction by the muscle cells of acetylcholine receptors bound by antibodies at the skeletal muscle motor endplate.

Explanation of Test

This measurement is considered to be the primary diagnostic test for MG in symptomatic patients. It also helps in managing response to immunosuppressive therapy.

Procedure

Obtain a 10-ml venous blood sample. Observe universal precautions.

Clinical Implications

1. The AChR antibodies are found in approximately 87% of persons with generalized MG; in 71% of persons with ocular MG; and 81% of persons in remission. These findings confirm the autoimmune nature of the disease.
2. Patients who have only eye symptoms tend to have lower titers than those with generalized myasthenia symptoms.

Interfering Factors

False-positive binding occurs in amyotrophic lateral sclerosis patients who have been treated with snake venom.

Patient Preparation

1. Explain test purpose. Assess for history of immunosuppressive drug treatment. Detection of acetylcholine receptor-binding antibody is infrequent in such cases.
2. Follow Chapter 1 guidelines for safe, effective, informed *pretest* care.

Patient Aftercare

1. Interpret test outcomes and possible need for other testing. Other tests now available to aid in the serologic diagnosis of MG include acetylcholine receptor-blocking antibodies, acetylcholine receptor-modulating antibody, and striational antibodies. These are ordered according to presentation of neurologic symptoms. All of these antibodies are less frequently detected in the early stages of MG (within 1 year of onset) and in patients treated with immunosuppressive drugs. None are found in cases of congenital MG.
2. See Chapter 1 guidelines for safe, effective, informed *posttest* care.

IgE ANTIBODY, SINGLE ALLERGEN, IRMA PANEL ●

Normal Values

Negative or positive for allergen-specific IgE by immunoradiometric assay (IRMA) and compared with a negative control tested simultaneously. *Example:* Positive = 251–2500% of negative control.

Background

A large number of substances have been found to have allergic potential. Measurable allergen-specific antibodies can be identified by an IRMA. The patient's serum should first be screened with a selected panel of five allergens and then followed, if appropriate, by an extended panel of additional allergens.

Explanation of Test

This study tests for reactions to certain respiratory and food allergy stimulants. The IRMA tests measure the increase and quantity of allergen-specific IgE antibodies and diagnoses an allergy to a specific allergen (eg, molds, weeds, foods, insects). These measurements are used in persons, especially children, with extrinsic asthma, hay fever, and atopic eczema, and they are an accurate and convenient alternative to skin testing. Although more expensive, they do not cause hypersensitivity reactions.

Additional antigens are continually being added, so up-to-date information should be sought. (Examples of categories include grasses, trees, molds, venoms, weeds, animal danders, foods, house dust, mites, antibiotics, and insects.)

Procedure

Obtain a 10-ml venous blood sample for each group of five allergens. Observe universal precautions.

Clinical Complications

1. Detection of an allergen-specific IgE antibody indicates immediate hypersensitivity to an allergen.
2. A positive IRMA is diagnostic of allergy to a particular allergen or allergens, irrespective of the level of total IgE.

Patient Preparation

1. Explain test purpose and procedure.
2. See Chapter 1 guidelines for safe, effective, informed *pretest* care.

Patient Aftercare

1. Interpret test outcomes and counsel appropriately concerning hypersensitivity, need for other tests, and lifestyle changes.
2. Follow Chapter 1 guidelines for safe, effective, informed *posttest* care.

CRYOGLOBULIN TEST ●

Normal Values

Negative for cryoglobulin.

If positive after 3 to 5 days at 4°C, immunofixation electrophoresis (IFE) of the cryoprecipitate is performed to identify the protein complex.

Background

Cryoimmunoglobulins are protein complexes that undergo reversible precipitation at low temperatures and redissolve on warming in the body or under laboratory conditions.

Explanation of Test

This test provides additional diagnostic information about certain disorders, such as malignant B-cell diseases, collagen disorders, acute and chronic infections, and primary cryoglobulinemia in persons with cold hypersensitivity. Detection of cryoglobulins is highly specific for immune complexes.

Procedure

Obtain a 15-ml venous blood sample. Observe universal precautions. Keep the specimen at 37°C until the cells are separated.

Clinical Implications

Disorders associated with cryoglobulinemia include

1. Malignant B-cell diseases (eg, multiple myeloma, Waldenstrom's macroglobulinemia, chronic lymphocytic leukemia)
2. Collagen diseases (eg, rheumatoid arthritis, Sjogren's syndrome, systemic lupus erythematosus)
3. Acute and chronic infections:

   - **a.** Syphilis
   - **b.** Subacute bacterial endocarditis
   - **c.** Infectious mononucleosis
   - **d.** Cytomegalovirus disease
4. Other disorders
   - **a.** Sarcoidosis
   - **b.** Acute poststreptococcal glomerulonephritis
   - **c.** Cirrhosis
   - **d.** Hemolytic anemia

Patient Preparation

1. Explain test purpose and procedure.
2. See Chapter 1 guidelines for safe, effective, informed *pretest* care.

Patient Aftercare

1. Interpret test results, counsel, and monitor appropriately for infections, collagen disorders, and malignant blood cell disease. Follow-up testing is usually needed.
2. Follow Chapter 1 guidelines for safe, effective, informed *posttest* care.

Patient Care for Collagen, Rheumatic, and Connective Tissue Diseases

PATIENT PREPARATION

Explain test purpose and procedure. A number of laboratory tests are ordered to diagnose complex problems, to assess and to monitor the course of collagen, rheumatic, and connective tissue disorders. These diseases include systemic lupus erythematosus (SLE), rheumatoid arthritis (RA), Sjogren's syndrome, systemic sclerosis, CREST syndrome, Raynaud's phenomenon sclerodactyly, telangiectasis, and mixed connective tissue disease (MCTD). Several of these tests are as follows:

1. Anticentromes antibody
2. Anti-dsDNA antibody
3. Antinuclear antibody
4. Anti-RNP antibody
5. Anti-Sm antibody
6. Anti-SSA antibody
7. Anti-SSB antibody
8. Anti-Scl-70 antibody
9. CH50 (total hemolytic complement)
10. C3 complement component
11. C4 complement component
12. C1 esterase inhibitor
13. Cryoglobulin test
14. Rheumatoid factor

Patient Aftercare

1. Interpret test results, monitor, and counsel about follow-up tests and treatment. These are chronic diseases that must be dealt with on a continuum and may require significant lifestyle changes. Repeat testing evaluates therapy effectiveness. Minor symptoms, in the absence of major involvement, are frequently treated with nonsteroidal anti-inflammatory drugs (NSAIDs), such as salicylates. Cutaneous manifestations respond to topical corticosteroid treatments. The short-acting corticosteroids (eg,

prednisone) are necessary if acute serologic changes and severe clinical manifestations appear. Short courses of moderate-dose corticosteroids suppress the symptoms of the acute disease, shorten time periods of exacerbation, normalize serologic parameters, and prevent or delay disease progression to its more serious stages. Evidence of rapid reduction of anti-dsDNA antibody levels following initiation of therapy suggests that nonimmune mechanisms operate to clear immune system aberrations. This is especially important for SLE, in which the accumulation of these immune complexes can lead to eventual renal failure.

2. Long-term, moderate to high dose corticosteroids are central regimens prescribed for diffuse proliferative glomerulonephritis as well as rheumatoid arthritis.
3. Corticosteroid dosage may be reduced and renal disease may be favorably managed by adding immunosuppressive drugs (cyclophosphamide or azathioprine). Infection secondary to immunosuppressive treatment is a leading cause of death for patients with SLE. Patient education plays a major role in prevention. Emphasize that the outlook is favorable for improved diagnosis, treatment, and understanding of these diseases.
4. Follow Chapter 1 guidelines for safe, effective, informed *posttest* care.

Patient Preparation and Aftercare

See special section on collagen, rheumatic, and connective tissue disease tests.

ANTIBODIES TO EXTRACTABLE NUCLEAR ANTIGENS (ENAs); **ANTIRIBONUCLEOPROTEIN** (RNP); **ANTI-SMITH** (SM); **ANTI-SJOGREN'S SYNDROME** (SSA AND SSB) ●

Normal Values

Negative by EIA for the following extractable nuclear antigens (ENAs): Anti-RNP, ribonucleoprotein; Anti-Sm, Smith; Anti-SSA/Ro, Sjogren's syndrome; Anti-SSB/La, Sjogren's syndrome.

Background

The ENAs, another group of nuclear antigens (nonhistone proteins) to which autoantibodies may develop, are so named because of their presence in saline solution extracts of certain nonhuman cells. The most common ENAs are ribonucleoprotein (RNP) and Smith (Sm). Antibodies to RNP are present in patients with a combination of overlapping rheumatologic symptoms, known as mixed connective tissue disease (MCTD).

Explanation of Test

These tests are indicated for differential diagnosis of systemic lupus erythematosus (SLE), scleroderma, rheumatoid arthritis, and Sjogren's syndrome. They are done to correctly identify a specific autoantibody directed against nuclear antigens composed of nonhistone proteins. All four of these antibodies will produce a finely speckled pattern of nuclear fluorescence in the ANA test. Anti-RNP detection is helpful in the differential diagnosis of systemic rheumatic disease and is a useful follow-up for collagen vascular autoimmune disorders. Also a follow-up for collagen vascular disorders, the test for anti-Sm is highly diagnostic of SLE. The SSA and SSB antibody detection is particularly useful when an "ANA-negative" case of SLE is expected.

Procedure

Obtain a 10-ml venous blood sample. Observe universal precautions.

Clinical Implications

1. A high level of RNP antibodies is an outstanding feature of MCTD.
2. Antibodies to the Sm antigen occur in SLE and are a specific marker for the disease.
3. The SSA/Ro and SSB/La antigens have a physical affinity for one another; patients frequently have antibodies to both. SSA antibodies may be found in Sjogren's syndrome alone or in Sjogren's syndrome associated with SLE. Persons with both Sjogren's and rheumatoid arthritis have neither SSA nor SSB antibodies. They tend to develop antibodies against the Epstein–Barr virus associated with rheumatoid arthritis nuclear antigen (RANA).

ANTISCLERODERMA (SCl-70) ANTIBODY TEST ●

Normal Value

Negative for antiscleroderma antibody by immunoblot assay.

Background

Scl-70 is a nuclear antigen that may cause autoantibodies to develop against it. It is a nonhistone protein.

Explanation of Test

This is a follow-up test for diagnosing vascular collagen diseases, especially for cases of suspected scleroderma. Scl-70 antibodies are seen in approximately 20% of patients with diffuse scleroderma and are highly specific for this disease. These antibodies produce a fine speckled pattern, with or without nucleolar staining, in the fluorescent ANA test.

Procedure

Obtain a 10-ml venous blood sample. Observe universal precautions.

Clinical Implications

The Scl-70 antibody is present in scleroderma, but rarely present in other rheumatic diseases (SLE, rheumatoid arthritis, and Sjogren's syndrome).

Patient Preparation and Aftercare

See special section on collagen, rheumatic, and connective tissue disease tests.

RHEUMATOID FACTOR, RHEUMATOID ARTHRITIS (RA) FACTOR ●

Normal Values

Nonreactive for RA factor: 0–39 IU/ml, based on rate nephelometry or latex agglutination
Weakly reactive: 40–79 IU/ml
Reactive: > 80 IU/ml

Background

The blood of many persons with rheumatoid arthritis contains a macroglobulin-type antibody, called *rheumatoid factor* (RF). Evidence indicates that rheumatoid factors are antigammaglobulin antibodies; however, until a specific antigen that produces RF is discovered, its exact nature can only be speculated. Even more uncertain is the role that RF plays in rheumatoid arthritis. Although RF may cause or perpetuate the destructive changes associated with rheumatoid arthritis, it also may be incidental to these changes, or it may even actually serve some beneficial purpose. RF is sometimes found in blood serum from patients with other diseases, even though RF incidence and values are higher in patients with rheumatoid arthritis.

Explanation of Test

This test diagnoses rheumatoid arthritis. It measures rheumatoid factors (antibodies directed against the Fc fragment of IgG). These are usually IgM antibodies, but may also be IgG or IgA.

Four of the following criteria must be met to diagnose rheumatoid arthritis:

Revised American College of Rheumatology Criteria for RA

1. Morning stiffness for at least 6 weeks.
2. Pain on motion or tenderness in at least one joint for at least 6 weeks.
3. Swelling in at least one joint for at least 6 weeks.
4. Swelling in at least one other joint for at least 6 weeks.
5. Symmetrical joint swelling with simultaneous involvement of the same joint on both sides of the body.
6. Subcutaneous nodules.
7. X-ray changes, including bony decalcification.

Procedure

Obtain a 10-ml venous blood sample. Observe universal precautions.

Clinical Implications

1. Whan a patient who tests positive improves, subsequent tests also remain positive (exception: if titers were initially low).
2. A positive RF test often supports a tentative diagnosis of early-age–onset rheumatoid arthritis (eg, versus rheumatic fever).
3. Rheumatoid factors frequently occur in a variety of other diseases, such as lupus erythematosus; endocarditis; tuberculosis; syphilis; sarcoidosis; cancer; viral infections; diseases affecting the liver, lung, or kidney; Sjogren's syndrome; and in patients with skin and renal allografts.
4. Absence of RF does not exclude the diagnosis or existence of rheumatoid arthritis.

Interfering Factors

The result is normally higher in older patients and in those who have received multiple vaccinations and transfusions.

Patient Preparation and Aftercare

See special section for collagen, rheumatic, and connective tissue disease tests.

ANTINUCLEAR ANTIBODY (ANA) TEST ●

Normal Values

Negative for ANA by indirect immunofluorescence (IFA).
If positive, pattern will be reported and serum will be titered.

Background

The diagnosis of SLE is difficult because clinical signs and symptoms are extremely varied and may mimic several connective tissue diseases, such as rheumatoid arthritis or other systemic autoimmune disorders. SLE is characterized by a profuse production of different autoantibodies, of which some are pathogenic. A multisystem disease, SLE can affect every organ system in the body (especially the kidney). It varies in its clinical manifestations in different persons or at different times. The IFA test for antinuclear antibodies (ANAs) is one of the most useful tests for SLE now available. ANAs are gamma globulins that react with cell nuclei of all organs, human or animal. ANAs usually belong to more than one immunoglobulin class. An effective fluorescent ANA test detects approximately 95% of SLE cases.

Explanation of Test

This test is used in the differential diagnosis of rheumatic diseases and to detect antinucleoprotein factors and patterns associated with certain autoimmune diseases. One particular antibody pattern is associated with SLE; another antibody pattern correlates with scleroderma, another with Sjogren's syndrome or with Raynaud's disease, and so forth. Although the ANA titer may not always correlate with the clinical disease picture, most SLE patients produce high ANA titers, with homogeneous and peripheral (RIM) staining patterns. Speckled and nucleolar patterns may be associated with SLE at lower frequencies.

Procedure

Obtain a 10-ml venous blood sample. Observe universal precautions.

Clinical Implications

1. The ANA test is positive at a titer of 1:20 or 1:40 (laboratory-dependent), with indirect immunofluorescence the most common test for ANA.
2. A positive result does not necessarily confirm a disease; ANAs at lower titers are present in some apparently normal persons.
3. Results of the percentage positive tests according to disease process are as follows: SLE and lupoid hepatitis = >95%; scleroderma = 60–70%; rheumatoid arthritis = 25%–30%; Sjogren's disease = 50%–60%; dermatomyositis = 10%–50%; polyarteritis = 10%.
4. A negative total antinuclear antibody test is strong evidence against the presence of SLE.

Interfering Factors

Certain drugs may cause positive ANA tests (eg, procainamide or hydralazine).

Patient Preparation

See special section for collagen, rheumatic, and connective tissue disease testing.

Patient Aftercare

1. See special section for collagen, rheumatic, and connective tissue disease testing.
2. Other confirmatory SLE tests include anti-dsDNA, CH50, and kidney or skin biopsy.
3. Follow-up tests for positive ANA include anti-double-stranded (ds)DNA antibodies to extractable nuclear antigens (anti-RNP, anti-Smith); anti-SSA, also known as Ro; anti-SSB, also known as La; antiscleroderma Scl-70; and anticentromere, also known as CREST antibody.

ANTI-dsDNA ANTIBODY TEST ●

Normal Values

Negative for anti-dsDNA: < 70 units by ELISA
Borderline: 70–200 units
Positive: > 200 units

Background

Although not completely understood, the primary mechanism of tissue injury in systemic lupus erythematosus (SLE) and related autoimmune disease is the formation of antigen–antibody immune complexes. Not all ANAs are pathogenic. For the few that are harmful, pathogenicity depends on the specific immunoglobulin class, ability to activate complement, size of the immune complex, and site of tissue deposition. For example, studies of immune complex-mediated tissue injury in the kidney have shown a clear relation between deposition of immune complexes and glomerular disease.

Explanation of Test

The anti-dsDNA test is done specifically to identify or differentiate native (double-stranded; ds) DNA antibodies, found in 40% to 60% of patients with SLE during the active phase of their disease, from other nonnative DNA antibodies, found in other rheumatic diseases. The presence of antibodies to dsDNA generally correlates with lupus nephritis. An anti-dsDNA test supports a diagnosis, monitors disease activity and response to therapy, and establishes a prognosis for SLE.

Procedure

Obtain a 10-ml venous blood sample. Observe universal precautions.

Clinical Implications

1. Anti-dsDNA concentrations may decrease with successful therapy and may increase with an acute recurrence of SLE.
2. DNA–anti-dsDNA immune complexes play a role in SLE pathogenesis through the deposit of these complexes within the kidney and other tissues.

Interfering Factors

The Farr assay, a radioimmunoassay method, detects both single-stranded (ss), as well as double-stranded (ds) DNA antibodies. Antibodies to ssDNA are nonspecific, but are associated with various other rheumatic diseases.

Patient Preparation and Aftercare

See special section for collagen, rheumatic, and connective tissue disease tests.

ANTICENTROMERE ANTIBODY TEST ●

Normal Values

Negative for anticentromere antibody by indirect immunofluorescence.
If positive, serum will be titered.

Explanation of Test

A variant of scleroderma, the CREST syndrome is characterized by calcinosis, Raynaud's phenomenon, esophageal dysfunction, sclerodactyly, and telangiectasia. Characteristically, anticentromere antibodies appear in approximately 90% of patients. This antibody is detected by using Hep-2 cells in various stages of cell division. The centromere region of the cell chromosomes will stain if an anticentromere antibody is present.

Procedure

Obtain a 10-ml venous blood sample. Observe universal precautions.

Clinical Implications

Positive results are associated with the CREST syndrome in scleroderma.

Patient Preparation and Aftercare

See special section on collagen, rheumatic, and connective tissue disease tests.

ANTICARDIOLIPIN ANTIBODY (aCL) TEST ●

Normal Values

Less than 23 g/L for IgG aCL antibodies based upon EIA.
Less than 11 mg/L for IgM aCL antibodies.

Background

Antiphospholipid antibodies react with most negatively charged phospholipids, including cardiolipin. Additionally, antiphospholipid antibodies in vitro are known to prolong phospholipid-dependent coagulation tests and have been historically referred to as the "lupus anticoagulant."

Explanation of Test

The test most commonly assesses risk of thrombosis in the presence of systemic lupus erythematosus (SLE).

Procedure

Obtain a 10-ml venous blood sample. Observe universal precautions.

Clinical Implications

1. Anticardiolipin antibodies (aCL) are frequently found with SLE and other autoimmune diseases. Elevated levels of aCL antibodies appear to be associated with venous or arterial thrombosis, thrombocytopenia, and recurrent fetal loss. The term "antiphospholipid syndrome" describes patients who present with these features in association with aCL antibodies or the lupus anticoagulant.

2. Patients with current or prior syphilis infections may have a false-positive result, without the risk of thrombosis.
3. Anticardiolipin antibodies can be transient during many infections. Repeat the test after 6 months.

Patient Preparation
1. Explain test purpose and procedure.
2. Follow guidelines in Chapter 1 for safe, effective, informed *pretest* care.

Patient Aftercare
1. Interpret test outcomes in light of the patient's history, physical findings, and other diagnostic procedures and results. If clinical findings suggest the presence of antiphospholipid antibodies and the absence of anticardiolipin antibodies, some recommend testing for the lupus anticoagulant to confirm the negative result. A patient is considered positive for antiphospholipid antibodies if one or both of the tests are positive.
2. See Chapter 1 guidelines for safe, effective, informed *posttest* care.

ANTI-INSULIN ANTIBODY TEST ●

Normal Values
Less than 3% binding of the patient's serum with labeled beef, human, and pork insulin.

Background
Persons with diabetes may form antibodies to the insulin they take and require larger doses because insulin is unavailable for glucose (metabolism) functions when the available insulin is partially (complexed) with these antibodies. Insulin antibodies (Ab) are immunoglobulins called *anti-insulin Ab;* they act as insulin-transporting proteins. The most common type of anti-insulin Ab is IgG, but it is found in all five classes of immunoglobulins in insulin-treated patients. These immunoglobulins, especially IgE, may be responsible for allergic manifestations; IgM may cause insulin resistance.

Explanation of Test
This insulin antibody level provides information for determining the most appropriate treatment for certain diabetic patients. It may focus on the reason for allergic manifestations. It can identify a state of insulin resistance, in which the daily insulin requirement exceeds 200 units for more than 2 days and may be associated with elevated anti-insulin antibody titers and insulin-binding capacity.

Procedure
Obtain a fasting, 2-ml venous blood sample. Observe universal precautions.

Clinical Implications

Anti-insulin antibody elevations are associated with insulin resistance and allergies to insulin.

Patient Preparation

1. Explain purpose of test. Fasting is required. Check with your laboratory for time frames.
2. Follow guidelines in Chapter 1 for safe, effective, informed *pretest* care.

Patient Aftercare

1. Interpret test outcomes. From antibody levels present and clinical findings, the dosage of insulin is changed to reduce or prevent further allergic manifestations or insulin resistance.
2. See Chapter 1 guidelines for safe, effective, informed *posttest* care.

ANTIMYOCARDIAL ANTIBODY TEST ●

Normal Values

Negative for antimyocardial antibody test by indirect immunofluorescence.
If positive, serum will be titered.

Background

There appears to be a significant association between the presence of antimyocardial antibodies and heart disease. These antibodies appear following cardiac surgery or myocardial infarction and may precede actual clinical evidence of myocardial injury.

Explanation of Test

This test is valuable in the differential diagnosis of coronary heart disease and for detecting minimal myocardial damage.

Procedure

Obtain a 5-ml venous blood sample. Observe universal precautions.

Clincal Implications

Antimyocardial antibodies are present

1. Following cardiac surgery
2. In myocardial infarction; less frequently with coronary insufficiency without infarction
3. In rheumatic fever
4. In chronic rheumatic diseases
5. In streptococcal infections

Patient Preparation

1. Explain test purpose.
2. Follow Chapter 1 guidelines for safe, effective, informed *pretest* care.

Patient Aftercare

1. Interpret test outcomes and monitor appropriately. Positive test results reveal minimal myocardial damage when other tests are inconclusive.
2. See Chapter 1 guidelines for safe, effective, informed *posttest* care.

ANTISPERM ANTIBODY TEST ●

Normal Values

Reported as percentage of sperm binding by immunobead technique.
More than 20% binding is usually required to lower patient's fertility.
Significance of percentage binding is inversely related to patient's sperm count; antibody class involved; site of sperm binding (sperm head, midpiece or tail).

Background

The majority of infertile men have blocking of the efferent testicular ducts. It is likely that (similar to vasectomy), reabsorption of sperm from blocked ducts results in the formation of autoantibodies to sperm.

Explanation of Test

This test detects sperm antibodies as part of infertility investigation. Antibodies directed toward various sperm antigens can produce reduced male fertility. However, the precise nature of the immune response against sperm antigens and the particular type of antibody responsible are unknown.

Procedure

A semen test sample is preferred for values. If semen procurement presents a problem for the male, a blood serum sample can be tested. For females, blood serum is preferred because of difficulty with cervical mucus collection.

Serum: 2.0 ml of blood. Send specimen *frozen* in plastic vial on dry ice.
Semen: Contents of semen ejaculate. Send specimen *frozen* in plastic vial on dry ice.
Cervical mucus: 1.0 ml of cervical mucus. Send specimen *frozen* in plastic vial on dry ice.

Clinical Implications

Antisperm antibodies are associated with

1. Blocked testicular efferent ducts.
2. Vasectomy: Antibodies and probable cellular immunity to sperm develop in most males as a result of the interaction of sperm antigens with the immune system.
3. In some studies, approximately 75% of women with primary infertility

had sperm agglutinins. However, 11% to 15% of *pregnant* women also had the same sperm antibody titers.

Clinical Alert

The potential adverse consequences of an immune sperm response include possible systemic effects in other organ systems and possible infertility after vasectomy reversal.

Patient Preparation

1. Explain test purpose and procedure. See details under Procedure for *Specimen Required.* Patient should be advised of the need for repeat testing.
2. See Chapter 1 guidelines for safe, effective, informed *pretest* care.

Patient Preparation

1. Interpret test results and counsel appropriately. It may be necessary to repeat this procedure on different sample types (eg, semen, blood) to establish a possible cause for infertility.
2. Follow Chapter 1 guidelines for safe, effective, informed *posttest* care.

ALPHA$_1$-ANTITRYPSIN (AAT) TEST

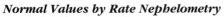

Normal Values by Rate Nephelometry

126–226 mg/dl

If result is $<$ 140 mg/dl, phenotype will be determined to confirm homozygous and heterozygous deficiencies.

Background

alpha$_1$-antitrypsin, a protein produced by the liver, inhibits the protease released into body fluids by dying cells. This protein deficiency is associated with pulmonary emphysema and liver disease. Human blood serum contains at least three inhibitors of protease. Two of the best known are alpha$_1$-antitrypsin and alpha$_2$-macroglobulin. Total antitrypsin levels in blood are composed of about 90% AAT and 10% alpha$_2$-macroglobulins.

Explanation of Test

This is a nonspecific method to diagnose inflammation, severe infection, and necrosis. AAT measurement is important for diagnosing respiratory disease and cirrhosis of the liver because of its direct relation to pulmonary and other metabolic disorders. Pulmonary problems, such as emphysema, occur when antitrypsin-deficient persons are unable to ward off the action of endoproteases. Those who are deficient in AAT develop emphysema at a much earlier age than other emphysema patients.

Procedure

Obtain a 10-ml venous blood sample. Observe universal precautions.

Clinical Implications

1. Interpretation of AAT levels is based on the following: high levels: generally found in normal persons; intermediate levels: found in persons with a predisposition to pulmonary emphysema; low levels: found in patients with obstructive pulmonary disease and in children with cirrhosis of the liver.
2. *Increased AAT levels* are seen in the following:
   - **a.** Acute and chronic inflammatory disorders
   - **b.** After injections of typhoid vaccine
   - **c.** Cancer
   - **d.** Thyroid infections
   - **e.** Oral contraceptive use
   - **f.** Stress syndrome
   - **g.** Hematologic abnormalities
3. *Decreased AAT levels* are associated with these following progressive diseases:
   - **a.** Adult early-onset, chronic pulmonary emphysema
   - **b.** Liver cirrhosis in children
   - **c.** Pulmonary disease
   - **d.** Severe hepatic damage
   - **e.** Nephrotic syndrome
   - **f.** Malnutrition

Interfering Factors

Serum levels may normally increase by 100% in pregnancy.

Patient Preparation

1. Explain test purpose and procedure. Fasting is required if the patient's history shows elevated cholesterol or triglyceride levels.
2. See Chapter 1 guidelines for safe, effective, informed *pretest* care.

Patient Aftercare

1. Interpret test results and counsel appropriately. Advise patients with decreased levels to avoid smoking and, if possible, occupational hazards, such as dust, fumes, and other respiratory pollutants.
2. Because AAT deficiencies are inherited, genetic counseling may be indicated. Follow-up AAT phenotype testing can be performed on family members to determine the homozygous or heterozygous nature of the deficiency.
3. Follow Chapter 1 guidelines for safe, effective, informed *posttest* care.

BLOOD BANKING OR IMMUNOHEMATOLOGY TESTS

OVERVIEW OF BLOOD BANKING OR IMMUNOHEMATOLOGY TESTS

These tests are done to prevent possible transfusion and transplant reactions; to identify potential problems, such as hemolytic disease of newborns; and to determine parentage. Immunohematology testing identifies highly reactive antigens and their antibodies present in nucleated blood cells.

DONATED BLOOD TESTING AND BLOOD PROCESSING

Testing of Blood Recipient and Donor Blood

All donated blood, as it is processed, must undergo several tests. These include tests for

1. ABO red cell groups
2. Rh factors
3. Antibody screen
4. Hepatitis B surface antigen (HBsAg)
5. Non-A, non-B hepatitis (hepatitis C)
6. Hepatitis C virus (anti-HVC)
7. Syphilis (VDRL)
8. Acquired immunodeficiency syndrome (HIV infection)
9. Adult T-cell leukemia/ lymphoma (HTLV-1)
10. Alanine aminotransferase (ALT)

Required testing for whole-blood or for packed red cells recipients include the following:

1. ABO red cell group
2. Rh factor
3. Antibody screen
4. Crossmatch for compatibility between donor's and recipient's cells and serum

Even though no crossmatch is needed for plasma administration, compatible ABO typing should be done. Platelets and granulocytes should be tested for HLA compatibility. *Histocompatibility locus A (HLA):* These antigens are found in blood cells and most tissues of the body. Because of previous transfusions or pregnancy, some patients will develop antibodies against these antigens and, if given incompatible blood, may have a transfusion reaction. Other donated blood-testing and processing considerations for autologous and directed donations, cytomegalovirus tests, and blood product irradiation are presented in the following list.

1. *Autologous donations* (blood recipient and donor are the same person) are blood products donated by patients for their own use. Many patients opt to donate their own blood before scheduled surgery because of the concern over transfusion-transmitted diseases.

2. *Homologous donations* (blood donor and blood recipient are not the same person) are blood products donated by one individual for use by other individuals.
3. *Directed donations:* Recipients choose the donors who will donate blood for their transfusions. Laws in several states declare that this request must be honored in nonemergency situations. Standards and testing procedures must be identical with those required for a homologous blood donor. (Autologous donors do not need to adhere to the same criteria as homologous blood donors.) The following list addresses some general guidelines for donating autologous blood.
   - **a.** There is no upper age limit, if healthy; lower age limit is 17.5 years and at least 110 lb (50 kg).
   - **b.** There are no weight requirements on the upper end.
   - **c.** Pregnant women can donate.
   - **d.** Hematocrit should be 33% or greater. If less than 33%, the patient's physician must approve the phlebotomy.
   - **e.** Normally, phlebotomy can be done at 3-day intervals; the final phlebotomy should be done at least 72 hours before the time of the scheduled surgery. Iron supplements may be prescribed to maintain adequate hemoglobin levels.
4. *Cytomegalovirus testing:* Cytomegalovirus (CMV) testing is done for those patients at risk for transfusion-associated CMV infections. These types of CMV infections were first seen as a mononucleosis syndrome after cardiopulmonary bypass surgery and were thought to be related to the use of fresh blood during the surgery. Clinical symptoms of transfusion-transmitted CMV infections include pneumonitis, hepatitis, retinitis, or disseminated infection. They generally occur in immunosuppressed patients, such as premature infants weighing less than 1200 g at birth, bone marrow and organ transplant patients, and certain immunocompromised oncology patients. Therefore, to prevent these infections, CMV antibody testing is done. Patients at risk should receive CMV-seronegative blood and blood products.
5. *Irradiation of blood products:* Sometimes, blood products are irradiated before transfusion for certain immunosuppressed patients. Graft-versus-host disease (GVHD) is a rare complication that follows transfusion of severely immunosuppressed patients. Graft-versus-host disease occurs if donor lymphocytes from blood or blood products engraft and multiply in a severely immunodeficient recipient. The engrafted lymphocytes react against host (recipient) tissues. Clinical symptoms include skin rash, fever, diarrhea, hepatitis, bone marrow suppression, and infection that frequently leads to death. GVHD can be prevented by irradiating blood products with 1500 to 5000 rad of cesium 137. This dose renders 85% to 95% of the lymphocytes in a unit of blood, platelet, or granulocyte concentrate incapable of engrafting; it does not affect red cells, platelets, or granulocytes.

BLOOD GROUPS; ABO RED CELL GROUPS

Normal Values

Antigen Present on Red Blood Cell	*Antibodies Present in Serum*	*Major Blood Group Designation*	*Distribution in the United States*
None	Anti-A, anti-B	O (universal donor)*	O 46%
A	Anti-B	A	A 41%
B	Anti-A	B	B 9%
AB	None	AB (universal recipient)†	AB 4%

*Named universal donor *because no antigens are present on red blood cells; therefore, the person is able to donate to all blood groups.*

†Named universal recipient *because no serum antibodies are present; therefore, the person is able to receive blood from all blood groups.*

Background

Human blood is grouped according to the presence or the absence of specific *blood group antigens* (ABO). These antigens, found on the surface of red blood cells, can induce the body to produce antibodies. (More than 300 distinct antigens have been identified.) Compatibility of the ABO group is the foundation for all other pretransfusion testing.

Explanation of Test

All blood donors and potential blood recipients need to be tested for blood type to prevent transfusion with incompatible blood products.

Specifically linked sugars determine the antigenic activities, named *A* and *B*. One sugar, *N*-acetylgalactosamine, gives the molecule A activity; another sugar, galactose, determines B activity. The backbone molecule (without galactose or *N*-acetylgalactosamine), has antigenic activity, termed *H*. This H substance, as well as H gene activity, is essential for the function of the ABO antigens. The following table lists the blood groups and their ABO antigens:

Blood Group	*ABO Antigen*
A	A
B	B
AB	A and B
O	Neither

In general, patients are transfused with blood of their own ABO group because antibodies against the other blood antigens may be present in the blood serum. These antibodies are designated anti-A or anti-B, based on the antigen they act against. Under normal conditions, a person's blood serum will *not* contain the antibody specifically able to destroy its antigen. For example, a person with antigen A will *not also* have anti-A antibodies in the serum; however, anti-B antibodies may be present. Therefore, antigen and antibody testing is necessary to confirm ABO grouping.

Clinical Alert

A transfusion reaction could be extremely serious and potentially fatal. Therefore, the blood group must be determined in vitro before any blood is transfused to another individual.

Before blood administration, two professionals (physicians or nurses) must check the recipient's blood group and type with the donor group and type to assure compatibility.

NOTE: *A blood group change or suppression may be induced by cancer or leukemia.*

Procedure

Obtain a 10-ml venous blood sample. Observe universal precautions.

Patient Preparation

1. Explain test purpose and procedure. Conditions that at some point may require transfusion include
   - **a.** Malignant tumors (leukemias)
   - **b.** Cardiac surgical procedures
   - **d.** Surgical hip procedures
   - **e.** Anemias
   - **f.** Certain obstetric or gynecologic procedures or complications
   - **g.** Bone and joint diseases
   - **h.** Lung disease
   - **i.** Kidney disease or genitourinary system surgical procedures
   - **j.** Massive trauma
   - **k.** Liver disease
   - **l.** Certain blood dyscrasias
2. See Chapter 1 guidelines for safe, effective, informed *pretest* care.

Patient Aftercare

1. Inform patient of blood group and interpret meaning. Rh-factors may have implications for the pregnant woman and fetus.

Incidence and Frequency of Blood Type and Rh Factors

Type and Rh Factor	*Incidence (How Many Have It)*	*Frequency of Occurrence (How Often) (%)*
O positive	1:3	37.4
O negative	1:15	6.6

(continued)

Incidence and Frequency of Blood Type and Rh Factors *(Continued)*

Type and Rh Factor	*Incidence (How Many Have It)*	*Frequency of Occurrence (How Often) (%)*
A positive	1:3	35.7
A negative	1:16	6.3
B postive	1:12	8.5
B negative	1:67	1.5
AB positive	1:29	3.4
AB negative	1:167	0.6

2. Follow Chapter 1 guidelines for safe, effective, informed *posttest* care.

Rh FACTORS; Rh TYPING

Normal Values: Incidence

White: 85% Rh-positive (have the Rh antigen)
15% Rh-negative (lack the Rh antigen)
Black: 90% Rh-positive (have the Rh antigen)
10% Rh-negative (lack the Rh antigen)

Background

Human blood is classified as Rh-positive or Rh-negative. This relates to the presence or the absence of the Rh antigen on the red cell membrane. The Rh antigen (now called Rh_o [D]) is, after the A and B antigens, the next most important antigen in transfusion practice.

Comparison of Terms Used in Rh System* Nomenclatures

Weiner	*Fisher–Race*
Rh_o	D
rh′	C
rh″	E
hr″	c
hr	e
hr	f (ce)
rh^G	G

*The term Rh factor, *without qualification,* means Rh_o (D = Rh:1). "Rh-positive" means RH_o (D) = positive.

Explanation of Test

The Rh system is composed of antigens tested for in conjunction with the ABO group. Rh_o (D) factor is often the only factor tested for. When this factor is absent, further typing is then done to identify any of the less common Rh factors present before the person is identified as "Rh-negative." Rh-negative individuals may develop antibodies against Rh-positive antigens if they are challenged through a transfusion of Rh-positive blood or through a fetomaternal bleed from an Rh-positive fetus.

Need for Blood Rh Typing

Blood Rh typing must be done because

1. Rh-positive blood administered to an Rh-negative person may sensitize the person to form anti-D (Rh_0).
2. Rh_0 D-positive blood administered to a recipient having serum anti-D (Rh_0) could be fatal.
3. One must identify RhIg (Rh immunoglobulin) candidates. Rh immunoglobulin is a concentrated solution of IgG anti-D (Rh_0) derived from human plasma. A 1-ml dose of RhIg contains 300 μg and is sufficient to counteract the immunizing effects of 15 ml of packed red cells or 30 ml of whole blood.
   - **a.** Rh-negative, pregnant women with Rh-positive partners may carry Rh-positive fetuses. Fetal cells may cross the placenta to the mother and cause production of antibodies in the maternal blood. The maternal antibody, in turn, may cross through the placenta into the fetal circulation and cause destruction of fetal blood cells. This condition, called *hemolytic disease of the newborn* (formerly called *erythroblastosis fetalis*), may cause reactions that range from anemia (slight or severe) to fetal death in utero. This condition can be prevented if an Rh-negative pregnant female receives an RhIg dose antepartum at 28 weeks' gestation and a postpartum injection of RhIg shortly after delivery of an RhD (Rh_0)-positive infant. Postpartum Rh immunization can occur, despite an injection of RhIg if more than 30 ml of fetal blood has entered the maternal circulation. The American Association of Blood Banks recommends that a postpartum blood specimen of all RhD (Rh_0)-negative women (those at risk of immunization) be examined to detect a fetal maternal hemorrhage larger than 30 ml.
   - **b.** Rh typing must also be done for patients who have had abortions or miscarriages.

Clinical Implications

1. The significance of Rh factors is based on their capacity to immunize as a result of receiving a transfusion or becoming pregnant. The Rh_0 (D) factor is by far the most antigenic; the other Rh factors are much less likely to produce isoimmunization. The following general conditions must be met for immunization to Rh factors to occur:
   - **a.** The Rh blood factor must be absent in the immunized person.
   - **b.** The Rh blood factor must be present in the immunizing blood.

- **c.** The blood factor must be of sufficient antigenic strength to produce a reaction.
- **d.** The amount of incompatible blood must be large enough to induce antibody formation.

Factors other than Rh_o (D) may induce formation of antibodies in Rh-positive persons, if the preceding conditions are met.

2. Antibodies for Rh′ (C) are frequently found together with anti-Rh_o (D) antibodies in the Rh-negative, pregnant woman whose fetus or child is type Rh-positive and possesses both factors.
3. With exceedingly rare exceptions, Rh antibodies do not form unless preceded by antigenic stimulation as occurs with
   - **a.** Pregnancy and abortions
   - **b.** Blood transfusions
   - **c.** Deliberate immunization, most commonly of repeated IV injections of blood for the purpose of harvesting a given Rh antibody

Patient Preparation

1. Explain purpose and procedure of Rh typing.
2. See Chapter 1 guidelines for safe, effective, informed *pretest* care.

Patient Aftercare

1. Interpret test outcome, inform and counsel about Rh type. Women of childbearing age may need special consideration. See page 592 for incidence of Rh type.
2. Follow Chapter 1 guidelines for safe, effective, informed *posttest* care.

Rh ANTIBODY TITER TEST ●

Normal Value

Normal is zero, no antibody present.

Explanation of Test

This antibody study determines the Rh-antibody level in an Rh-negative or pregnant woman whose partner is Rh-positive. If the Rh-negative woman is carrying an Rh-positive fetus, the antigen from the fetal blood cells causes antibody production in the mother's serum. The firstborn child usually shows no ill effects; however, with subsequent pregnancies, the mother's serum antibodies increase and eventually destroy the fetal red blood cells (hemolytic disease of the newborn).

Procedure

Obtain a 10-ml venous blood sample from the mother. Observe universal precautions.

Clinical Implications

If the Rh-antibody titer in the pregnant woman is higher than 1:64, an intrauterine exchange transfusion may be considered.

Patient Preparation

1. Explain test purpose and procedure.
2. See Chapter 1 guidelines for safe, effective, informed *pretest* care.

Patient Aftercare

1. Interpret test outcome and counsel appropriately.
2. Follow Chapter 1 guidelines for safe, effective, informed *posttest* care.

ROSETTE TEST, FETAL RED CELLS (FETAL–MATERNAL BLOOD)

Normal Values

Negative for fetal blood loss; no fetal RBCs in maternal blood.

Explanation of Test

This test detects fetal cells in the maternal circulation. The detection of fetal erythrocytes is important for diagnosing anemia of the newborn when it is suspected that a severe fetal red cell loss has occurred and when serious risk of the mother becoming immunized against the fetal red cell groups occurs or is anticipated. In these instances, the mother's blood sample should be collected immediately after delivery to be examined for fetal cells.

The rosette test is 97% accurate for detecting a fetomaternal bleed that exceeds 30 ml of whole blood.

Procedure

A 7-ml venous blood EDTA sample is obtained from the mother shortly after delivery and examined for rosettes or mixed field agglutinates. The amount of fetal blood that has escaped into the maternal circulation can be roughly calculated using this formula:

$$\text{Milliliters of fetal blood} = \%\ \text{HgF cells} \times 50$$

Clinical Implications

1. When the test sample contains few or no RhD-positive fetal cells, rosetting or agglutination is absent, and the fetomaternal bleed (fetal blood loss) is less than 30 ml, one dose of parenteral RhoGAM (RhIg) will prevent immunization. If the fetal blood loss into the maternal circulation exceeds 35 ml, more than one vial of RhoGAM will be required. One vial of RhoGAM will neutralize about 30 to 35 ml of Rh-positive blood.
2. When rosetting is observed, a fetomaternal bleed of greater than 30 ml is possible. A quantitative test can determine the RhoGAM dosage necessary to prevent future complications.

Patient Preparation

1. Explain test purpose and procedure.
2. See Chapter 1 guidelines for safe, effective, informed *pretest* care.

Patient Aftercare

1. Interpret test outcome. Counsel relative to RhoGAM administration and follow-up maternal testing.
2. Follow Chapter 1 guidelines for safe, effective, informed *posttest* care.
3. The efficiency of RhoGAM is judged by the disappearance of hemoglobin F–containing cells after its administration. If the fetal cells have not disappeared 12 to 24 hours after the first RhoGAM dose, more RhoGAM is required.

> **Clinical Alert**
>
> An Rh_o (D) immune globulin screen can be done to determine need for antepartum and postpartum RhoGAM. Screening includes ABO, Rh typing, and microscopic Du antibody tests.

KLEIHAUER–BETKE TEST OR FETAL HEMOGLOBIN STAIN

Normal Values

Negative: No Rh_o (O) cells in maternal circulation.

Explanation of Test

The Kleihauer–Betke test is a quantitative test to determine the amount of fetomaternal hemorrhage in an RhD-negative mother and the amount of RhIg (RhoGAM) necessary to prevent future complications. The test is done after full-term delivery if newborn anemia is present or when the mother is Rh-negative or Du-negative.

Procedure

A 7-ml maternal venous blood EDTA sample is obtained immediately after delivery. The specimen should be examined immediately or else refrigerated. Amniotic fluid also may be tested.

Clinical Implications

1. Results indicate moderate to great fetomaternal hemorrhage (50%–90% of fetal RBCs contain HgF).
2. With full-term delivery, newborn RBCs must be Rh_o (D)-*positive,* and the direct antiglobulin test (for anti-Rh_o (O) must be *negative* for the mother to be a candidate for RhIg (Rh_oGAM).

Patient Preparation

1. Explain test purpose and procedure.
2. See Chapter 1 guidelines for safe, effective, informed *pretest* care.

Patient Aftercare

1. Interpret test outcomes and counsel parents appropriately relative to fetal bleed and RhIg (RhoGAM) to suppress the immunization of fetal red cells or whole-blood hemorrhage (Table 8-5).

   Vials of RhIg = ml of fetal blood/30

   Many recommend doubling the calculation of RhIg. The method of calculating fetal blood is not entirely accurate. The results of undertreatment are serious, but the effects of overtreatment are minor
2. See Chapter 1 guidelines for safe, effective, informed *posttest* care.

CROSSMATCH (COMPATIBILITY TEST) ●

Normal Values

Compatibility: No clumping or hemolysis when serum and cells are appropriately mixed and incubated. The major crossmatch shows compatibility between recipient serum and donor cells; the minor crossmatch shows compatibility between recipient cells and donor serum.

Background

The primary purpose of the crossmatch, or compatibility test, is to prevent a possible transfusion reaction. It consists of the *major crossmatch* and, infrequently, the *minor crossmatch*.

1. Major crossmatch detects antibodies in the recipient's serum that may

TABLE 8-5
Recommendations for Dose of RhIG in Massive Fetomaternal Blood Based on the Acid Elution Test

	Fetomaternal Hemorrhage Volume (ml whole blood)		
Fetal cells (%)	*Average*	*Range**	*Vials of RhIG to Inject*
0.3–0.5	20	<50	2
0.6–0.8	35	15–80	3
0.9–1.1	50	22–110	4
1.2–1.4	65	30–140	5
1.5–2.0	88	37–200	6
2.1–2.5	115	52–250	6

*The range provides for the poor precision of the acid separation elution test. These recommendations are based on one vial needed for each 15 ml of red blood cells or 30 ml of whole blood.

damage or destroy the cells of the proposed donor (Table 8-6). Of the two tests, the major crossmatch is the more important.

2. Minor crossmatch detects antibodies in the donor's serum capable of affecting the red blood cells of the recipient. Because donor antibodies will be greatly diluted in vivo by the recipient's plasma, these antibodies are considered to be of minor importance.
3. The type and screen determines the ABO and Rh_o (D) type as well as the presence or absence of unexpected antibodies from the recipient. The type and screen is a safe alternative for the routine type and crossmatch ordered preoperatively for cases that may, but usually do not, require transfusion (eg, hysterectomy or cholecystectomy). If blood is needed, a major crossmatch must be done before transfusion.

TABLE 8-6
Antibodies Found in Crossmatching

Blood Grouping System	*Antibody*	*Description*
Rh-hr	Anti-D	Rh1 May cause severe hemolytic disease of newborn
	Anti-C	Rh2 Often found with anti-D, -Ce(rh_i) or -C^w
	Anti-E	Rh3 Often found with anti-c
	Anti-c	Rh4 Often found with anti-E
	Anti-e	Rh5 Often found with anti-C
	Anti-C^w	Rh8
	Anti-V	Rh10 Alternative antigen names: ce^s hr^v
Kell	Anti-K	K1 Some non-red cell immune Occasional Kell system antibodies may not react
	Anti-k	K2 Antigen may be depressed by the presence of Kp^a
	Anti-Kp^a	K3 Few non-red cell immune
	Anti-Kp^b	K4
	Anti-Js^a	K6 Few non-red cell immune
	Anti-Js^b	K7
Duffy	Anti-Fy^a	Some antibodies exhibit dosage.
	Anti-Fy^b	Some antibodies may bind complement.

(continued)

TABLE 8-6 *(Continued)*

Blood Grouping System	Antibody	Description
Kidd	Anti-Jk^a	Antibodies may exhibit dosage. May cause severe delayed hemolytic transfusion reactions.
Kidd	Anti-Jk^b	Antibody titers may drop rapidly below detectable levels. Antibodies may require anti-C3 for detection.
Lutheran	Anti-Lu^a Anti-Lu^b	Antibody gives mixed-field–like agglutination
MN	Anti-M	Common antibody Seldom clinically significant or implicated in HDN May be pH-dependent or exhibit dosage
	Anti-N	Rare antibody Rarely causes HDN Formaldehyde-induced anti-N commonly found in dialysis patients
	Anti-S	Antibody may be enhanced if incubated below 37°C before AHG.
	Anti-s	
	Anti-U	Autoanti-U identified as rare cause of WAIHA
Lewis	Anti-Le^a	Frequently found in serum of pregnant women
	Anti-Le^b	Neutralized by soluble antigen
	-Le^{bh}	Anti-Le^b often found with anti-Le^a
	-Le^{bL}	Anti-Le^b usually made by Le(a−b−) individuals
P	Anti-P_1	Antigen strength variable; neutralized by soluble antigen
	Anti-P	Biphasic hemolytic IgG autoantibody in PCH Alloantibody is usually potent IgM hemolysin.
	Anti-PP_1P^k (Tj^a)	
Xg	Anti-Xg^a	X-linked
Colton	Anti-Co^a Anti-Co^b	Rare antibodies
Dombrock	Anti-Do^a	Incidence of Do^a lower in blacks, American Indians, and Orientals
	Anti-Do^b	Infrequently reported antibodies
Diego	Anti-Di^a	Di^a antigen frequency higher in Orientals and American Indians
	Anti-Di^b	
Wright	Anti-Wr^a	IgM and IgG forms of antibody reported Frequently occurring antibody

(continued)

TABLE 8-6 *(Continued)*

Blood Grouping System	Antibody	Description
Vel	Anti-Vel	Antibodies usually IgM
		Antigen strength variable
		Binds complement
Sid	Anti-Sid^a	Antigen weaker during pregnancy
		Wide variation of antigen expression
		Agglutinates have refractile, mixed-field appearance.
HLA-associated	Anti-Bg$_a$	Antigen strength variable
	-Bg$_b$	Antibodies often found in multitransfused or multiparous patients
	-Bg$_c$	
	-B$_g$	Antibodies characteristically weakly reactive
		Bg/HLA associations: Bg^a/HLA-B7, Bg^b/HLA-B17, Bg^c/HLA-A28
Cartwright	Anti-Yt^a	Antibody not uncommon in Yt(a−) individuals
	Anti-Yt^b	Rare antibody usually found in combination with other antibodies
HTLA (high-titer, low-avidity)	Anti-CH^a	Antigen strength variable
	-Rg^a	Antibodies characteristically weakly reactive
	-Kn^a	
	-McC^a	
	-Yk^a	
	-Cs^a	
	-Gy^a	
	-Hy	
	-JMH	
I	Anti-I	Most frequent cold autoagglutination
		Anti-I in CHD has wide thermal range, high titer; binds complement; seen as alloantibody in i adults
	Anti-i	Antibody seen in serum of patients with infectious mononucleosis
		Rare cause of CHD
		Antigen very weakly expressed on the cells of most adults

(Adapted from Baxter Healthcare Corporation, Dade Division, Miami, FL, Baxter Healthcare Corporation, 1987)

Explanation of Test

Crossmatching must be done to detect different types of antibodies, such as high-protein medium-acting antibodies, saline-acting antibodies, antibodies recognizable only with the antiglobulin technique.

Clinical Alert

Even the most carefully performed crossmatch will not detect all possible incompatible sources.

Procedure

Obtain a 10-ml venous blood sample. Observe universal precautions.

Clinical Implications

1. A *transfusion reaction* occurs when incompatibile blood is transfused, specifically if antibodies in the recipient's serum cause rapid red blood cell destruction in the proposed donor unit.
   - **a.** Certain antibodies, although not causing immediate red cell destruction and transfusion reaction, nevertheless, may reduce the normal life span of transfused incompatible cells; this may necessitate subsequent transfusions.
   - **b.** Obviously, the patient will derive the most benefit from red cells that survive longest.
2. The probable benefits of each blood transfusion must be weighed against the risks; these include
   - **a.** Hemolytic transfusion reactions owing to infusion of incompatible flood (can be fatal)
   - **b.** Febrile or allergic reactions
   - **c.** Transmission of infectious disease (eg, hepatitis)
   - **d.** Stimulation of antibody production, which could complicate later transfusions or childbearing

Clinical Alert

1. The most common cause of hemolytic transfusion reaction is the administration of incompatible blood to the recipient because of faulty matching in the laboratory, improper patient identification, or incorrect labeling of donor blood. If a transfusion reaction is suspected, discontinue the transfusion and notify the blood bank and attending physician immediately.
2. Assess for the following *symptoms* of transfusion reaction:
   - **a.** Fever
   - **b.** Chills
   - **c.** Chest pain
   - **d.** Hypotension
   - **e.** Nausea
   - **f.** Dyspnea
   - **g.** Shock
   - **h.** Oliguria

(continued)

(Clinical Alert continued)

- **i.** Back pain
- **j.** Feeling of heat along vein being transfused
- **k.** Constricting chest and lumbar back muscles
- **l.** Facial flushing
- **m.** Hemoglobinuria
- **n.** Oozing blood from wounds
- **o.** Anemia
- **p.** Allergic reactions such as local erythema hives and itching

3. After massive blood transfusions, test for

- **a.** Hypocalcemia
- **b.** Potassium intoxication
- **c.** Increased blood ammonia
- **d.** Increased oxygen affinity
- **e.** Hypothermia (from blood)
- **f.** Hemosiderosis

4. Document transfusion reaction signs and symptoms; notify the blood bank of reaction, and carry out follow-up interventions.

Types of Transfusion Reactions

ACUTE HEMOLYTIC TRANSFUSION REACTION (HTR)

HTR reaction is triggered by an antigen–antibody reaction and activates the complement and coagulation systems. These are most always due to ABO incompatibility because of misidentification that results in the patient receiving incompatible blood. Symptoms: fever, chills, backache, vague uneasiness, and red urine. HTR reactions are potentially fatal.

BACTERIAL CONTAMINATION

Bacteria may enter the blood during phlebotomy. These microbes will multiply faster in components stored at room temperature than in refrigerated components. Although rare, bacteria in blood or its components can cause a septic transfusion reaction. Symptoms include high fever, shock, hemoglobulinuria, DIC, and renal failure. Such reactions can be fatal.

FEBRILE NONHEMOLYTIC REACTION (FNH)

FNH reactions are defined as a temperature increase of 1°C or more. They are seldom dangerous and may be caused by an antibody–antigen reaction.

ANAPHYLACTIC REACTIONS

1. Anaphylactic reactions occur after infusion of as little as a few milliliters of blood or plasma.
2. Anaphylaxis is characterized by coughing, bronchospasm, respiratory distress, vascular instability, nausea, abdominal cramps, vomiting, diarrhea, shock, and loss of consciousness.
3. Some reactions occur in IgA-deficient patients who have developed anti-IgA antibodies after immunization through previous transfusion or pregnancy.
4. These reactions can be prevented by giving IgA-deficient blood components.

(continued)

Types of Transfusion Reactions *(Continued)*

CUTANEOUS HYPERSENSITIVITY REACTIONS

Urticarial reactions are very common, second in frequency only to febrile nonhemolytic reactions and are usually characterized by erythema, hives, and itching. Allergy to some soluble substance in donor plasma is suspected.

NONCARDIOGENIC PULMONARY REACTIONS (NPR)

Symptoms of NPR include chills, fever, cyanosis, and hypotension. These are possibly reactions between the donor's leukocyte antibodies and the recipient's leukocytes. NPR produces white cell aggregates that become trapped in the pulmonary microcirculation. The finding on chest x-ray films are typical of acute pulmonary edema. If subsequent transfusions are needed, leukocyte-reduced red cells may prevent NRA reactions.

CIRCULATORY OVERLOAD

Rapid increases in blood volume are not tolerated well by patients with compromised cardiac or pulmonary function. Symptoms of circulatory overload include coughing, cyanosis, orthopnea, difficulty in breathing, and a rapid increase in systolic blood pressure.

Patient Preparation

1. Explain purpose and procedure of crossmatching.
2. See Chapter 1 guidelines for safe, effective, informed *pretest* care.

Patient Aftercare

1. Interpret test outcome and counsel patient concerning potential transfusion reactions.
2. Follow Chapter 1 guidelines for safe, effective, informed *posttest* care.

COOMBS ANTIGLOBULIN TEST ●

Normal Values

Direct Coombs test: negative for red blood cells
Indirect Coombs test: negative for serum

Explanation of Test

The Coombs test shows the presence of antigen–antibody complexes through the *direct* method; it detects antibodies that react only through a potentiating medium, by the *indirect* method. The *direct Coombs* test detects antigen–antibody complexes on the red blood cell membrane (*in vivo*) as well as red blood cell sensitization. It is diagnostic for

1. Hemolytic disease of the newborn in which the red cells of the infant are sensitized and exhibit antigen–antibody complexes *in vivo*.
2. Acquired hemolytic anemia when an antibody is produced that coats the patient's own cells (autosensitization *in vivo*)
3. Transfusion reaction because the patient may have received incompatible blood which, in turn, has sensitized the patient's own red cells.
4. Red blood cell sensitization caused by drugs. The *indirect Coombs* test detects serum antibodies, reveals maternal anti-Rh antibodies during pregnancy, and can detect incompatibilities not found by other methods.

Procedure

Obtain a 10-ml venous blood sample. Observe universal precautions.

Clinical Implications

1. The *direct Coombs test* is *positive* in the presence of
   - **a.** Autoimmune hemolytic anemia (most cases)
   - **b.** Transfusion reactions
   - **c.** Cephalothin therapy (75% of cases)
   - **d.** Drugs, such as α-methyldopa (Aldomet), penicillin, insulin
   - **e.** Hemolytic disease of newborn
   - **f.** Paroxysmal cold hemoglobinurea
2. The direct Coombs test is *negative* in nonautoimmune hemolytic anemias.
3. The *indirect Coombs test* is *positive* in the presence of specific antibodies, usually from a previous transfusion or pregnancy; nonspecific antibodies, as in cold agglutination disease or drug-induced hemolytic anemia.

Interfering Factors

Several drugs may cause the direct Coombs test to be positive.

Clinical Alert

Antibody identification is performed when results of the antibody screen or direct antiglobulin tests are positive and unexpected blood group antibodies need to be classified. Antibody identification tests are an important part of pretransfusion testing so that the appropriate antigen-negative blood can be transfused. These tests are also helpful for diagnosing hemolytic disease of the newborn and autoimmune hemolytic anemia. A 7-ml venous blood sample with added EDTA and 20 ml of clotted blood are studied. Notify the laboratory of diagnosis, history of recent and past transfusions, pregnancy, and any drug therapy.

Patient Preparation

1. Explain purpose and procedure of Coombs test.
2. See Chapter 1 guidelines for safe, effective, informed *pretest* care.

Patient Aftercare

1. Interpret test outcome and counsel appropriately. Hemolytic disease of newborn (HDN) occurs when the mother is Rh-negative and the fetus is Rh-positive. Diagnosis is derived from the following information: mother is Rh (–), the newborn is Rh (+), the direct Coombs test is (+). Newborn jaundice results from Rh incompatibility.
2. Follow Chapter 1 guidelines for safe, effective, informed *posttest* care.

LEUKOAGGLUTININ TEST ●

Normal Values

Negative for leukoagglutinins.

Background

Leukoagglutinins are antibodies that react with white blood cells and sometimes cause febrile, nonhemolytic transfusion reactions. Patients who exhibit this type of transfusion reaction should receive leukocyte-poor blood for any subsequent transfusions.

Explanation of Test

This study is done when a blood reaction occurs, even though compatible blood has been given. The donor plasma contains an antibody that reacts with recipient white cells to produce an acute clinical syndrome of fever, dyspnea, cough, pulmonary infiltrates, and in more severe cases, cyanosis and hypertension. Patients immunized by previous transfusions, pregnancy, or during allografts often experience these febrile, nonhemolytic transfusion reactions because of incompatible transfused leukocytes. This type of reaction must be confirmed (as compared with hemolytic reactions) before additional transfusions can be safely administered.

Procedure

Obtain a 10-ml venous blood sample. Observe universal precautions.

Clinical Implications

1. Agglutinating antibodies may appear in the donor's plasma.
2. When the agglutinating antibody appears in the recipient's plasma, febrile reactions are common; however, pulmonary manifestations do not occur.
3. Febrile reactions are more common in pregnant women and those individuals with a history of multiple transfusions.

Clinical Alert

1. Febrile reactions can be prevented by separating out white cells from the donor blood before transfusion.
2. Patients whose blood contains leukoagglutinins should be instructed that they generally need to be transfused with leukocyte-poor blood to minimize these reactions.

Patient Preparation

1. Explain test purpose and procedure.
2. See Chapter 1 guidelines for safe, effective, informed *pretest* care.

Patient Aftercare

1. Interpret test outcome and counsel patient concerning future transfusion precautions.
2. Follow Chapter 1 guidelines for safe, effective, informed *posttest* care.

PLATELET ANTIBODY DETECTION TESTS

Normal Values

PLAI: negative platelet hyperlysibility: negative
ALTP: negative drug-dependent platelet antibodies: negative
PAIgG: negative

Explanation of Test

Platelet antibody detection studies are used to diagnose posttransfusion purpura, alloimmune neonatal thrombocytopenic purpura, idiopathic thrombocytopenia purpura, paroxysmal hemoglobinuria, and drug-induced immunologic thrombocytopenia.

Procedure

A 10- to 30-ml venous blood sample is required

Blood specimen requirements

30 ml of venous blood when platelet count is 50,000 to 100,000/mm^3
20 ml of venous blood when platelet count is 100,000 to 150,000/mm^3
10 ml of venous blood when platelet count is > 150,000/mm^3

Interfering Factors

Alloantibodies formed in response to previous blood transfusions during pregnancies may produce positive reactions. Such antibodies are usually specific for human leukocyte antigens (HLA) found in platelets and other cells. Whenever possible, obtain samples for platelet antibody testing before transfusing.

Clinical Implications

1. Antibodies to platelet antigens are of two types: autoantibodies develop in response to one's own platelets, as in idiopathic thrombocytopenia purpura, and alloantibodies develop following exposure to foreign platelets after a transfusion.
2. Antiplatelet antibody, usually having anti-PLAI specificity, occurs in posttransfusion purpura.
3. A persistent or rising antibody titer during pregnancy is associated with neonatal thrombocytopenia.
4. PLAI incompatibility between mother and fetus appears to account for more than 60% of alloimmune neonatal thrombocytopenic purpura. A finding of a PLAI-negative mother and a PLAI-positive father provides presumptive diagnostic evidence.
5. Platelet-associated IgG antibody is present in 95% of idiopathic (autoimmune) thrombocytopenic purpura (both acute and chronic) cases. Patients responding to steroid therapy or undergoing spontaneous remission show increased circulatory times that correlate with decreased PAIgG levels.
6. The platelet hyperlysibility assay measures the sensitivity of platelets to lysis. This test is positive in, and specific for, paroxysmal hemoglobinuria.
7. In drug-induced immunologic thrombocytopenia, antibodies that react only in the presence of the inciting drug can be detected. Quinidine, quinine, chlordiazepoxide, sulfa drugs, and diphenylhydantoin most commonly cause this type of thrombocytopenia. Gold-dependent antibodies and heparin-dependent platelet IgG antibodies can be detected by direct assay. (Approximately 1% of persons receiving gold therapy develop thrombocytopenia as a side effect.) Thrombocytopenia is also a well-known side effect of heparin.

NOTE: *Platelet compatibility typing is done to assure that hemostatically stable platelets can be transfused (eg, for aplastic anemia and malignant disorders). This is important because most patients repeatedly transfused with platelets from random donors become partially or totally refractory to further platelet transfusion because of alloimmunization.*

Platelet typing also provides diagnostic evidence of posttransfusion purpura. Platelets are routinely typed for PLAI, HLA-A2, and PLEI. Those matched for HLA antigens generally produce satisfactory posttransfusion improvement. A standard platelet count performed 1 hour after the end of a fresh platelet concentrate transfusion is a sensitive indicator for the presence or absence of clinically important antibodies against HLA antigens.

Patient Preparation

1. Explain test purpose and procedure.
2. See Chapter 1 guidelines for safe, effective, informed *pretest* care.

Patient Aftercare

1. Interpret test outcomes, counsel, and monitor appropriately for bleeding tendencies. Assess for prescribed medications as cause of purpura.
2. Follow Chapter 1 guidelines for safe, effective, informed *posttest* care.

HUMAN LEUKOCYTE ANTIGEN (HLA) TEST ●

Normal Values

Requires clinical correlation.

Background

The major histocompatibility antigens of humans belong to the HLA system. They are present on all nucleated cells, but can be detected most easily on lymphocytes. Each antigen results from a gene that shares a locus on the chromosome with another gene, one paternal and one maternal (two alleles). More than 27 of these antigens have been identified. The HLA complex, located in the short arm of chromosome 6, is a major histocompatibility complex in humans that is responsible for many important immune functions.

Explanation of Test

This test determines the leukocyte antigens present on human cell surfaces. When tissue or organ transplants are contemplated, HLA typing identifies the degree of histocompatibility between donor and recipient. By matching donors and potential recipients with compatible lymphocytes and similar HLA types, it is possible to prolong transplant survival and to reduce rejection episodes. The HLA also aids in diagnosis of parentage as well as certain rheumatoid diseases, particularly ankylosing spondylitis. HLA-B27, one of the HLA antigens, is found in 90% of the patients. Generally, the presence of a certain HLA antigen may be associated with increased susceptibility to a specific disease; however, it does not mandate that that person will develop the disease.

Procedure

Obtain a 10- to 24-ml heparinized venous blood sample. Observe universal precautions. The patient's HLA type is determined by testing the patient's lymphocytes against a panel of defined HLA antiserums directed against the currently recognized HLA antigens. The HLA antigens are identified by letter and number. When viable human lymphocytes are incubated with a known HLA cytotoxic antibody, an antigen–antibody complex will be formed on a cell surface. The addition of serum that contains complement kills the cells, which are then recognized as possessing a defined HLA antigen.

Clinical Implications

1. Association between particular HLA antigens and certain disease states includes

- **a.** Ankylosing spondylitis (HLA-B27)
- **b.** Multiple sclerosis (HLA-B27 + Dw2 + A3 + B18)
- **c.** Myasthenia gravis (HLA-B8)
- **d.** Psoriasis (HLA-A13 + B17)
- **e.** Reiter's syndrome (B27)
- **f.** Juvenile insulin-dependent diabetes (Bw15 + B8)
- **g.** Acute anterior uveitis (B27)
- **h.** Graves disease (B27)
- **i.** Juvenile rheumatoid arthritis (B27)
- **j.** Celiac disease (B8)
- **k.** Dermatitis herpetiformis (B8)
- **l.** Autoimmune chronic active hepatitis (B8)

2. Four groups of cell surface antigens, HLA-A, HLA-B, HLA-C, and HLA-D, constitute the strongest barriers to tissue transplantation.
3. In parentage determination, if a reputed father presents a phenotype (genotype completely determined by heredity; two haplotypes or gene clusters, one from father and one from mother) with no haplotype or antigen pair identical with one of the child's, he is excluded as the supposed father. If one of the reputed father's haplotypes (gene clusters) is the same as one of the child's, he *may be* the father. The chances of his being accurately identified as the father increase in direct proportion to the rarity of the presenting haplotype in the general population. Put another way, if the haplotype is very common, there is an increased probability that another man with the same haplotype may also be the father. When the frequence of a haplotype is known, the probability that the nonexcluded man is the father can be calculated. However, the degree of certainty diminishes as the incidence of the haplotype increases.

Patient Preparation

1. Explain test purpose and procedure.
2. See Chapter 1 guidelines for safe, effective, informed *pretest* care.

Patient Aftercare

1. Interpret test outcomes and counsel appropriately. HLA testing is best used as a diagnostic adjunct and should not be considered as diagnostic in and of itself. Explain the need for possible further testing.
2. Follow Chapter 1 guidelines for safe, effective, informed *posttest* care.

● TUMOR MARKERS

Physical examination and standard radiologic techniques can usually detect tumors 1 cm in volume. A tumor mass of this size would have completed 30 doublings (two-thirds of its growth) and would contain a billion (10^9) cells. Tumor cells capable of forming metastases are likely to be released into either the bloodstream or the regional lymphatics. Thus, tumor testing has focused on identifying certain tumor-related substances that might allow early

TABLE 8-7
Tumor Markers

Tumor markers are substances produced and secreted by tumor cells and found in serum of persons with cancer. This table includes tumor-specific or tumor-associated antigens (proteins and oncofetal antigens), enzymes and hormones. Refer to Chapters 6 and 8 for complete listing of normal values, clinical implications and safe, effective, informed patient preparation and aftercare.

Name of Test Clinical Marker in Current Use and Selected Normal Values	Type of Cancer in Which Tumor Marker May Be Found	Conditions Other Than Cancer That Are Associated With Abnormal Values
ENZYMES		
1. Prostatic acid phosphatase (PAP). Increased values owing to increased metabolism and catabolism of cancer cells—levels increase with stage of cancer and age of individual. NL <4 Adult: 0–3.1 mg/ml Child: 8.6–12.6 U/ml Newborn: 10.4–16.4 U/ml	1(a) Carcinoma of prostate with the following elevation: carcinoma with no metastasis 10–20%; metastasis with one 20–40%; metastases with bone involvement 70–90% (usually osteoblastic) (b) in 3/4 patients arises in posterior lobe of prostate (c) used to monitor therapy with antineoplastic drugs (d) leukemia (hairy-cell); (e) cancer metastatic to bone (osteoblastic lesions)	1(a) Noncancer prostatic condition, prostate palpation, hyperplasia, infection of prostate following cystostomy, prostate surgery, and chronic prostatitis (b) Other—Gaucher's disease (lipid storage disease), Nieman-Pick disease, Paget's disease, osteoporosis, renal osteopathy, hepatic cirrhosis, pulmonary embolism and hyperparathyroidism
2. Lactate dehydrogenase (LDH); increased isoenzymes I and II	2(a) Neuroblastomic carcinoma of testes. Elevated in 60% of those with stage 3 testicular cancer—serial LDH may help to detect recurrence of cancer (b) Ewing's sarcoma (c) Acute lymphocytic leukemia; (d) Non-Hodgkin's lymphoma	2. Cellular injury/hemolysis, myocardial infarction, hepatic diseases; see Cardiac Enzyme Tests

3. Neuron-specific enolase (NSE): normal staining. Produced by neurons and neuroendocrine cells of the central and peripheral nervous system	3. NSE increases: (a) neuroblastomas; (b) APUD system tumor—small cell lung cancers, pancreatic islet cell, medullary thyroid carcinoma. (c) Wilm's tumor and pheochromocytoma	
4. Alkaline phosphatase (ALP) originates in osteoblasts, lining of hepatobiliary tree and intestinal tract and placenta Adults: 30–85 U/ml Child: <2z-85–235 U/ml 2-21z: 30–200 U/ml	4. Increases—osteosarcoma, hepatocellular, metasatic to liver, primary or secondary bone tumors	4. Increase—Paget's disease, nonmalignant liver disease, normal pregnancy, healing fractures, hyperparathyroidism. Decrease—hypoparathyroidism, malnutrition, scurvy, pernicious anemia
5. Other enzymes: γ-glutamyl transpeptidase, muramidase, creatinine, phosphokinase isoenzyme (CPK-BB), β-glucurmidase, terminal deoxynucleotidyl transferase, ribonuclease, histaminase (medullary cancer of thyroid), amylase, and cystine aminopeptidase		
HORMONES		
1. Human chorionic gonadoptropin (HCG) produced by placental syncytiotrophoblast—not usually found in sera of healthy, nonpregnant persons. Male: <2.5 IU/L Postmenopausal: <9.0 IU/L Pregnancy: peaks at 10 weeks gestation	1. Increase—gestational trophoblastic tumors, seminomatous and nonseminomatous testes cancer, ovarian tumors, pancreatic islet-cell cancer, liver (21%), stomach (22%), and less valuable with lung and lymphoproliferative disease	1. Increase—gestational trophoblastic neoplasms (hydatiform mole) neoplasm of stomach, colon, pancreas, lungs and liver, multiple pregnancy. Decrease—ectopic pregnancy and abortion

(continued)

TABLE 8-7 *(Continued)*

Name of Test Clinical Marker in Current Use and Selected Normal Values	*Type of Cancer in Which Tumor Marker May Be Found*	*Conditions Other Than Cancer That Are Associated With Abnormal Values*
2. Calcitonin (CT) malignant C-cell tumor produces increase CT levels. <14–19 pg/ml	2. Increase—metastatic breast greatly elevated, limited in primary small tumor burden breast cancer as levels lower, lung, pancreas, hepatoma and renal cell carcinoid	2. Increase—Zollinger–Ellison syndrome, pernicious anemia, chronic renal failure, pseudohypoparathyroidism, apudomas, alcoholic cirrhosis, Paget's disease, pregnancy, and benign breast or ovarian disease. Decrease—with therapy and a rise after therapy suggests progressive disease
3. Other Hormones: ACTH (lung—oat cell), PTH (lung—epidermoid), insulin (lung), glucagon (pancreas), gastrin (stomach and other carcinomas), prostaglandins and erythropoietin (kidney).		
ONCOFETAL ANTIGENS		
1. Alphafetoprotein (AFP) produced by fetal liver, yolk sac, and intestinal epithelium. Disappears from blood soon after birth and not present in healthy individuals, 10 ng/ml	1. Inceases—primary hepatocellular cancer, embryonal cell (nonseminomatous germ cell) testicular tumors, yolk sac ovarian tumors, teratocarcinoma, gastric, pancreatic, colonic, breast, renal, and lung	1. Increase—fetal distress and death, neural tube defects, viral hepatitis, primary biliary cirrhosis, partial hepatectomy, ataxic-telangiectasia, Wiskott–Aldrich syndrome, multiple pregnancy and abortion

2. Carcinoembryonic antigen (CEA). Initially isolated in endodermally derived adenocarcinoma and fetal gastrointestinal tissue 0–2.5 mg/ml; up to 10 ng/ml in smokers	2. Increases—colon (especially metastatic or recurrence), pancreas, lung, stomach, metastatic breast, ovary, bladder, limbs, neuroblastoma, leukemia, thyroid, and osteogenic carcinoma. Useful to monitor therapy with antineoplastic drugs and following surgery of neoplasma—not a screening test for cancer	2. Increase—inflammatory bowel disease, rectal polyps, active ulcerative colitis, pancreatitis, alcoholic cirrhosis, peptic ulcers, cholecystitis, chronic renal failure, pulmonary emphysema, bronchitis, pulmonary infections and fibrocystic breast disease. Most levels decline with remission of disease
PROTEINS		
1. CA 15-3 antigen <22 U/ml (breast-cystic fluid protein-BCFP)	1. Increase—greatly elevated in metastatic breast—limited in small tumor burdening breast cancer. Decrease—with therapy and increased rise after therapy suggests progressive disease	1. Increases—benign breast or ovarian disease
2. $beta_2$-Microglobulin (HLA antigen system) 4–12 mg/nl	2. Increase—multiple myeloma, other B-cell neoplasms, lung cancer, hepatoma, breast cancer	2. Increase—ankylosing spondylitis and Reiters syndrome
3. Prostatic-specific antigen (PSA)—more sensitive than PAP—correlates with stage of disease. 0–4 ng/ml	3. Increase—prostate cancer the higher the level, the greater the tumor burden. Successful surgery, chemotherapy or radiation cause marked reduction in levels	3. Increase—benign prostatic hypertrophy, prostate massage, prostate surgery, and prostatitis
4. CA 19-9 carbohydrate antigen, <37 U/ml	4. Increase—pancreas and hepatobiliary cancer, primarily mild elevation—gastric and colorectal cancer	4. Increase—pancreatitis, cholecystitis, cirrhosis, gallstones, and cystic fibrosis (minimal elevations)
5. CA 125 (ovarian cancer) (glycoprotein) 0–35 U/ml	5. Increase—epithelial ovary, fallopian tube, endometrium, endocervix, pancreas, and liver. Less increase—colon, breast, lung, and gastrointestinal	5. Increase—pregnancy, endometriosis, pelvic inflammatory disease, menstruation, acute and chronic hepatitis, ascites, peritonitis, pancreatitis, and GI disease, Meig's syndrome, pleural effusion and pulmonary disease

(continued)

TABLE 8-7 *(Continued)*

Name of Test Clinical Marker in Current Use and Selected Normal Values	***Type of Cancer in Which Tumor Marker May Be Found***	***Conditions Other Than Cancer That Are Associated With Abnormal Values***
6. Tissue polypeptide antigen (TPA); 80–100 U/L in serum—may also be detected in urine, washings and effusions	6. Increase—gastrointestinal, genitourinary tract, breast, lung, thyroid	6. Increase—hepatitis, cholangitis, cirrhosis, pneumonia, or urinary tract infections
7. Immunoglobulins—monoclonal proteins (M proteins), immunoglobulins that are produced by B lymphocytes; Absent: Refer to serum protein electrophoresis (SPEP) or urine protein electrophoresis (UPEP)	7. Multiple myeloma, macroglobulinemia, amyloidosis, B-cell lymphoma, multiple solid tumors	7. Cold agglutinin disease, Sjogren's syndrome, Gaucher's disease, lichen myxedematosus, cirrhosis, renal failure, and sarcoid
8. Other antigens: colon mucoprotein antigen (CMA), colon-specific antigen (CSA), zino glycinate marker (ZGM-colon), pancreatic oncofetal antigen (POA), S-100 protein (malignant melanoma), sialoglycoprotein (wide variety of cancers), B-protein (wide variety of antigens), and "Tennessee" antigen glycoprotein (wide variety of cancers).		

detection of malignancy, determination of prognosis, and evaluation of tumor burden (size, location, encroachment on other tissues or organs).

Tumor markers include genetic markers (abnormal chromosomes or oncogenes), enzymes, hormones, oncofetal antigens, glycoproteins, tumor antigens on cell surfaces, and substances produced in response to tumor growth (eg, cell reactive protein, circulating immune complexes, and prostate-specific antigen). Tumor markers (other than those identified in Table 8-7) are used and developed to obtain greater sensitivity and specificity about tumor activity. In general, these markers lack specificity for cancer; none is pathognomonic for any one type of neoplasm. Diagnosis still derives from comprehensive patient history, physical examination, and diagnostic testing. Tumor marker studies do not replace biopsy and pathologic tissue examination, but they are helpful for detecting tumors, checking for disease recurrence or progression, and assessing therapeutic effectiveness. Table 8-7 displays clinical markers in current use.

BIBLIOGRAPHY

Abbas AK et al: Cellular and Molecular Immunology, 2nd ed, Philadelphia, WB Saunders, 1994

Barrett JT: Medical Immunology: Text and Review. Philadelphia, FA Davis, 1991

Beneson A et al: HIV Testing: Model Performance Evaluation Program. Atlanta, Centers for Disease Control, 1990

Bridges AJ et al: Antinuclear antibody testing in a referral laboratory. Laboratory Medicine, 24(6):345–349, June 1993

Check I et al: Flow cytometry for cell surface phenotyping. Clinical Chemistry Newsletter, April 1991

Domato JJ, O'Bryan B: Resolution of indeterminate HIV-I test data using the Department of Defense HIV-I testing program. Laboratory Medicine, 22(2):107–113, February 1994

Englehard VH: How cells process antigens. Scientific American 270(4):54–61, August 1994

Harrison H et al: Serum protein electrophoresis: Basic principles, interpretations, practical considerations and new techniques. ASCP Check Sample, PTS 98-98, 1993

Henry JB (ed): Todd, Sanford, Davidsohn's Clinical Diagnosis and Management by Laboratory Methods, 18th ed. Philadelphia, WB Saunders, 1990

Jackson M et al: Viral hepatitis, anatomy of a diagnosis. American Journal of Nursing, January: 43–48, 1994

Kallestad Diagnostics, Inc: Assay summary. Cardiolipin. January 1991

Kallestad Diagnostics, Inc: Autoantibodies to nuclear antigens: An update. Reference from workshop, June 1990

Kantor FS: Disarming Lyme disease. Scientific American 27(5):34–39, September 1994

Mainous AG, Hagen MD: Public awareness of prostate cancer and the prostate-specific antigen test. Cancer Practice 2(3):217–221, May–June 1994

Miller LE et al: Manual of Laboratory Immunology, 2nd ed, Philadelphia, Lea & Febiger, 1991

Leavelle DE (ed): Interpretive Handbook: Interpretive Data for Diagnostic Laboratory Tests. Rochester, MN, Mayo Medical Laboratories, 1990

Ndimbia OK, Riddle PB: Serological assessment of the prospective organ donor. Laboratory Medicine 24(2):103–106, February 1993

Nichols Institute: Assay Summary, Soluble amyloid beta protein precursor. October, 1993

Sager D et al: Assays for rheumatoid factor: A review of their utility and limitations in clinical practice. Laboratory Medicine, 23(1):15–18, January 1992

Sheehan C: Clinical Immunology: Principles and Laboratory Diagnosis. Philadelphia, JB Lippincott, 1990

Takaichi Y et al: The significance of antithyroglobulin and antithyroidal microsomal antibodies in patients with hyperthyroidism due to Graves' disease treated with antithyroidal drugs. Journal of Clinical Endocrinology and Metabolism 68:1097–1100, 1989

Walker RH: American Association of Blood Banks, 11th ed, Technical Manual. Arlington, VA, American Association of Blood Banks, 1993

Wilson M, Arrowood MJ: Diagnostic parasitology: Direct detective methods and serodiagnosis. Laboratory Medicine 24(3):145–149, March 1993

1994 Revised Guidelines for the Performance of $CD4^+$ T-cell determinations in persons with human immunodeficiency virus (HIV) infection. US Department of Health and Human Services, Public Health Service, Centers for Disease Control and Prevention, Atlanta, GA, March 4, 1994

9

Nuclear Medicine Studies

OVERVIEW OF NUCLEAR STUDIES

Radionuclide studies are performed in a department of nuclear medicine. The success of a particular study depends on the existence of detectable differences in the concentrations of administered radioactive materials in normal and abnormal tissue in areas of the body under study.

Radionuclide imaging is used mainly to allow visualization of organs and regions within organs that cannot be seen on a simple x-ray film. Space-occupying lesions, especially tumors, stand out particularly well. Generally, these lesions are represented by areas of reduced radioactivity; however, in some instances, such as in bone scanning, areas of increased activity represent pathology.

Radionuclide describes an atom with an unstable nucleus within its orbital electrons. In an attempt to reach stability, the radionuclide emits one or more types of radiation, the most common examples being alpha particles, beta particles, and gamma electromagnetic radiation. In nuclear medicine, with the exception of therapy, gamma radiation is used in diagnostic procedures. Gamma radiation is easy to detect and is the least ionizing type.

Principles of Nuclear Imaging Studies

In general, gamma rays are used for imaging organ systems and provide an indication of how well an organ system functions. Computerized radiation detection equipment, particularly *scintillation detectors,* detect gamma rays by giving off a light flash, or scintillation. The imaging device outlines and photographs the organ under study and provides information on its size, shape, position, and functional activity. With a computer receiving digital signals converted from the scintillations, some measurements are obtained in nuclear cardiology, such as ejection fractions.

The radioactive materials used in nuclear medicine in diagnostic imaging are called *radiopharmaceuticals,* which distribute throughout tissues, organs, and organ systems, depending on their tissue specificity and how they are administered. Within these organs, the radioactive material shows distributions in normal tissue that differ from those in diseased tissue.

There are two major types of radiopharmaceutical uptake. The first is known as a *hotspot,* in which an increased area of uptake of the radiopharmaceutical is compared with its normal distribution (the bone scan is an example.) The other type is a *coldspot,* in which an area of decreased uptake of the radiopharmaceutical is compared with the background (liver and lung scanning are examples).

In the nuclear medicine *in vitro* laboratory, radionuclides are used in numerous ways. They may be tagged to proteins and used in competitive protein-binding studies. They also may be labeled with antibodies or antigens and used in radioimmunoassay (RIA) studies. Radioimmunoassay methods have a high degree of sensitivity and specificity to detect substances within the body in trace quantities. This may be as low as a picogram or one-trillionth of a gram. The type of substances detected include hormones, antibiotics, carcinogens, drugs, vitamins, and immunoglobulins.

Imaging Used in Nuclear Medicine

Today several types of imaging devices are used in the field of nuclear medicine. The most basic imaging device is the gamma camera. This instrument is placed over the target area, where it views the entire field at once. For routine imaging it does not move, nor does it require the patient to move. A picture is constructed similar to that used in time photography. This is referred to as static imaging. Depending on the organ, various static images are obtained (anterior, posterior views) as established by protocols. At times, extra static images or "spot" views may be required. Dynamic imaging is another type, in which a computer takes a rapid series of images while the radiopharmaceutical flows through the organ of interest. One image, for example, may be acquired in 25 milliseconds. Whole-body imaging occurs when the patient lies on a table, and the table moves slowly until the entire patient has been viewed by the camera. In some systems, the table remains stationary while the camera scans over the patient. The major limitation of the gamma camera is that it is two-dimensional and suffers from a lack of depth perception.

Today, gamma cameras have achieved the third dimension through single-photon emission computed tomography (SPECT). (Tomography is the process of obtaining a picture of a specific segment or slice in the body.) Along with improvements in radiopharmaceuticals, SPECT has increased the specificity, sensitivity, and diagnostic ability of nuclear medicine imaging. Another form of tomographic imaging is positron emission tomography (PET) (see Part 3 for discussion).

The computed results of nuclear imaging may be recorded in the following ways:

1. Gray-scale photographic images: These are recorded on special single-emulsion film; the varying count rate appears as lighter or darker shades of gray, thus using the complete spectrum of the gray scale.
2. Color imaging: Color imaging involves a more complicated procedure than those described for gray-scale and usually requires some sort of computer processing.
3. Cine mode: By linking a computer to the scintillation camera, sequential pictures (or frames) are obtained and stored. After computer data processing, the frames are viewed in a cinematic mode, in which the movement of the radiopharmaceuticals portrays a specific organ's function.

Part 1

Nuclear Scans

General Procedure for Nuclear Medicine Scans

1. A radiopharmaceutical is administered orally or intravenously to the patient. At times, other drugs may be given to enhance the effects of radiopharmaceuticals, depending on the physiology involved.
2. A sufficient time interval is allowed for the radioactive material to follow its specific metabolic pathway in the body and to concentrate in the specific tissue to be studied.
3. An imaging device records the position and concentration of the radiation that emerges from the radionuclide. A computer is used to process the recorded radiation in many nuclear medicine exams.
4. The total length of examining time depends on the following:
   - **a.** Radiopharmaceutical used and time variable to allow for concentration in tissues
   - **b.** Type of imaging equipment used
   - **c.** Patient positioning
   - **d.** Different or additional views based on patient history and nuclear medicine protocols

Benefits and Risks

Benefits and risks should be explained before testing. Patients retain the radioactivity for relatively short periods. The radioactive energy does dissipate on its own, and some of the radiation will be eliminated in urine and feces.

Technetium (^{99m}Tc), which is the most commonly used tracer, is significantly reduced in 6 hours and is virtually gone from the patient's body in 24 hours. Other tracers, such as iodine, indium, and thallium, take approximately 13 hours to 8 days, respectively, for half of the energy to dissipate.

Patients need to know that once the energy has been eliminated, they are no longer carrying the radioactivity. A radiation hazard to the patient always exists. In all radionuclide procedures, the value and importance of the information gained must be weighed against the potential hazard of radiation to the patient. If a radionuclide study will advance the solution of a difficult problem, or provide information that cannot be obtained in any other way, then it should be done. For example, some of the following factors may be considered:

1. In almost all instances, radionuclide imaging exposes the patient to less radiation than would be received undergoing a similar procedure with diagnostic x-ray studies.
2. With a nuclear medicine scan, metastatic disease to the bone can be

found 6 months to a year before it can be detected with the usual bone radiograph.

Clinical Considerations

The following information should be obtained before diagnostic testing:

1. Menstrual history of women of childbearing age: Pregnancy is a contraindication to radionuclide studies.
2. Whether a mother is breastfeeding her baby: This is very important because radionuclide studies are contraindicated in nursing mothers. The mother may be advised to stop nursing for a set time period (eg, 2 to 3 days with ^{99m}Tc).
3. History of allergies: Certain patients may have adverse allergic reactions to some of the radionuclides and other drugs used in various procedures as required (see each procedure for the types of drugs used).
4. Knowledge of recent exposure to radionuclides: A history of any recent examination in which radionuclides were administered should be recorded because a previous study could seriously interfere with the clinician's interpretation of the current study.
5. Presence of any prostheses in the body: These must be recorded on the patient's history because certain devices can shield the gamma energy. Also, patient's jewelry or any kind of metal will interfere with a nuclear medicine exam.
6. Current medication, treatment, or diagnostic measures (eg, telemetry, oxygen, urine collection, and intravenous lines).
7. Age and current weight: This information is used to calculate the amount of the radioactive substance to be administered before imagery. If the patient is younger than 18, notify the examining department before testing. This information is vital for a technologist to perform any nuclear medicine procedure.
8. Other special considerations related to the patient's well-being should be communicated to the examining department, such as
   - **a.** Transportation needs, such as cart, wheelchair
   - **b.** An intravenous or nasogastric tube
   - **c.** If patient is diabetic (also, see item 3)
   - **d.** Pertinent medications
   - **e.** Any special patient restrictions or necessary physical supports/restraints to help in mobility and positioning

Clinical Alert

Premenopausal women should be advised to practice effective birth control during the testing period. These tests may be harmful to a fetus. Nuclear medicine needs to be notified if the patient may be pregnant or is breastfeeding.

Standard Precautions, Pretest Care for Nuclear Scans

1. Explain nuclear scan purpose, procedure, benefits, and risks.
2. Assess for allergy to radioactive medications such as iodine.
3. Inform patient that nuclear medicine procedures provide less radiation exposure than most x-ray examinations. Reassure that test is safe and painless. Side effects, such as nausea, are minimal.
4. Inform patient that procedure is performed in department of nuclear medicine and that procedure lasts about 1 hour.
5. Have the patient appropriately dressed, usually in robe and slippers. It is important that there be no metal objects on the patient during the procedure.
6. Obtain an accurate weight because this is the basis for the radiopharmaceutical dose to be administered.
7. In general, signed consent forms are not required, unless required by the FDA, or if the patient undergoes physical stress.
8. If a female patient is premenopausal, instruct patient to use effective birth control while being tested because the test may be harmful to the fetus.
9. Fetal radiation should be avoided whenever possible. The radiation dose to the fetus from nuclear scan is equal to the radiation required for one abdominal x-ray study.

Clinical Alert

1. Nuclear medicine procedures are contraindicated in pregnancy and lactation.
2. These precautions are to be followed for radionuclide laboratory procedures in Part 2 and PET scans in Part 3 of this chapter.

Standard Precautions and Posttest Care for Nuclear Scans

1. Advise pregnant staff and visitors to avoid prolonged contact with the patient for 24 to 48 hours after administration of radioactive medication.
2. Use routine disposal procedures for body fluids and excretions unless patient also is receiving therapeutic doses of radiation therapy.
3. Document assessment of patient, how the patient tolerated the procedure, and total examining time. Record any problems that may have occurred during the procedure.
4. Monitor injection site for signs of bruising, hematoma, infection, discomfort, and irritation.

Clinical Alert

These precautions are also to be followed for radionuclide laboratory procedures in Part 2 and PET scans in Part 3 of this chapter.

● CARDIAC STUDIES

MYOCARDIAL PERFUSION SCAN ●

Normal Values

Normal stress test: electrocardiogram and blood pressure normal.
Normal myocardial perfusion under both stress and rest conditions.

Explanation of Test

Technetium Tc99m sestamibi (Cardiolite) and thallium 201 (^{201}Tl) are the radioactive imaging agents used in conjunction with a treadmill stress electrocardiographic (ECG) test to diagnose ischemic heart disease and allow differentiation of ischemia and infarction. It will reveal wall motor defects and heart pump performance during increased oxygen demands. These scans are also done before and after streptokinase treatment for coronary artery thrombosis. Thallium 201 is a physiologic analogue of potassium. The myocardial cells extract potassium, as do other muscle cells.

The ^{99m}Tc sestamibi is taken up by the myocardium through passive diffusion followed by active uptake within the mitochondria. Unlike thallium, technetium does not undergo any significant redistribution. Therefore, there are some procedural differences.

Myocardial activity is also dependent on blood flow. Consequently, when the patient is injected during peak exercise, the normal myocardium will have much greater activity than the abnormal myocardium. Thus, coldspots indicate a decrease or absence of flow.

A completely normal stress study may eliminate the need for cardiac catheterization in the evaluation of chest pain and nonspecific abnormalities of the ECG. The use of SPECT imaging can more accurately localize regions of ischemia.

Persantine (dipyridamole; DPY) administration is indicated in persons unable to exercise to achieve desired cardiac stress and maximum cardiac vasodilation. This medication has an effect similar to that of exercise on the heart.

Persons who are candidates are those with lung disease, peripheral vascular disease with claudication, amputation, spinal cord injury, multiple sclerosis, morbid obesity, and patients taking β-adrenergic blockers.

Dipyridamole stress testing is also valuable as significant predictors of cardiovascular death, reinfarction, and risk of postoperative ischemia events; this test can also be used in reevaluation of unstable angina.

Procedure

THALLIUM

1. While using a treadmill, the patient undergoes a cardiac stress test.
2. When the cardiologist has determined that the patient has reached maximum heart stress (10 to 20 minutes), an injection of radioactive thallium is given. The patient then lies down on the scanning table.

3. The scanning begins within 5 minutes. Usually, three static views are taken or SPECT imaging is performed.
4. A repeat scan is done approximately 3 to 4 hours later at rest to check redistribution.

NOTE: *Some nuclear medicine procedures require the patient to return 24 hours later for a reinjection of thallium, followed by rest imaging.*

SESTAMIBI

1. The patient is injected and scanned 15 minutes for the resting phase.
2. Four hours later, the patient undergoes cardiac stress testing as in the thallium procedure. The patient is given a second injection and scanning begins within 15 minutes.
3. Usually, 3 static views are taken or SPECT imaging is performed.

NOTE: *Some nuclear medicine departments will*

1. Do the stress phase 24 hours following rest imaging.
2. Do a combination of radiopharmaceuticals for stress and rest.

DIPYRIDAMOLE

1. Dipyridamole is infused intravenously over a 4-minute period before administration of either radiopharmaceutical.
2. The DPY may be given orally in some instances.
3. Under certain conditions, the DPY procedures can be done at bedside. When tomographic views are obtained in the nuclear medicine department, results are more sensitive and specific.

Clinical Implications

1. A test that is abnormal during exercise, but remains normal at rest, indicates ischemia.
2. The scan for infarction will remain abnormal after rest.
3. Hypertrophy produces an increase in uptake.
4. The progress of disease can be estimated.
5. The location and extent of myocardial disease can be assessed.
6. Specific and significant abnormalities in the stress ECG are usually indications for cardiac catheterization or further studies.

Interfering Factors

1. Inadequate cardiac stress.
2. For dipyridamole
   a. The major disadvantage of DPY is the lack of information that would be provided by the ECG response to exercise.
   b. Injection of DPY in the upright or standing positions or with isometric handgrip may increase myocardial uptake.

Patient Preparation

1. Explain test purpose and procedure, benefits, and risks. See standard nuclear scan pretest precautions on page 622.
2. Before the stress test is begun, an intravenous line is started, and ECG leads and blood pressure cuff are attached.
3. Advise the patient that the exercise stress period will be continued for 45 to 60 seconds after injection to allow the thallium to be cleared during a period of maximum blood flow.
4. No discomfort is experienced during the thallium series test (only feelings associated with stress testing).
5. Fasting is necessary for at least 2 hours, and no smoking is permitted for 2 hours before and during the entire thallium stress test.
6. With sestamibi, patients should drink milk or eat a light, fatty meal 15 minutes after each injection.
7. For dipyridamole administration:
   a. Patients should be fasting for at least 6 hours and avoid caffeine for at least 24 hours.
   b. Blood pressure, heart rate, and ECG are monitored for any changes during dipyridamole infusion. Aminophylline will be given if vital signs change radically.
8. See Chapter 1 additional guidelines for safe, effective, informed *pretest* care.

Clinical Alert

1. The stress study is contraindicated on patients who
   a. Have a combination of right and left bundle-branch block
   b. Have left ventricular hypertrophy
   c. Are using digitalis and quinidine
   d. Are hypokalemic (because the results are difficult to evaluate)
2. Contraindications to dipyridamole imaging are severe coronary artery disease, angina at rest, and arrhythmia.
3. Adverse short-term effects of DPY occur in 30% to 40% of patients and include nausea, headache, dizziness, facial flush, vomiting, angina, ST-segment depression, and ventricular arrhythmia.

Patient Aftercare

1. Observe patient for possible reaction to dipyridamole injection.
2. Interpret test outcomes and counsel appropriately.
3. Refer to nuclear scan posttest precautions on page 622.
4. Follow Chapter 1 guidelines for safe, effective, informed *posttest* care.

MYOCARDIAL INFARCTION SCAN

Normal Values

Normal distribution of the radiopharmaceutical in sternum, ribs, and other bone structures. No myocardial uptake.

Explanation of Test

Technetium Tc99m stannous pyrophosphate (PYP) is the radioactive-imaging agent used to demonstrate the general location, size, and extent of myocardial infarction 24 to 96 hours after suspected myocardial infarction and as an indication of myocardial necrosis, to differentiate between old and new infarcts. In some instances, the test is sensitive enough to detect an infarct 12 hours to 7 days after its occurrence. Acute infarction is associated with an area of increased radioactivity or hotspot on the myocardial image. This test is useful when ECG and enzyme studies are not definitive. Myocardial infarction imaging is commonly done the day before heart surgery and again postoperatively.

Procedure

1. This myocardial scan involves a 2–4 to 6-hour waiting period for the patient after the intravenous injection of the radionuclide. During this waiting period, the radioactive material will accumulate in the heart muscle.
2. The imaging period takes 15 to 30 minutes, during which time the patient must lie quietly on an examining table. The patient is rotated for different views.

Clinical Implications

1. When a scan is entirely normal in a person admitted with a diagnosis of "rule out myocardial infarction," this is an indication that an acute infarction is not present.
2. Myocardial uptake of the PYP is compared with the ribs (2+) and sternum (4+). Higher uptake levels (4+) reflect greater myocardial damage.
3. Larger defects have a much poorer prognosis than small defects.

Interfering Factors

1. Gated and PYP studies will interfere with other nuclear tests, such as liver, bone, or lung scan, if they are done on the same day.
2. False-positive infarct avid (PYP) scans can occur in chest wall traumas, recent cardioversion, and unstable angina.

Patient Preparation

1. Tests can be done at bedside in the acute phase of infarction if equipment is available.
2. Explain nuclear scan purpose, procedure, benefits, and risks. Refer to general procedure description of benefits and risks; clinical considera-

tions and standard precautions; and pretest care for nuclear scans on page 622.
3. Imaging must occur within a 12-hour to 7-day period following the onset of infarct symptoms. Otherwise, false-negative results may be reported.
4. See Chapter 1 for additional guidelines for safe, effective, informed *pretest* care.

Patient Aftercare

1. Interpret test outcome and monitor appropriately. If heart surgery is needed, counsel concerning follow-up testing after surgery.
2. Refer to standard precautions, posttest care for nuclear scans on page 622.
3. Follow additional guidelines in Chapter 1 for safe, effective, informed *posttest* care.

MULTIGATED ACQUISITION (MUGA) **SCAN** ●

Normal Values

Normal cardial wall motion and ejection fractions under conditions of stress and rest. If administered, normal cardiac response to nitroglycerin.
Normal nitroglycerin test: blood pressure within expected limits.

Explanation of Test

This method is similar to routine imaging, except that scintillation events are distributed into not one, but multiple images during acquisition. *Gated* refers to the synchronizing of the imaging equipment and computer with the patient's ECT so that images are free of motion or blur.

Once injected, the distribution of the radiopharmaceutical is regulated by synchronizing the recording of cardiac images with the ECG. This technique provides a means of obtaining information about cardiac output, end systolic volume, end diastolic volume, ejection fraction, ejection velocity, and regional wall motion of the ventricles. By using a computer, wall motion of the ventricles can be portrayed in a cinematic mode to visualize contraction and relaxation. This method of determining heart wall motion and ejection fraction (that portion of the ventricular volume ejected in systole) could be measured only by angiography before use of this technique. This scan may also be performed with stress testing and to see the effect of drug intervention (using nitroglycerin) on heart performance.

Procedure for MUGA

1. This scan may be performed with or without stress testing and is usually performed in conjunction with heart wall motion study.
2. This test could be performed at bedside if necessary.
3. The patient's own red blood cells become labeled with ^{99m}Tc stannous pyrophosphate.
4. An ECG is required to be set up on the patient because the patient's R-

wave signals the computer and camera to take several image frames for each cardiac cycle.

5. The patient is scanned immediately after radiopharmaceutical labeling.

Procedure for Nitroglycerin Testing

1. Cardiologist should be present.
2. A resting MUGA is done for a baseline study.
3. Nitroglycerin is given, another scan is taken, nitroglycerin is given again, and scans are taken until the level of blood pressure desired by the cardiologist is reached.
4. Total study time is 1.5 hours.

Clinical Implications

Abnormal MUGA studies are associated with

1. Congestive cardiac failure
2. Change in ventricular function owing to infarction
3. Persistent arrhythmias from poor ventricular function
4. Regurgitation owing to valvular disease
5. Ventricular aneurysm formation

Interfering Factors

1. Long-acting nitrates affect coronary blood flow. For this reason, such medications should be discontinued 8 to 12 hours before testing.
2. Inability to attain reliable ECG connection.

Patient Preparation

1. Explain nuclear scan purpose, procedure, benefits, and risks. Refer to general procedures, description of benefits, risks and clinical considerations on pages 620–621.
2. An ECG is required before imaging if stress testing is required; a 24-hour fast is recommended, and the patient may be either supine or seated on a bicycle ergometer.
3. Follow standard precautions, *pretest* care for nuclear scans on page 622.
4. See Chapter 1 for additional guidelines on safe, effective, informed *pretest* care.

Patient Aftercare

1. Interpret MUGA outcomes and monitor appropriately.
2. Resume medications.
3. Refer to standard precautions, *posttest* care for nuclear scans on page 622.
4. Follow basic Chapter 1 guidelines for safe, effective, informed *posttest* care.

CARDIAC FLOW STUDIES; FIRST-PASS; AND SHUNT SCANS

Normal Values

Normal wall motion and ejection fraction.
Normal pulmonary transit times and normal sequence of chamber filling.

Explanation of Test

The cardiac flow study is useful in the determination of both right and left ventricular ejection fractions. Although not required, it is preferred to have the patient monitored by ECG after injection. The camera traces the flow of the radioactivity in its "first pass" through the cardiac chambers in several rapid images (0.025 to 0.5 seconds each).

This angiographic study of the chambers of the heart using jugular vein injection of ^{99m}Tc is also helpful in the study of heart chamber disorders, especially in the investigation of left-to-right and right-to-left shunts. Children are the usual candidates for this procedure.

Procedure

1. A 3-way stopcock with saline flush is used for radionuclide injection in the antecubital fossa. The radionuclide is injected in the external jugular vein to ensure a compact bolus for a shunt evaluation.
2. The patient lies on his or her back with the head slightly raised.
3. The total patient time is approximately 20 to 30 minutes; the actual scan time is 5 minutes.
4. A resting MUGA is performed with *each* shunt study.

Clinical Implications

1. Abnormal first-pass ejection fraction values are associated with
   - **a.** Congestive heart failure
   - **b.** Change in ventricular function owing to infarction
   - **c.** Persistent arrhythmias from poor ventricular function
   - **d.** Regurgitation owing to valvular disease
   - **e.** Ventricular aneurysm formation
2. Abnormal heart shunts reveal
   - **a.** Left-to-right shunt
   - **b.** Right-to-left shunt
   - **c.** Mean pulmonary transit time
   - **d.** Tetrology of Fallot (seen more often in children)

Interfering Factors

There should not be any other detectable radioactivity in patients.

Patient Preparation

1. Explain nuclear scan purpose, procedure, benefits, and risks.
   First pass: An IV line is required to be set up with a 3-way stopcock.
   Shunt: A jugular IV line may be required to be set up, which is usually done by a physician.

2. See Chapter 1 for additional guidelines for safe, effective, informed *pretest* care.
3. Refer to general procedures, description of benefits, risks, clinical considerations, standard nuclear scan pretest precautions on pages 620–622.
4. Obtain signed, witnessed consent form if stress testing is to be done.

Patient Aftercare

1. Interpret test outcomes, monitor, and counsel appropriately.
2. Refer to standard nuclear scan posttest precautions on page 622.
3. Follow basic Chapter 1 guidelines for safe, effective, informed *posttest* care.

ENDOCRINE STUDIES

THYROID SCAN

Normal Values

Normal or evenly distributed concentration of radioactive iodine; normal size, position, shape, site, weight, and function of thyroid; absence of nodules.

Explanation of Test

This test systematically measures the uptake of radioactive iodine (either ^{131}I or ^{123}I) by the thyroid. It is requested for the evaluation of thyroid size, position, and function and used in the differential diagnosis of masses in the neck, base of the tongue, or mediastinum. Thyroid tissue can be found in each of these three locations. In many instances, ^{99m}Tc may be used in place of iodine for visualizing the thyroid.

Benign adenomas may appear as nodules of increased uptake of iodine ("hot" nodules), or they may appear as nodules of decreased intake ("cold" nodules). Malignant areas generally take the form of cold nodules. The most important use of thyroid scans is the functional assessment of these thyroid nodules.

Iodine (and, consequently, radioiodine) is actively transported by the thyroid gland, where it is incorporated into the production of thyroid hormone. The radioactivity of the gland is scanned by a gamma camera, and this information is then transformed into a film, thereby outlining the normal thyroid and demonstrating any areas of abnormality.

A thyroid scan performed with iodine is usually done in conjunction with a radioactive iodine uptake study, which is usually performed at 6 and 24 hours postdose when ^{131}I is used. The uptake and scan are performed the same day when ^{123}I is used (one 24-hour uptake may still be required with ^{123}I). For a complete thyroid workup, thyroid hormone levels are usually measured by taking a blood specimen and performing radioimmunoassay tests as directed by the physician. Some physicians also may require a thyroid ultrasound examination as part of a complete workup.

Procedure

1. The patient either swallows radioactive iodine in a tasteless capsule or a liquid or has the radionuclide injected intravenously (for ^{99m}Tc).
2. Usually, the neck area is counted for uptake 6 or 24 hours later (or both). The area is scanned at 24 hours when ^{131}I is used and at 2 to 6 hours when ^{123}I is used.
3. The patient lies on his or her back on the examining table with the neck hyperextended.
4. Normal scan time is 20 minutes.

Clinical Implications

1. Cancer of the thyroid most often presents itself as a nonfunctioning cold nodule, which indicates a focal area of decreased uptake.
2. Some abnormal results are
   - **a.** Hyperthyroidism, represented by an area of diffuse increased uptake
   - **b.** Hypothyroidism, represented by an area of diffuse decreased uptake
   - **c.** Graves' disease, represented by an area of diffuse increased uptake
   - **d.** Autonomous nodules, represented by focal area of increased uptake
   - **e.** Hashimoto's disease, represented by mottled areas of decreased uptake

Interfering Factors

1. Thyroid scans must be completed before radiographic examinations using contrast medicine (intravenous pyelogram, gallbladder, cardiac catheterization, and myelograms) are performed.
2. If possible, any medication containing iodine should not be given until thyroid scans are concluded. Notify the attending physician if thyroid studies have been ordered, together with interfering radiographs or medications.

Limitations of Test

Measurements of free serum thyroxine (free T_4) and free triiodothyronine (free T_3) by RIA are much more reliable tests for function of the thyroid.

Patient Preparation

1. Instruct the patient about nuclear scan purpose, procedure, and special restrictions. Refer to general procedures, description of benefits, risks, and clinical considerations, standard nuclear scan pretest precautions on pages 620–622.
2. Because the thyroid gland responds to small amounts of iodine, the patient may be requested to refrain from iodine intake for at least 1 week

before the test. Patients should consult with a physician first. Restricted items include the following:

a. Certain thyroid drugs
b. Weight-control medicines
c. Multiple vitamins
d. Some oral contraceptives
e. Gallbladder and other radiographic dyes containing iodine
f. Cough medicine
g. Iodine-containing foods, especially kelp, and "natural" foods

3. Alleviate any fears the patient may have about radionuclide procedures.
4. See Chapter 1 guidelines for safe, effective, informed *pretest* care.

Clinical Alert

1. Thyroid scans are contraindicated in pregnancy. Thyroid testing in pregnancy is limited to blood testing.
2. This study should be completed before thyroid-blocking contrast agents for radiographs are administered and before thyroid or iodine drugs are given.
3. Occasionally, scans are done purposely with iodine or some thyroid drug in the body. In these cases, the doctor is testing the thyroid response to drugs. These stimulation and suppression scans are usually done to determine the nature of a particular nodule and to determine if the tissue is functioning or nonfunctioning.

Patient Aftercare

1. If iodine has been administered, observe patients for iodine allergic precautions as needed.
2. Refer to standard nuclear scan posttest precautions on page 622.
3. Interpret test outcomes and counsel appropriately.
4. Follow Chapter 1 guidelines for safe, effective, informed, *posttest* care.

ADRENAL GLAND SCAN

Normal Values

No evidence of tumors or hypersecreting hormone sites.

Normal salivary glands, urinary bladder, and vague shape of liver and spleen can be seen.

Explanation of Test

Nuclear medicine evaluation of the adrenal gland is divided into two different components: cortex and medulla. Because the demand for adrenal cortical imaging is limited and radiopharmaceuticals are difficult to obtain, the scope of adrenal imaging is limited to the medulla.

The purpose of imaging the adrenal medulla is to obtain images that aid in identifying sites of certain tumors that produce excessive amounts of catecholamines. Pheochromocytomas develop in cells that make up the adrenergic portion of the autonomic nervous system. Many of these well-differentiated cells are found in adrenal medullas. Adrenergic tumors have been called *paragangliomas* when found outside the adrenal medulla, but many refer to all neoplasms that secrete norepinephrine and epinephrine as pheochromocytomas. Because the only definite and effective therapy is surgery to remove the tumor, identifying the site using this test, as well as CT scans and ultrasound, is an essential goal of treatment.

Procedure

1. The radionuclide iobenguane (^{131}I) ($^{131}MIGB$) is injected intravenously.
2. Scans will be done on the 2nd, 3rd, and 4th days in most instances (day 1 being the day of injection). Occasionally, only 1 day of imaging will be necessary, whereas in a few patients, imaging will be required on the 6th and 7th days. Scanning will be done from the urinary bladder to the mastoid area when searching for a primary tumor.
3. Generally, three views are sufficient for a search: (1) anterior display of the pelvis and lower abdomen; (2) posterior display of abdomen and lower chest; and (3) upper chest and head. If metastasis is suspected, then the upper legs, the humeri, and all of the head are examined as well.
4. Scanning time each day is approximately 30 minutes.

Clinical Implications

1. Abnormal results give substance to the "rough rule of 10." This means that
   - **a.** Ten percent are in children.
   - **b.** Ten percent are familial.
   - **c.** Ten percent are bilateral in the adrenal glands.
   - **d.** Ten percent are malignant.
   - **e.** Ten percent are multiple, in addition to bilateral, tumors.
   - **f.** Ten percent are extrarenal.
2. Over 90% of primary pheochromocytomas occur in the abdomen.
3. Pheochromocytomas in children often represent a familial disorder.
4. Bilateral adrenal tumors often indicate a familial disease and vice versa.
5. Multiple extrarenal pheochromocytomas are often malignant.
6. The presence of two or more pheochromocytomas almost always indicates malignant disease.

Interfering Factors

Barium interferes.

Patient Preparation

1. Explain nuclear scan purpose, procedure, benefits, and risks. Radioactive exposure is comparable with that of a computed tomography (CT) scan of the adrenal glands or conventional radiograph of the kidneys and adrenal glands. Obtain patient's signed legal consent form.

2. To prevent uptake of radioactive iodine by the thyroid gland, Lugol's solution or potassium iodine will be given for a time before the test as well as after the test. For example, a common protocol is 2 days before injection of radionuclide and 10 days after the injection.
3. Refer to general procedures, description of benefits, risks, and clinical considerations and standard nuclear scan pretest precautions on pages 620–622.
4. See Chapter 1 basic guidelines for safe, effective, informed *pretest* care.

Patient Aftercare

1. Interpret test outcomes and counsel appropriately about the need for possible follow-up tests. Follow-up tests include
   - **a.** Kidney and bone nuclear scans to give further orientation to abnormalities discovered in ^{131}MIBG tests.
   - **b.** CT scans if MIBG scans have failed to locate the tumor.
   - **c.** Ultrasound of pelvis if the tumor produces urinary symptoms.
2. Refer to standard nuclear scan posttest precautions on page 622.
3. Follow Chapter 1 guidelines for safe, effective, informed *posttest* care.

PARATHYROID SCAN ●

Normal Values

No areas of increased perfusion or uptake in parathyroid and thyroid.

Explanation of Test

This test is primarily done for presurgical localization of parathyroid adenomas in clinically proved cases of primary hyperparathyroidism. It is helpful in demonstrating intrinsic or extrinsic parathyroid adenoma. Two tracers, thallium and technetium, are injected 5 to 10 minutes before imaging.

Procedure

1. The radionuclide thallium is injected, and 15 minutes later, imaging is done. This image is stored in the computer.
2. Without moving the patient, technetium is injected and, after 10 minutes, a second image is obtained and computerized. Computer processing involves subtracting the technetium-visualized thyroid structures from the thallium accumulation in a parathyroid adenoma.
3. Total examination time is 30 to 45 minutes.

NOTE: *Certain camera/computer systems permit simultaneous imaging of both radiopharmaceuticals.*

Interfering Factors

Recent ingestion of iodine in food or medication and recent tests with iodine content may reduce the effectiveness of the study.

Clinical Implications

Abnormal concentrations reveal parathyroid adenoma, both intrinsic and extrinsic, but cannot differentiate between benign and malignant parathyroid disease

Clinical Considerations

Pregnancy is a relative contraindication. However, if primary hyperparathyroidism is suspected and surgical exploration is essential before delivery, the study may be performed.

Patient Preparation

1. Explain purpose, procedure, benefits, and risks of parathyroid scan.
2. Assess for the recent intake of iodine. However, this finding is not a specific contraindication to performing the study.
3. The thyroid should be carefully palpated because thallium may accumulate in thyroid adenomas.
4. Refer to general procedures, description of benefits, risks, clinical considerations and standard nuclear scan pretest precautions on pages 620–622.
5. See Chapter 1 basic guidelines for safe, effective, informed *pretest* care.

Patient Aftercare

1. Refer to standard nuclear scan posttest precautions on page 622.
2. Interpret test outcome and monitor appropriately.
3. Follow Chapter 1 guidelines for safe, effective, informed *posttest* care.

● GENITOURINARY STUDIES

RENAL BLOOD FLOW SCAN ●

Normal Values

Normal blood flow in both kidneys through the arterial, capillary, and venous phases.

Explanation of Test

This test is performed to evaluate renal blood flow, renal mass vascularity, the efficacy of renal transplants, and arteriovenous malformations. The patient is injected with a bolus of radioactivity, and images are obtained in a series (1 to 5 seconds are common for each frame). Computers are used to generate time–activity curves for each kidney and aorta. Unilateral and bilateral disease can be assessed.

Procedure

1. The patient is injected through an intravenous line with a 3-way stopcock and saline flush attached.

2. Imaging begins immediately after injection while the patient is in the camera's field of view.
3. A computer is then used to process the images.
4. This procedure is often performed in conjunction with a renogram and renal structural imaging.

Clinical Implications

1. Computer-generated curves provide analyses that aid in the determination of unilateral or bilateral disease.
2. Increased blood flow to a vascular tumor can be visualized.
3. Decreased blood flow is observed with renal transplant rejection.

Interfering Factors

There should be no other detectable radioactivity in the patient.

Patient Preparation

1. Explain nuclear scan purpose, procedure, benefits, and risks.
2. An intravenous line with 3-way stopcock is set up before imaging.
3. The patient is either seated or lying in the supine position for the procedure.
4. Refer to standard nuclear scan pretest precautions on page 622.
5. See Chapter 1 guidelines for safe, effective, informed *pretest* care.

Patient Aftercare

1. Interpret test outcomes and counsel appropriately.
2. Refer to standard nuclear scan posttest precautions on page 622.
3. Follow Chapter 1 guidelines for safe, effective, informed *posttest* care.

RENAL STRUCTURAL SCAN ●

Normal Values

Normal size, shape, position, and function of kidneys.

Explanation of Test

This test is done to determine anatomic outlines in each kidney. It is also used to detect renal masses and to localize the kidney before needle biopsy. It can reveal positive evidence of renal disease when other tests are normal. The scan will also reveal lesions produced by vascular occlusion in the kidney. Parenchymal, tubular, and glomerular function can be ascertained with various renal imaging agents. Radioactive substances such as ^{99m}Tc, succimer (DMSA), glucoheptonate (GH), or pentetic acid (DTPA) are injected intravenously and a short time later will be concentrated and held in the kidneys. Technetium Tc99m DMSA and ^{99m}Tc GH are used primarily for anatomic visualization, whereas ^{99m}Tc DTPA is used to demonstrate glomerular filtration. Scanning will demonstrate the size, shape, and position of the kidneys as well as the distribution of the radioisotope in the kidneys. Renal scans and renograms can be done simultaneously, giving both morphologic and functional data about the kidneys. The iodine-sensitive or azotemic patient who cannot tolerate an intravenous pyelogram can be evaluated in this way. In many instances, this study will be accompanied by a diagnostic ultrasound procedure.

Procedure

1. Scanning of the kidney area is done 30 minutes to 1 hour after the intravenous injection of the radionuclide. A renal blood flow and a 10-minute postinjection static film are taken in the sitting position.
2. Scans of the kidneys are then repeated at a later time, or may be done at several different time intervals, after the initial injection. This will depend on the patient's condition and the pharmaceutical used.
3. The patient must remain still during the delayed scans for 30 minutes or more, and usually, a prone position is used for this part of the procedure. Most often, both kidneys are scanned at the same time; however, they can be done separately.
4. In many nuclear medicine departments, this information is then processed by computer for further interpretation.

Clinical Implications

1. Abnormal results indicate
   - **a.** Space-occupying "cold" or nonfunctioning areas caused by tumors, cysts, or abscesses
   - **b.** Congenital abnormalities
   - **c.** Nonfunctioning kidneys
   - **d.** Infarction
   - **e.** Status of postrenal transplant
   - **f.** Severe renal insufficiency
2. In patients with uremia, the size, shape, and location of the kidneys can be demonstrated when no visualization occurs in the intravenous pyelogram.

Patient Preparation

1. Explain the nuclear scan purpose, procedure, benefits, and risks.
2. Alleviate any fears the patient may have about radionuclide procedures.
3. Refer to general procedures, description of benefits, risks, clinical considerations, and standard nuclear scan pretest precautions on pages 620–622.
4. See Chapter 1 basic guidelines for safe, effective, informed *pretest* care.

Patient Aftercare

1. Interpret test outcomes and monitor appropriately.
2. Refer to standard nuclear scan posttest precautions on page 622.
3. Follow Chapter 1 guidelines for safe, effective, informed *posttest* care.

RENOGRAM; KIDNEY FUNCTION SCAN ●

Normal Values

Right and left kidney blood flow is equal in both kidneys.
In 10 minutes, 50% of the radioactivity should be excreted.

Explanation of Test

This test is done to study the function of both kidneys and is used to detect renal parenchymal or vascular disease as well as defects in excretion. Radiopharmaceuticals used in the renogram are ^{99m}Tc-DTPA, [^{131}I]Hippuran or ^{99m}Tc-mertiatide (MAG-3), which permit visualization of renal clearance.

Each radiopharmaceutical is processed differently through the kidneys and is quantitatively analyzed, providing the following information:

^{99m}Tc-DTPA	Glomerular filtration rate (GFR)
[^{131}I]Hippuran	Effective renal plasma flow (ERPF)
^{99m}Tc-mertiatide	MAG-3 clearance

The quantitative values are normalized to the body's surface area. The placement of the radiation detectors over the kidneys permits the monitoring of the uptake and the disappearance of the radioactivity. This information is usually displayed with a chart recording or entered into a computer. The shape of this wave may be correlated with several measures of renal function such as tubular secretion and excretion.

Indications for Testing

1. To detect the presence or absence of unilateral kidney disease
2. For long-term follow-up of patients with hydroureteronephrosis
3. To study the hypertensive patient to determine a renal basis for the disease
4. To study the azotemic patient and the patient in whom urethral catheterization is contraindicated or impossible
5. To evaluate obstruction in the upper urinary tract
6. To study the kidney first when an intravenous pyelogram cannot be done because of allergy to iodine
7. To assess renal transplant efficacy

Procedure

1. The patient is usually placed in an upright position in front of the camera.
2. The radiopharmaceutical is injected intravenously. An intravenous diuretic also may be administered.
3. Imaging with the camera is started immediately after injection.
4. A urine sample or a blood specimen may be obtained at the end of the

procedure. Bladder catheterization is necessary in persons with suspected distal ureteral obstruction.

5. Total examination time is approximately 30 minutes.
6. The renogram is often performed in conjunction with nuclear medicine tests of renal function.

Clinical Alert

A renogram may be performed in pregnant women when it is imperative that renal function be ascertained.

Clinical Implications

Abnormal pattern results may be indicative of

1. Hypertension
2. Obstruction by stones or tumors
3. Renal failure
4. Decreased renal function
5. Diminished blood supply
6. Renal transplant rejection

Interfering Factors

Antihypertensive medications may interfere with the test results.

Patient Preparation

1. Explain nuclear scan purpose, procedure, benefits, and risks. Refer to general precautions, description of procedure, benefits, risks, clinical considerations, and standard nuclear scan pretest precautions on pages 620–622.
2. The patient should eat and be well hydrated with two to three glasses of water (unless contraindicated) before undergoing the scan (10 ml of water per kilogram of body weight).
3. Some patients may be given a diuretic to differentiate between nonobstructed dilation with slow renal clearance and a mechanical obstruction.
4. See Chapter 1 guidelines for safe, effective, informed *pretest* care.

Patient Aftercare

1. Encourage fluids and frequent bladder emptying to promote excretion of radioactivity.
2. Interpret test outcomes and counsel appropriately.
3. Refer to standard nuclear scan *posttest* precautions on page 622.
4. Follow Chapter 1 guidelines for safe, effective, informed *posttest* care.

Clinical Alert

1. The test should not be done immediately after an intravenous pyelogram because the patient needs to be at least normally hydrated.
2. Severe impairment of renal function or massive enlargement of the collecting system may impair drainage, even without true obstruction.

TESTICULAR (SCROTAL) SCAN

Normal Values

Normal blood flow to scrotal structures, with even distribution and concentration of radiopharmaceutical.

Explanation of Test

This test is performed on an emergency basis in the evaluation of acute, painful testicular swelling. It also is used in the differential diagnoses of torsion of acute epididymitis and in the evaluation of injury, trauma, tumors, and masses. The radiopharmaceutical [^{99m}Tc]pertechnetate is used before imaging. The images obtained differentiate lesions associated with increased perfusion from those that are primarily ischemic.

Procedure

1. The patient lies on his back under the nuclear camera. The penis is gently taped back onto the lower abdominal wall.
2. A small tracer dose of radionuclide is injected intravenously.
3. Imaging is performed in two phases: first as a dynamic blood flow study of the scrotum and second, as an assessment of distribution of radiopharmaceutical in the scrotum.
4. Total examining time is 30 to 45 minutes.

Clinical Implications

1. Abnormal concentrations reveal
   a. Tumors
   b. Hematomas
   c. Infection
   d. Torsions (with reduced blood flow)
2. The nuclear scan is most specific soon after the onset of pain, before abscess is a clinical consideration.

Patient Preparation

1. Explain the purpose, procedure, benefits, and risks of the test. There is no discomfort involved in testing.
2. If the patient is a child, a parent should accompany the boy. The examining department prefers the father.

3. The penis is taped to the lower abdominal wall.
4. Refer to standard nuclear scan *pretest* precautions on page 622.
5. See Chapter 1 guidelines for safe, effective, informed *pretest* care.

Patient Aftercare

1. Refer to standard nuclear scan *posttest* precautions on page 622.
2. Interpret test outcome and monitor appropriately.
3. Follow Chapter 1 guidelines for safe, effective, informed *posttest* care.

● GASTROINTESTINAL STUDIES

HEPATOBILIARY (GALLBLADDER) SCAN ●

Normal Values

Following the intravenous administration of the radionuclide, the substance will be excreted rapidly from the blood by the polygonal cells of the liver. The transit through the liver cells to the biliary tract is rapid (15 to 30 minutes), and significant uptake occurs in the normal gallbladder. Normal distribution patterns are visualized in the biliary system.

Explanation of Test

This study, using ^{99m}Tc-labeled iminodiacetic acid (IDA) agents (eg, ^{99m}Tc-disida or disofenin tracers), is done to visualize the gallbladder and determine patency of the biliary system.

Radionuclides have a short transit time through the liver, with the advantage of a low radiation dose, but the scan must be done quickly because the radioactivity excreted by the hepatic parenchymal cells is concentrated in the gallbladder and excreted into the gastrointestinal tract. A series of images traces the excretion of the radioactivity. Through computer analysis, the activity in the gallbladder is quantitated in each image, and the amount ejected is calculated (ejection fraction).

Indications for Testing

1. Evaluate cholecystitis
2. Differentiate between obstructive and nonobstructive jaundice
3. Investigate persons with upper abdominal pain
4. Biliary assessment postsurgery and evaluation of biliary atresia

Procedure

1. The radionuclide is injected intravenously.
2. Imaging starts immediately after injection, and a series of images are taken at 10- to 15-minute intervals for as long as 60 to 90 minutes.

3. In the event of biliary obstruction, delayed views may be obtained at 4 and 24 hours.
4. Computer assessments of the images are made and quantitative measurements, such as a gallbladder EF, are performed.
5. In some patients, cholecystokinine (CCK) is administered to help differentiate difficult to determine situations (acute versus chronic cholecystitis). The CCK can be given in lieu of performing the 4-hour scan.

Clinical Implications

1. Abnormal concentration patterns will reveal unusual bile communications.
2. Determine if the jaundiced patient is a surgical or nonsurgical candidate.
3. Gallbladder visualization excludes the diagnosis of acute cholecystitis with a high degree (close to 100%) of certainty.

Interfering Factors

1. Patients with high serum bilirubin levels (> 10 mg/dl) may have less reliable test results.
2. Patients receiving total parenteral nutrition (TPN) or those with long-term fasting may not have gallbladder visualization.

Patient Preparation

1. Explain nuclear scan purpose, procedure, benefits, and risks.
2. The patient should fast for at least 2 hours before testing and prolonged fasting (> 24 hours) is to be avoided.
3. Discontinue opiate- or morphine-based pain medications 2 to 6 hours before the test.

   Refer to general procedures, description of benefits, risks, clinical considerations, and standard nuclear scan *pretest* precautions on pages 620–622.
5. See Chapter 1 basic guidelines for safe, effective, informed *pretest* care.

Patient Aftercare

1. Interpret test outcome and monitor appropriately.
2. Refer to standard nuclear scan *posttest* precautions on page 622.
3. Follow Chapter 1 guidelines for safe, effective, informed *posttest* care.

PAROTID (SALIVARY) **GLAND SCAN** ●

Normal Values

No evidence of tumor type activity or blockage of ducts.
Normal size, shape, and position of glands.

Explanation of Test

This study is helpful in the evaluation of swelling masses in the parotid region. It is done to detect blocked ducts of the parotid and submaxillary glands and tumors of parotid or salivary glands, and to diagnose Sjogren's syndrome in rheumatoid arthritis. The radionuclide injected intravenously is [^{99m}Tc]pertechnetate. One of the limitations of the test is that it cannot furnish an exact preoperative diagnosis.

Procedure

1. Radionuclide (^{99m}Tc) is injected intravenously. Scanning is done immediately. There are three phases to imaging: blood flow, uptake or trapping mechanism, and secreting capability.
2. The patient is examined in a sitting position.
3. Pictures of the gland are taken every few minutes for 30 minutes (two anteroposterior and one oblique).
4. If a secretory function test is being done to detect blockage of the salivary duct, three-fourths of the way through the test the patient is asked to suck on a lemon slice. If the salivary duct is normal, it will cause the gland to empty. This is not done in tumor detection.
5. Total test time is 45 to 60 minutes.

Clinical Implications

1. The reporting of a hot nodule amidst normal tissue that accumulates the radionuclide is associated with tumors of the ducts, as in
   - **a.** Warthin's tumor
   - **b.** Oncocytoma
   - **c.** Mucoepidermoid tumor
2. The reporting of a cold nodule amidst normal tissue that does not accumulate the radionuclide is associated with
   - **a.** Benign tumors, abscesses, or cysts, which are indicated by smooth, sharply defined outlines
   - **b.** Adenocarcinoma, which is indicated by ragged, irregular outlines
3. The reporting of diffuse decreased activity, such as an obstruction, chronic sialadenitis, or Sjogren's syndrome.
4. The reporting of diffuse increased activity, such as acute parotitis.

Patient Preparation

1. Explain nuclear scan purpose, procedure, benefits, and risks.
2. There is no pain or discomfort involved.
3. Lemon may be given to the patient to stimulate parotid secretion.
4. Refer to general procedures, description of benefits, risks, clinical considerations, and standard nuclear scan *pretest* precautions on pages 620–622.
5. See Chapter 1 basic guidelines for safe, effective, informed *pretest* care.

Patient Aftercare

1. Interpret test outcome and monitor appropriately.
2. Refer to standard nuclear scan *posttest* precautions on page 622.
3. Follow Chapter 1 guidelines for safe, effective, informed *posttest* care.

GASTROESOPHAGEAL REFLUX SCAN

Normal Values

A normal gastroesophageal reflux scan will show less than 4% gastric reflux across the esophageal sphincter.

Explanation of Test

After oral administration of radioactive medication (^{99m}Tc sulfur colloid) in orange juice, the patient is immediately scanned to verify that all the liquid is in the stomach. With an abdominal binder applied, further images are obtained at 0, 20, 40, 60, 80, and 100 mm Hg. A computer is used to calculate the percentage reflux into the esophagus for each image.

Procedure

1. The patient is given the radioactive medication in 150 ml of orange juice followed by 150 ml 0.1 *N* HCl.
2. An immediate image is taken to verify complete swallowing.
3. Additional images are obtained at different pressures as applied by the abdominal binder.
4. Images are obtained as quickly as possible (30 seconds each) to minimize patient discomfort.

Clinical Implications

More than 4% reflux at any pressure level is abnormal. The percentage reflux is used to evaluate patients before and after surgery for gastroesophageal reflux.

> **Clinical Alert**
>
> Patients who have esophageal motor disorders, hiatal hernias, or swallowing difficulties should have an endogastric tube inserted for the procedure.

Interfering Factors

Upper gastrointestinal procedures performed in radiology may interfere with this method.

Patient Preparation

1. Explain nuclear scan purpose, procedure, benefits, and risks.
2. Refer to general procedures, description of benefits, risks, clinical considerations, and standard nuclear scan *pretest* precautions on pages 620–622.

3. The patient should fast overnight.
4. Oral intake of the orange juice and 0.1 *N* HCl may be uncomfortable for the patient.
5. An abdominal binder is placed around the patient and inflated to different pressures.
6. A supine position is maintained through the imaging procedure.
7. Should reflux occur at lower pressures, an additional 30 ml of water is given to clear the esophagus.
8. See Chapter 1 basic guidelines for safe, effective, informed *pretest* care.

Patient Aftercare

1. Patients having endogastric tubes will need to have the tube removed after the procedure.
2. Refer to standard nuclear scan *posttest* precautions on page 622.
3. Interpret test outcome and monitor appropriately.
4. Follow Chapter 1 guidelines for safe, effective, informed *posttest* care.

GASTRIC EMPTYING SCAN ●

Normal Values

Normal half-time clearance ranges are:

45–110 minutes for solids
10–65 minutes for liquids

Explanation of Test

Gastric-emptying imaging is used to assess gastric motility disorders and patients with unexplained nausea and vomiting. The emptying of food by the stomach is a complex process and is controlled by food composition (fats and carbohydrates), form (liquid or solid), hormones (gastrin and cholecystokinin secretion), and nervous innervation. Because the clearance of liquids and solids vary, the imaging procedure traces both food forms. Indications for imaging are both mechanical and nonmechanical gastric motility disorders. Mechanical disorders include peptic ulcerations, gastric surgery, trauma, and cancer. Nonmechanical disorders include diabetes, uremia, anorexia nervosa, certain drugs (opiates), and neurologic disorders.

Procedure

1. The fasting patient consumes the solid phase (^{99m}Tc sulfur colloid usually in scrambled eggs or oatmeal) followed by the liquid phase (^{111}In DTPA in 300 ml water).
2. The patient is imaged immediately in the supine position.
3. Subsequent images are obtained every 15 minutes for the next 2 hours. Each image takes only 60 seconds to obtain.

4. Computer processing is used to determine the half-time clearance for both liquid and solid phases.

Clinical Implications

1. Slow or delayed emptying results are usually seen in
   a. Peptic ulceration
   b. Diabetes
   c. Smooth-muscle disorders
   d. Following radiation therapy
2. Accelerated emptying is often visualized in
   a. Zollinger–Ellison syndrome
   b. Certain malabsorption syndromes
   c. Following gastric or duodenal surgery

Interfering Factors

1. Administration of certain medications (gastrin, cholecystokinin) will interfere with emptying.
2. The liquid phase may interfere with the solid phase.

Patient Preparation

1. Explain purpose, procedure, benefits, and risks.
2. Refer to general procedures, description of benefits, risks, clinical considerations, and standard nuclear scan precautions on pages 620–622.
3. The patient should fast for 8 hours.
4. Some procedures require oral intake of both liquid and solid phases; other procedures require only the solid phase.
5. The patient is requested to sit up between each image.
6. See Chapter 1 guidelines for safe, effective, informed *pretest* care.

Patient Aftercare

1. The patient may eat and drink normally.
2. Interpret test outcomes and counsel appropriately.
3. Refer to standard nuclear scan *posttest* precautions on page 622.
4. Follow Chapter 1 basic guidelines for safe, effective, informed *posttest* care.

LIVER SCAN

Normal Values

Normal size, shape, and position within the abdomen.
Normal size of cardiac impression on liver.
Normally functioning liver and reticuloendothelial system.

Explanation of Test

This test is used to demonstrate the functions, anatomy, and size of the liver. Alterations in function may indicate an obstruction, hepatitis, hepatic abscesses, and the cause of jaundice. It is helpful in determining the cause of right upper quadrant pain and in the detection of metastatic disease, cirrhosis, ascites, infarction caused by trauma, and liver damage from radiation therapy. The majority of liver scans continue to be performed as part of a search for metastatic disease and in the differential diagnosis of jaundice.

A radioactive material, ^{99m}Tc-labeled sulfur colloid, is injected intravenously. Liver imaging is done using SPECT, which gives a three-dimensional result of the radiopharmaceutical distributions. The ^{99m}Tc labeled to a patient's own red blood cell is the radiopharmaceutical most specific for detection of hemangioma in the liver.

Liver–Lung Combination Scan

There may be times when a liver–lung scan may be ordered in combination with a white blood cell or gallium scan to identify tumor masses or abscess formation in the subdiaphragmatic area. Procedure and patient preparation are the same as for a liver scan and lung scan.

Limitations of Test

This procedure provides limited information on hepatic parenchymal cell function.

Procedure

1. The chosen pharmaceutical is injected intravenously.
2. After administration of the radionuclide, the patient lies on his or her back on an examining table for anterior pictures to determine liver uptake.
3. The entire study usually takes 60 minutes from injection to finish.
4. The spleen is usually scanned when performing a liver scan.
5. The hepatobiliary scan assesses parenchymal cell function.

Clinical Implications

Abnormal liver scan patterns occur in

1. Cirrhosis
2. Hepatitis
3. Trauma
4. Hepatomas
5. Sarcoidosis
6. Metastasis
7. Cysts
8. Perihepatic abscesses
9. Hemangiomas
10. Adenomas
11. Ascites

Patient Preparation

1. Explain purpose, procedure, benefits, and risks.
2. Refer to general procedures, description of benefits, risks, clinical considerations, and standard nuclear scan *pretest* precautions on pages 620–622.
3. See Chapter 1 guidelines for safe, effective, informed *pretest* care.

Patient Aftercare

1. Refer to standard nuclear scan *posttest* precautions on page 622.
2. Interpret test outcome and monitor appropriately.
3. Follow Chapter 1 basic guidelines for safe, effective, informed *posttest* care.

SPLEEN SCAN

Normal Values

Normal size of spleen, cell function, and blood flow to spleen.
The amount of uptake in the spleen should always be less than the liver.

Explanation of Test

This examination is performed to demonstrate anatomic changes in the reticuloendothelial cells of the spleen. Spleen imaging is accomplished by the use of a radioactive nuclide colloid such as ^{99m}Tc sulfur colloid. The amount of this pharmaceutical taken up by the spleen is dependent on the blood flow to the spleen and its cell function. Resulting images allow the examiner to determine the size and condition of the spleen. This scan also may be used to demonstrate space-occupying lesions or accessory spleens, to visualize the infiltration of Hodgkin's or metastatic disease, and to evaluate trauma cases to rule out infarct. This procedure is performed in conjunction with a liver scan. Spleen imaging may be performed using SPECT.

Clinical Alert

1. It is essential that the nuclear medicine department know the purpose of the examination.
2. Additional views may be required for accurate diagnosis, as in trauma and suspected infarct.

Procedure

1. Obtain and record patient history.
2. The radiopharmaceutical is injected intravenously.
3. A 10- to 20-minute wait is required to allow the injected radiopharmaceutical to be absorbed into the reticuloendothelial cells.
4. A minimum of three views are obtained. On some occasions, additional oblique views may be required.
5. Total examining time is approximately 60 minutes from injection to conclusion. The time involved will vary depending on the patient's ability to cooperate and the size and condition of the spleen. The ability of the cells to accumulate the radiopharmaceutical will also affect the imaging time.

Clinical Implications

Abnormal concentrations reveal

1. Unusual splenic size
2. Infarction
3. Ruptured spleen
4. Accessory spleen
5. Tumors
6. Metastatic spread
7. Leukemia
8. Hodgkin's disease

Spleens larger than 14 cm are abnormally enlarged; those less than 7 cm are abnormally small. Areas of absent radioactivity or holes in the spleen scans are associated with abnormalities that displace or destroy normal splenic pulp.

Interfering Factors

1. Possible artifacts may occur if the images are taken immediately after the administration of barium for radiologic colon examinations. Barium is a dense material and may attenuate some of the gamma radiation from ^{99m}Tc sulfur colloid, which is the pharmaceutical most often used.
2. About 30% of persons with Hodgkin's disease with spleen involvement will have a normal spleen scan.

Patient Preparation

1. Explain the purpose, procedure, benefits, and risks of the test.
2. Obtain a thorough history.
3. Whenever possible, schedule the scan before any test using barium as a contrast.
4. Refer to general procedures, description of benefits, risks, clinical considerations, and standard nuclear scan *pretest* precautions on pages 620–622.
5. The test can be performed in a trauma case or when a ruptured spleen is suspected, at bedside, or in the emergency room.
6. See Chapter 1 basic guidelines for safe, effective, informed *pretest* care.

Patient Aftercare

1. Refer to standard nuclear scan *posttest* precautions on page 622.
2. Interpret test outcome and monitor appropriately.
3. Follow Chapter 1 guidelines for safe, effective, informed *posttest* care.

GASTROINTESTINAL BLOOD LOSS SCAN ●

Normal Values

No sites of active bleeding.

Explanation of Test

This test is very sensitive in the detection and location of acute gastrointestinal bleeding that occurs distal to the ligament of Treitz. (Gastroscopy is the procedure of choice in diagnosing upper gastrointestinal bleeding.) Before the refining of this diagnostic technique, barium enemas were used to identify lesions that reflect the site of bleeding, but these examinations are not specific and frequently miss small sites of bleeding, such as that caused by diverticular disease and angiodysplasia. This scan is also indicated for detection and localization of recent hemorrhage, both peritoneal and retroperitoneal.

Technetium Tc 99m sulfur colloid is the radiopharmaceutical of choice for suspected active bleeding. Because liver and spleen rapidly clear this agent from the vasculature, the detection of bleeding by extravasation of the radiopharmaceutical into the bowel occurs. For intermittent bleeding, use of ^{99m}Tc-labeled red blood cells is more practical in delayed imaging up to 24 hours after injection.

Procedure

1. Radiopharmaceutical ^{99m}Tc sulfur colloid or ^{99m}Tc-labeled red blood cells are injected.
2. Imaging is begun immediately and continued every few minutes. Images are obtained anteriorly over the abdomen at 5-minute intervals for 30 to 60 minutes. If the study is negative at 1 hour, delayed images can be obtained at 2, 6, and sometimes 24 hours later, when necessary, to identify the location of difficult to determine bleeding sites.
3. Total examining time varies.

Clinical Alert

1. This test is contraindicated in those who are hemodynamically unstable. In these instances, angiography or surgery should be the procedure of choice.
2. Assess patients for signs of active bleeding during the examining period. The procedure will be performed by the department of nuclear medicine any time during a 24-hour period.

Clinical Implications

Abnormal concentration of red blood cells with areas of radioactivity greater than the background activity is associated with

1. Approximate geographic location of active GI bleeding, both peritoneal as well as retroperitoneal.
2. Nongastrointestinal sites of hemorrhage, such as in the lungs, can also be identified up to 24 hours postinjection.

Interfering Factors

The presence of barium in the GI tract may obscure the bleeding site. This is because of the high density of barium and the inability of the technetium to penetrate the barium.

Patient Preparation

1. Explain the purpose and procedure, benefits, and risks of the GI blood loss scan.
2. Determine whether the patient has received barium as a diagnostic agent in the last 24 hours. If the presence of barium in the GI tract is questionable, an abdominal radiograph may be ordered.
3. Advise the patient that delayed images may be necessary. Also, if active bleeding is not seen on initial scans, additional images must be obtained for as long as 24 hours after injection, whenever the patient has clinical signs of active bleeding.
4. Refer to general procedures, description of benefits, risks, and clinical considerations, and standard nuclear scan *pretest* precautions on pages 620–622.
5. See Chapter 1 basic guidelines for safe, effective, informed *pretest* care.

Patient Aftercare

1. Refer to standard nuclear scan *posttest* precautions on page 622.
2. Interpret test outcome and monitor appropriately.
3. Follow Chapter 1 guidelines for safe, effective, informed *posttest* care.

● NEUROLOGIC STUDIES

BRAIN SCAN ●

Normal Values

Normal extracranial and intracranial blood flow.

Normal distribution, with highest uptake in the gray matter, basal ganglia, thalamus, and peripheral cortex; central white matter and ventricles show less activity.

Explanation of Test

Radionuclide brain imaging using ^{99m}Tc-labeled complexes, such as DTPA and pertechnetate, were used for the diagnosis of pathologic abnormalities such as tumors, cerebrovascular aneurysms, and hematomas. With the advent of computed tomography (CT) and magnetic resonance imaging (MRI), this form of imaging has generally become obsolete. However, when coupled with the radionuclide angiogram, technetium-labeled complexes have clinical usefulness in children in such cases as hydrocephalus, encephalitis, and brain death.

Recent developments in radiopharmaceuticals and SPECT have rejuvenated brain imaging. Technetium Tc 99m exametazime is the radiopharmaceutical used to cross the blood–brain barrier. Iofetamine I123 was the first agent used to cross the blood–brain barrier, but it is being replaced by the technetium complexes. The blood–brain barrier is not a specific anatomic structure but a complex system including capillary endothelium with closed intracellular clefs, a small or absent extravascular fluid space between endothelium and glial sheaths, and the membrane of the neurons themselves. Further, SPECT technology allows for numerous slices, providing depth resolution from different angles. These developments have permitted nuclear medicine to evolve into a physiologic and functional neuroimaging modality. Although PET scanning is more effective in functional diagnosis, SPECT is less expensive and more available.

Procedure

1. The radionuclide is injected intravenously.
2. Imaging usually begins immediately after administration and takes about 1 hour to complete.
3. With the patient in the supine position, SPECT images are obtained around the circumference of the head.
4. With administration of iodoiophetamines, some departments require a dark and quiet environment.

> **Clinical Alert**
>
> Assess for medication history of monoamine oxidase (MAO) inhibitors. Iofetamine I123 should not be used during or 14 days after administration of MAO inhibitors.

Clinical Implications

1. Abnormal patterns are indicative of altered radionuclide distribution in cases such as
   - **a.** Alzheimer's disease
   - **b.** Stroke
   - **c.** Dementia
   - **d.** Seizure disorders
   - **e.** Epilepsy
   - **f.** Systemic lupus erythematosus
   - **g.** Huntington's disease
   - **h.** Parkinson's disease
   - **i.** Psychiatric diagnosis (schizophrenia)
2. The cerebral blood flow in the presence of brain death will show a very distinct image of no tracer uptake in the anterior or middle cerebral arteries or the cerebral hemisphere, along with the presence of uptake in the scalp.

Interfering Factors

1. Any patient motion, such as coughing or leg movement, can alter cerebral alignment.
2. Sudden distractions or loud noises can alter the distribution of [^{123}I]iofetamine.

Patient Preparation

1. Explain the purpose, procedure, benefits, and risks of a brain scan.
2. Reassure the patient that the test is safe, nontoxic, and painless.

3. Refer to general procedures, description of benefits, risks, clinical considerations, and standard nuclear scan *pretest* precautions in pages 620–622.
4. Because precise head alignment is crucial, advise the patient to remain quiet and still.
5. Obtain a careful neurologic history before testing.
6. See Chapter 1 basic guidelines for safe, effective, informed *pretest* care.

Patient Aftercare

1. Refer to standard nuclear scan *posttest* precautions on page 622.
2. Interpret test outcome and monitor appropriately.
3. Follow Chapter 1 basic guidelines for safe, effective, informed *posttest* care.

CISTERNOGRAPHY (CEREBROSPINAL FLUID FLOW SCAN) ●

Normal Values

Unobstructed cerebrospinal fluid (CSF) flow and normal reabsorption.

Explanation of Test

This study, in which a radionuclide (usually ^{111}In-labeled DTPA) is injected by lumbar puncture, is a sensitive indicator of altered flow and reabsorption of CSF. In the treatment of hydrocephalus, it aids in the selection of the type of shunt and pathway, as well as in the prognosis of both shunting and hydrocephalus.

Procedure

1. A sterile lumbar puncture is performed after the patient has been positioned and prepared (see pp. 279–282 for procedure). At this time, a tracer dose of radionuclide is injected into the cerebrospinal circulation.
2. The patient must lie flat after the puncture; the length of time depends on the physician's order.
3. Imaging will be done at 2 to 6 hours after injection, then again at 24 hours, 48 hours, and 72 hours in some cases.
4. Examining time is 1 hour for each scan.

Clinical Implications

Abnormal filling patterns reveal

1. Hydrocephalus
2. Subdural hematoma
3. Spinal mass lesions
4. Posterior fossa cysts
5. Parencephalic and subarachnoid cysts
6. Shunt patency
7. Diagnosis and localization of rhinorrhea and otorrhea

Patient Preparation

1. Explain the purposes, procedures, benefits, and risks for both lumbar puncture and cisternography.

2. Refer to general procedures, description of benefits, risks, clinical considerations, and standard nuclear scan *pretest* precautions on pages 620–622.
3. Advise the patient that it may take as long as 1 hour for each scan.
4. The patient must be taken by cart to the nuclear medicine department for the first scan because of the preceding lumbar puncture.
5. See Chapter 1 basic guidelines for safe, effective, informed *pretest* care.

Patient Aftercare

1. Follow instructions for lumbar puncture (see p. 282) and standard nuclear scan *posttest* precautions on page 622.
2. Be alert to complications of lumbar puncture, such as meningitis, allergic reaction to anesthetic, bleeding into spinal canal, herniation of brain tissue, and mild to severe headaches.
3. Interpret test outcome and monitor appropriately.
4. Follow Chapter 1 basic guidelines for safe, effective, informed *posttest* care.

● TUMOR AND INFLAMMATORY PROCESS STUDIES

GALLIUM (^{67}Ga) SCANS (LIVER, BONE, BRAIN, BREAST SCANS) ●

Normal Value

No evidence of tumor-type activity.

Explanation of Test

This test is used to detect the presence, location, and size of tumors, adhesions, abscesses, and inflammation in body cavities, primarily in the liver, bone, brain, and breast.

> **NOTE:** *WBCs labeled with ^{99m}Tc and ^{111}In are more specific for abscess and inflammatory imaging.*

It is most useful in differentiating malignant from benign lesions and determining the extent of invasion of known malignancies. The lymph nodes are also scanned for involvement. These studies are used to help stage bronchogenic cancer, Hodgkin's and non-Hodgkin's lymphomas. Gallium scans also may be used to record tumor regression following radiation or chemotherapy, thereby noting the body response to therapy. The radionuclide injected intravenously is gallium citrate (^{67}Ga).

Areas of the body most often examined by this method are the lymph system, liver, bone, brain, and breast. Only 5% pathologic activity is necessary for detection by this technique, whereas 45% activity is required for radiographic examination. The underlying mechanism for the uptake of ^{67}Ga is not well understood. Uptake in some neoplasms may depend on the presence of transferrin receptors in tumor cells, but this is only speculation. Once gallium enters a tissue, it remains there.

Procedure

1. If imaging of the abdomen is to be performed, a laxative is usually given the evening before the scanning.
2. Laxatives, suppositories, tap water enemas, or a combination thereof, are often ordered before scanning. The patient may eat breakfast the day of imaging.
3. The radionuclide is injected 24 to 72 hours before imaging.
4. The patient must lie quietly without moving during the scanning procedure. Anterior and posterior views of the entire body are done.
5. Additional imaging may be done at 24-hour intervals to differentiate normal bowel activity from pathologic concentrations.

Clinical Implications

1. An abnormal gallium concentration usually implies the existence of underlying disease, as in
   a. Malignancy, especially lung, testes, and mesothelioma
   b. Stages of lymphomas, Hodgkin's disease, melanoma, hepatoma, soft-tissue sarcomas, primary tumors of bone and cartilage, neuroblastomas, and leukemia
   c. Abscesses
   d. Tuberculosis
   e. Thrombosis
   f. Sarcoidosis
2. Further diagnostic studies are usually done to distinguish benign from malignant lesions.
3. Tumor uptake of ^{67}Ga varies with tumor type, among persons with tumors of some histologic types, and even with tumor sites in a given patient.
4. Tumor uptake of ^{67}Ga may be significantly reduced following effective treatment.
5. Although ^{111}In white blood cell imaging is more specific for abscess localization, gallium imaging is still used as a multipurpose screening procedure.

Interfering Factors

1. A negative study cannot be definitely interpreted as ruling out the presence of disease (40% false-negative results in gallium studies).
2. It is difficult to detect a single, solitary nodule, such as in adenocarcinoma. Lesions smaller than 2 cm can be detectable. Tumors near the liver are difficult to detect, as is interpretation of ileac nodes.
3. Because gallium does collect in the bowel, there may be an abnormal concentration in the lower abdomen; therefore, enemas are ordered before testing.

4. Degeneration or necrosis of tumor and antineoplastic drugs immediately before scans cause false-negative results.

Patient Preparation

1. Explain the purpose, procedure, benefits, and risks of gallium scan.
2. Reassure the patient that there is no pain involved, except for an intravenous injection.
3. Alleviate any fear the patient may have about radionuclide procedures.
4. Usually, no change in eating habits is necessary before testing. However, some departments expect their patients to eat a low-residue lunch and clear liquid supper the day before examination.
5. Refer to general procedures, description of benefits, risks, clinical considerations, and standard nuclear scan *pretest* precautions on pages 620–622.
6. The usual preparation includes oral laxatives beginning on the day of injection and continuing until imaging is completed, or enemas or suppositories before the examination. These preparations clean normal gallium activity from the bowel.
7. Actual scanning time is 45 to 90 minutes.
8. See Chapter 1 basic guidelines for safe, effective, informed *pretest* care.

Patient Aftercare

1. Refer to standard nuclear scan *posttest* precautions on page 622.
2. Interpret test outcome and monitor appropriately.
3. Follow Chapter 1 guidelines for safe, effective, informed *posttest* care.

Clinical Alert

Breastfeeding should be discontinued for at least 4 weeks following testing.

WBC SCAN (INFLAMMATORY IMAGING)

Normal Values

Normal value occurs in the liver, spleen, and bone marrow. There are no signs of leukocyte localization outside of the reticuloendothelial system.

Explanation of Test

This test, in which a sample of the patient's own leukocytes (white blood cells) has been isolated, labeled with indium oxine, and reinjected, is used for the localization of abscess formation. The study is indicated in persons with signs and symptoms of a septic process, fever of unknown origin, and suspected intra-abdominal abscess. It is also helpful in determining the cause of complications of surgery, injury, or inflammation of the GI tract and pelvis. The test results are based on the fact that any collection of labeled white cells outside the liver, spleen, and functioning bone marrow indicates an abnormal area to which the white blood cells are being attracted. This procedure is 90% sensitive and 90% specific for inflammatory disease or abscess formation.

Procedure

1. A venous blood sample of 40 ml is obtained to isolate and label the white blood cells. The laboratory process takes about 3 hours to complete.
2. The white blood cells are labeled with radioactive ^{111}In and injected intravenously.
3. After a waiting period, the patient returns for imaging at 24 and 48 hours.
4. Imaging time is about 1 hour each time.

Clinical Implications

Abnormal concentrations indicate

1. Abscess formation
2. Acute and chronic osteomyelitis and infection of orthopedic prostheses
3. Active inflammatory bowel disease
4. Postsurgical abscess sites and wound infections

Interfering Factors

1. False-negative reactions are known to occur when the chemotactic function of the white blood cell has been altered, as in hemodialysis, hyperglycemia, hyperalimentation, steroid therapy, and long-term antibiotic therapy.
2. Gallium scans up to 1 month earlier can interfere.
3. False-positive scans occur in the presence of GI bleeding and in upper respiratory infections and pneumonitis when patients swallow purulent sputum.

See Standard Considerations, Patient Preparation and Aftercare on pages 620–622.

> **Clinical Alert**
>
> If the patient does not have an adequate number of white blood cells, then donor cells can be used. It is possible in some instances to do a successful study in persons who have fewer than 1000 white blood cells per centimeter.

MONOCLONAL ANTIBODY (ONCOSCINT) **SCAN**

Normal Values

Distribution occurs in the normal liver, spleen, bone marrow, and bowel.

Explanation of Test

This test is used to detect the location and size of known extrahepatic malignancies. It is most useful with ovarian or colorectal carcinoma. The test is not used to serve as a screening technique. The radiopharmaceutical is indium In111 satumomab pendetide (OncoScint), which is derived from the mouse immune system. The procedure can be used for disease staging, pre- and postsurgical evaluation, and radiation therapy efficacy. Patients with rising serologic tumor marker titers are primary candidates for initial imaging.

Procedure

1. The patient is slowly injected with the radiopharmaceutical over a period of 5 minutes.
2. Optimal images are obtained on the patient between 2 and 4 days after injection (additional images may be obtained at 24 hours and at 5 days). Check with your diagnostic department.
3. The patient is placed in the supine position during the scanning period. Either a series of stationary images or SPECT imaging is performed.

Clinical Implications

1. Abnormal distributions are found in ovarian and colorectal cancer. Any changes in the distribution provide evidence of the effectiveness of surgery or therapy.
2. Abnormal results have been observed in nonspecific areas, such as inflammatory bowel disease, colostomy sites, and postoperative bowel adhesions.
3. A patient's medical history should be carefully reviewed before a diagnosis is made.

Interfering Factors

Radioactivity in the bowel may interfere with colorectal assessment. Follow-up imaging is useful after a cathartic and to clarify equivocal findings.

Patient Preparation

1. Explain imaging purpose, procedure, benefits, and risks.
2. Refer to general procedures, description of benefits, risks, clinical considerations, and standard nuclear scan *pretest* precautions on pages 620–622.
3. An intravenous line is established before radiopharmaceutical injection.
4. If indicated by the nuclear medicine department, a cathartic may be required to resolve bowel activity from abnormal pathology.

Patient Aftercare

1. Refer to standard nuclear scan *posttest* precautions on page 622.
2. Interpret test outcome and monitor appropriately.
3. Observe the patient for 1 hour after injection of ^{111}In satumomab pendetide for antibody reactions (eg, chills, fever, nausea).
4. Some patients may develop human mouse antibody (HAMA) titers after OncoScint injection.
5. Follow Chapter 1 guidelines for safe, effective, informed *posttest* care.

Clinical Alert

1. Human mouse antibody titers may result in falsely elevated immunoassay levels for CA125 and carcinoembryonic antigen (CEA).
2. No other medications should be injected into the intravenous line used for radiopharmaceutical injection.

GENERAL STUDIES

LUNG SCANS; VENTILATION AND PERFUSION

Normal Values

Normal functioning lung.
Normal pulmonary vascular supply.
Normal gases exchanged.

Explanation of Test

Lung scan is done for three major purposes: to detect the percentage of the lungs functioning normally; to diagnose and locate pulmonary emboli; and to assess the pulmonary vascular supply by providing an estimate of regional pulmonary blood flow. It is a simple method for following the course of embolic disease because an area of ischemia will persist after apparent resolution on a radiograph of the chest. With pulmonary emboli, the blood supply beyond an embolus is restricted. Imaging will reveal poor or no visualization of the affected area. Only three tests are positive immediately following pulmonary embolus: pulmonary arteriogram, measurement of physiologic dead space, and lung scan. Assessment of the adequacy of pulmonary artery perfusion in areas of known disease also can be done reliably. As soon as a pulmonary embolism is suspected, a ventilated perfusion study should be considered and, if possible, should be performed within 2 days of the acute event.

There are two types of lung scans: (1) the ventilation scan, in which the movement of air or lack of air in the lungs may be demonstrated. As an alternative, droplets of radioactive material can be administered by a positive-pressure ventilator. The aerosol is then breathed through a mouthpiece or face mask. (2) The perfusion scan, in which the blood supply to the tissues in the lungs can be demonstrated. Technetium Tc 99m aerosols, krypton 81m, or xenon 113 gas is used in the ventilation lung scan. When inhaled, radioactive gas follows the same pathway as the air in normal breathing. In some pathologic conditions affecting ventilation, there will be significant alteration in the normal ventilation process. The ventilation scan is performed with the lung perfusion scan and is important in the diagnosis of pulmonary emboli. When the ventilation scan is performed in conjunction with the lung perfusion scan, it is helpful in diagnosing bronchitis, asthma, inflammatory fibrosis, pneumonia, chronic obstructive pulmonary disease, and lung cancer.

The lung perfusion study is usually performed after the ventilation scan. Following the intravenous injection of a macroaggregated albumin (MAA) labeled with technetium, assessment of pulmonary vascular supply is done by scanning.

Certain limitations exist with these tests. With a positive chest film and a positive scan, the differential possibilities are multiple: pneumonia, abscess, bullae, ateliosis, and carcinoma, among others. A pulmonary arteriogram is still necessary before an embolectomy can be attempted.

Clinical Alert

Pulmonary perfusion imaging is contraindicated in patients with primary pulmonary hypertension or right-to-left heart shunts.

Procedure

1. The patient breathes for approximately 4 minutes through a closed, nonpressurized ventilation system. During this time, a small amount of radioactive gas will be administered into the system.
2. Breath-holding will be required for a brief period some time during the examination.
3. The examining time is 10 to 15 minutes. When performed with a lung perfusion scan, 30 to 45 minutes is the testing time (used in differential diagnosis of embolism).
4. The perfusion scan immediately follows the ventilation study.

Clinical Implications

Abnormal ventilation and perfusion patterns may indicate the possibility of

1. Tumors
2. Emboli
3. Pneumonia
4. Atelectasis
5. Bronchitis
6. Asthma
7. Inflammatory fibrosis
8. Chronic obstructive pulmonary disease
9. Lung cancer

Interfering Factors

1. False-positive scans occur in vasculitis, mitral stenosis, pulmonary hypertension, and when tumors obstruct a pulmonary artery with airway involvement.
2. During the injection of MAA, care must be taken that the patient's blood does not mix with the radiopharmaceutical in the syringe. Otherwise, hotspots will be seen in the lungs.

Patient Preparation

1. Explain the purpose, procedure, benefits, and risks of the test.
2. Alleviate any fears the patient may have concerning nuclear medicine procedures.
3. It is important that a record of a recent radiograph of the chest be available.
4. The patient must be able to follow directions for breathing and holding his or her breath, including breathing through a mouthpiece or into a face mask.
5. Refer to general precautions, description of benefits, risks, clinical considerations, and standard nuclear scan *pretest* precautions on pages 620–622.
6. See Chapter 1 guidelines for safe, effective, informed *pretest* care.

Patient Aftercare

1. Refer to standard nuclear scan *posttest* precautions on page 622.
2. Interpret test outcome and monitor appropriately.
3. Follow Chapter 1 guidelines for safe, effective, informed *posttest* care.

BONE SCAN ●

Normal Values

No areas of greater or lesser concentration of radioactive material in bones.

Explanation of Test

This test is used primarily to evaluate and follow persons with known or suspected metastatic disease, and the majority of bone scans continue to be done for this reason. Breast, prostate, lung tumors, and lymphomas tend to metastasize to bone. Bone scans will demonstrate lesions 3 to 6 months before they appear in radiographs.

This scan is commonly used in the evaluation of patients with unexplained bone pain and of patients with primary bone tumors, arthritis, osteomyelitis, abnormal healing of fractures, fractures, shin splints, and compression fractures of the vertebral column. It is also used for patients with chronic renal failure in whom it is necessary to detect soft-tissue calcification and in pediatric patients with hip pain (Legg–Calve–Perthes disease). It is also done to identify suitable bone biopsy sites, to evaluate those areas difficult to demonstrate radiographically, such as the sternum and the scapula, and to help determine the age and metabolic activity of traumatic injuries and infection.

Other indications are to evaluate candidates for knee and hip prostheses, to diagnose aseptic necroses and vascularity of the femoral head, and for presurgical assessment of viable bone tissue when amputation is necessary. Evaluation of prosthetic joints and internal fixation devices that are suspected of becoming loose or infected is also done.

This test is also done to confirm the clinical impression of internal derangement of the temporomandibular joint (TMJ). The TMJ is the most actively used joint in the body. Single-photon emission computed tomography has a sensitivity of 94% and a specificity of 70%.

A bone-seeking radiopharmaceutical is used to image the skeletal system. An example would be ^{99m}Tc-labeled phosphate injected intravenously. Imaging usually begins 2 to 3 hours after injection. The examiner will look for the distribution and concentration of the pharmaceutical in the bone. Abnormalities, such as increased blood flow to bone and increased metabolism, will concentrate the radiopharmaceutical at a higher or lower rate than the normal bone. The radiopharmaceutical mimics calcium physiological function; therefore, it will concentrate more heavily in the areas of increased metabolic activity.

Procedure for Bone Scan

1. Radioactive ^{99m}Tc phosphate is injected intravenously.
2. A 2- to 3-hour waiting period is necessary for the radiopharmaceutical concentrate in the bone. During this time, the patient may be asked to drink 4 to 6 glasses of water.
3. Before the scan begins, the patient is asked to urinate because a full bladder will mask the pelvic bones.
4. The scan takes about 30 to 60 minutes to complete. The patient must be still during scanning. The table or the scanner will slowly move the patient under and over a sensitive radiation detector.
5. Additional spot views of specific bone structure may be performed, or SPECT may be done as an option.

Clinical Alert

1. For osteomyelitis, an immediate dynamic flow procedure of blood perfusion is performed.
2. For TMJ scanning, SPECT imaging is performed, as well as the lateral planes.

Interfering Factors

1. False-negative bone scans occur in multiple myeloma of bone. When this condition is known or suspected, the scan is an unreliable indicator of skeletal involvement.
2. Patients with follicular thyroid cancer may harbor metastatic bone marrow disease, but these lesions are often missed by scans.

Clinical Implications

1. Abnormal concentrations indicate the following:
   a. Very early bone disease and healing. This is detected by radioisotopic

scan long before it is visible on radiographs. The latter are positive for bone lesions only after 30% to 50% decalcification (bone calcium decreased) has occurred.

2. Many disorders can be detected, but not differentiated, by this test (eg, cancer, arthritis, benign bone tumors, fractures, osteomyelitis, Paget's disease, and aseptic necroses). The findings must be interpreted in the light of the whole clinical picture because any process inducing an increased calcium excretion rate will be reflected by an increased uptake in the bone.
3. Breast cancer-positive bone scan finding in the preoperative period depends on the staging of the disease, and these scans are recommended before initial therapy. *Stages 1 and 2:* 4% will have positive bone scan. *Stage 3:* 19% will have positive bone scan. Yearly bone scans should be done for follow-up.
4. Multiple myeloma is the only tumor that shows better detectability with a plain radiograph than with a radionuclide scan.
5. Multiple focal areas of increased activity in the axial skeleton are commonly associated with metastatic bone disease. The reported percentage of solitary metastatic lesions varies on a site-by-site basis. With a single lesion in the spine or pelvis, the cause is more likely to be metastatic disease than one occurring in the extremities or ribs.
6. Increased uptake with hot areas associated with increased osteoblastic activity about the margins of a displaced joint occur in TMJ disk displacement, bite abnormality, and congenital deformity of the mandible.

Clinical Alert

1. The flare phenomenon occurs in patients with metastatic disease who are receiving a new therapy. In some persons, the bone scan may show increased activity or new lesions in persons with clinical improvement. It is due to a healing response in prostate and breast cancer within the first few months of a new treatment. These lesions should show marked improvement on scans 3 to 4 months later.
2. Radiographic correlation is necessary to rule out a benign process when solitary areas of increased or decreased uptake occur.
3. The TMJ examination should be deferred in women who are pregnant or who are breastfeeding infants.

Patient Preparation

1. Instruct the patient about the purpose and procedure of the test and his or her involvement. Alleviate any fears concerning the procedure. Advise the patient that frequent drinking and activity in the first 6 hours help reduce excess radiation to the bladder and gonads.

2. The patient can be up and about during the waiting period.
3. If the patient is in pain or debilitated, assist him or her to void before the test. Otherwise, give a reminder about emptying the bladder before the test.
4. A sedative should be ordered and administered to any patient who will have difficulty lying quietly during the scanning period.
5. Refer to general procedures, description of benefits, risks, clinical considerations, and standard nuclear scan *pretest* precautions on pages 620–622.
6. See Chapter 1 basic guidelines for safe, effective, informed *pretest* care.

Patient Aftercare

1. Advise the patient to empty his or her bladder when imaging is completed to decrease radiation exposure time.
2. Refer to standard nuclear scan *posttest* precautions on page 622.
3. Interpret test outcome and monitor appropriately.
4. Follow Chapter 1 guidelines for safe, effective, informed *posttest* care.

^{131}I TOTAL-BODY SCAN ●

Normal Value

No functioning extra thyroid tissues outside of the thyroid gland.

Explanation of Test

This study, using ^{131}I or ^{123}I, is done to search for any functioning thyroid tissue anywhere in the body. It is helpful in determining the presence of metastatic thyroid cancer and the amount and location of residual tissue following thyroidectomy. The procedure is occasionally performed in conjunction with thyroid therapy using ^{131}I for thyrocarcinoma.

Procedure

1. Radionuclide is administered orally in a capsule form.
2. Imaging will take place 24 to 72 hours after administration.
3. Imaging can take as long as 2 hours to perform.
4. Sometimes, thyroid-stimulating hormone (TSH) is administered intravenously before the radionuclide is given. This stimulates any residual thyroid tissue so it will take up enough ^{131}I or ^{123}I to be detected.

Clinical Implications

1. Abnormal uptake of iodine reveals areas of extra thyroid tissue, such as
   a. Stroma ovarii
   b. Substernal thyroid
   c. Sublingual thyroid
2. Residual tissue following thyroidectomy
3. Metastatic thyroid cancer

Clinical Alert

1. When possible, this test should be performed before any other radionuclide procedures and before using any iodine contrast medium, surgical preparation, or other form of iodine.
2. The test is most effective when endogenous TSH levels are high, to stimulate radionuclide uptake by metastatic neoplasm.

Patient Preparation

1. Explain the purpose, procedure, benefits, and risks of total body scan.
2. Advise the patient that the imaging process may take a long time. If iodine allergies are suspected, observe the patient during and after testing for possible reactions.
3. Refer to general procedures, description of benefits, risks, clinical considerations, and standard nuclear scan *pretest* precautions on pages 620–622.
4. See Chapter 1 guidelines for safe, effective, informed *pretest* care.

Patient Aftercare

1. Refer to standard nuclear scan *posttest* precautions on page 622.
2. Interpret test outcome and monitor appropriately.
3. Follow Chapter 1 basic guidelines for safe, effective, informed *posttest* care.

Part Two

Radionuclide Laboratory Procedures (Other Than Radioimmunoassay [RIA] Studies)

Overview of Laboratory Procedures

Minute quantities of radioactive materials may be detected in blood, feces, urine, other body fluids, and glands. Very small amounts of radioactive substances may be administered to patients, and then their body fluids and glands may be examined in the laboratory for concentrations of radioactivity.

One procedure checks the ability of the body to absorb the administered radioactive compound. An example of this type of study is the Schilling test.

Another procedure, such as radioactive iodine uptake or blood volume determination, tests the ability of the body to localize or dilute the administered radioactive substance.

Part 2 of this chapter includes a sampling of tests that employ the use of radionuclides in the study of disease. Imaging may or may not be required as part of these procedures.

SCHILLING TEST

Normal Values

Excretion of 7% or more of test dose of cobalt-tagged vitamin B_{12} in urine.

Explanation of Test

This 24-hour urine test is used to diagnose pernicious anemia (one form of macrocytic anemia) and malabsorption syndromes. It is an indirect test of intrinsic factor deficiency. This test evaluates the body's ability to absorb vitamin B_{12} from the GI tract and is based on the anticipated urinary excretion of radioactive vitamin B_{12}. The procedure may be done in two stages: stage I without intrinsic factor; stage II with intrinsic factor. The second occurs only when an abnormal first stage occurs.

In stage I, the fasting patient is given an oral dose of vitamin B_{12} tagged with radioactive cobalt (^{57}Co). An intramuscular injection of vitamin B_{12} is given to saturate the liver and serum protein-binding sites, which allows radioactive vitamin B_{12} to be excreted in the urine. A 24-hour urine specimen is then collected.

The amount of the excreted radioactive B_{12} is determined and expressed as a percentage of the given dose. Normal persons will absorb and, therefore, excrete as much as 25% of the radioactive B_{12}. Patients with pernicious anemia absorb little of the oral dose and, thus, have little radioactive material to excrete in the urine.

Procedure

1. The patient must fast for 12 hours before the test. (Intake of food is delayed 3 hours after vitamin B_{12} doses are administered.)
2. A tasteless capsule of radioactive B_{12}, labeled with ^{57}Co, is administered orally by a nuclear medical technologist.
3. Then a nonradioactive B_{12} is given by intramuscular injection by a registered nurse or nuclear medical technologist.
4. Total urine is collected for 24 or 48 hours from the time the patient receives the injection of vitamin B_{12}.
   - **a.** Obtain a special 24-hour urine container from the laboratory. No preservative is required.
   - **b.** Ensure that there is no contamination of the urine with stool.
   - **c.** Follow the procedure for 24-hour urine collection (see Chap. 3).
   - **d.** In presence of renal disease, one 48-hour collection may be necessary.

Clinical Implications

1. An abnormally low value (eg, < 7%) or borderline (7% to 10%) allows two interpretations:
   a. Absence of intrinsic factor
   b. Defective absorption in the ileum
2. When the absorption of radioactive vitamin B_{12} is low from the first stage, the test must be repeated with intrinsic factor (stage II) to rule out intestinal malabsorption (confirmatory Schilling test).
   a. If the urinary excretion then rises to normal levels, it indicates a lack of intrinsic factor, suggesting the diagnosis of pernicious anemia.
   b. If the urinary excretion does not rise, malabsorption is considered the cause of the patient's anemia.

NOTE: *A dual radionuclide method is an alternative method in which both stages are performed at the same time.*

Interfering Factors

1. Renal insufficiency may cause reduced excretions of radioactive vitamin B_{12}. If renal insufficiency is suspected, a 48- to 72-hour urine collection is advised because eventually nearly all the absorbed material will be excreted, and urine specific gravity and volume are checked.
2. The patient should not undergo diagnostic procedures that interfere with B_{12} absorption.
3. The single most common source of error in performing the test is *incomplete collection of urine.* Some laboratories may require a 48-hour collection to allow for a small margin of error.
4. Urinary excretion of B_{12} is depressed in elderly patients, diabetics, patients with hypothyroidism, and those with enteritis.
5. Fecal contamination in the urine will lead to false results and will invalidate the test.

Patient Preparation

1. Explain the purpose, procedure, benefits, and risks of the test.
2. Refer to general procedures, description of benefits, risks, clinical considerations, and standard nuclear scan *pretest* precautions on pages 620–622.
3. A random sample urine specimen is usually obtained before the B_{12} doses are administered.
4. Give a written reminder to the patient about fasting and collection of a 24-hour urine specimen. Water is permitted during the fasting period.
5. Food and drink are permitted 3 hours after the doses of vitamin B_{12} are given. The patient is encouraged to drink as much as can be tolerated during the entire test.
6. Be certain the patient receives the nonradioactive B_{12}. If the intramuscular dose of vitamin B_{12} is not given, the radioactive vitamin B_{12} will be found in the liver instead of the urine.
7. See Chapter 1 basic guidelines for safe, effective, informed *pretest* care.

Clinical Alert

1. No laxatives are to be used during the test.
2. Bone marrow aspiration should be done before the Schilling test because the vitamin B_{12} administered in the test will destroy the diagnostic characteristics of the bone marrow.

Patient Aftercare

1. Assess for compliance with 24-hour urine collection protocols. (See Chap. 3 for specifics of urine collection.)
2. Refer to standard nuclear scan *posttest* precautions on page 622.
3. Interpret test outcome and monitor appropriately.
2. Follow Chapter 1 guidelines for safe, effective, informed *posttest* care.

TOTAL BLOOD VOLUME DETERMINATION; PLASMA VOLUME; RED CELL VOLUME

Normal Values

Total blood volume:	55–80 ml/kg
Red cell volume:	20–35 ml/kg (greater in men than in women)
Plasma volume:	30–45 ml/kg

NOTE: *Because adipose tissue has a sparser blood supply than lean tissue, the patient's body type can affect the proportion of blood volume to body weight, which is why test findings should always be reported in milliliters per kilogram.*

Explanation of Test

The purpose of this test is to determine circulating blood volume, to help evaluate the bleeding or debilitated patient, and to determine the origin of hypotension in the presence of anuria or oliguria when dehydration may be the cause. This determination is one way to monitor blood loss during surgery; it is used as a guide in replacement therapy following blood or body fluid loss and in the determination of whole-body hematocrit. The results are useful in determining the most appropriate blood component for replacement therapy (eg, whole blood, plasma, or packed red cells).

Total blood volume determinations are of value in the following situations:

1. To evaluate GI and uterine bleeding.
2. To aid in the diagnosis of hypovolemic shock.
3. To aid in the diagnosis of polycythemia vera.
4. To determine the required blood component for replacement therapy, as in persons undergoing surgery.

These tests will reveal an increased or a decreased plasma volume or red cell mass. A sample of the patient's blood is mixed with a radioactive substance, incubated at room temperature, and reinjected. Another blood sample is obtained 15 minutes later. The most commonly used tracers in blood volume determination are serum albumin tagged with ^{131}I or ^{125}I and patient or donor red blood cells tagged with ^{51}Cr. The combination of procedures, or total blood volume, is the only true blood volume. Other volume studies are plasma volume and ^{51}Cr red cell volume, which may be done separately.

The plasma volume is used to establish a vascular baseline, to determine changes in plasma volume before and after surgery, and to evaluate fluid and blood replacement in GI bleeding and burn and trauma cases.

The ^{51}Cr-labeled red cell volume study is done to see what percentage of the circulating blood is composed of red cells. This procedure is performed in connection with red cell survival, GI blood loss, or ferrokinetic studies.

Procedure

1. Record the patient's height and current weight.
2. Venous blood samples are obtained, and one sample is mixed with a radionuclide.
3. Fifteen to 30 minutes later, the blood is reinjected.
4. About 15 minutes later, another venous blood sample is obtained.

Clinical Implications

1. A normal total blood volume with a decreased red cell content indicates the need for a transfusion of packed red cells.
2. Polycythemia vera may be differentiated from secondary polycythemia.
   a. Increased total blood volume owing to an increased red cell mass suggests polycythemia vera. The plasma volume is most often normal.
   b. Normal or decreased total blood volume owing to a decreased plasma volume suggests secondary polycythemia. The red cell volume is most often normal.

Clinical Alert

If intravenous blood component therapy is ordered for the same day, the blood volume determination should be done before the intravenous line is started.

Patient Preparation

1. Explain the purpose, procedure, benefits, and risks of test.
2. The patient should be weighed just before the test if possible.
3. Refer to general procedures, description of benefits, risks, clinical considerations, and standard nuclear scan *pretest* precautions on pages 620–622.
4. See Chapter 1 basic guidelines for safe, effective, informed *pretest* care.

Patient Aftercare

1. Refer to standard nuclear scan *posttest* precautions on page 622.
2. Interpret test outcome and monitor appropriately.

3. Follow Chapter 1 basic guidelines for safe, effective, informed *posttest* care.

RED BLOOD CELL (RBC) SURVIVAL TIME TEST ●

Normal Values

Normal half-time ^{51}Cr red blood cell survival is approximately 25 to 35 days.
Chromium 51 in stool: < 3 ml/24 hr

Explanation of Test

This blood test has its greatest use in the evaluation of known or suspected hemolytic anemia and is also indicated when there seems to be an obscure cause for anemia, to identify accessory spleens, and to determine abnormal red cell production or destruction. A sample of the patient's red blood cells is mixed with a radioactive substance (^{51}Cr), incubated at room temperature, and reinjected. Blood specimens are drawn at the end of a 24-hour period and at regular intervals for at least 3 weeks. After counting the specimens, the results are plotted, and the red cell survival time is calculated. Results are based on the fact that disappearance of radioactivity from the circulation corresponds to the disappearance of the red blood cells, thereby determining overall erythrocyte survival.

Scanning of the spleen is often done as part of this test. Red blood cell survival is usually ordered in conjunction with blood volume determination and radionuclide iron uptake and clearance tests. When stool specimens are collected for 3 days, the test is often referred to as the gastrointestinal blood loss test, which is different from the nuclear scan study on page 649.

Procedure

1. A venous blood sample of 20 ml is obtained.
2. Ten to 30 minutes later, the blood is reinjected after being tagged with a radionuclide, ^{51}Cr.
3. Blood samples are usually obtained the first day, again at 24, 48, 72, and 96 hours, then at weekly intervals for 3 weeks. Time may be shortened, depending on the outcome of the test. As part of this procedure, a radioactive detector may be used over the spleen, sternum, and liver to assess the relative concentration of radioactivity in these areas. This external counting helps determine if the spleen is taking part in excessive sequestration of red blood cells as a causative factor in anemia.
4. In some instances, a 72-hour stool collection may be ordered to detect GI blood loss. At the end of each 24-hour collection period, the total stool is to be collected by the department of nuclear medicine. This test can be completed in 3 days.

Clinical Implications

1. Shortened red cell survival may be the result of blood loss, hemolysis, and removal of red blood cells by the spleen, as in

a. Chronic granulocytic leukemia
b. Hemolytic anemia
c. Hemoglobin C disease
d. Hereditary spherocytosis
e. Pernicious anemia
f. Megaloblastic anemia of pregnancy
g. Sickle cell anemia
h. Uremia

2. Prolonged red cell survival time may be the result of abnormality of red cell production as in thalassemia minor.
3. If hemolytic anemia is diagnosed, further studies are needed to establish whether red blood cells have intrinsic abnormalities, or whether the anemia results from immunologic effects of the patient's plasma.
4. Results will be normal in
   a. Hemoglobin C trait
   b. Sickle cell trait
5. Half of the radioactivity of plasma may not disappear for 7 to 8 hours.

Patient Preparation

1. Explain the purpose and procedure of the test. Emphasize that this test requires a minimum of 2 weeks of the patient's time, with trips to the diagnostic facility for venipunctures.
2. If stool collection is required, advise the patient of the importance of saving all stool and that stool be free of urine contamination (see stool chapter).
3. Refer to general procedures, description of benefits, risks, clinical considerations, and standard nuclear scan *pretest* precautions on pages 620–622.
4. See Chapter 1 basic guidelines for safe, effective, informed *pretest* care.

Clinical Alert

1. The test is usually contraindicated in an actively bleeding patient.
2. Record and report signs of active bleeding.
3. Transfusions should not be given when the test is in progress. If it is necessary to do so, notify the nuclear medicine department to terminate the test.

Patient Aftercare

1. Refer to standard nuclear scan *posttest* precautions.
2. Interpret test outcome and monitor appropriately.
3. Follow Chapter 1 guidelines for safe, effective, informed *posttest* care.

RADIOACTIVE IODINE (RAI) UPTAKE TEST

Normal Values

1% to 13% absorbed by thyroid gland after 2 hours
5% to 20% absorbed by thyroid gland after 6 hours

15% to 40% absorbed by thyroid gland after 24 hours
Values are laboratory-dependent.

Explanation of Test

This direct test of the function of the thyroid gland measures ability of the gland to concentrate and retain iodine. When radioctive iodine is administered, it is rapidly absorbed into the bloodstream. This procedure measures the rate of accumulation, incorporation, and release of iodine by the thyroid. The rate of absorption of the radioactive iodine (which is determined by an increase in radioactivity of the thyroid gland) is a measure of the ability of the thyroid gland to concentrate iodide from the blood plasma. The radioactive isotopes of iodine usually used are either ^{131}I or ^{123}I.

This procedure is indicated in the evaluation of hypothyroidism, hyperthyroidism, thyroiditis, goiter, pituitary failure, and posttreatment evaluation. The patient who is a candidate for this test may have a lumpy or swollen neck or complain of pain in the neck, be jittery and ultrasensitive to heat, or may be sluggish and ultrasensitive to cold. The test is more useful in the diagnosis of hyperthyroidism than in hypothyroidism.

Procedure

> **NOTE:** *The test is usually done in conjunction with a thyroid scan (page 630) and assessment of thyroid hormone blood levels (see Chapter 6).*

1. A fasting state is preferred. A good history and listing of all medications are a must for this test. (The history should also include nonprescription medications and patient dietary habits.)
2. A liquid form or a tasteless capture of radioiodine is administered orally. The patient is usually instructed not to eat for 1 hour after administration of radioiodine.
3. The amount of radioactivity is measured by a scan of the radioactivity in the thyroid gland 2, 6, and 24 hours later. There is no pain or discomfort involved.
4. The patient will have to return to the laboratory at the designated time because the exact time of measurement is crucial in determining uptake.

Clinical Alert

1. This test is contraindicated in pregnant or lactating women, in children, in infants, and in those individuals with iodine allergies.
2. Whenever possible, this test should be performed before any other radionuclide procedures are done, before any iodine medications are given, and before any radiographs using iodine contrast medium are done.

Clinical Implications

1. Increased uptake (eg, 20% in 1 hour, 25% in 6 hours, 45% in 24 hours) suggests hyperthyroidism but is not diagnostic for it.
2. Decreased uptake (eg, 0% in 2 hours, 3% in 6 hours, 10% in 24 hours) may be caused by hypothyroidism but is not diagnostic for it.
   a. If the administered iodine is not absorbed, as in severe diarrhea or intestinal malabsorption syndromes, the uptake may be low even though the gland is functioning normally.
   b. Rapid diuresis during the test period may deplete the supply of iodine, causing an apparently low percentage of iodine uptake.
   c. In renal failure, the uptake may be high even though the gland is functioning normally.

Interfering Factors

1. The chemicals, drugs, and foods that interfere with the test by *lowering uptake* are the following:
   a. Iodized foods and iodine-containing drugs, such as Lugol's solution, expectorants, cough medicines, saturated solutions of potassium iodide (SSK), and vitamin preparations that contain minerals (1 to 3 weeks time for the effect of these substances in the body).
   b. Radiographic contrast media, such as Diodrast (iodopyracet), Hypaque (sodium diatrizoate), Renografin, Lipoidal, Ethiodol, Pantopaque (iophendylate), Telepaque (iopanoic acid), 1 week to a year or more in duration. Consult with nuclear medicine laboratory for specific times.
   c. Antithyroid drugs, such as propylthiouracil and related compounds (2 to 10 days' duration).
   d. Thyroid medications such as Cytomel, desiccated thyroid, thyroxine Synthroid (1 to 2 weeks' duration).
   e. Miscellaneous drugs—thiocyanate, perchlorate, nitrates, sulfonamides, tolbutamide (Orinase), corticosteroids, PAS, isoniazid, phenylbutazone (Butazolidin), thiopental (Pentothal), antihistamines, ACTH, aminosalicylic acid, amphenone, cobalt, and coumarin anticoagulants. Consult with the diagnostic department for duration times, which may vary.
2. The compounds and conditions that interfere by *enhancing uptake* are as follows:
   a. TSH
   b. Pregnancy
   c. Cirrhosis
   d. Barbiturates
   e. Lithium carbonate
   f. Phenothiazines (1 week)
   g. Iodine-deficient diets
   h. Renal failure

Patient Preparation

1. Explain the purpose and procedure of the test, which takes 24 hours to complete. Assess and record pertinent dietary and medication history. Inform about interfering factors.
2. Advise that iodine intake is restricted for at least 1 week before testing.

3. Refer to general procedures, benefits, risks, clinical considerations, and standard nuclear scan *pretest* precautions on pages 620–622.
4. See Chapter 1 basic guidelines for safe, effective, informed *pretest* care.

Patient Aftercare

1. Resume medications and normal diet.
2. Refer to standard nuclear scan *posttest* precautions on page 622.
3. Interpret test outcome and monitor appropriately.
4. Follow Chapter 1 basic guidelines for safe, effective, informed *posttest* care.

THYROID-STIMULATING HORMONE (TSH) TEST ●

Normal Values

TSH: less than 5μU/ml (laboratory-dependent)

In normal persons, TSH, T_4, and RAI uptake are increased within 8 to 10 hours after TSH is given.

Explanation of Test

This test measures the response of the thyroid gland to an injection of TSH. This examination is used in conjunction with the RAI uptake test. It is done to differentiate primary from secondary hypothyroidism, to determine the level of thyroid gland activity, especially borderline thyroid function, and to evaluate thyroid hormone therapy. It is indicated in the evaluation of hypopituitarism and to demonstrate the presence of normal suppressed thyroid tissue in persons with autonomous hyperfunctioning nodules. The thyroid gland may have impaired RAI uptake because of intrinsic disease (primary hypothyroidism) or insufficient stimulation by the pituitary gland (secondary hypothyroidism). Patients who have a decreased amount of functioning thyroid gland, as in subtotal thyroidectomy, radiation therapy, or thyroiditis, may have a normal RAI uptake and still fail to respond to TSH stimulation. Such persons have a low thyroid reserve and need continued observation to prevent myxedema.

Procedure

1. *Day 1:* Patient receives 10 units TSH intramuscularly.
2. *Day 2:* Background counts over thyroid are taken and 10 more units of TSH are administered intramuscularly. Radioactive iodine is also given at this time (either ^{123}I or ^{131}I may be used).
3. Patient returns in 2 to 6 hours for uptake.
4. *Day 3:* A 24-hour thyroid uptake and thyroid scan are performed.

Clinical Alert

The TSH should be administered by a physician because the patient may have a reaction to this hormone.

Clinical Implications

1. No response to TSH is seen in the following conditions:
   a. Primary untreated hypothyroidism (increase ranges from 3 times normal to 100 times normal in severe myxedema).
   b. Chronic Hashimoto's thyroiditis.
2. The TSH-positive response is seen in the following conditions:
   a. Pituitary hypothyroidism, secondary hypothyroidism
   b. Hypothalamic hypothyroidism, tertiary hypothyroidism

Interfering Factors

Iodine intake will invalidate uptake results. Also, see *Interfering Factors* for the RAI uptake test.

Patient Preparation

1. Explain the purpose and procedure of the test, which takes several days to complete. Check with the appropriate department for the protocols to be used. Also, refer to general procedures, description of benefits, risks, clinical considerations, and standard *pretest* nuclear scan precautions on pages 620–622.
2. Advise that iodine intake is restricted for at least 1 week before testing.
3. Inform the patient that TSH is given intramuscularly.
4. See Chapter 1 guidelines for safe, effective, informed *pretest* care.

Patient Aftercare

1. Refer to standard nuclear scan *posttest* precautions on page 622.
2. Observe for reaction to TSH administration.
3. Interpret test outcome and monitor appropriately.
4. Follow Chapter 1 guidelines for safe, effective, informed *posttest* care.

PERCHLORATE SUPPRESSION STUDY/IODINE WASHOUT TEST ●

Normal Values

In normal persons, the uptake of radioactive iodine will not change appreciably following the administration of perchlorate.

Explanation of Test

The perchlorate test is used to evaluate patients with suspected Hashimoto's disease or to demonstrate an enzyme deficiency within the thyroid gland. The procedure is used to identify defects in the iodide organification process within the thyroid. This study is based on the fact that potassium perchlorate competes with and displaces the iodide ions that are not organified. Iodide is a compound of iodine. Iodine is concentrated within the thyroid gland and quickly becomes bound to the protein thyroglobulin after becoming organified. The administration of perchlorate will stop any further trapping of iodide, as well as the release of any unbound iodide, within the thyroid gland, thus stopping the normal process. When iodine is trapped within the gland, it is enzymatically combined with amino acids to form thyroxine, and the perchlorate will not remove the iodine from the gland. Patients with an enzyme deficiency will show a drop in their uptake greater than 15% after the administration of perchlorate.

Procedure

1. A complete patient history is taken.
2. Body background is measured for residual radiation by imaging.
3. A small tracer dose of radioactive iodine is administered orally (either ^{123}I or ^{131}I may be used).
4. An uptake is performed at 1 and 2 hours after administration.
5. After the 2-hour uptake is performed, the patient is given 400 mg to 1 g of potassium perchlorate orally.
6. Uptakes are performed every 15 minutes for the first hour postdose perchlorate and then 30 minutes thereafter for the next 2 to 3 hours.
7. Uptakes performed after the administration of perchlorate are compared with the 2-hour uptake before perchlorate.
8. The results are recorded on linear graph paper as counts over the thyroid versus time in minutes of the uptake.

Clinical Implications

Abnormal results reveal

1. Enzyme deficiency within a thyroid gland
2. Hashimoto's disease

NOTE: *Both disease processes will interfere with the organification process.*

Interfering Factors

See the RAI uptake test.

Patient Preparation

1. Explain the purpose, procedure, and time frames of the test.
2. The patient should be fasting for this procedure.
3. Advise the patient that no form of iodine should be ingested for at least 1 week before testing; this includes medications, foods, and contrasts used in radiographs.
4. Refer to general procedures, benefits, risks, clinical considerations, and standard nuclear scan *pretest* precautions on pages 620–622.

Patient Aftercare

1. Refer to standard nuclear scan posttest precautions on page 622.
2. Interpret test outcomes and monitor for Hashimoto's disease and thyroid gland enzyme deficiency.
3. Follow Chapter 1 guidelines for safe, effective, informed *posttest* care.

^{131}I THYROID CYTOMEL SUPPRESSION TEST

Normal Values

Euthyroid patients with normal thyroid uptakes can expect a depression of the second uptake of at least 50% following Cytomel administration.

Explanation of Test

This test measures the response of the thyroid metabolic system to the administration of oral triiodothyronine (Cytomel). The uptake of iodine by a normal thyroid gland will decrease following the administration of oral triiodothyronine.

A patient who has a high initial uptake because of iodine deficiency, dyshormonogenesis condition, or who is recovering from a subacute thyroiditis, will have a sharp decline, usually about one-half the baseline value, after the administration of Cytomel. Some patients will not be suppressed by the administration of Cytomel. In most instances, those patients will be hyperthyroid because of a toxic goiter (Graves' disease), a toxic multinodular goiter, or a toxic autonomously functioning thyroid adenoma. In some instances, a nonhypothyroid patient will not suppress after administration of Cytomel. An example would be a person with euthyroid Graves' disease.

Procedure

1. A careful patient history must be taken before the administration of Cytomel.
2. If the physician agrees that the Cytomel will not have an adverse effect, the patient is started on a regimen for a period of 5 to 10 days.
3. The patient must return to the nuclear medicine department 1 day before the last dose of Cytomel is taken.
4. On that day, a body background sample is taken for residual radioactive iodine from the previous uptake and recorded.
5. A new tracer dose of radioactive iodine is given and amount, date, and time are recorded (either ^{123}I or ^{131}I may be used).
6. The patient returns after the last dose of Cytomel is taken, and an uptake is performed (2- and 6-hour uptakes are usual after radioiodine is given).

Clinical Implications

1. The euthyroid patient who is iodine-deficient will normally have a high uptake initially and a decreased second uptake following the administration of Cytomel.
2. A patient with a hyperthyroid condition demonstrating a high initial uptake will show no appreciable change on the second uptake following the administration of Cytomel.
3. Other abnormal findings include
   a. TSH-dependent tissue will be suppressed.
   b. Autonomous nodules will not be suppressed.
   c. Patients with thyroid cancer may or may not be suppressed.

d. Thyroid tissue destroyed as a result of therapy or disease will remain unchanged.
e. A scan of the thyroid performed before and after the administration of Cytomel will demonstrate an autonomous nodule or tissue because it is unaffected by TSH.

Patient Preparation

1. Explain the purpose and procedure of the test, including the time involved and the proper administration of Cytomel. Assess for allergy to iodine.
2. Advise the patient not to consume any products containing iodine or take any medication that would affect this study.
3. Refer to general procedures, benefits, risks, clinical considerations, and standard nuclear scan *pretest* precautions on pages 620–622.
4. See Chapter 1 basic guidelines for safe, effective, informed *pretest* care.

Patient Aftercare

1. Refer to standard nuclear scan *posttest* precautions on page 622.
2. Observe for adverse reactions to Cytomel or iodine.
3. Interpret test outcome and monitor appropriately.
4. Follow Chapter 1 guidelines for safe, effective, informed *posttest* care.

Part Three

Positron Emission Tomography: Pet Scans

Normal Values

Normal patterns of tissue metabolism based on oxygen, glucose, and fatty acid utilization, and protein synthesis.

Normal blood flow and tissue perfusion can be visualized.

Explanation of Test

Positron emission tomography (PET) is the combined use of positron-emitting isotopes and emission-computed tomography to measure regional tissue function (see p. 619 for SPECT). Like a CT scan, the PET scanner, which is shaped like a giant tire, does transverse imaging. The injected or inhaled radionuclide will emit radioactivity in the form of positrons that are detected and transformed into a visual display by a computer. Oxygen 15, nitrogen 13, carbon 11, and fluorine 18 are common radioactive nuclides used in PET procedures. Fluorine 18 is often used for several reasons. Its half-life is long enough to trace a biochemical reaction in a person. It is capable of being labeled to a variety of carriers. The molecules allow greater imaging flexibility. Fluorine 18 is primarily administered in a glucose form called fluorodeoxyglucose (FDG).

The PET studies are noninvasive tests used most commonly to determine physiologic function of the brain and heart. However, the technique is applicable to the examination of all parts of the body for the diagnosis and staging of disease and monitoring therapy. Unlike MR and CT scans, PET can provide physiologic, anatomic, and biochemical data. Although PET is more sensitive than SPECT, it is considerably more expensive. At this time, use of the PET is mainly in large medical centers with a large number of experimental studies being done.

Uses of PET

Positron emission tomography may be used for a variety of physiologic activities, including blood flow and tissue metabolism.

Procedures

1. Patient procedures vary and the total time to perform a single scan takes from 1 to 2 hours.
2. The patient is positioned on a table and positioned within scanner. Before administration of radiopharmaceutical, a background transmission scan is performed. In certain procedures, this may be optional.
3. The radioactive drug is administered intravenously. The patient must wait 30 to 45 minutes in department, usually remains on table, and then the area of interest is scanned.

BRAIN IMAGING

Clinical Implications

1. In *epilepsy,* focal areas with increased metabolism have been seen during actual stage of epilepsy, and decreased oxygen utilization and blood flow during interictal stage. (PET become an alternative to depth electrode implants.)
2. In *stroke,* an extremely complex pathophysiologic picture is being revealed: anaerobic glycolysis, depressed oxygen utilization, and decreased blood flow.
3. In *dementia,* decreased glucose consumption (hypometabolic activity) is revealed by PET imaging. Positron emission tomography is used to differentiate Alzheimer's disease and other types of dementia, such as Huntington's disease and Parkinson's disease.
4. In *schizophrenia,* some studies using labeled glucose indicate reduced metabolic activity in the frontal region. The PET scans can also distinguish the developmental stages of cranial tumors and give information about operability of such tumors.

5. In *brain tumors,* data have been collected concerning oxygen use and blood flow relationships for these tumors. Gliomas have relatively good perfusion in comparison with their decreased oxygen utilization. The high uptake of radiopharmaceutical in gliomas is reported to correlate with the tumor's histological grade.

Interfering Factors

Excessive anxiety can alter test results when brain functioning is being tested. Tranquilizers cannot be given before the test because they alter glucose metabolism.

Patient Preparation for Brain PET Scan

1. Instruct the patient about PET scan purpose, procedure, and special requirements. Refer to general procedures, description of benefits, risks, clinical considerations, and standard nuclear scan test precautions on pages 620–622.
2. Advise patient that lying as still as possible during scan is necessary. However, patient is not to fall asleep nor count to pass the time.
3. During the scan, it is important to maintain a quiet environment.
4. See Chapter 1 guidelines for safe, effective, informed *pretest* care.

CARDIAC IMAGING

Clinical Implications

1. In cardiology, PET imaging provides measurements of blood flow and myocardial perfusion. These measurements are used to detect
   a. Coronary artery disease, which is characterized by areas of decreased blood flow or perfusion, or both ([^{13}N]ammonia is used).
   b. For the detection of transient ischemia, both stress and rest images are performed (see *Nuclear Medicine Cardiac Stress Testing*).
   c. In addition to blood flow and perfusion, the metabolism of the myocardium can be assessed for viability; FDG is ideal for this purpose.
2. A high rate of glucose consumption is required to meet the energy needs of the heart. Myocardial cells that do not show higher rates of glucose metabolism in areas of decreased blood flow, indicate myocardial tissue that is no longer viable.

Patient Preparation for Heart PET Scan

1. Instruct the patient about PET scan purpose, procedure, and special requirements. Refer to general procedures, description of benefits, risks, clinical considerations, and standard nuclear scan *pretest* precautions on pages 620–622.
2. An intravenous line may need to be established. Fasting, smoking restrictions, and certain medications may be required before imaging. Consult with the referring physician or the nuclear imaging department.

3. It may be necessary to place ECG leads on patient. See *Nuclear Medicine Cardiac Patient Preparation for Stress Testing.*
4. See Chapter 1 guidelines for safe, effective, informed *pretest* care.

TUMOR IMAGING

Clinical Implications

1. Measurements of glucose—fluorodeoxyglucose (FDG)—metabolism is used to determine tumor growth. Because small amounts of FDG can be visualized, early tumor detection is possible before structural changes occur as detected by MR or CT. Tumor grading can be assessed by the rate of increases in glucose metabolism. In cases of suspected tumor recurrence after therapy, PET differentiates any new growth from necrotic tissue.
2. PET is used to distinguish between recurrent, active tumor growth and necrotic masses in soft tissue, which is difficult for MR and CT methodologies to differentiate.

Patient Preparation for Tumor Imaging PET Scans

1. Refer to general procedures, description of benefits, risks, clinical considerations, and standard nuclear scan test precautions on pages 620–622.
2. No special preparation is needed.
3. See Chapter 1 guidelines for safe, effective, informed *pretest* care.

Patient Aftercare for All PET Scans

1. Interpret test outcome and monitor appropriately.
2. Refer to standard nuclear scan *posttest* precautions on page 622.
3. Follow Chapter 1 guidelines for safe, effective, informed *posttest* care.

BIBLIOGRAPHY

Baum S et al: Atlas of Nuclear Medicine Imaging. New York, Appleton & Lange, 1993

Bernier DR, Christina PE, Langa JK et al: Nuclear Medicine Technology and Techniques, 3rd ed. St. Louis, CV Mosby, 1994

D'Agincourt L: PET's diagnostic prowess widens its clinical appeal. Diagnostic Imaging 11(10):90–99, October 1989

Early PJ, Sodee DB: Principles and Practice of Nuclear Medicine, 2nd ed. St. Louis, CV Mosby, 1995

Freeman LM (ed): Advances in functional neuroimaging. Mediphysics 1(20), 1988; 1(4), 1988; 2(3), 1989

George MS, Ring HA, Costa DC, Ell PJ, Kouris K, Jarritt PH: Neuroactivation and neuroimaging with SPECT. New York, Springer-Verlag, 1991

McDonagh A: Getting your patient ready for a nuclear scan. Nursing '91 21(2):53–57, February 1991

Mettler FA, Gulberteau MJ: Essentials of Nuclear Medicine Imaging, 3rd ed. Philadelphia, WB Saunders, 1991

OncoScint CR/OV Satumomab Pendetide, Knoll Pharmaceutical Company and Cytogen Corporation, 1993

Plankey EL, Plankey MW: Prep talk: A nuclear approach to cancer detection. AJR 9(6):June 1990

Porth CM: Pathophysiology: Concepts of Altered Health States, 3rd ed. Philadelphia, JB Lippincott, 1990

Weikart C: New eye into the heart. Registered Nurse, October, 1993

10

X-Ray Studies

OVERVIEW OF X-RAY STUDIES

General Principles

X-ray studies, also known as *radiographs* or *roentgenograms,* are used to examine soft and bony tissues of the body. X-rays (roentgen rays) are very short wavelength electromagnetic vibrations produced when fast-moving electrons collide with substances in their pathways. They are similar to light rays, except x-ray wavelengths are only 1/10,000 the length of visible light rays. Because of this short wavelength, x-rays can penetrate very dense substances to produce images or shadows that can then be recorded on photographic film. The basic principle of radiography rests with the fact that differences in density between various body structures produce images of varying light or dark intensity on the x-ray film, much like the negative print of a photograph. Dense structures appear white, whereas air-filled areas are black.

During x-ray examinations, a high-voltage electric current passes through a tungsten "target" in a vacuum tube. Less than 1% of the high-speed electrons (cathode rays) are actually transformed into x-rays; the rest of this energy changes into heat.

X-rays travel in straight lines at the speed of light (86,000 miles/sec). When the x-ray beam passes through matter, some of its intensity is absorbed. The more dense the matter is, the greater the degree of x-rays absorbed. Photographic film is affected by x-rays in the same way it is affected by light. The sensitive silver film emulsion undergoes a chemical change when it is exposed to x-radiation. Subsequent processing results in an image that is a composite of black, white, and various tones of gray, which represent varying degrees of tissue density through which the x-ray beams have passed. Modern x-ray equipment allows use of high-resolution techniques, video-screens, digital magnetic records, and laser printers that produce much sharper pictures of bones and organs than could be obtained in the past.

USE OF CONTRAST MEDIA

Many radiographic techniques use the natural contrasts and varying densities that exist in body tissue—air, water (in soft tissue), fat, and bone. The lungs and gastrointestinal tract normally contain air or gases. Other body structures are encased in a fatty envelope. Bone contains naturally occurring mineral salts. However, at times, diagnosis of certain pathologic conditions requires that visualization of details that cannot be revealed through plain film radiography be highlighted by the presence of *contrast media* in the area. These contrast substances can be administered through oral, rectal, or injectable routes.

The ideal contrast medium should be relatively harmless, inert, and should not interfere with any physiologic functions. It may be classified as either radiopaque (not permitting the transmission of x-rays) or radiolucent (permitting partial transmission of x-rays). Ultimately, one must always be alert to the possibility of a reaction, and emergency supplies and equipment should be readily available.

The following contrast media are used routinely in radiographic studies:

1. Barium sulfate (radiopaque)
   a. Used for gastrointestinal studies
   b. Prepared as a colloidal suspension
   c. Effectively delineates small, filling defects
2. Organic iodides (radiopaque)
   a. Examples: sodium diatrizoate, meglumine diatrizoate, metrizamide, and "nonanoic" agents
   b. Used for studies of the kidney, liver, blood vessels, urinary bladder, and urethra
   c. Includes a water-soluble iodide used in myelography
3. Iodized oils (radiopaque): Used in myelography, bronchography, and lymphangiograms
4. Oxygen, helium, air, carbon dioxide, nitrous oxide, and nitrogen (radiolucent): Used for visualization of joints, subarachnoid space, pleural space, peritoneal cavity, and pericardial space

ADVERSE REACTIONS TO CONTRAST MEDIA

The ingestion of contrast media can sometimes cause allergic reactions that can range from mild (nausea and vomiting) to severe anaphylaxis (cardiovascular collapse and central nervous system depression, leading to death if untreated).

Table 10-1 lists the range of possible adverse reactions to iodine contrast media.

Clinical Considerations When Iodine Contrast Media Are Used

1. The highest frequency of side effects occurs in patients aged 20 to 49 years; the lowest frequency is in those older than 70 years of age.
2. Patients who are allergic to iodine contrast media must have this information documented in their healthcare records. Subsequent reactions can occur because the risk for these increases three to four times after a reaction (the second reaction may not necessarily be more severe). The patient must be made aware of the implications for this situation.
3. Check the patient's fasting status before x-rays are begun. Except in an extreme emergency, iodine contrast media should never be administered intravenously sooner than 90 minutes after the patient has eaten. In most instances, the patient should be on nothing by mouth (NPO) status the night before any radiographic testing using an iodine contrast medium is done.
4. Death from an allergic reaction can occur if severe symptoms go untreated. Staff in attendance must be qualified to administer cardiopulmonary resuscitation, should it be necessary. Emergency equipment and supplies must be readily available.

TABLE 10-1
Signs, Symptoms, and Incidence of Reactions to Iodine Contrast Media

Cardiovascular	*Respiratory*	*Cutaneous*	*Gastrointestinal*	*Neurologic*	*Urinary*
Pallor	Sneezing	Erythema	Nausea	Anxiety	Flank pain
Diaphoresis	Coughing	Feeling of warmth	Vomiting	Headache	Hematuria
Tachycardia	Rhinorrhea	Parotitis	Metallic taste	Dizziness	Oliguria
Bradycardia	Wheezing	Urticaria	Abdominal cramps	Agitation	Albuminuria
Palpitations	Acute asthma attack	Pruritus	Diarrhea	Vertigo	WBCs in blood
Arrhythmia	Laryngospasm	Pain at injection site	Paralytic ileus	Slurred speech	Acute renal failure
Acute pulmonary edema	Cyanosis	Angioneurotic edema		Disorientation	
	Laryngeal edema			Stupor	
Shock	Apnea			Coma	
Congestive heart failure	Respiratory arrest			Convulsions	
Cardiac arrest					

All Iodine Contrast Reactions	*Incidence (%)*
MINOR REACTIONS REQUIRING NO TREATMENT Nausea, vomiting, mild urticaria, rash, dizziness, lightheadedness	1:20 (5)
INTERMEDIATE REACTIONS THAT REQUIRE TREATMENT, NO HOSPITALIZATION, NOT LIFE-THREATENING Extensive urticaria, facial and laryngeal edema, bronchospasm, dyspnea, mild chest pain, headache, chills and fever	1:100(1)
SEVERE REACTIONS THAT REQUIRE HOSPITALIZATION AND ARE LIFE-THREATENING Laryngeal and pulmonary edema, hypotension, circulatory collapse, severe angina, myocardial infarction, cardiac arrhythmia, convulsion, coma, respiratory arrest	1:2000 (0.05)
CARDIAC ARREST	1:6000 (0.017)
DEATH	1:40,000 (0.0025)

5. Promptly administer antihistamines per physician's order if mild to moderate reactions to iodine contrast substances occur.
6. When coordinating x-ray testing that uses a contrast medium, keep in mind that studies using iodine or barium should be scheduled at different times.
7. Some physiologic change can be expected whenever an iodine contrast substance is injected, as in an intravenous pyelogram (IVP). Physiologic responses to iodine given intravenously include hypotension, tachycardia, or arrhythmias. For this reason, always check the blood pressure, pulse, and respiration before and after these tests.
8. If possible, after the test, large amounts of oral fluids should be taken to promote frequent urination. This flushes the iodine out of the body.
9. Possible contraindications to the administration of iodine contrast substances include:
   - **a.** Sickle cell anemia—use may increase sickling effect
   - **b.** Syphilis—use may lead to nephrotic syndrome
   - **c.** Long-term steroid therapy—iodine substance may render part of the drug inactive
   - **d.** Pheochromocytoma—may produce a sudden, potentially fatal, rise in blood pressure
   - **e.** Hyperthyroidism
   - **f.** Chronic obstructive pulmonary disease (COPD)
   - **g.** Multiple myeloma
   - **h.** Acute asthma
   - **i.** History of renal failure
   - **j.** Pregnancy

Clinical Alert

1. Careful patient preparation can prevent the need to repeat the procedure.
2. No contrast medium is without risk for causing reactions. Benefit versus risk must be considered. For example, in a workup to detect cancer, the benefits of early detection far outweigh the dangers of cumulative x-ray radiation exposure. The patient needs to know this; in fact, this information must be given because the patient has a legal right to this knowledge.
3. Never inject iodized oils or barium into the bloodstream.

Clinical Considerations When Barium Contrast Is Used

There is always some risk when introducing barium sulfate or a similar contrast medium into the gastrointestinal tract.

1. Barium radiography may interfere with many other abdominal examinations. A number of studies, including other x-rays, tests using iodine, ul-

trasound procedures, radioisotope studies, tomograms, computed scanning, and proctoscopy must be scheduled before barium studies. Consult with the x-ray department for the proper sequencing of barium studies.

2. Emphasize that a laxative should be taken after a procedure is completed when barium sulfate is used.
3. Elderly, inactive persons should be checked for impaction if they fail to defecate within a reasonable length of time. The first sign of impaction in the elderly may be fainting.
4. Observe and record findings about stool color and consistency for at least 2 days to determine if barium has been evacuated. Stools will be light in color until all barium has been expelled. Outpatients should be given a written reminder to inspect stools for at least 2 days.
5. If possible, avoid giving narcotics, especially codeine, when barium x-rays are ordered because these drugs, in and of themselves, can cause constipation.
6. Barium may aggravate acute ulcerative colitis or can cause a bowel obstruction that may be partial or complete.
7. Barium should *not* be used for intestinal study when a bowel perforation is suspected because leakage of barium through a perforation can cause peritonitis. Iodinated contrast media should be used when perforations are suspected.

There are special clinical considerations for ostomy patients undergoing bowel preparation for gastrointestinal studies: Communication should be tailored to achieve the most optimal outcomes. In most cases, the standard dietary and medication restrictions will apply, but modifications involving mechanical bowel cleansing with enemas and physiologic cleansing with laxatives may need to be made.

Clinical Alerts for Patients With Ostomies

1. Enemas and laxatives should not be given to a person with an ileostomy in preparation for x-rays or endoscopy because this puts the person with an ileostomy at risk for dehydration and electrolyte imbalance. On the other hand, a person with a sigmoid colostomy needs enemas before x-rays or endoscopy. Consequently, it is very important to identify the type of surgical procedure the patient has had. Moreover, not all colostomies need irrigation. For example, the person with an ascending right-sided colostomy will normally pass a liquid, pasty stool, high in water content and digestive enzymes; such a patient may have only laxatives ordered.
2. Notify the radiology department that the person has an ostomy.
3. Advise all patients to bring extra ostomy supplies and pouches with them for use after the procedure is completed.

See page 711 for specifics regarding barium enema preparation for those patients with ostomies.

Computed Tomography (CT): Overview

Computed tomography (CT), also called *CT scanning, computerized tomography,* or *computerized axial tomography* (CAT), produces x-rays similar to those used in conventional radiography taken with a special scanner system. Conventional x-rays pass through the body and produce an image of bone, soft tissues, and air on film. With CT scans, a computer provides rapid complex calculations that determine the extent to which tissues absorb multiple x-ray beams. CT is unique because it can produce cross-sectional images ("slices") of anatomic structures without superimposing tissues on each other. Additionally, CT can discern the different characteristics of tissue structures within solid organs.

Spiral CT scanners are one of the latest innovations. This modification of the conventional CT technique employs continuous scanning and produces a spiral, three-dimensional raw data set that allows for three-dimensional reconstruction to make CT angiography possible.

Digital Radiography and Fluorography: Overview

Digital radiography is a computer-based imaging modality with exceptionally high spatial resolution. A conventional x-ray beam is capable of producing far more information about body structure and physiology than is possible to record on x-ray film. Some of this information is lost in the transfer. The lost information involves compression of three-dimensional data to two dimensions; decrease in spatial resolution; reduction in visualization of soft tissue, organs, and vascular structures; and the inability to transfer accurate information about blood flow, blood volume, and ejection fractions. However, this information can be regained, to a great extent, by digital radiography. Images may be computer-enhanced or otherwise manipulated. Digital data storage permits instant retrieval of radiologic images for study or review.

Digital Subtraction Imaging: Overview

Digital subtraction angiography (DSA) is a computerized method of studying arterial anatomy that produces images free of superimposed surrounding osseous structures. Basically, a fluoroscopic image is converted from analog (continuous variable data) to digital (discrete data) form. The image is then digitally stored as a matrix (signals transformed into lattice-work image) with a varying number of picture elements (pixels). After each image is converted to digital form, the first image or mask is subtracted from the object image, pixel by pixel. As in computed tomography, the number of pixels into which the image is divided influences the quality of the image. This quality is influenced by the sophistication of the computer used and the speed at which the images can be processed.

LIMITATIONS

1. Patient reaction risk can be about the same as that of conventional techniques that require contrast medium administration.
2. To examine the abdomen and lower extremities, larger-field size usually requires multiple injections of contrast medium.

ADVANTAGES

1. Doses of contrast medium required by standard angiography can be reduced considerably for DSA. Risks associated with toxicity and injury to the blood vessels also may be lessened.
2. Contrast medium can be infused through a smaller-bore catheter (5 vs 8 French). This reduces the likelihood of complications so that this procedure may often be amenable to an outpatient setting.
3. Permanent recordings are entered on disks within a very short time period (< 1 minute).
4. Degree of arterial occlusion (in percentages) can be measured.
5. High-quality, computer-enhanced images translated into real-time values can be instantly replayed on a video monitor. This information also can be taped onto and stored on standard video cassettes.
6. DSA can enhance standard arteriograms. For example, small blood vessel images, hard to visualize with a standard arteriogram, can be easily captured and visualized with DSA.

Magnetic Resonance Imaging (MR, MRI): Overview

Magnetic resonance (MR), formerly called nuclear magnetic resonance (NMR), is a noninvasive, nonionic technique that produces cross-sectional images of the human anatomy through exposure to magnetic energy sources but *without using radiation*. Although not an actual radiographic procedure, this versatile device is used to differentiate tissues in healthy and diseased states. For example, MRI can differentiate normal brain gray matter from white matter based on typical differences in water content of these different tissues. Or, in patients with multiple sclerosis, the normal fatty tissue around nerve fibers has deteriorated: MRI can readily demonstrate this. Additionally, MRI is useful in detecting tumors, infection sites, and more recently, in performing angiographic studies of selected vasculature with a process known as magnetic resonance angiography (MRA).

The MRI machines are essentially large magnets fitted with a group of field control coils. Atomic nuclei, when placed in a magnetic field and stimulated by a particular radiofrequency, emit measurable radio signals that are influenced by the type and the condition of tissue that contains these nuclei. These radio signals are detected and converted to a visual display on a computer monitor or etched on magnetic tape for later playback on a videoscreen. (See Chap. 15 for complete explanation of testing.)

Angiography: Overview

Angiography uses x-ray examinations to study the vascular structures of the body. It involves injection of an organic contrast solution (such as iodine) through a catheter inserted into the femoral artery or, less frequently, the brachial artery. The catheter is selectively placed into the artery under fluoroscopic visualization by the radiologist performing the examination. After satisfactory x-ray films have been obtained, the catheter is removed, and direct pressure is held on the puncture site until bleeding is controlled (usually several minutes). The patient usually remains at complete flat bed rest for at least 6 hours after the procedure. During this time, flexion or bending of the joint adjacent to the puncture site is restricted.

The nomenclature of the studies is derived from the vascular structure studied and the study method used. *Arteriography* refers to contrast dye studies of arterial vessels. Venous structures may also be visualized, as these procedures progress. *Venography* is the contrast dye study of peripheral or central veins. *Lymphography* studies lymph vessels and nodes. *Angiocardiography* investigates the interior of the heart and adjacent great vessels, such as the pulmonary arteries. *Aortography* refers to a contrast study of aortic segments, such as the thoracic aorta (*thoracic aortography*), the abdominal aorta (*abdominal aortography*), or the lumbar corta (*lumbar aortography*).

Types of Angiogram Studies

Name	*Structure Studied*
Arteriography	Arteries
Venography	Peripheral or ventral veins
Lymphography	Lymph vessels and nodes
Angiocardiography	Interior heart and adjacent vessels
Aortography	Thoracic, abdominal, lumbar aorta

Angiographic examinations also can be named for the route used to inject the contrast dye. For example, *renal arteriography* is performed by inserting a catheter into the abdominal aorta and then directing it into the renal artery. During *peripheral arteriography,* the dye is injected directly into the vessel being studied (eg, femoral artery). If done through the venous route, a large bolus of contrast medium is directly injected into a peripheral vein (eg, venous aortography). As the dye flows through the right side of the heart, lungs, and left side of the heart, x-ray films are taken to track the flow of dye through these structures.

INDICATIONS FOR ANGIOGRAPHY

1. Examination of cervical carotid arteries
2. Evaluation of intracranial arteries
3. Before performing transsphenoidal hypophysectomy
4. Postoperative evaluation
5. Detection of superior sagittal sinus thrombosis
6. Identification of renal and iliac arteries in relation to an abdominal aortic aneurysm
7. Accurate screening examination for renovascular hypertension. In this instance, the study can be performed before a routine IVP; it uses the same dose of contrast material.
8. Periodic reevaluation of arterial angioplasty
9. Evaluation of vascular integrity in the presence of traumatic lesions
10. Evaluation of vascular grafts for patency

Clinical Alert

1. The catheter puncture site **must be observed frequently** and closely for hemorrhage or hematoma formation. These can be serious complications and require **immediate attention** should they occur. **Many of these patients have been receiving anticoagulants preprocedure.**
2. Vital signs, puncture site assessment, and neurovascular assessments may need to be done as frequently as every 15 minutes for the first few hours after the procedure. Neurovascular assessments include evaluation of color, motion, sensation, capillary refill time, pulse quality, and temperature (warm or cool) of the affected extremity. Compare the affected with nonaffected extremity.
3. Review the chart or question the patient or physician about deficits that were present before the procedure to establish baseline levels of circulatory function. Report postprocedure changes immediately.
4. The affected extremity must **not** be bent for several hours, and the patient must lie flat, except for a pillow under the head. Do not raise the head of the bed or cart because this can put a strain on a femoral puncture site. The patient may turn if the affected extremity is maintained in a straight position. If needed, a "fracture" bedpan can lessen strain on a groin site.
5. If bleeding or hematoma occurs, apply pressure to the site. Sometimes "sandbags" may be applied to the puncture site as a routine part of postprocedural protocols.
6. Maintain a functional intravenous access site. Usually, the patient will return to the nursing unit with an IV in place.
7. A Doppler device may reveal audible pulse sounds if pulses are nonpalpable.
8. Sudden onset of pain, numbness or tingling, greater degree of coolness, decreased or absent pulses, or blanching color of an extremity are always cues to notify the physician immediately. These signs can signal arterial occlusion, which may require rapid surgical intervention.

RISKS OF RADIATION

Exposure of the human body to x-rays carries with it certain risks. Genetic alterations may occur if reproductive organs are exposed to radiation. The reproductive cells (specifically, the DNA within the chromosomes) may undergo mutations. These mutations can then cause genetic changes in the exposed person's offspring. Somatic changes (those that occur in body tissue other than the reproductive cells) may also occur in other types of tissue receiving excessive or repeated doses of radiation.

The dangers of exposure to radiation arise both from the absorption of relatively large amounts of radiation over a short time period, and also from cumulative effects of smaller amounts received over longer time periods. Moreover, the cumulative effects of radiation may not become evident for several years. For example, radiation can be the cause of cancer that develops many years after exposure.

During the first trimester of pregnancy, the fetus is especially at risk for genetic alterations. Precautions must be taken to prevent or minimize radiation exposure to the uterus. (See Tables 10-2, 10-3, and 10-4).

Safety Measures

Certain precautions must be taken to protect patients, medical and nursing personnel, and other technical staff from unnecessary exposure to radiation.

GENERAL PRECAUTIONS

1. Staff in the radiology department should wear lead aprons and gloves if indicated, when not within a shielded booth during x-ray exposures. Patients should be shielded appropriately insofar as the procedure allows.

TABLE 10-2
Estimated Mean Dose to Uterus/Embryo From Common X-Rays and Scans*

Beam Radiation	*Dose Equivalent (rem)*
Skull	<0.01
Chest	<0.01
Upper GI series	0.048
Barium enema	0.822
Cholecystogram	<0.02
Intravenous pyelogram	0.814
Abdomen, KUB	0.263
Lumbosacral spine	0.639
Pelvis	0.194
Hip	0.128
Radionuclide Scans	***Dose Equivalent (rem)***
Liver (4 mCi ^{99m}Tc)	0.028
Bone (20 mCi ^{99m}Tc)	0.500
Gallium (5 mCi ^{67}Ga)	1.250
Thyroid (5 mCi ^{99m}Tc)	0.135

*For the type of radiation used in common x-rays and radionuclide scans, rads and rems are interchangeable. Radiation dose absorbed by the body is measured in rems or rads (mrem or mrad). These dose equivalents are the upper limits of radiation that should not be exceeded for uterus/embryo.

TABLE 10-3
Estimated Genetic Effects of Radiation‡

Genetic Disorder	Incidence (Per Million Liveborn Offspring)	Additional Effects of Exposure of 1 rem per Generation*	
		First Generation	Later Generations
AUTOSOMAL DOMINANT DISORDER			
Severe	2500	5–20	25
Mild	7500	1–15	75
X-linked	400	<1	<5
Recessive	2500	<1	Very slow increase
CHROMOSOMAL DISORDER			
Translocation	600	<5	Slight increase
Trisomes	3800	<1	<1
Congenital Abnormalities	20,000–30,000	10	10–100
OTHER COMPLEX DISORDERS			
Heart disease†	600,000	Unknown	Unknown
Cancer	300,000	Not estimated	Not estimated

*Radiation dose absorbed by body is measured in rems or rads. Terms are interchangeable. Double the dose for chronic exposure of 100 rem.

†No implication is made that any form of heart disease is caused by radiation exposure. The effects (if any) are analogous to environmental risk factors and contribute to (along with other mutations expressed in later generations) the genetic component of susceptibility.

‡The genetically significant dose (GSD) to the U.S. population from x-ray diagnostics has increased approximately 50% over the last 15 years. The GSD is estimated to be 30 mrad per lifetime. More recent calculations include greater numbers of spinal x-rays owing to inclusion of chiropractic data. Also, the total number of diagnostic x-rays has increased approximately 32%. About two-thirds of this increase is due to femal exposure for lumbar spine and barium enema procedures and male exposure to hip and pelvic area x-rays.

(From Beir V: Health Effects of Exposure to Low Levels of Ionizing Radiation. Washington, DC, National Academy Press, 1990.)

TABLE 10-4
Understanding Radiation Risks; Gonad and Bone Marrow Radiation Exposure Doses From Common X-Ray Procedures

Gonad dose is defined as the estimated amount of radiation absorbed by the ovaries and testes for each of these common procedures. Exceeding this dose may produce altered genetic effects (genetically significant dose, GSD). *Bone marrow dose* is defined as the esimated amount of radiation absorbed by bone marrow.

Relatively High Gonad Dose: Adult (over 100 mrad)	***Moderate Gonad Dose: Adult (10–100 mrad)***	***Low Gonad Dose: Adult (less than 10 mrad)***
Lumbar spine, lumbosacral vertebrae	Men: stomach, upper gastrointestinal tract	Head (including cervical spine)
Pelvis	Cholecystography, cholangiography	Dental (full mouth)
Hip and femur (upper third)	Femur (lower two-thirds)	Arm (including forearm and hand)
Urography	Dorsal spine, abdomen	Bony thorax (ribs, sternum, clavicle, shoulder)
Retrograde pyelography		Dorsal spine
Urethrocystography		Lower leg, foot
Lower gastrointestinal tract		Chest (heart, lung)
Abdomen Obstetric abdomen Pelvimetry Hysterosalpingography Women: gallbladder, small bowel, and upper gastrointestinal		
Pelvimetry	Retrograde pyelography	Femur, hip
Lower gastrointestinal tract	Urethrocystography	Head, chest, heart, lung
Urography	Hysterosalpingography Stomach and upper gastrointestinal tract Lumbar or dorsal spine, lumbosacral spine Pelvis, abdomen Cholecystography Cholangiography, bony thorax (ribs, sternum, clavicle, shoulder)	Dental (full mouth)

(From National Council on Radiation Protection and Measurement. Exposure of the U.S. Population from Diagnostic Medical Radiation. Bethesda, MD, 1989) NCR Report No. 180.

2. The x-ray tube housing should be checked periodically to detect radiation leakage and to indicate when repairs or adjustments need to be done.
3. The patient's medical records should be reviewed for radiation therapy history.
4. X-ray tubes should have adequate layers of aluminum to filter out excess radiation while still providing detailed images.
5. Fast film and high-resolution screens produce quality results.
6. X-ray size must be carefully adjusted so that no more tissue than necessary is exposed to the x-rays. Collimators (shutters), cones, or lead diaphragms can assure proper sizing and x-ray exposure area.
7. The gonads should be shielded on both female and male patients of childbearing age unless the examination involves the abdomen or gonad areas.

PRECAUTIONS TO BE USED WITH PREGNANT PATIENTS

1. Women of childbearing age who could possibly be in the first trimester of pregnancy should *not* have x-ray examinations involving the trunk or pelvic regions. A brief menstrual history should be obtained to determine if a possible pregnancy exists. If pregnancy is possible, a pregnancy test should be done before proceeding with x-ray examination.
2. All pregnant patients, no matter what trimester, should avoid radiographic, fluoroscopic, and serial film studies of the pelvic region, lumbar spine, and abdomen if at all possible.
3. Should x-ray studies be necessary for obstetric reasons, *repeat films* should not be done.
4. If x-ray studies of nonreproductive tissues are necessary (eg, dental x-rays), the abdominal and pelvic regions should be shielded with a lead apron.

Responsibilities in Ordering and Scheduling X-Ray Examinations

Correct and complete information should be entered on the requisition for x-ray studies. Explain the purpose and procedure of the x-ray examination. Written instructions may be helpful to the patient.

When a complete genitourinary–gastrointestinal (GU/GI) workup is scheduled, the sequence of x-ray procedures should follow a definite order:

First day: IVP and barium enema
Second day (or subsequent day): upper GI series

Barium studies should be scheduled *after*

1. Abdominal or pelvic ultrasound examination
2. Lumbar–sacral spine x-rays
3. Pelvic x-rays

4. Hysterosalpingogram
5. Intravenous pyelogram (IVP)

As a general rule, examinations that *do not* require contrast should *precede* examinations that *do* require contrast. All examinations that require *iodine contrast* should be completed before those that require *barium* contrast. In addition, examinations that require *iodine contrast* must *precede* nuclear medicine examinations that require radioactive iodine administration (thyroid scans).

Other x-ray examinations that do not require preparation can be performed at any time. Such examinations include

Chest x-ray
X-rays of the head, spine and extremities
Noncontrast abdomen x-rays (eg, KUB, abdomen series)
Mammograms

CHEST RADIOGRAPHY

Normal Values

Normal appearing and positioned chest, bony thorax (all bones present, aligned, symmetrical, and normally shaped), soft tissues, mediastinum, lungs, pleura, heart, aortic arch, and certain abdominal arteries.

Explanation of Test

The chest x-ray is the most frequently requested radiograph. It is used to diagnose cancer, tuberculosis and other pulmonary diseases, and disorders of the mediastinum and bony thorax. The chest x-ray can provide a record of the sequential progress or development of a disease. It can also provide valuable information about the condition of the heart, lungs, gastrointestinal tract, and thyroid gland. A chest x-ray must be done after the insertion of chest tubes or subclavian catheters to determine their anatomic position as well as detection of possible pneumothorax related to the insertion procedure. In addition, positions of other devices, such as nasogastric or enteric feeding tubes, can be landmarked and readjusted if necessary.

Procedure

1. Routine chest radiography consists of two images: a frontal view (anteroposterior; AP) and a left lateral view. It is usually performed with the patient in a standing position. Upright chest films are of utmost importance (films taken in supine position will not demonstrate fluid levels). This observation is especially important when testing patients on bed rest.
2. Street clothing covering the chest is removed to the waist. Only cloth or

paper hospital gowns free of buttons and snaps may be worn during the x-ray. Jewelry must be removed.

3. Monitoring cables and patches should not obscure the chest area if possible.
4. The patient is instructed to take a deep breath and to exhale; then to take another deep breath and to hold it while the x-ray image is "shot." After the x-ray is completed, the patient may breathe normally.
5. The procedure takes only a few minutes.

Clinical Implications

1. Abnormal chest x-ray results indicate the following lung conditions:
   - **a.** Presence of foreign bodies
   - **b.** Aplasia
   - **c.** Hypoplasia
   - **d.** Cysts
   - **e.** Lobar pneumonia
   - **f.** Bronchopneumonia
   - **g.** Aspiration pneumonia
   - **h.** Pulmonary brucellosis
   - **i.** Viral pneumonia
   - **j.** Lung abscess
   - **k.** Middle lobe syndrome
   - **l.** Pneumothorax
   - **m.** Pleural effusion
   - **n.** atelectasis
   - **o.** Pneumonitis
   - **p.** Congenital pulmonary cysts
   - **q.** Pulmonary tuberculosis
   - **r.** Sarcoidosis
   - **s.** Pneumoconiosis (eg, asbestosis)
   - **t.** Coccidioidomycosis
   - **u.** Westermark's sign indicates decreased pulmonary vascularity, sometimes thought to suggest pulmonary embolus.
2. Abnormal conditions of the bony thorax include
   - **a.** Scoliosis
   - **b.** Hemivertebrae
   - **c.** Kyphosis
   - **d.** Trauma
   - **e.** Sarcoma
   - **f.** Bone destruction or degeneration
   - **g.** Osteoarthritis
   - **h.** Osteomyelitis
3. Cardiac enlargement is visible.

Interfering Factors

An important consideration in interpreting chest radiographs is to ask whether the film is in "full inspiration." Certain disease states do not allow the patient to fully inhale. The following conditions may alter the ability to breathe properly and should be considered when evaluating radiographs:

1. Obesity
2. Severe pain
3. Congestive heart failure
4. Scarring of lung tissues

Patient Preparation

1. No special preparation is required. However, the patient should be given a brief explanation of the purpose and procedure of this test and assured that there will be no discomfort.
2. Remove all jewelry and other ornamentation in the chest area before the x-ray.

3. Remind the patient of the need to remain motionless and to follow all breathing instructions during the procedure.
4. See Chapter 1 guidelines for safe, effective, informed *pretest* care.

Clinical Alert

A portable x-ray machine may be brought to the nursing unit if the patient may not be transported. The nurse may need to assist x-ray personnel in positioning the patient and film. It is the x-ray technologist's responsibility to clear all unnecessary personnel from the radiation field before x-ray exposure.

Patient Aftercare

1. Interpret test outcomes and monitor for pulmonary disease and chest disorders.
2. Follow Chapter 1 guidelines for safe, effective, informed *posttest* care.

CHEST TOMOGRAPHY

Normal Values

Same as chest x-ray.

Explanation of Test

Tomography (computed tomography; CT) is a special radiographic procedure that produces images of a specific plane of the body, free from other superimposed structures. Chest tomograms (CT) are particularly useful in the study of patients with pulmonary tuberculosis, thoracoplasty, or lung abscess. They can also outline detailed anatomy of the lung, mediastinum, and other thoracic structures as well as outlining vascular patterns in emphysema, pulmonary hypertension, and other pulmonary vascular abnormalities.

Procedure

1. Remove street clothing and jewelry or other ornamentation to the waist. A hospital gown may be worn.
2. Position the patient on the movable x-ray exam table. Measure the patient's chest area to define boundaries of the anatomic region to be studied. Sometimes ink marks placed on the patient's skin identify specific areas of interest.
3. After determining proper image plans and other technical factors, a number of x-ray exposures are made.
4. Ask the patient to hold a deep inspiration while each of the x-rays are taken.

Clinical Implications

Abnormal results may reveal the following:

1. Cavities and nodular infiltration associated with tuberculosis but not visible on routine x-ray films
2. Bronchiectasis associated with tuberculosis
3. Outline of tumor in bronchogenic carcinoma
4. Calcium in small parenchymal nodules
5. Site of bronchial occlusion

Interfering Factors

These are the same as the foregoing for chest x-ray films.

Patient Preparation

1. No dietary alterations are necessary. However, explain the purpose and procedure of this test and assure the patient that no discomfort will be felt.
2. All jewelry and ornamentation in the chest area must be removed before the x-ray examination.
3. Instruct the patient on holding still and following breathing instructions during the procedure.
4. See Chapter 1 guidelines for safe, effective, informed *pretest* care.

Patient Aftercare

1. Interpret test outcomes and monitor for lung disease and pulmonary vascular abnormalities..
2. Follow Chapter 1 guidelines for safe, effective, informed *posttest* care.

PARANASAL SINUSES RADIOGRAPHY AND TOMOGRAPHY (CT; CAT) ●

Normal Values

Normal sinuses are radiolucent (allow x-rays to pass through—show up dark on film) because of their air content. The paranasal sinuses are paired cavities lined by mucous membranes that arise as outpouchings from the nasal fossa and extend into the maxillary, ethmoid, sphenoid, and frontal bones. They are named according to the bones in which they develop.

Explanation of Test

Radiographs of the sinuses can detect unilateral or bilateral diseases. Tomograms of the sinuses are usually done to outline foreign bodies, to determine the presence or extent of bony tumor involvement, and to determine the extent and location of fractures of the bony walls of the sinuses and the nasal bones.

Procedure

1. If possible, have the patient sit upright. This will allow determination of sinus fluid levels when present.
2. A comfortably padded vice headbrace that restricts movement is applied to the patient's head.
3. Several x-rays are taken with the patient's head in different positions.
4. The radiographic exam takes approximately 15 to 20 minutes to complete. Allow additional time for tomographic imaging.

Clinical Implications

Abnormal results reveal the following:

1. Acute sinusitis
2. Chronic sinusitis
3. Cysts (retention and nonsecreting)
4. Mucocele
5. Polyps
6. Tumors of the bone and soft tissue
7. Allergic reactions
8. Trauma
9. Foreign bodies

Patient Preparation

1. No dietary preparation is required. However, a brief explanation of the purpose and procedure of this test should be given. Assure the patient that no discomfort will be felt.
2. All dentures, partials, jewelry, and other ornamentation in the head and neck area must be removed before the study.
3. Instruct the patient to hold still during the procedure.
4. See Chapter 1 guidelines for safe, effective, informed *pretest* care.

Patient Aftercare

1. Interpret test outcomes, counsel, and monitor for sinus disorders and trauma.
2. Follow Chapter 1 guidelines for safe, effective, informed *posttest* care.

ORTHOPEDIC RADIOGRAPHY

Normal Values

Normal osseous and soft-tissue structures.

Explanation of Test

Orthopedic radiography examines a particular bone, group of bones, or joint. The bony or osseous system presents five functions of radiologic significance: structural support of the body, locomotion, red marrow storage, calcium storage, and protection of underlying soft tissue and organ structures.

Optimal results from orthopedic x-ray examinations depends on proper immobilization of the part being studied. To produce a thorough image of the body part, at least two and sometimes more projections are required. These are usually taken at angles of 90° to one another (eg, anteroposterior and lateral views).

To examine more complex structures, such as the spine and skull, or to examine a structure in greater detail, several projections from various angles may be required.

Procedure

1. Dietary restrictions are not necessary.
2. The patient assumes the positions most favorable to capturing the best images. However, the degree of patient mobility and physical condition may also need to be considered. Typically, the anatomic structures being studied are examined from several angles and positions. This may require the examiner to physically manipulate the body area into a position that will allow optimal visualization.
3. Jewelry, zippers, snaps, monitoring cables, and so forth, interfere with proper visualization. These objects must be removed from the visual field if possible. Skull x-rays require removal of dentures and partials.
4. Surgical-type hardware used to stabilize a traumatized area must sometimes be removed. This should be done only under the direction of the attending physician.

Clinical Implications

Abnormal results may reveal the following:

1. Fractures
2. Dislocations
3. Arthritis
4. Osteoporosis
5. Osteomyelitis
6. Degenerative joint disease
7. Hydrocephalus
8. Sarcoma
9. Abscess and aseptic necrosis
10. Paget's disease
11. Gout
12. Acromegaly
13. Metastatic processes
14. Myeloma
15. Osteochondrosis, for example,
    a. Legg–Calve–Perthes disease
    b. Osgood–Schlatter disease
16. Bone infarcts
17. Histiocytosis X
18. Bone tumors (benign and malignant)
19. Foreign bodies

Interfering Factors

Radiography of the lumbosacral spine, coccyx, or pelvis must be completed before barium studies because residual barium may interfere with proper visualization. Jewelry and accessories, heavy clothing, metallic objects, zippers, buttons, snaps, cables, and other monitoring equipment and supplies can interfere with optimal views and need to be removed before the exam.

Patient Preparation

1. Explain the purpose and procedure of the test. No preparation or dietary restrictions are necessary.
2. Assure the patient that the procedure in and of itself causes no pain. However, necessary manipulation of the body may cause discomfort. If appropriate, pain medication may be administered before the procedure.
3. Advise the patient that all dentures, partials, jewelry, and other ornamentation worn in the anatomic area being examined must be removed before the study. If possible, simple clothing should be worn and the previously mentioned items should be left at home or in the patient's room.
4. Emphasize the importance of not moving the body during the procedure unless specifically instructed otherwise. Movement will distort or "blur" the image and will often require repeat films.
5. See Chapter 1 guidelines for safe, effective, informed *pretest* care.

Patient Aftercare

1. Interpret test outcomes and monitor for fractures, dislocations, and other orthopedic disorders. Counsel about need for follow-up procedures.
2. Follow Chapter 1 guidelines for safe, effective, informed *posttest* care.

Clinical Alert

1. Orthopedic radiography also can provide information about soft-tissue structures, such as swelling or calcifications. However, radiography alone cannot provide data about the condition of cartilage, tendons, or ligaments.
2. Portable x-ray machines can be taken to the nursing unit if the patient cannot be transported to the radiology department. Nursing personnel may need to assist in the process. The x-ray technologist is responsible for clearing all unnecessary personnel from the immediate radiation field before "shooting the film."

ABDOMINAL PLAIN FILM OR KUB (KIDNEY, URETERS, BLADDER); "SCOUT FILM;" "FLAT PLATE"

Normal Values

Normal abdominal structures.

Explanation of Test

This radiographic study does *not* use contrast media. It is done to aid in the diagnosis of intra-abdominal diseases, such as nephrolithiasis, intestinal obstruction, soft tissue masses, or ruptured viscus. It may be the preliminary step in evaluating the gastrointestinal tract, the gallbladder, or the urinary tract, and it is done before IVP or other renal studies. Abdominal films may provide information on the size, shape, and position of the liver, spleen, and kidneys.

Procedure

1. The patient wears a hospital gown. All metallic objects must be removed from the abdominal area.
2. The patient lies in a flat supine position on the x-ray table. A second film may be taken with the patient standing or sitting.
3. If the patient cannot sit or stand, a position on the left side with the right side up will need to be assumed.

Clinical Implications

Abnormal results reveal the following:

1. Calcium deposits in blood vessels and lymph nodes, cysts, tumors, or stones
2. Ureters not clearly defined, although calculi may be visualized within the ureters.
3. The urinary bladder can often be identified by the shadow it casts, especially in the presence of high specific gravity urine.
4. Abnormal kidney size, shape, and position
5. Appendicolithiasis
6. Foreign bodies
7. Abnormal fluid; ascites
8. Large tumors and masses (ovarian or uterine) if they displace normal bowel configurations
9. Abnormal gas distribution associated with bowel perforation or obstruction
10. Fusion anomalies
11. "Horseshoe"-shaped kidneys

Interfering Factors

1. Barium may interfere with optimal visualization. Therefore, this exam should be done before barium studies.
2. A flat plate of the abdomen does not detect free air.

Patient Preparation

1. Explain the purpose and procedure of the test. Normal diet may be taken unless contraindicated. Assure the patient that the procedure in itself is not painful.
2. Remove belts, zippers, jewelry, and other ornamentation from the abdominal area.
3. Instruct the patient to remain still and to follow breathing instructions.
4. See Chapter 1 guidelines for safe, effective, informed *pretest* care.

Clinical Alert

1. Abdominal plain films are not appropriate for certain conditions, such as esophageal varices or bleeding peptic ulcer.
2. A portable x-ray machine may be brought to the nursing unit if the patient cannot be moved. Assist with positioning as necessary. The x-ray technologist is responsible for clearing all unnecessary personnel from the radiation field before the x-ray is taken.

Patient Aftercare

1. Interpret test outcomes and monitor for intra-abdominal disease.
2. Follow Chapter 1 guidelines for safe, effective, informed *posttest* care.

STOMACH; GASTRIC RADIOGRAPHY (INCLUDING UPPER GI EXAMINATION)

Normal Values

Normal stomach size, contour, motility, and peristaltic activity.

Explanation of Test

Gastric radiography visualizes the form, position, mucosal folds, peristaltic activity, and motility of the stomach and upper gastrointestinal (GI) tract. An upper GI series includes the esophagus, duodenum, and upper portion of the jejunum.

Preliminary films without the use of a contrast medium are useful in detecting perforation, presence of radiopaque foreign substances, gastric wall thickening, and displacement of the gastric air bubble, which may indicate a mass external to the stomach.

Oral contrast substances such as barium sulfate or diatrizoate meglumine (Gastrografin) will highlight such things as hiatal hernia, pyloric stenosis, gastric diverticulitis, presence of undigested food, gastritis, congenital anomalies (eg, dextroposition or duplication), or diseases of the stomach (eg, gastric ulcer, cancer, and stomach polyps).

Procedure

1. Change from street clothing into a hospital gown. Jewelry and other ornamentation must be removed.
2. Instruct the patient to swallow the barium after the patient is properly positioned in front of the fluoroscopy machine. Some changes of position may be necessary during the procedure. A motorized tabletop will shift the patient from an upright to a supine position when appropriate. Fluoroscopy allows visualization and filming of actual activity taking place.

3. Following fluoroscopic examination, several conventional x-ray films are taken. The patient will need to breath-hold during each exposure.
4. Exam time may be 20 to 45 minutes.

Clinical Implications

Abnormal x-ray results reveal the following:

1. Congenital anomalies
2. Gastric ulcer
3. Carcinoma of stomach
4. Gastric polyps
5. Gastritis
6. Foreign bodies
7. Gastric diverticula
8. Pyloric stenosis
9. Reflux and hiatal hernia
10. Volvulus of the stomach

NOTE: *Normal contours may be deformed by intrinsic tumors or consistent filling defects as well as by stenosis in conjunction with dilation.*

Interfering Factors

1. If the patient is debilitated, proper examination may be difficult; it may be impossible to adequately visualize the stomach.
2. Retained food and fluids interfere with optimal film clarity.

Patient Preparation

1. Explain purpose and procedure of the test. (See barium contrast test precautions.) Written instructions on pretest preparation are helpful.
2. Complete fasting from food and fluids is required from midnight until the examination is completed.
3. Instruct the patient to hold still and follow breathing instructions during the procedure.
4. See Chapter 1 guidelines for safe, effective, informed *pretest* care.

Patient Aftercare

1. Pretest diet and activity may be resumed. Provide food and fluids.
2. Administer laxatives as ordered. If barium sulfate or diatrizoate meglumine has been taken, a laxative should be taken.
3. Observe and record stools for color and consistency. Monitor evacuation of barium. Counsel that follow-up procedures may be necessary.
4. Follow Chapter 1 guidelines for safe, effective, informed *posttest* care.

SMALL INTESTINE RADIOGRAPHY AND FLUOROSCOPY

Normal Values

Normal small intestine contour, position, and motility.

Explanation of Test

These small intestine studies, usually scheduled in conjunction with upper GI series, are done to diagnose small bowel diseases (eg, ulcerative colitis, tumors, active bleeding, or obstruction). A contrast material, such as barium sulfate or meglumine diatrizoate, will highlight Meckel's diverticulum, congenital atresia, obstruction, filling defects, regional enteritis, lymphoid hyperplasia, tuberculosis of small intestine (malabsorption syndrome), sprue, Whipple's disease, intussusception, and edema.

The mesenteric small intestine begins at the duodenojejunal junction and ends at the ileocecal valve. The mesenteric small intestine is not routinely included as part of an upper GI study.

Procedure

1. The patient needs to change into a hospital gown after removing street clothes and accessories. A preliminary plain-film study is done with the patient on the examining table.
2. Then, while standing in front of the fluoroscopy machine, the patient swallows the prescribed amount of chalky contrast material.
3. This is followed by timed films usually taken every 30 minutes.
4. The examination is not complete until the ileocecal valve has filled with contrast material. This may take several minutes (for those patients having a bypass) or up to several hours.

Clinical Implications

Abnormal results indicate

1. Anomalies of small intestine
2. Errors of rotation
3. Meckel's diverticulum
4. Atresia
5. Neoplasms
6. Regional enteritis (Crohn's disease)
7. Tuberculosis
8. Malabsorption syndrome
9. Intussusception
10. Roundworms (ascariasis)
11. Intra-abdominal hernias

Interfering Factors

1. Delays in small intestine motility can be due to
   a. Morphine use
   b. Severe or poorly controlled diabetes
2. Increases in motility in the small intestine can be due to
   a. Fear or anxiety
   b. Excitement
   c. Nausea
   d. Pathogens
   e. Viruses
   f. Diet such as very high fiber

Patient Preparation

1. Explain the purpose and procedure of the test. Refer to barium contrast test precautions (see pages 687–688). Written reminders for pretest instructions are helpful, especially diet limitations.
2. Maintain total fast from midnight until the examination is completed.
3. Do not administer laxatives or enemas to a patient with an ileostomy.
4. Instruct the patient about the need to hold still and to follow breathing instructions during the procedure.
5. See Chapter 1 guidelines for safe, effective, informed *pretest* care.

Patient Aftercare

1. Resume pretest diet and activity. Assist patient if necessary.
2. Administer laxatives if ordered. If a barium sulfate swallow has been done, a laxative should be taken. However, do not give laxatives to a patient with an ileostomy unless specifically ordered.
3. Monitor stools for color and consistency.
4. Counsel about motility disorders and other small intestine abnormalities. Follow-up procedures may be necessary.
5. Follow Chapter 1 guidelines regarding safe, effective, informed *posttest* care.

COLON RADIOGRAPHY; BARIUM ENEMA; AIR-CONTRAST STUDY ●

Normal Values

Normal colon position, contour, filling, movement time, and patency.

Explanation of Test

This fluoroscopic and filmed examination of the large intestine (colon) allows visualization of the position, filling, and movement of contrast medium through the colon. It can reveal the presence or absence of diseases, such as diverticulitis, cancer, polyps, colitis, obstruction, or active bleeding. Barium or diatrizoate meglumine (Hypaque) is instilled into the large intestine through a rectal tube inserted into the colon. The radiologist, with the aid of the fluoroscope, observes the barium as it flows through the large intestine. X-ray films are taken at the same time.

For a satisfactory examination, the colon must be thoroughly cleansed of fecal matter. This is most important. Accurate identification of small polyps is possible only in a clean bowel. Stool presence can also make the search for bleeding sources much more difficult.

If polyps are suspected, an air-contrast colon examination may be done. The procedure is basically the same as for the barium enema. However, more complex radiographs need to be taken with the patient in several different positions. A "double contrast" mixture of air and barium is instilled into the colon under fluoroscopic visualization.

Procedure

1. Initially, the patient lies on his or her back while a preliminary x-ray film is made.
2. The patient then lies on his or her side, while barium is administered by rectal enema fashion (through the rectum and up through the sigmoid, descending, transverse, and ascending colon, to the ileocecal valve).
3. Following fluoroscopy, which includes several "spot films, " conventional x-ray films are taken. After these are completed, the patient is free to expel the barium. After evacuation, another film is made.

Clinical Implications

1. Abnormal results indicate
   a. Lesions or tumors (benign)
   b. Obstructions
   c. Megacolon
   d. Fistulae
   e. Inflammatory changes
   f. Diverticulae
   g. Chronic ulcerative colitis
   h. Stenosis
   i. Right-sided colitis
   j. Hernias
   k. Polyps
   l. Intussusception
   m. Carcinoma
2. Appendix size, position, and motility can also be evaluated; however, a diagnosis of acute or chronic appendicitis *cannot* be made from x-ray findings. Instead, typical signs and symptoms of appendicitis provide the most accurate data for this diagnosis.

Interfering Factors

A poorly cleansed bowel is the most common interfering factor. Fecal matter interferes with accurate and complete visualization. Therefore, it is imperative that proper bowel cleansing be conscientiously carried out, lest the procedure need repeating.

Patient Preparation

Preparation involves a three-step process over a 1- to 2-day period; this includes (1) diet restrictions; (2) physiologic cleansing of large bowel by means of oral laxatives; and (3) mechanical cleansing with enemas. Twelve- to 18-hour protocols are common. Follow institutional protocols.

1. Explain the purpose and procedure of the test. Patients may be apprehensive or embarrassed. Include a family member in this process if it appears likely that the patient will need assistance with preparation. Explain need to cooperate to expedite the procedure. Emphasize that the actual time frame when the colon is full is quite brief.
2. A written reminder about the following may be helpful:
   a. Only a clear liquid diet should be taken before testing (according to protocols).
   b. Stool softeners, laxatives, and enemas need to be taken to assure bowel cleanliness necessary for optimal visualization. Agents such as X-Prep, citrate of magnesia, and bisacodyl assist in emptying the ascending and right-to-midtransverse colon (proximal large bowel). Enemas cleanse the left transverse, descending, sigmoid colon, and rectum. Suppositories also empty the rectum.
   c. Fast from food and fluids are prescribed before the test. Remain NPO after midnight until the test is completed. Oral medications should be held unless specifically ordered otherwise.
3. Refer to barium contrast test precautions on pages 687–688.
4. See Chapter 1 guidelines for safe, effective, informed *pretest* care.

Patient Aftercare

1. Resume pretest activity and diet. Assist the patient if necessary. This bowel examination can be very exhausting. Patients may be weak, thirsty, hungry, and tired. Provide a calm restful environment to promote return to normal status.
2. Laxatives should be administered for at least 2 days after these studies or until stools return to normal. Instruct the patient to assess stools during this time. Stools will be light-colored until all barium has been expelled. Outpatients should be given a written reminder to inspect stools for 2 days.
3. Follow Chapter 1 guidelines for safe, effective, informed *posttest* care.

Clinical Alert

1. Multiple enemas given before the procedure, especially to a person at risk for electrolyte imbalances, could induce a rather rapid hypokalemia. Enema fluid, if not expelled within a reasonable time, can be absorbed through the bowel wall and deposited in the interstitial spaces and, eventually, within extracellular spaces.
2. Caution should dictate administration of cathartics or enemas in the presence of acute abdominal pain, ulcerative colitis, or obstruction. Consult with the physician or radiology department and consider the following points:
   a. Introducing large quantities of water into the bowel of patients with megacolon should be avoided because of the potential danger of water intoxication. In general, patients with toxic megacolon should *not* receive enemas.
   b. In the presence of colon obstruction, large water volumes from enemas may be reabsorbed and impaction may occur.
   c. Rectal obstruction will make it difficult or impossible to give cleansing enemas because the solution will not be able to enter the colon. Consult the physician or radiology department.
3. Strong cathartics administered in the presence of obstructive lesions or acute ulcerative colitis can present hazardous or life-threatening situations.
4. Be aware of complications that can occur when barium sulfate or other contrast media are introduced into the GI tract. For example,barium may aggravate acute ulcerative colitis or cause a progression from partial to complete obstruction. Also, barium should not be given as contrast for intestinal studies when a bowel perforation is suspected. Leakage of barium through the perforation may cause peritonitis. Iodinated contrast substances should be used if perforation is suspected.
5. The NPO orders include oral medications except where specified otherwise.

Special Considerations for Children or Elderly Adults Receiving Barium Enemas

1. Because a successful examination of the large intestine depends on the ability of the bowel to retain contrast medium during visualization and filming, special techniques are used for infants and young children or the infirm or uncooperative adult patient.
2. After inserting a small enema tip into the rectum, the infant's buttocks are gently taped together to prevent leakage of contrast material during the study.
3. For the older patient, a special retention enema tip may be used. This device resembles a regular enema tip, but it can be inflated (much like an indwelling urinary catheter) after insertion into the rectum. Once the examination is done, the retention balloon is deflated and the tip removed.

Special Considerations for Barium Enema in the Presence of a Colostomy

1. See pages 687–688 for assessment criteria.
2. Laxatives can be taken.
3. Suppositories are of no value.
4. Follow physician's diet orders.
5. If irrigation is necessary, a preassembled colostomy irrigation kit or a soft, no. 28 standard tip Foley catheter attached to a disposable enema bag may be used.
6. If both loops of a double-barreled colostomy are irrigated, the irrigation solution may be expelled through the rectum as well as the stoma.
7. Advise the patient that a Foley catheter is used to introduce the barium into the stoma.
8. The patient should bring supplemental colostomy supplies to the radiology department for posttest use.

Aftercare of Patients With Stomas

1. Persons with descending or sigmoid colostomies may need a normal saline or tap water irrigation to wash out the barium.
2. Advise those who normally irrigate the colostomy to wear a disposable pouch for several days until all the barium has passed.

T-TUBE CHOLANGIOGRAPHY; BILIARY DUCT RADIOGRAPHY ●

Normal Values

Patent common bile duct.

Explanation of Test

Intravenous cholangiogram studies the biliary ducts. It is usually performed if the gallbladder is not visualized following an oral choledochogram. An intravenous injection of contrast is tracked by radiographic and tomographic means.

T-tube cholangiography is done during or after gallbladder surgery to evaluate the patency of the hepatic and common bile ducts before removal of the T-tube (a T-tube is a self-retaining drainage tube that is sometimes inserted into the common bile duct during surgery). An iodine contrast dye is injected into the T-tube and a fluoroscopic examination is made. Postoperatively, this test is usually done about 10 days after surgery.

Procedure

For T-tube cholangiogram

1. The patient lies on the x-ray table as an iodine contrast medium is injected into the T-tube.
2. Normally, no pain or discomfort should be felt. However, some persons may feel pressure with injection.
3. After the procedure, the T-tube should be unclamped and allowed to drain freely unless otherwise ordered. This minimizes prolonged, irritating contact of residual contrast in the bile duct.

Clinical Implications

Abnormal results will reveal stenosis obstruction, or choledocholithiasis (bile duct calculi) of the common bile duct.

Patient Preparation

1. Explain the purpose and procedure of the test. Assure the patient that the procedure is not painful, but some discomfort or pressure may be felt when the contrast is injected.
2. Street clothing and accessories, such as jewelry, must be removed before the study. Provide a gown for patient use.
3. Stress the importance of remaining still and following breathing instructions during the procedure.
4. Refer to iodine test precautions.
5. Omit food and fluid before the examination. Check institutional protocols for specific dietary and fluid restrictions. A laxative may be ordered the evening before the exam.
6. Inform the patient and family that an IV cholangiogram can be a lengthy procedure of 2 or more hours.
7. See Chapter 1 guidelines for safe, effective, informed *pretest* care.

Patient Aftercare

1. Posttest nausea, vomiting, and a transient elevated temperature may occur as a reaction to the iodine contrast.
2. Document observations and notify physician if necessary.
3. Follow Chapter 1 guidelines for safe, effective, informed *posttest* care.

Clinical Alert

1. Persistent fever, especially if associated with chills, may indicate bile duct inflammation.
2. Follow-up care: Monitoring for hemorrhage, pneumothorax, or peritonitis is necessary after percutaneous transhepatic cholangiography. Unusual pain or tenderness, difficulty breathing, or change in vital signs may signal these complications.

Other Tests for Biliary System Examinations

Intravenous cholangiography: Radiographic visualization of the large hepatic ducts and the common ducts by means of intravenous injection of a contrast medium.

Operative cholangiography: Cannulation and injection of contrast medium into the exposed cystic duct or common bile duct during surgery.

Percutaneous transhepatic cholangiography: A needle or small-diameter catheter is percutaneously introduced into the liver and the bile duct. Following injection of the contrast agent, hepatic and common ducts should be visualized. The dilated biliary tree can be shown up to the point of obstruction (usually in the common duct). This procedure is frequently done for jaundiced patients whose liver cells are unable to properly transport oral or IV contrast agents.

T-tube (or postoperative) cholangiography: see page 711

Intravenous cholecystography: Radiographic visualization of the gallbladder after intravenous injection of a contrast agent

Oral cholecystography: Radiographic visualization of the gallbladder after oral injection of an opaque medium

Endoscopic retrograde cholangiopancreatography (ERCP): This endoscopic procedure uses an injection of contrast substance to evaluate the patency of pancreatic and common bile ducts, the duodenal papilla, and the normalcy of the gallbladder (see Chapter 12)

ESOPHAGEAL RADIOGRAPHY

Normal Values

Normal size, contour, swallowing, peristalsis, and movement of material through the esophagus.

Explanation of Test

Usually, the esophagus is examined in conjunction with an examination of the stomach, duodenum, and upper jejunum. In common terminology, this examination is referred to as an *upper GI series*. However, the esophagus also may be examined separately if specific complaints focus on this area.

This x-ray and fluoroscopic examination visualizes esophageal position, patency, and contour. Technique varies according to such factors as the presence or absence of a lesion and the degree of obstruction. Preliminary films without use of contrast media identify opaque foreign bodies in the neck and thorax, displacement of trachea, or air or fluid in mediastinal tissues or pleural cavities.

Oral contrast medium, such as barium sulfate or diatrizoate meglumine, permits visualization of the esophageal lumen. Many x-ray departments use a very viscous barium preparation that resembles toothpaste to fully coat the esophageal walls. Swallowing small cotton pledgets soaked in barium is useful when the esophagus is being examined for the presence of small or sharp foreign bodies, such as fish bones. Congenital esophageal abnormalities can also be detected by this method. Sclerodermal esophageal abnormalities, diverticulae, cancer, inflammatory strictures, and spasms can also be identified. Although difficult to identify, esophageal varices, if present, indicate cirrhosis of the liver.

Procedure

1. The patient removes street clothing and accessories and wears a hospital gown.
2. As the patient stands in front of the fluoroscope and swallows barium (a chalky-tasting contrast media) the movement of the barium through the esophagus is visualized and recorded. Body position may be adjusted as the motorized x-ray table moves the patient from an upright to supine position.
3. Following actual fluoroscopic examination, conventional x-ray films are taken. It will be necessary for the patient to hold his or her breath during exposures.

Clinical Implications

1. Abnormal results indicate
   - **a.** Congenital esophageal abnormalities
   - **b.** Esophageal alterations associated with scleroderma
   - **d.** Cancer
   - **e.** Stricture associated with inflammation and spasm
   - **f.** Acute ulcerative esophagitis
   - **g.** Chronic fibrosing esophagitis
   - **h.** Peptic ulcer of the esophagus
   - **i.** Achalasia (cardiospasm)
   - **j.** Chalasia (cardioesophageal relaxation
   - **k.** Polyps
   - **l.** Foreign bodies
   - **m.** Rupture
   - **n.** Paralysis
2. Esophageal varices may be difficult to identify; if present, they indicate cirrhosis of the liver.

Patient Preparation

1. Explain the purpose and procedure of the test. A written reminder may be helpful. Because barium has a chalky taste, it is often flavored.

2. No food or liquids are permitted from midnight until the examination is completed.
3. Refer to barium contrast test precautions on pages 687–688. Stress the importance of holding still and following breathing instructions during the procedure.

Patient Aftercare

1. Resume diet and activity, as ordered.
2. If barium has been taken, a laxative should be administered after the examination is completed.
3. Check stool for barium (color and consistency) to determine that all barium has been evacuated.
4. Follow Chapter 1 guidelines for safe, effective, informed *posttest* care.

INTRAVENOUS UROGRAPHY (IVU); **EXCRETORY UROGRAPHY OR IV PYELOGRAPHY** (IVP) ●

Normal Values

1. Normal size, shape, and position of the kidneys, ureters, and bladder. Normal kidneys are approximately as long in dimension as three and one-half vertebral bodies. Therefore, kidney size is estimated in relation to this rule of thumb.
2. Normal renal function
   a. Two to five minutes after the injection of contrast material, the kidney outline will appear on x-ray film. Threadlike strands of contrast material will appear in the calyces.
   b. When the second film is taken 5 to 7 minutes after contrast injection, the entire renal pelvis will be visualized.
   c. The last films taken will show the ureters and bladder as the contrast material makes its way into the lower urinary tract.
3. No evidence of residual urine should be found on the postvoid film.

Explanation of Test

Intravenous urography is one of the most frequently ordered tests in cases of suspected renal disease or urinary tract dysfunction.

> **NOTE:** *An IVU is indicated during the initial investigation of any suspected urologic problem, especially to diagnose kidney and ureter lesions and impaired renal function.*

The term *intravenous urogram* is preferred to *intravenous pyelogram* (IVP) because urogram implies visualization of the entire urinary tract, whereas pyelogram refers specifically to visualization of the kidneys. An intravenous radiopaque iodine contrast substance is injected. The contrast substance concentrates in the urine. Following this, a series of x-ray films are made at predetermined intervals over the next 20 to 30 minutes. A final postvoid film is taken after the patient empties the bladder.

Films show kidney size, shape, and structure; ureters; bladder; and the degree to which the bladder can empty. Renal function is reflected by the length of time it takes the contrast material to first appear and then to be excreted by each kidney. Kidney disease, ureteral or bladder stones, and tumors can be detected with IVU.

Tomography also may be done in conjunction with IVU to obtain better visualization of renal lesions. This obviously increases examination time. If kidney tomography (CT or CAT) or nephrotomograms are ordered separately, the procedure and preparation are the same as for IVU.

Procedure

1. A preliminary x-ray film is taken with the patient in a supine position to assure that the bowel is empty and kidney location can be visualized.
2. The intravenous contrast material is injected, usually into the antecubital vein.
3. During and following the intravenous contrast injection, alert the patient that they may experience warmth, flushing of the face, salty taste, and nausea.
   - **a.** Should these sensations occur, instruct the patient to take slow, deep breaths. Have an emesis basin and tissue wipes available. Use universal precautions when handling secretions.
   - **b.** Assess for other untoward signs, such as respiratory difficulty, diaphoresis, numbness, palpitations, or urticaria. Be prepared to respond with emergency drugs, equipment, and supplies. The items should be readily available.
4. Following injection of the contrast material, at least three x-ray films are taken at predetermined intervals.
5. After these films are taken, instruct the patient to void before the final film is taken to determine the ability of the bladder to empty.

Clinical Implications

1. Abnormal IVU findings may reveal the following:
   - **a.** Altered size, form, and position of the kidneys, ureters, and bladder
   - **b.** Duplication of the pelvis or ureter
   - **c.** The presence of only one kidney
   - **d.** Hydronephrosis
   - **e.** A supernumerary kidney
   - **f.** Renal or ureteral calculi (stones)
   - **g.** Tuberculosis of the urinary tract
   - **h.** Cystic disease
   - **i.** Tumors
   - **j.** The degree of renal injury subsequent to trauma
   - **k.** Prostate enlargement (male)
   - **l.** Enlarged kidneys suggesting obstruction or polycystic disease
   - **m.** Evidence of renal failure in the presence of normal-sized kidneys that suggests an acute rather than chronic disease process
   - **n.** Irregular scarring of the renal outlines, suggesting chronic pyelonephritis
2. A time delay in radiopaque contrast visualization is indicative of renal

dysfunction. No contrast visualization may indicate very poor renal function or no function.

Interfering Factors

1. Feces or intestinal gas will obscure urinary tract visualization.
2. Retained barium can obscure optimal views of the kidneys. (For this reason, barium tests should be scheduled after IVU when possible.)

Patient Preparation

1. Explain the purpose and procedure of the test. A written reminder may be helpful.
2. Observe iodine contrast test precautions. Determine allergies to contrast substances.
3. Because a relative state of dehydration is necessary for contrast material to concentrate in the urinary tract, instruct the patient to abstain from *all* food, liquid, and medication (if possible) for 12 hours before examination. Remaining NPO after the evening meal will meet this criteria.

   NOTE: *Elderly or debilitated patients with poor renal reserves may not tolerate these dehydration protocols (NPO, laxatives, enemas). In such instances, consult with the radiologist or the patient's physician to ascertain the proper route to follow.*

   For infants and small children, NPO time usually varies from 6 to 8 hours pretest. If in doubt, verify protocols with radiologist or attending physician.
4. Usually, the patient takes a laxative the evening before the examination and receives an enema the next morning.
   - **a.** Patients with intestinal disorders such as ulcerative colitis should be given a cathartic only with specific physician orders.
   - **b.** Elderly patients may need assistance to the bathroom. Be alert for signs of weakness and stress.
5. Children younger than 7 years of age should not be given pretest cathartics or enemas. Should the preliminary x-ray film show intestinal gas obscuring the kidneys, a few ounces of infant formula or carbonated drink may relieve the concentration of gas at that particular location.
6. Check stool and abdominal distention to evaluate for possible barium retention if used in previous studies. Additional bowel preparation may be necessary.
7. See Chapter 4 for assessment criteria.
8. See Chapter 1 guidelines for safe, effective, informed *pretest* care.

Patient Aftercare

1. Resume prescribed diet and activity after the examination.
2. Teach and encourage the patient to drink sufficient fluids to replace those lost in pretest phase.

3. Encourage rest, as needed, following the examination. Instruct the patient to "let their body tell" about rest needs.
4. Observe and document mild reactions to the iodine material, which may include hives, skin rashes, nausea, or swelling of the parotid glands (iodinism). Notify the physician if the signs and symptoms persist. Oral antihistamines may relieve more severe symptoms.
5. Follow Chapter 1 guidelines for safe, effective, informed *posttest* care.

Clinical Alert

1. Contraindications to an IVU or IVP include
   a. Hypersensitivity or allergy to iodine preparations
   b. Combined renal and hepatic disease
   c. Oliguria
   d. Renal failure: most radiology departments require recent creatinine test levels to determine whether to administer contrast materials. Generally, creatinine levels higher than 1.5 mg/dl raise suspicion, and signal the need for repeat of lab work. A BUN level above 40 mg/dl also may contraindicate use of iodine contrast.
   e. Multiple myeloma, unless the patient can be adequately hydrated during and after the study
   f. Advanced pulmonary tuberculosis
   g. Patients receiving drug therapy for chronic bronchitis, emphysema or asthma
2. Some physiologic changes can be expected from radiopaque iodine injections. Hypertension, hypotension, tachycardia, arrhythmias, or other electrocardiographic (ECG) changes fall into this category.
3. An iodine-based contrast medium is given with caution in the presence of hyperthyroidism, asthma, hay fever, or other allergies.
4. Observe for anaphylaxis or severe reactions to iodine, as evidenced by shock, respiratory distress, precipitous hypotension, fainting, convulsions, or actual cardiopulmonary arrest. Resuscitation supplies and equipment should be readily available.
5. In all cases except emergencies, a contrast medium should not be injected sooner than 90 minutes after eating.
6. Intravenous iodine can be highly irritating to the intimal layer of the veins and may cause painful vascular spasm. In this case a 1% procaine IV injection may relieve vascular spasm and pain. Sometimes local vascular irritation is severe enough to induce thrombophlebitis. Warm or cold compresses to the area may relieve pain. However, these do not prevent sloughing. The attending

(continued)

(Clinical Alert continued)

physician should be notified. Anticoagulant therapy may need to be instituted.

7. Local reactions to iodine may be evidenced by extensive redness, swelling, and pain at the injection site. Even a small amount of iodine contrast entering subcutaneous tissues can cause tissue sloughing, which may require skin grafting. Radiographic evidence of iodine contrast leakage within soft tissues surrounding the injection site confirms extravasation. Treatment may include a local infiltration of hyaluronidase, but this can vary.

RETROGRADE PYELOGRAPHY

Normal Values

Normal ureter and kidney contours and size.

Explanation of Test

Retrograde pyelography generally confirms intravenous urogram (IVU) findings and is indicated when IVU yields insufficient results because of kidney nonvisualization (congenital kidney absence), decreased renal blood flow that impairs renal function, obstruction, kidney dysfunction, presence of calculi, or patient allergy to intravenous contrast material. This x-ray examination of the upper urinary tract begins with cystoscopy to introduce ureteral catheters up to the level of the renal pelvis. Following this, iodine contrast is injected into the ureteral catheter and films are then taken. The chief advantage of retrograde pyelography lies in the fact that the contrast substance can be directly injected under controlled pressure so that optimal visualization is achieved. Renal function impairment does not influence the degree of visualization.

Procedure

1. The examination is usually done in the surgical department in conjunction with cystoscopy.
2. Sedation and analgesia may precede insertion of a local anesthetic into the urethra (see under *Cystoscopy*). General anesthesia may be required if the patient will not be able to fully cooperate with the procedure.

Clinical Implications

Abnormal results reveal

1. Intrinsic abnormality of ureters and kidney pelvis such as congenital defects
2. Extrinsic abnormality of the ureters such as obstructive tumor or stones

Interfering Factors

Because barium may interfere with test results, these studies must be done before barium x-rays are administered.

Patient Preparation

1. Explain the purpose and procedure of the test.
2. The patient or other authorized person must sign and have witnessed a legal consent form before examination.
3. Follow iodine contrast test precautions.
4. Fast from food and fluids after midnight before the test.
5. Administer cathartics, suppositories, or enemas as ordered.
6. See Chapter 1 guidelines for safe, effective, informed *pretest* care.

Patient Aftercare

1. Observe for allergic reaction to iodine contrast.
2. Check vital signs frequently for first 24 hours. Follow institutional protocols if general anesthetics were administered.
3. Record accurate urine output and appearance for 24 hours following procedure. Hematuria or dysuria may be common after the examination. If hematuria does not clear and dysuria persists or worsens, notify the physician. Instruct the patient to do the same.
4. Administer analgesics as necessary. (Discomfort may be present immediately following the examination and may require a prescriptive analgesic if not controlled otherwise, eg, codeine.)
5. Follow Chapter 1 guidelines for safe, effective, informed *posttest* care.

Clinical Alert

Renal function tests of blood and urine must be completed before this examination is done.

Other Tests Used to Examine the Urinary System

Excretion urography or intravenous pyelography (IVP): After injection of an intravenous contrast agent, the collecting system (calyces, pelvis, and ureter) of each kidney is progressively opacified. Radiographs are made at 5- to 15-minute intervals until the urinary bladder is visualized.

Drip infusion pyelography: This is a modification of conventional pyelography. An increased volume of contrast agent is administered by continuous intravenous infusion.

Cystography: The urinary bladder is opacified by means of a contrast agent instilled through a urethral catheter. After the patient voids, air may be introduced into the bladder to obtain a double contrast study.

Retrograde cystourethrography: After catheterization, the bladder is filled to capacity with a contrast agent and radiography visualizes the bladder and urethra.

Voiding cystourethrography: After contrast material has been instilled into the urinary bladder, films are made of the bladder and urethra during the process of voiding.

LYMPHANGIOGRAPHY

Normal Values

Normal lymphatic vessels and nodes.

Explanation of Test

Lymphangiography examines the lymphatic channels and lymph nodes by means of radiopaque iodine contrast oil injected into the small lymphatics of the foot. This test is commonly ordered for patients with Hodgkin's disease or cancer of the prostate to check for nodal involvement. Lymphangiography is also indicated to evaluate edema of an extremity without known cause, to determine the extent of adenopathy, to stage lymphomas, and to localize affected nodes as part of surgical or radiotherapeutic treatment.

Procedure

1. The patient is positioned supine on the x-ray table.
2. A blue dye is injected intradermally between each of the first three toes of each foot to stain the lymphatic vessels.
3. After the site is infiltrated with local anesthetic, a 1- to 2-in. incision is made on the dorsum of each foot.
4. The lymphatic vessel is identified and cannulated to faciliate extremely *low*-pressure injection of the iodine contrast medium.
5. When the contrast medium reaches the level of the third and fourth lumbar vertebrae (as seen on fluoroscopy), the injection is discontinued.
6. Abdominal, pelvic, and upper body films demonstrate the lymphatic vessels filling.
7. A second set of films is obtained in 12 to 24 hours to demonstrate filling of the lymph nodes.
8. The nodes in the inguinal, external iliac, common iliac, and periaortic areas, as well as the thoracic duct and supraclavicular nodes, can be visualized.
9. When a lymphatic of the hand is injected, the axillary and supraclavicular nodes should be visible.
10. Because the contrast dye remains present in the nodes for 6 months to 1 year after lymphangiography, repeat studies can be done to track disease activity and to monitor treatment without the need to repeat contrast injection.
11. The patient may need to have additional films taken.

Clinical Implications

Abnormal results indicate

1. Retroperitoneal lymphomas associated with Hodgkin's disease

2. Metastasis to lymph nodes
3. Abnormal lymphatic vessels

Patient Preparation

1. Explain the purpose and procedure of the test. Obtain a signed, witnessed consent form.
2. See iodine contrast test precautions on page 685.
3. Take food, fluids, and medications as per routine.
4. Instruct the patient that they may feel some discomfort when the local anesthetic is injected into the feet.
5. Administer oral antihistamines per physician orders if allergy to the iodized contrast agents is suspected.
6. See Chapter 1 guidelines regarding safe, effective, informed *pretest* care.

Patient Aftercare

1. Check and record the patient's temperature every 4 hours for 48 hours postexamination.
2. Provide restful environment if needed.
3. If ordered, elevate the legs to prevent swelling.
4. Watch for complications such as delayed wound healing, infection, leg edema, allergic dermatitis, headache, sore mouth and throat, skin rashes, transient fever, lymphangitis, and oil embolism.
5. See Chapter 1 guidelines for safe, effective, informed *posttest* care.

Clinical Alert

1. Lymphangiography is usually contraindicated in
   a. Known iodine hypersensitivity
   b. Severe pulmonary insufficiency
   c. Cardiac disease
   d. Advanced renal or hepatic disease
2. The major complication of the procedure relates to contrast media embolization into the lungs. This will diminish pulmonary function temporarily and, in some patients, may produce lipid pneumonia. The patient may require aggressive respiratory management if this complication is life-threatening.

MAMMOGRAPHY; BREAST RADIOGRAPHY

Normal Values

Essentially normal breast tissue: calcification, if present, should be evenly distributed—normal ducts with gradual narrowing ductal system branches.

Explanation of Test

Soft-tissue mammography visualizes the breast tissue on photographic film and detects small abnormalities that could warn of cancer. Its primary use is to screen for and discover cancers that escape detection by other means, such as palpation. Typically, cancers smaller than 1 cm cannot be detected by routine clinical examination or self-breast examinations. Because the average breast cancer has probably been present for some time before it reaches the clinically palpable 1-cm size, the prognosis for cure is excellent if detected in this preclinical or presymptomatic phase.

The low-energy x-ray beam used for this procedure is applied to a tightly restricted area and consequently does not produce significant radiation exposure to other areas of the body. Therefore, it is quite acceptable from a radiation safety standpoint to recommend routine screenings. Diagnosis by mammography is based on the radiographic appearance of gross anatomic structures. Benign heart lesions tend to push breast tissue aside as they expand, whereas malignant lesions may invade surrounding breast tissue. Although false-negative and false-positive readings may occur, mammography does enjoy a very high degree of accuracy.

Most breast lumps are not malignant. Many are benign cysts. For women older than age 40, the benefits of using low-dose mammography to find early, curable cancers outweigh possible risk from radiation.

Likelihood of Breast Cancer

By Age	*Odds*
25	1:19,608
30	1:2,525
35	1:622
40	1:217
45	1:93
50	1:50
55	1:33
60	1:24
65	1:17
70	1:14
75	1:11
80	1:10
85	1:9
95 and older	1:8

National Cancer Institute

The American College of Radiology (ACR) accredits mammography services. To earn accreditation, mammograms must be performed by specially trained and credentialed radiographers and the films must be interpreted by radiologists who meet criteria for continuing education in mammography. Additionally, the ACR has stringent standards for equipment, film quality, and radiation dose. Select health insurers require mammographic services to be performed at an ACR-accredited institution.

Indications for Mammography

1. To detect clinically nonpalpable breast cancers in women older than age 40, younger women at high risk, or those having a history of breast cancer
2. When signs and symptoms of breast cancer are present
   a. Skin changes (eg, "orange peel" skin associated with inflammatory type cancer)
   b. Nipple or skin retraction
   c. Nipple discharge or erosion
3. Breast pain
4. "Lumpy" breast; multiple masses or nodules
5. Pendulous breasts that are difficult to examine
6. Survey of opposite breast after mastectomy
7. Patients at risk for having breast cancer (eg, having family history of breast cancer)
8. Adenocarcinoma of undetermined origin
9. Previous breast biopsy
10. To examine biopsy samples of breast tissue
11. Follow-up studies for questionable mammographic images

NOTE: *The American Cancer Society recommends a baseline mammogram for all women between 35 and 40 years of age, an annual or biannual mammogram for ages 40 to 49, and a yearly mammogram after 50 years of age.*

Procedure

1. Ask the patient to identify the affected breast area (Fig. 10-1).
2. Expose the breast and rest it on a film holder. Position the moveable paddle over the breast so that the paddle compresses the breast tissue. Smooth out all skin folds and wrinkles. This maneuver is critically important since inadequate compression will produce a suboptimal image (only specially trained technologists usually perform mammograms).
3. Two views of each breast are usually taken. When digital mammography is done, images appear on a videomonitor, rather than film. Image can be technically enhanced for better visualization of an area.
4. Before or following the x-ray examination, the technologist will visually observe and manually palpate the breasts.
5. Total examining time is about 1/2 hour.

Clinical Alert

1. Computer-ordered diagnosis is a new detection technique. Software that acts like a second opinion scans the image and notes suspicious areas that a radiologist could miss.
2. Most radiologists double-read all mammograms.
3. Comparison with old mammograms is very important.

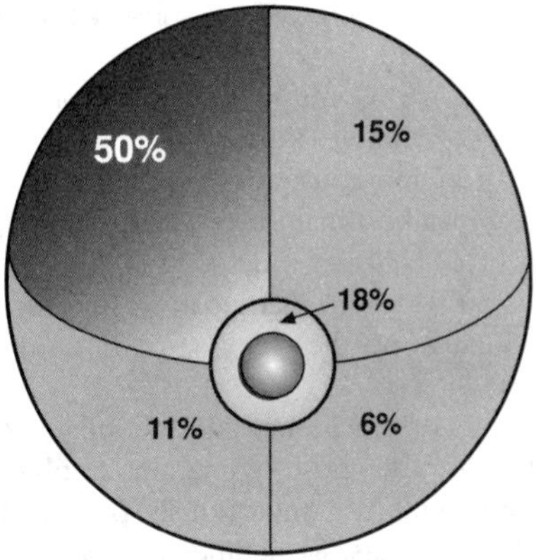

FIGURE 10-1
Half of all breast cancers develop in the upper outer section. (Source: Department of Health and Human Services, 1994)

Clinical Implications

1. Abnormal findings reveal
  a. Benign breast mass: on mammogram it appears as a round, smooth mass with definable edges. If calcifications are present, they are usually coarse.
  b. Cancerous mass: on mammogram it appears as an irregular shape with extensions into adjacent tissue. Increased numbers of blood vessels are present. Primary and secondary signs of breast cancer are apparent.

2. Speculated mass, on occasion, may be smooth and regular.

3. Calcifications present in the malignant mass (duct carcinoma) or in adjacent tissue (lobular carcinoma) are described as innumerable punctate calcifications resembling fine grains of salt, or rodlike calcifications that appear thin, branching, and curvilinear.

4. The likelihood of malignancy increases with a greater number of calcifications in a cluster. However, a cluster with as few as three calcifications, particularly if they are irregular in shape or size, can occur in cancer.

5. Typical parenchymal patterns:
  N_1: Normal
  P_1: Mild duct prominence on less than one-quarter of the breast
  P_2: Marked duct prominence
  DY: Dysplasia: Some diagnosticians believe that the person who exhibits dysplasia is 22 times more likely to develop breast cancer than the person with normal results.

6. Findings of breast cancer when contrast is injected are associated with extravasation of contrast, filling defects, obstruction, or irregular narrowing of ducts.

   a. Intraductal papilloma: Contrast mammography (ductograms, galactograms) is a most valuable aid for diagnosing intraductal papillomas. Mammary duct injection is used when cytologic examination of breast fluid or discharge is abnormal. In contrast mammography, after careful cannulation of a discharging duct, about 1 ml of a radiopaque substance, such as 50% sodium diatrizoate is injected into the breast duct with a blunt 25-gauge needle.

7. Difficult diagnoses
   a. Colloid (gelatinous or mucinous) and medullary (circumscribed) carcinomas are difficult to diagnose by mammography.
   b. Soft tissue mammography is notoriously poor in localizing nonpalpable intraductal papillomas. Sometimes the calcifications of cancer and sclerosing adenosis may be indistinguishable, particularly if the adenosis is not bilateral.

Patient Preparation

1. Explain the purpose, procedure, benefits, and risks of mammograms. Mammography is the single best method for detecting breast cancer while still in a curable stage. Some discomfort is to be expected when the breast is compressed.
2. Instruct the patient not to apply deodorant, perfume, powders, or ointment to the underarm area on the day of the examination. Skin residue from these preparations can obscure optimal visualization.
3. Advise the patient to wear separates, rather than a dress, because clothing must be removed from the upper body.
4. Suggest that patients who have painful breasts refrain from caffeine, such as found in coffee, tea, cola, and chocolate, for 5 to 7 days before testing.
5. See Chapter 1 guidelines for safe, effective, informed *pretest* care.

Patient Aftercare

1. Interpret test outcomes and counsel appropriately. If a biopsy is necessary, see procedures for biopsy using x-ray technology.
2. Follow Chapter 1 guidelines for safe, effective, informed *posttest* care.

Clinical Alert

1. A mammogram detects abnormalities that could *warn* of cancer. The actual diagnosis of cancer is made by biopsy (only one in five biopsies tests positive for cancer).
2. Several methods provide a breast tissue sample necessary for cancer diagnosis. Two of these are stereotactic core biopsy and surgical biopsy.

Procedure for Stereotactic X-Ray Guided Core Biopsy

1. A local anesthetic and a sedative are administered.
2. The patient lies on the abdomen, allowing the breast to protrude through opening in a special table.
3. Two stereoview mammograms are taken allowing precise positioning of hollow-core needle.
4. Needle shoots into the breast at precise locations. Multiple (core) tissue samples are taken because tumors have both benign and malignant areas.
5. Breast is cleansed and sterile dressing applied.

Procedure for Needle X-Ray Localization and Surgical Biopsy

This is a two-step process involving x-ray and surgery.

1. A local anesthetic and sedative are administered. In some instances, general anesthesia is used.
2. With breast x-rays as a guide, a needle is inserted that holds a fine wire. When the needle point is at the tip of the x-ray-defined abnormality, the guidewire is released. It stays there until the surgeon (guided by the wire) removes it along with the abnormal tissue.

COMPUTED TOMOGRAPHY (CT) **OF THE BRAIN/HEAD** (COMPUTERIZED AXIAL TOMOGRAPHY [CAT]); **BRAIN SCAN** ●

Normal Values

No evidence of tumor, other pathology, or fracture.

Typically, low-density tissue areas appear black, whereas higher density tissues appear as shades of gray. The lighter the shading, the higher the density.

Explanation of Test

Computed tomography of the head is a relatively simple x-ray examination done by means of a special scanning machine to evaluate suspected intracranial lesions. (See page 689 for CT explanation.) A narrow beam of attenuated x-rays that allows little internal radiation scatter is transmitted through the specific body area being evaluated and is measured by special detectors. A computer rapidly processes complex calculations and determines the degree of multiple x-ray beams not absorbed by the tissues in their path. The results form a cross-sectional picture of the anatomic head structure that includes the internal cranial structure, brain tissue, and surrounding cerebrospinal fluid (CSF). This axial image of the head is similar to one's view of the head if one looks down through the top of the head.

The CT method measures the attenuation coefficient of tissue that reflects the electron density as well as the elemental composition of the tissue being studied. When more phosphorus is present in gray matter than in white matter (a change in elemental composition), there is a difference in attenuation coefficient for low-energy x-rays, even though these tissues are of the same density. Because clotted blood, cystic fluid, bone, CSF, and air exhibit different coefficients, it is possible to demonstrate the anatomic distributions of these different tissues.

By rotating the x-ray source around the head, it is possible to obtain and process several attenuation readings. These clearly detailed cross-sectional images are displayed on a screen, photographed, and reproduced on x-ray film. In preparation for the procedure, the patient's head is immobilized in the scanner so that no movement can take place. Then, the head is scanned in successive cross-sectional "slices" so that a permanent record (x-ray) can be made and later studied. It follows that the patient must be relatively calm and able to remain quiet during the test. Destructive, atrophic, space-occupying intracranial lesions, and congenital abnormalities, such as hydrocephalus, may be diagnosed. A CT scan can demonstrate minor differences in density and composition. Consequently, it can differentiate tumors from soft tissues, air space from CSF, and normal blood from clotted blood. Disruptions in permeability, such as a break in the blood–brain barrier, resulting in the accumulation of IV contrast material can also be demonstrated by the basal increase of attenuation coefficients.

In interpreting the scan, structures are identified by appearance, shape, size, symmetry, and position. Usually, a space-occupying lesion will show characteristic displacement or deformity of some part of the ventricular system. Scans can be done in different planes and can produce thinner "slices" if necessary, such as for the evaluation of small, intracranial structures, including the pituitary gland, optic nerves, and ossicles in the middle ear.

Procedure

1. During the test, the patient must lie perfectly still on a motorized table, with the head comfortably immobilized. The table is moved into a donut-shaped frame called a gantry. X-ray tubes situated within this gantry actually move around the patient in circular fashion.
2. If tissue density enhancement (a questionable area needs further clarification) is desired, an iodinated radiopaque substance can be injected intravenously. Some patients experience nausea and vomiting after receiving this contrast dye.
3. Additional pictures are taken during contrast injection.
4. During and following the intravenous injection, the patient may experience warmth, flushing of the face, salty taste, or nausea. Encourage the patient to deep-breathe. An emesis basin should be readily available.
5. Watch for other untoward signs, such as respiratory difficulty, diaphoresis, numbness, or palpitations.

Clinical Implications

TISSUES WITH INCREASED DENSITY

Tissue abnormalities can be identified by observing tissue-density alterations in the scan pictures. The presence of calcium adds to increased lesion density. Meningiomas and low-grade astrocytomas may show up as white areas on the films because of their high tissue density. Calcium also collects in angiomas, aneurysms, and degenerative and infected tissue. Hematoma can be easily distinguished. In the presence of intracranial hemorrhage, once clotting has occurred, serum is absorbed and tissue density becomes much higher than normal. Hemoglobin and calcium ions influence density increases. Preoperatively, the ability to pinpoint the location of the lesion, its size, relation to other structures, or the extent of edema lessens the risks associated with neurosurgical procedures. In the case of subarachnoid hemorrhage, scans can locate the source of bleeding. When multiple aneurysms exist, scans provide a means of identifying or confirming these aneurysms. Computed scanning provides an easy method of identifying trauma-induced extradural, subdural, or intracerebral hematomas and edema.

TISSUES EXHIBITING DECREASED DENSITY

Decreased tissue density evident on scanning is caused by many pathologic conditions. Cell structure breakdown during infarctions, infections, tumor necrosis, cyst formation, degenerative processes, benign cysts, and edema are pathologic processes that reduce tissue density. These areas appear darker on the scan pictures.

TISSUES REQUIRING CONTRAST MEDIA

Lesions that have the same tissue density as that of adjacent normal brain tissue are difficult to differentiate on the routine scan. Consequently, the basis for using contrast enhancement is that the breakdown of the blood–brain barrier that occurs in the presence of abnormal lesions permits small amounts of contrast substances to pass into abnormal brain tissue. Contrast enhancement is indicated when tumors, multiple sclerosis, aneurysm, or vascular abnormality are evident, or when the patient presents with a history of headache and seizures.

Interfering Factors

1. A false-negative CT scan may occur in the presence of hemorrhage. As hematomas age, their appearance on CT scans changes from high-intensity to low-intensity levels, partly because older hematomas become more transparent to x-rays.
2. Patient movement will negatively affect image quality and accuracy.

Patient Preparation

1. Explain test purpose and procedure. Provide written instructions. Reinforce knowledge concerning possible adverse effects, such as radiation exposure or allergy to iodine contrast media. The amount of x-ray exposure for this examination is about the same as that received during a routine skull x-ray.
2. Refer to iodine contrast test precautions on page 685.
3. Generally, the patient should fast 2 to 3 hours before the test if contrast

study is planned. Prescribed medications can be taken before CT studies. Diabetics should take their insulin and be allowed to eat.

4. Reassure the patient that scanning produces no greater radiation than conventional x-ray studies.
5. Check for allergies. Nausea and vomiting, warmth, and flushing of the face may signal a possible iodine allergy. See pages 685–687 for additional assessment criteria.
6. Reassure the patient prone to claustrophobia that claustrophobic fear of the scanner is common. Pictures of actual introduction to the scanner may alleviate these fears.
7. Administer analgesics and sedatives, especially to minimize pain and unnecessary movement.
8. See Chapter 1 guidelines for safe, effective, informed *pretest* care.

Patient Aftercare

1. Determine whether an iodine contrast substance was used. If used, observe and record information about these reactions if they occur. Mild reactions to symptoms may include hives, skin rashes, nausea, swelling of parotid glands (iodism), or most serious of all, anaphylaxis.
2. Notify the physician immediately if allergic reactions occur. Antihistamines may be necessary to treat symptoms.
3. Documentation should include assessment of information needs, instructions given, time examination was completed, patient response to the procedure, and allergic reactions should these occur.
5. Follow Chapter 1 guidelines for safe, effective, informed *posttest* care.

COMPUTED TOMOGRAPHY (CT) OF THE BODY; COMPUTERIZED AXIAL TOMOGRAPHY (CAT) BODY SCAN ●

Normal Values

No apparent tumor or pathology: on CT scans, air appears black, bone appears white, soft tissue appears in varied shades of gray. Shade patterns and their correlation to different tissue densities, together with the added dimensions of depth, identify normal body structures and organs.

Explanation of Test

Body imaging gives detailed cross-sectional images of the chest, abdomen, spine, and extremities. When used to evaluate neoplastic and inflammatory disease, CT data acquisition can be rapidly sequenced to evaluate blood flow and to determine vascularity of a mass. This technique, known as *dynamic CT scanning* requires the administration of IV contrast. In addition, CT can detect intervertebral disk disease, herniation, and soft tissue damage to ligaments within joint spaces.

Conventional x-ray machines produce a "flat" picture with organs in the front of the body that appear to be superimposed over organs toward the back of the body. The result is a two-dimensional image of the three-dimensional body. CT imaging produces many cross-sectional anatomic views, without superimposing structures. The new spiral CT scanners show promise for CT angiography and for three-dimensional reconstruction techniques.

Procedure

1. In most laboratories, CT abdominal examination is preceded by having the patient drink a special contrast preparation several minutes before the commencement of the study. This contrast material outlines the bowel so it can be more readily differentiated from other structures.
2. The patient lies supine on a motorized couch that moves into a donut-shaped frame, called a gantry. X-ray tubes within the gantry move around the patient as the pictures are taken. These films are projected onto a monitor screen at the same time.
3. The patient should lie without moving and be able to follow breathing instructions.
4. Should a questionable area need further clarification, iodine contrast substance is injected intravenously and more pictures are taken. Of note, all patients having pelvic CT scans are given a barium contrast enema. Furthermore, all female patients undergoing pelvic CT scans may require insertion of a vaginal tampon to delineate the vaginal wall.
5. The patient may experience warmth, flushing of the face, salty taste, and nausea with IV injection of the contrast material. Slow, deep breaths may alleviate these symptoms. Have an emesis basin available as a precaution. Watch for other untoward signs, such as respiratory difficulty, heavy sweating, numbness, palpitations, or progression to an anaphylactic reaction. Resuscitation equipment and drugs should be readily available. Notify the physician immediately.

Clinical Implications

Abnormal CT scan findings reveal

1. Tumors, nodules, and cysts
2. Ascites
3. Abscessed or fatty liver
4. Aneurysm of abdominal aorta
5. Lymphoma
6. Enlarged lymph nodes
7. Pleural effusion
8. Cancer of pancreas
9. Retroperitoneal lymphadenopathy
10. Abnormal collection of blood, fluid or fat
11. Skeletal bone metastasis
12. Cirrhosis of liver
13. Fractures
14. Soft tissue or ligament damage

Interfering Factors

1. Retained barium can obscure organs in the upper and lower abdomen. (Barium tests should be scheduled to *follow* a CT scan when possible.)
2. Inability of the patient to lie quietly. Movement will produce less than optimal pictures.

Patient Preparation

1. Explain the purpose and procedure of the test. Written explanations may be helpful. Benefits and risks of the test should be explained to the patient before the procedure.
2. Refer to iodine and barium contrast test precautions on pages 685–688.
3. Prescribed medications can be taken before CT studies. Diabetics should take their insulin and be allowed to eat. The CT scanning time can be adjusted so that the examination does not interfere with a patient's medication.
4. Inform the patient that an iodine contrast substance may be administered before and during the examination. Determine allergy to iodine. See pages 685–688 for additional assessment criteria. Pelvic CT examinations usually require both intravenous and rectal administration of contrast material.
5. Abdominal cramping and diarrhea may occur; therefore, drugs such as glucagon, Lipomul, or Donnatal will be ordered to decrease these side effects.
6. Solid foods are usually held on the day of the examination until test completion. Clear liquids may be taken up to 2 hours before examination. If in doubt, check with the diagnostic department for specific protocols. The patient with diabetes may need to adjust insulin dose and diet pretest. For CT of the abdomen, the patient is usually NPO.
7. Instruct patients that they may experience warmth, flushing of the face, salty metallic taste, and nausea or vomiting if IV iodine is administered.
8. Claustrophobic sensations while in the CT scanner are common. Show the patient a picture of the scanner.
9. Sedation and analgesics may help the patient lie quietly during the test.
10. See Chapter 1 guidelines for safe, effective, informed *pretest* care.

Patient Aftercare

1. Observe and document the following reactions to iodine contrast material: hives, skin rashes, nausea, swelling of parotid glands (iodism), or anaphylactic reaction.
2. Notify the physician immediately if symptoms are serious.
3. Antihistamines may relieve the more severe symptoms.
4. Document preparation and instructions given to the patient or significant others, the time the procedure was completed, patient's response to the procedure, and any allergic reactions, together with subsequent treatment.
5. Follow Chapter 1 guidelines for safe, effective, informed *posttest* care.

DIGITAL SUBTRACTION ANGIOGRAPHY (DSA) (TRANSVENOUS DIGITAL SUBTRACTION) ●

Normal Values

Normal carotid arteries, vertebral arteries, abdominal aorta and its branches, renal arteries, and peripheral arteries.

Explanation of Test

Digital angiography is a computer-based imaging method of performing vascular studies that require catheterization of certain venous or arterial vessels. Vasculature studied includes the carotid vessels; intracranial vessels; those vessels originating from the aortic arch; abdominal vessels including celiac, renal, and mesenteric branches; and other peripheral vessels. Digital subtraction angiography began as an intravenous technique, but because of its limitations, other methods of iodine contrast administration have been instituted. For example, intra-arterial injection can be used for detailed visceral studies. The presence of the contrast material blocks the path of x-rays and makes the blood vessels visible on x-ray film. Basically, an image taken just before contrast injection is subtracted from that taken when the contrast material is actually within the vascular system. The resulting image shows only the distribution of the contrast substance. Digital subtraction is used to isolate a clinically relevant subset of information and is particularly useful in preoperative and postoperative evaluations for vascular and tumor surgery.

In addition to reducing the risk associated with arterial puncture, the procedure precludes the potential trauma and embolic complications associated with arterial catheterization. Because arterial punctures are not always necessary, this test may be routinely performed on an outpatient basis with considerably less risk and at lower cost than conventional angiography.

Visualization of the carotid and vertebral vasculature is possible in those patients with a history of stroke, transient ischemic attacks, bruit, or subarachnoid hemorrhage. The procedure may be used as an adjunct to CT scanning and may be performed just before the CT scan in cases in whom there is evidence of an aneurysm, vascular malformation, or hypervascular tumor.

Procedure

1. The antecubital area of the right arm is prepared and injected with a local anesthetic. The basilic vein may be easier to cannulate than the cephalic vein. For some studies, the femoral vein is used.
2. The catheter and guidewire within the catheter are usually advanced into the superior vena cava or right atrium of the heart. The guidewire is removed, and the catheter is connected to a power injector that administers iodine under pressure, in defined quantities, and at prescribed intervals. X-ray images are then taken and stored on digital or film media.
3. Once the procedure is terminated, the catheter is removed.
4. A dressing is placed over the venous insertion site and manual pressure is applied to the puncture site for about 5 minutes, or until bleeding stops. A more permanent pressure dressing is then taped in place. This may usually be removed in 24 hours.
5. Monitor frequently for hemorrhage or hematoma formation.

Clinical Implications

1. Abnormal results reveal the following:
   - **a.** Arterial stenosis
   - **b.** Large aneurysms

c. Large jugular tumors or other masses
d. Total occlusion of arteries
e. Thoracic outlet syndrome
f. Large or central pulmonary emboli
g. Vascular parathyroid adenoma
h. Pheochromocytoma
i. Ulcerative plaque
j. Tumor circulation

2. Abnormalities that may be identified with about 65% accuracy include the following:
   a. Total occlusion of internal carotid arteries
   b. Vessel ulcers without web stenosis or thrombosis
   c. Aortic arch occlusion
   d. Subclavian steal
   e. Meningiomas

Interfering Factors

1. Because this examination is very sensitive to physical movement, motion artifact will produce poor images. Consequently, uncooperative or agitated patients cannot be studied. Even the act of swallowing results in unsatisfactory images. Measures to reduce swallowing, such as breath-holding, using a bite block, or exhaling through a straw, do not always yield satisfactory results.
2. Vessel overlap of external and internal carotid arteries makes it almost impossible to obtain a select view of a specific carotid artery because contrast fills both arteries almost simultaneously.

Clinical Alert

Tests should be used cautiously in those patients with renal insufficiency or unstable cardiac disease. Assess for contraindications to the iodinated contrast drug listed on page 687.

Patient Preparation

1. Explain the purpose and procedure of the test and document instructions given. Reinforce explanation dealing with test benefits and risks. This method of testing is decidedly less risky and produces less radiation exposure than conventional arteriography.
2. The patient must be coherent and cooperative and able to hold the breath and remain absolutely still when so instructed.
3. A legal consent form must be properly signed and witnessed.
4. Refer to iodine contrast test precautions.
5. Determine allergies, especially those to iodine or other contrast media. See pages 684–687 for additional assessment criteria.
6. In many instances, glucagon is intravenously administered just before abdominal examinations. This serves to reduce motion artifacts by stopping peristalsis.

7. No food or fluids should be taken within 2 hours before the study to minimize vomiting if an iodine contrast reaction occurs.
8. The few risks include such things as venous thrombosis or infection. When dye is administered through the venous route, the arteries, which are normally under higher pressure than the veins, can clear contrast dye through the process of normal circulation. For the same reason, there is less risk of loosening plaque.
9. Of benefit is that all arteries in a specific area can be visualized on one series of exposures. This overview gives the advantage of being able to evaluate the entire blood supply to a given area at one time. In contrast, during routine angiography, only one specific artery at a time can be visualized.
10. See Chapter 1 guidelines for safe, effective, informed *pretest* care.

Patient Aftercare

1. Check vital signs frequently. Report unstable signs to the physician.
2. Observe the catheter insertion site for signs of infection, hemorrhage, or hematoma. Use sterile aseptic technique at all times. Monitor neurovascular status of extremity. Report problems to the physician promptly.
3. Observe the allergic reactions to iodine. Mild side effects include nausea, vomiting, dizziness, or urticaria. Also, watch for other complications, such as abdominal pain, hypertension, congestive heart failure, angina, myocardial infarction, or anaphylaxis. In susceptible persons, renal failure may occur because higher doses of contrast materials are given compared with those of conventional arteriograms. Resuscitation equipment and supplies should be readily available. Promptly report these conditions to the physician.
4. Instruct the patient to increase fluid intake at least to 2000 ml during the 24 hours after the procedure to facilitate excretion of the iodine contrast substance.
5. Interpret test outcomes and monitor appropriately.
6. Follow Chapter 1 guidelines for safe, effective, informed *posttest* care.

ARTHROGRAPHY; JOINT RADIOGRAPHY ●

Normal Values

Normal filling of encapsulated joint structures, joint space, bursae, menisci, ligaments, and articular cartilage.

Explanation of Test

Arthrography involves multiple x-ray examinations of encapsulated joint structures following injection of contrast agents into the joint capsular space. Arthrography is done in cases of persistent unexplained joint discomfort. Even though the knee is the most frequently studied joint, the shoulder, hip, elbow, wrist, and temporomandibular joints also may be similarly examined using local anesthetics under aseptic conditions.

Procedure

1. The patient is positioned on the back on the examining table.
2. The skin around the joint is surgically prepared and draped.
3. A local anesthetic is then injected into tissues around the joint. It is usually unnecessary to anesthetize the actual joint space.
4. Effusion fluids in the joint, if present, are aspirated. Then, the contrast agents (gas, water, or soluble iodine) are injected. After the needle is removed, the joint is manipulated to ensure even distribution of the contrast material. In some cases, the patient may need to walk or exercise the joint for a few minutes.
5. During the examination, several positions are assumed to obtain varied x-ray views of the joint.
6. A special frame may be attached to widen the joint space for a better view. Pillows and sandbags also may be used to position the joint properly.

Clinical Implications

Abnormal results reveal

1. Arthritis
2. Dislocation
3. Ligament tears
4. Rotator cuff rupture
5. Synovial abnormalities
6. Narrowing of joint space
7. Cysts

Patient Preparation

1. Explain the purpose and procedure of the test. Advise that some discomfort is normal during contrast dye injection and during joint manipulation.
2. In most instances, a properly signed and witnessed consent form is required.
3. Refer to iodine test precautions on pages 685–687. Check for known allergies to iodine or other contrast substances.
4. See Chapter 1 guidelines for safe, effective, informed *pretest* care.

Patient Aftercare

1. The joint should be at rest for 12 hours.
2. An elastic bandage may be applied to the knee joint for several days after the exam.
3. Ice can be applied to the area if swelling occurs. Pain can usually be controlled with a mild analgesic.
4. Cracking or clicking noises in the joint may be heard for 1 or 2 days following the test. This is normal. Notify the physician if crepitant noises persist or increased pain, swelling, or restlessness occurs.
5. Follow Chapter 1 guidelines for safe, effective, informed *posttest* care.

MYELOGRAPHY

Normal Values

Normal lumbar or cervical myelogram.

Explanation of Test

Myelography is a radiographic study of the spinal subarachnoid space in which iodine contrast material is introduced into that space so the spinal cord and nerve roots are outlined and dura mater distortions may be detected.

The test is done to detect neoplasms, ruptured intravertebral disks, or extraspinal lesions such as arthritic stenosis or ankylosing spondyloses. This examination is also indicated when compression of the spinal or posterior fossa neural structure or nerve roots is suspected. The test is frequently done before surgical treatment for a ruptured vertebral disk or release of stenosis. Symptoms may include unrelieved back pain, pain radiating down the leg, absent or abnormal ankle and knee reflexes, claudication of neurospinal origin, or past history of cancer, with loss of mobility or bladder control.

Often, myelograms are performed in conjunction with spinal CT scans. Myelograms fall into three categories: positive contrasts using water-soluble iodine; use of iodized oil; and negative air contrast. Water-soluble iodine contrast is the most commonly used medium for myelograms. Both water-soluble and air contrast are followed by CT scanning, to improve visualization. In low-dose myelograms, a very small amount of water-soluble contrast is injected and immediately followed by scanning. An air myelogram is often a last resort examination but can be the test of choice for persons too large for a conventional CT myelogram, for those in traction, or those patients with unstable spinal fractures.

Procedure

1. The test is usually done in the x-ray department, with the patient positioned on the abdomen during the procedure.
2. The puncture area is prepared and draped.
3. The procedure is the same as that for lumbar puncture (see Chapter 5), except for the injection of the contrast substance and fluoroscopic x-ray films. With the use of water-soluble contrast, a narrow-bone needle (22-gauge) may be used. A lumbar puncture is done when lumbar defect is suspected; a cervical puncture is done for a suspected cervical lesion. In children, the level at which the lumbar puncture is performed is much lower than the level in adults to avoid puncturing the spinal cord. Depending on the contrast substance used, it may be removed (oil) or may be left to be absorbed (water or air).
4. The table is tilted during the procedure to achieve optimal visualization. Shoulder and foot braces help maintain correct position.

Clinical Implications

Abnormal results reveal distorted outlines of the subarachnoid space that indicate the following:

1. Ruptured intervertebral disk
2. Compression and stenosis of spinal cord
3. Landmarking the exact level of intravertebral tumors
4. Spinal canal obstruction
5. Avulsion of nerve roots

Patient Preparation

1. Explain the purpose, procedure, benefits, and risks of the test. Explain that some discomfort may be felt during the procedure. Disadvantages of water and air contrast include poor visualization and painful headache (air contrast) because of the difficulty in controlling the gas introduced into the area. Oil contrast substances can cause tissue irritation or be poorly absorbed from the subarachnoid space. Oil may still be visible on x-ray examination for up to 1 year following the original examination. About one in 20 examinations use oil; air is rarely used. Refer to iodine contrast test precautions if iodine is used.
2. A legal consent form must be properly signed and witnessed before the test.
3. Explain that the examination table may be tilted during the test, but that the patient is securely fastened and will not fall off the table.
4. Most diagnostic departments require the patient to refrain from eating for approximately 4 hours before testing. Clear liquids may be permitted and even encouraged to lower the incidence of headaches after the test. Check with radiology department and physician for specific orders.
5. A myelogram usually produces slight discomfort. However, if the patient has trouble moving, a pain reliever may be necessary to allow easier positioning and movement during the test.
6. See Chapter 1 guidelines for safe, effective, informed *pretest* care.

Patient Aftercare

1. Bed rest is necessary for several hours after testing. If a water-soluble contrast is used, the head of the bed should be elevated at 45° for 8 to 24 hours after the procedure. The patient is also advised to lie quietly. This position will reduce upward dispersion of the contrast medium and will keep it out of the head, where it may cause headache. If oil contrast dye is used, the patient will usually need to be prone for 2 to 4 hours, and then to remain on the back for another 2 to 4 hours. If the entire amount of oil contrast has not been withdrawn at the end of the procedure, the head will need to be elevated to prevent the oil from flowing into the brain.
2. Encourage fluid intake to hasten absorption of residual contrast material, to replace CSF, and to reduce risk of headache.

3. Check for bladder distention and adequate voiding, especially if metrizamide has been used.
4. Check vital signs frequently (at least every 4 hours) for the first 24 hours after the examination.
5. Follow Chapter 1 guidelines for safe, effective, informed *posttest* care.

Clinical Alert

1. Observe the patient for possible complications such as nausea, headache, fever, seizure, paralysis, arachnoiditis (inflammation of the spinal cord coverings), change in level of consciousness, drowsiness, stupor, neck stiffness, and sterile meningitis reaction (severe headache, symptoms of arachnoiditis, slow-wave patterns on electroencephalogram).
2. Alteration of CSF pressure may cause an acute exacerbation of symptoms that may require immediate surgical intervention. Lumbar punctures should not be done unless absolutely necessary.
3. This test is to be avoided unless there is a reason to suspect a lesion. Multiple sclerosis, for example, may be worsened by this procedure.
4. Determine whether water-soluble, oil, or air contrast was used for the procedure, because aftercare interventions will differ.
5. If nausea or vomiting occurs after the procedure and a water-soluble contrast has been used, do not administer phenothiazine antiemetics such as prochlorperazine (Compazine).

DENTAL RADIOGRAPHY

Normal Values

Normal mandible, maxilla, temporomandibular joints, maxillary sinuses, and primary or permanent dentition.

Explanation of Test

Dental x-rays screen and diagnose causes of pain and other symptoms related to the teeth, jaws, and temporomandibular joints, as well as follow-up for dental therapy. Many different types of dental radiographs are available because of the complex tissue density found within the human masticatory system. The x-rays are categorized by the location at which the film is placed during the procedure. *Intraoral* refers to films taken inside the mouth; *extraoral* x-rays are taken outside the oral cavity. The most common x-rays taken are the bite wing and the periapical, both of which are intraoral. A list of various types of dental x-rays include the following:

INTRAORAL (TAKEN INSIDE MOUTH)

1. Bite wing shows coronal portion of the tooth; also done for caries detection; shows bite correlation between upper and lower teeth.
2. Periapical shows x-ray of the whole tooth and immediate surrounding area
3. Occlusal shows chewing surfaces and curve of mandibular molar teeth.

EXTRAORAL (TAKEN OUTSIDE THE MOUTH)

1. Lateral skull projection (transcranial; TMJ screen)
2. Lateral sinus projection (sinus view)
3. Posteroanterior skull projection
4. Posteroanterior mandibular projection
5. Posteroanterior maxillary projection (TMJ, bones of the maxillary area)
6. Posteroanterior frontal sinus projection
7. Bregma–Mentum sinus projection (sinus view)
8. Inferosuperior zygomatic arch sinus projection (zygomatic bone, sinus)
9. Panarex (full mouth x-ray)
10. Tomography (CT)
11. Arthrography

Procedure

1. When taking x-rays inside the mouth, the patient is seated upright and the film and holder are placed in the mouth. The patient may bite on the holder or may anchor it with a finger to keep it in place. A lead apron with a cervical collar is draped over the patient's torso and neck area.
2. Different designs of film holders facilitate the proper alignment for correct x-ray tube orientation. There are also many different types of extraoral films that can be taken, each with their own procedures. For example, with the lateral skull projection, the patient sits upright and the film packet is placed on one side of the head. The x-ray source is placed on the opposite side. In other instances, such as x-rays outside the mouth, the x-ray machine rotates around the face.

Clinical Alert

Previous extensive radiation therapy or a current state of pregnancy may present contraindications to dental x-rays. Consult the patient's physician if in doubt.

Clinical Implications

1. Abnormal results reveal the following:
   a. Dentition
      (1) Changes in number of teeth
      (2) Changes in shape of teeth
      (3) Changes in pulp canal
      (4) Miscellaneous other teeth lesions

b. Radiolucent lesions of the jaw
   (1) Lesions at the tooth apex
   (2) Midline tooth lesions
   (3) Lesions in place of a missing tooth
   (4) Lesions around the crown of an impacted tooth
   (5) Bubblelike radiolucencies
   (6) Other multiple, but different radiolucent lesions
   (7) Lesions that destroy the cortical plate of the tooth

3. Mixed lesions (radiopaque and radiolucent)
4. Salivary gland lesions
5. Soft-tissue lesions
6. Temporomandibular joint abnormalities

Interfering Factors

Certain factors can interfere with proper visualization:

1. Braces and retainers
2. Partials and dentures
3. Restorations
4. Jewelry, such as earrings
5. Bony growths on the inside of the mandible and the midline of the hard palate (tori); excess deposits of bone

Patient Preparation

1. Explain purpose, benefits, risks, (minimum radiation exposure) and procedures. Stress the importance of holding still and breathing through the nose to lessen the gag reflex.
2. Assist patient to rinse mouth before procedure.
3. Assess for contraindications and interfering factors.
4. See Chapter 1 guidelines for safe, effective, informed *pretest* care.

Patient Aftercare

1. Evaluate x-rays and explain abnormalities. Comparison with a normal x-ray may be beneficial.
2. Follow Chapter 1 guidelines for safe, effective, informed *posttest* care.

HYSTEROSALPINGOGRAM; UTERINE AND FALLOPIAN TUBE RADIOGRAPHY ●

Normal Values

Normal intrauterine cavity; patent fallopian tubes.

Explanation of Test

Hysterosalpingography involves radiographic visualization of the uterine cavity and the fallopian tubes to detect abnormalities that may be the cause of infertility or other problems. Normally, contrast dye introduced into the uterine cavity will travel through the fallopian tubes and "spill" into the peritoneal cavity, where it will be naturally resorbed.

Procedure

1. The patient removes all clothing and puts on a hospital gown. The bladder should be emptied before the study begins.
2. The patient lies supine on the x-ray table in a lithotomy position. Preliminary pelvic x-ray films may be taken.
3. The radiologist or gynecologist introduces a speculum into the patient's vagina and inserts a cannula through the cervical canal. The iodinated contrast agent is administered into the uterus through this cannula.
4. The speculum is removed (unless it is radiolucent), and both fluoroscopic and conventional filming are done.

Clinical Implications

Abnormal findings include

1. Bicornuate uterus or other uterine cavity anomalies
2. Tubal tortuosity
3. Tubal obstruction evidenced by failure of the contrast dye to spill into the peritoneal cavity on one or both sides. Bilateral tubal obstruction causes infertility.
4. Scarring and evidence of old pelvic inflammatory disease.

Patient Preparation

1. Explain purpose and procedure of the test. Some institutions require a properly signed and witnessed surgical permit.
2. Refer to iodine contrast test precautions on pages 685–687.
3. Verify date of last menstrual period to assure that the patient is not pregnant.
4. Advise that some discomfort may be experienced, but this subsides quickly.
5. Suggest that the patient bring along sanitary napkins to wear because some spotting and contrast dye discharge may occur.
6. See Chapter 1 guidelines for safe, effective, informed *pretest* care.

Clinical Alert

Pregnancy and active pelvic inflammatory disease are contraindications to hysterosalpingogram.

Patient Aftercare

1. Monitor patient discomfort and administer analgesics as ordered.
2. Instruct the patient to report heavy vaginal bleeding or abnormal discharge, unusual pain, or fever to the referring physician.
3. Interpret test outcomes and counsel about infertility problems.
4. Follow Chapter 1 guidelines for safe, effective, informed *posttest* care.

BIBLIOGRAPHY

American College of Radiology: List of Accredited Mammography Facilities. Reston, VA, American College of Radiology, 1992

Andolina VF: Mammographic Imaging: A Practical Guide. Philadelphia, JB Lippincott, 1992

Ballinger PW: Merrill's Atlas of Roentgenographic Positions and Standard Radiologic Procedures, Vols. 1–3, 7th ed. St. Louis, CV Mosby, 1991

Bier V: Health Effects of Exposure to Low Levels of Imaging Radiation. Washington, DC, National Academy Press, 1990

Bontrager KL: Textbook of Radiographic Positioning and Related Anatomy, 3rd ed. St. Louis, CV Mosby, 1993

Bush WH: Urologic Imaging and Interventional Techniques. New York, Urban & Schwarzenber, 1989

Eastman-Kodak: Dental Radiography and Photography, Vol. 57 (1-4), 1985

Gore RM: Textbook of GI Radiology. Philadelphia, WB Saunders, 1994

Hoffman DA et al: Effects of imaging radiation on the developing embryo and fetus: A review. HHS Publication No. FDS 81-8170

Juhl JH, Crumny AB: Paul and Juhle. Essentials of Radiologic Imaging. Philadelphia, JB Lippincott, 1993

Kaut C: MRI Workbook for Technologists. New York, Raven Press, 1992

Kricun ME (ed): Imaging of Bone Tumors. Philadelphia, WB Saunders, 1993

Leiner S: Recurrent urinary tract infections in otherwise healthy adult women: Rationale strategies for workup and management. Nurse Practitioner 20(2) 48–55, February 1995.

Mace JD: Radiographic Pathology for Technologists, 2nd ed. St. Louis, CV Mosby, 1994

Monroe D: Patient teaching for x-ray and other diagnostics (cardiac cath). RN 54(2):44–46, February 1991

Monroe D: Patient teaching for x-ray and other diagnostics (ERCP and oral cholecystogram). RN 53(4):52–56, April 1990

Newhouse JH: Understanding MRI. Boston, Little, Brown & Co, 1991

NRCP: Exposure of the MS population from diagnostic medical radiation. Baltimore, National Council on Radiation Protection and Measurements, May 1989

Pinnar J: Patient teaching for x-ray and other diagnostics (thallium and stress tests). RN 54(3):32–36, March 1991

Seeram EL: Computerized Tomography: Physical Principles, Clinical Applications and Quality Control. Philadelphia, WB Saunders, 1994

Skucas J (ed): Radiographic Contrast Agents, 2nd ed. Rockville, MD, Aspen, 1989

Taveras JM: Radiology—Diagnosis, Imaging, Intervention, Vol. 1. Philadelphia, JB Lippincott, 1994

Torres LS: Basic Medical Techniques and Patient Care for Radiologic Technologists, 4th ed. Philadelphia, JB Lippincott, 1993

11

Cytology and Genetic Studies

CYTOLOGIC STUDIES

OVERVIEW OF CYTOLOGIC STUDIES

Exfoliated cells in body tissues and fluid are studied to count and determine the type of cells present, and to diagnose malignant and premalignant conditions. The staining technique developed by Dr. George N. Papanicolaou has been especially useful in diagnosis of malignancy, and it is now routinely used in the cytologic study of the female genital tract, as well as in many types of nongynecologic specimens.

Some cytologic specimens (eg, smears of the mouth, genital tract, and nipple discharge) are relatively easy to obtain for study. Other samples are from less accessible sources (eg, amniotic fluid, pleural effusions, and cerebrospinal fluid), and special techniques, such as fine-needle aspiration (see p. 746), are required for collection. Tissue samples obtained in surgery are also examined, and skin biopsies for fibroblast culture are done. In all studies, the source of the sample and its method of collection must be noted so that the evaluation can be based on complete information.

Specimens for cytologic study are usually composed of many different cells. Some are normally present, whereas others indicate pathologic conditions. Under certain conditions, cells observed as normal in one sample may be indicative of an abnormal state when observed elsewhere. All specimens are examined for the number of cells, cell distribution, surface modification, size, shape, appearance and staining properties, functional adaptations, and inclusions. The cell nucleus is also examined. Any increases or decreases from normal values are noted.

Gynecologic specimens are smeared and fixed in 95% alcohol. (Some types of spray fixative are also available.) Nongynecologic specimens are generally collected without preservative, and they must be handled carefully to prevent drying or degeneration. Check with your individual laboratory for collection requirements. It is important that all cytologic specimens are sent to the laboratory as soon as they are obtained to prevent disintegration of cells or any other process that could cause alteration of the material for study.

Clinical Alert

1. The test is only as good as the specimen received.
2. Specimens collected from patients in isolation should be clearly labeled on the specimen container and requisition form with appropriate warning stickers. The specimen container should then be placed in two protective bags before transporting it to the laboratory.

(continued)

(Clinical Alert continued)

2. The Occupational Safety and Health Administration (OSHA) requires that all specimens be placed in a secondary container before transporting them to the laboratory. Most laboratories prefer plastic biohazard bags. Requisitions should be kept on the outside of the bag, or in a separate compartment in the biohazard bag, if available.

In practice, cytologic studies will be commonly reported as

1. Inflammatory
2. Benign
3. Atypical
4. Suspicious for malignancy
5. Positive for malignancy (in situ versus invasive)

Histology

Material submitted for tissue examination may be classified according to the histologic or cellular characteristics. A basic method for classifying cancer according to the histologic or cellular characteristics of the tumor is Broder's classification of malignancy.

Grade I: Tumors showing a marked tendency to differentiate; 75% or more of cells differentiated

Grade II: 75% to 50% of cells differentiated, slight to moderate dysplasia and metaplasia

Grade III: 50% to 25% of cells differentiated, marked dysplasia, marked atypical, and cancer in situ

Grade IV: 25% to 0% of cells differentiated

The TNM system is a method of identifying tumor stages according to spread of the disease. This system evolved from the work of the International Union Against Cancer and the American Joint Committee on Cancer. In addition, the TNM system further defines each specific type of cancer, such as breast, head, or neck. This staging system (on pp. 747–748), which is employed for previously untreated and treated cancers, classifies the primary site of cancer and its extent and involvement, such as lymphatic and venous invasion.

CYTOLOGIC STUDY OF FINE-NEEDLE ASPIRATION ●

Normal Value

Negative: no abnormal cells present.

Explanation of Test

Fine-needle aspiration is a method of obtaining diagnostic material for cytologic study that causes a minimal amount of trauma to the patient.

Bacteriologic studies also may be done on material obtained during fine-needle aspiration. Unfixed material, either left in the syringe or on a needle rinsed in sterile saline, may be taken to the microbiology department for study.

*TNM System**

Three capital letters are used to describe the extent of the cancer:

T: *P*rimary tumor
N: *R*egional lymph nodes
M: *D*istant metastasis

Chronology of Classification
c: Clinical–diagnostic
p: Postsurgical treatment—pathologic
r: Retreatment
a: Autopsy

This classification is extended by the following designations:

T Subclasses (Extent of Primary Tumor)
TX: Tumor cannot be adequately assessed
T0: No evidence of primary tumor
Tis: Carcinoma in situ
T1, T2, T3, T4: Progressive increase in tumor size and involvement

N Subclasses (Involvement of Regional Lymph Nodes)
NX: Regional lymph nodes cannot be assessed clinically
N0: Regional lymph node metastasis
N1, N2, N3, N4: Increasing degrees of demonstrable abnormality of regional lymph nodes

Histopathology
GX: Grade cannot be assessed
G1: Well-differentiated grade
G2: Moderately well-differentiated grade
G3: Poorly differentiated grade
G4: Undifferentiated

Metastasis
MX: The minimum requirements to assess the presence of distant metastasis cannot be met
M0: No evidence of distant metastasis
M1: Distant metastasis present
Specify sites of metastasis

*Adapted from Beahrs OH, Myers MH (eds): Manual for Staging of Cancer, 4th ed. Philadelphia, JB Lippincott, 1992.

The category M1 may be subdivided according to the following notations:

Pulmonary:	PUL	Hepatic:	HEP
Osseous:	OSS	Brain:	BRA
Lymph nodes:	LYM	Skin:	SKI
Bone marrow:	MAR	Peritoneum:	PER
Pleura:	PLE	Other:	OTH

In certain sites further information on the primary tumor may be recorded under the following headings:

Lymphatic Invasion (L)
LX: Lymphatic invasion cannot be assessed
L0: No evidence of lymphatic invasion
L1: Lymphatic invasion

Venous Invasion (V)
VX: Venous invasion cannot be assessed
V0: No venous invasion
V1: Microscopic venous invasion
V2: Macroscopic venous invasion

Residual Tumor (R)
This information does not enter into establishing the stage of the tumor but should be recorded for use in considering additive therapy. When the cancer is treated by definitive surgical procedures, residual cancer, if any, is recorded.

Residual Tumor Following Surgical Treatment
RX: Residual tumor at primary site cannot be assessed
R0: No residual tumor
R1: Microscopic residual tumor
R2: Macroscopic residual tumor
M: Symbol—in parentheses indicates multiple tumors
Y: Symbol—Y prefix indicates classification occurring with intense multi-modality therapy
r: Symbol—r prefix indicates recurrent tumors after a disease-free interval

Procedure

1. Superficial or palpable lesions may be aspirated without radiologic aid, but nonpalpable lesions are aspirated with radiographic aid for needle placement.
2. After the needle is properly positioned, the plunger of the syringe is retracted to create negative pressure. The needle is moved up and down and sometimes at several different angles. The plunger of the syringe is released, and the needle is removed.
3. The material obtained is expressed onto slides that are then smeared to-

gether and fixed immediately. The needle may be rinsed in sterile saline or 50% alcohol for further studies.

Clinical Implications

Abnormal results are helpful in identifying

1. Infectious processes: The infectious agent may be seen, or characteristic cellular changes may indicate the infectious agent that is present.
2. Benign conditions: Some characteristic cellular changes may be present, indicating the presence of a benign process.
3. Malignant conditions, either primary or metastatic: If the disease is metastatic, the findings may be reported as consistent with the primary malignancy.

Patient Preparation

1. Explain the purpose and procedure, benefits, and risks. Although a local anesthetic is generally used, the procedure will cause some discomfort, and this should not be minimized. If the approach involves passing near a rib, the pain may be greater because of the sensitivity of the bone and is not a cause for alarm. Unexpected pain may induce a vasovagal or other undesirable response. Besides vasovagal responses, risks may include infection, hematoma, or hemorrhage, depending on the site aspirated.
2. See guidelines in Chapter 1 for safe, effective, informed *pretest* care.

Patient Aftercare

1. Monitor for signs of inflammation and use site care infection control measures. Pain may be common in sensitive areas, such as the breast, nipple, and scrotum. Specific problems vary depending on site aspirated (ie, hemoptysis following a lung aspirate).
2. Counsel about follow-up procedures for infectious and malignant conditions.
3. Follow guidelines in Chapter 1 for safe, effective, informed *posttest* care.

Clinical Alert

1. Traumatic complications are rare. Fine-needle aspiration of the lung infrequently results in pneumothorax. Local extension of the malignancy is a consideration, but studies have shown this to be an extremely rare occurrence.
2. A negative finding on a fine-needle aspirate does not rule out the possibility that a malignancy is present. The cells aspirated may have been from a necrotic area of the tumor or a benign area adjacent to the tumor.

CYTOLOGIC STUDY OF LIVER BIOPSIES

Normal Values

Negative for malignant or other abnormal cells and tissues.

Explanation of Test

Cellular material from the liver may be useful in evaluating the status of the liver in diffuse disorders of the parenchyma and the diagnosis of space-occupying lesions. Liver biopsy is especially useful when the clinical findings and laboratory test portions are not diagnostic (when the aspartate transaminase [AST] level is 10 to 20 times less than the upper defined limit and the alkaline phosphatase [ALP] level is less than 3 times the limit), and when the diagnosis or etiology cannot be established by other means (enlarged liver of unknown origin and systemic disease affecting the liver, such as military tuberculosis).

Procedure

1. See section on fine-needle biopsy on page 746.
2. The test is done at the bedside under local anesthesia. Specimens may be obtained using ultrasound radiologic guidance and a tissue core biopsy needle, such as the Menghini needle, which will provide histologic and cytologic material, or one may use a fine-needle aspirate needle, which will obtain cytologic material only.
3. Tissue specimens are generally placed in 10% formalin for fixation. Check with your laboratory for specific instructions for handling special cases (ie, liver biopsies for copper levels).
4. Touch prints on glass slides may be made before fixation to be submitted for cytologic evaluation. Needle rinses in 50% alcohol or saline may provide helpful diagnostic material as well.
5. Direct slides from needle aspirates may be made, with the slides being fixed immediately in 95% alcohol. See Chapter 12 on endoscopic examination and liver biopsy.

Clinical Implications

Abnormalities in test results of liver biopsies may be helpful in detecting the following:

1. Benign disorders, such as
   - **a.** Metabolic disorders
     - **(1)** Fatty metamorphosis
     - **(2)** Hemosiderosis
     - **(3)** Accumulation of bile (may be due to hepatitis, obstructive jaundice, or malignancy)
     - **(4)** Diabetes
   - **b.** Hepatic cirrhosis
   - **c.** Abscess
   - **d.** Hepatic cysts (congenital or hydatid)

2. Malignant processes, such as
   a. Primary tumors of the liver
      (1) Hepatocellular carcinoma
      (2) Cholangiocarcinoma
   b. Metastatic tumors

Interfering Factors

The reported effectiveness of liver aspirates or biopsies varies in the limited published information. Because a very small fragment of tissue, often partially destroyed, is taken in a random manner from a large organ, localized disease is easily missed.

1. False-negative samples may be due to
   a. Sampling error: Detection rate of liver metastases is approximately 50% to 70% with blind biopsy and about 85% (range 67% to 96%) using ultrasound guidance. Also, many *diseases* produce nonspecific changes that may be spotty, healing, or minimal.
   b. Degeneration or distortion caused by faulty preparation of specimen.
2. False-positive results may be due to misinterpretation of markedly reactive hepatocytes.

Patient Preparation

1. Explain the purpose of the test, the nature of the procedure, and the benefits and risks. The procedure usually causes minimal discomfort, but only for a short while. Explain that the doctor will inject a local anesthetic into the skin. Remember to ask if the patient has ever had a reaction to any numbing medicines.
2. The patients should be NPO for 4 to 6 hours before the procedure. The patient will be asked to lie on his or her back with right arm above the head. During the biopsy, the patient should take a deep breath in, blow the air out, and hold his or her breath.
3. Risks include a small, but definite, risk of intra-abdominal bleeding and bile peritonitis. Percutaneous liver biopsy results in complications in only about 1% of cases.
4. See guidelines in Chapter 1 for safe, effective, informed *pretest* care.

Patient Aftercare

See section on fine-needle aspirations. Other instructions for aftercare may include the following:

1. Strict bed rest for at least 6 hours is generally ordered, with observation for 24 hours.
2. Assess the patient's pulse, blood pressure, and respiration every 15 minutes for the first hour, every 30 minutes for the next 2 hours, once in each of the next 4 hours, and then every 4 hours until his or her condition is stable.

3. Notify the doctor if the patient's blood pressure differs markedly from baseline or if he or she is in severe pain.
4. Keep the patient NPO for 2 hours, then the previous diet can be resumed.
5. After 6 hours, a blood hematocrit is generally ordered to rule out internal bleeding.
6. The patient should be warned not to cough hard or strain for 2 to 4 hours following the procedure. Heavy lifting and strenuous activities should be avoided for about a week.
7. Follow the guidelines in Chapter 1 for safe, effective, informed *posttest* care.

Clinical Alert

Contraindications to percutaneous liver biopsy include

1. A prothrombin time in the anticoagulant range (2 to 3 seconds over control values)
2. Other bleeding disorders
3. A platelet count of fewer than 50,000 mm^3
4. Marked ascites
5. Suspected vascular tumor of the liver
6. Infection of the biliary tract or subdiaphragmatic or right hemothoracic infection.
7. Inability of the patient to cooperate during the procedure
8. See section on fine-needle aspirations on page 746.

CYTOLOGIC STUDY OF THE RESPIRATORY TRACT

(See also Chap. 7, under *Respiratory Tract Cultures.*)

Normal Value

Negative.

Explanation of Test

The lungs and the passages that conduct air to and from the lungs form the respiratory tract, which is divided into the upper and lower respiratory tracts. The upper respiratory tract consists of the nasal cavities, the nasopharynx, and the larynx; the lower respiratory tract consists of the trachea and the lungs. Cytologic studies of sputum and bronchial specimens are quite important as diagnostic aids because of the frequency of cancer of the lung and the relative inaccessibility of this organ. Also detectable are cell changes that may be related to the future development of malignant conditions and to inflammatory conditions.

Sputum is composed of mucus and cells. It is the secretion of the bronchi, lungs, and trachea and, therefore, is obtained from the lower respiratory tract (bronchi and lungs). Although sputum is ejected through the mouth, it originates in the lower respiratory tract. Saliva produced by the salivary glands in the mouth is *not* sputum. A specimen can be correctly identified as sputum in microscopic examination by the presence of dust cells (carbon dust-laden macrophages). Although the glands and secretory cells in the mucous lining of the lower respiratory tract produce up to 100 ml of fluid daily, the healthy person normally does not cough up sputum.

Procedures

FOR OBTAINING SPUTUM

1. The preferred material is an early-morning specimen. Three specimens are usually collected on three separate days.
2. The patient must inhale air to the full capacity of the lungs and then exhale the air with an expulsive deep cough.
3. The specimen should be coughed directly into a wide-mouthed clean container containing 50% alcohol. (Some cytology laboratories prefer the specimen to be fresh if it will be delivered to the laboratory immediately.)
4. The specimen should be covered with a tight-fitting clean lid.
5. The specimen should be labeled with the patient's name, age, date, diagnosis, and number of specimens (1, 2, or 3) and immediately sent to the laboratory.

FOR OBTAINING BRONCHIAL SECRETIONS

Bronchial secretions are obtained during bronchoscopy (see Chap 12). Diagnostic bronchoscopy involves removal of bronchial secretions and tissue for cytologic and microbiologic studies. Secretions obtained are collected in a clean container and taken to the cytology laboratory. If microbiologic studies are ordered, the container *must* be sterile.

FOR OBTAINING BRONCHIAL BRUSHINGS

Bronchial brushings are obtained during bronchoscopy. The material collected can be smeared directly on all-frosted slides and immediately fixed, or the actual brush may be place in a container of 50% ethyl alcohol or saline (check with the laboratory for their preference) and delivered to the cytology laboratory.

FOR BRONCHOPULMONARY LAVAGE

Bronchopulmonary lavage may be used to evaluate patients with interstitial lung disease. Saline is injected into the distal portions of the lung and aspirated back through the bronchoscope into a specimen container. This essentially "washes out" the alveoli. The fresh specimen should be brought directly to the laboratory. A total cell count and a differential cell count are performed to determine the relative numbers of macrophages, neutrophils, and lymphocytes.

Clinical Implications

Abnormalities in sputum and bronchial specimens may sometimes be helpful in detecting the following:

1. Benign atypical changes in sputum, as in
   a. Inflammatory diseases
   b. Asthma (Creola bodies, Curschmann's spirals, and eosinophils may be found, but they are not diagnostic of the disease.)
   c. Lipid pneumonia. (Lipophages may be found, but they are not diagnostic of the disease.)
   d. Asbestosis (ferruginous or asbestos bodies)
   e. Viral diseases
   f. Benign diseases of lung, such as bronchiectasis, atelectasis, emphysema, and pulmonary infarcts
2. Metaplasia, which is the substitution of one adult cell type for another: Severe metaplastic changes are found in patients with
   a. History of chronic cigarette smoking
   b. Pneumonitis
   c. Pulmonary infarcts
   d. Bronchiectasis
   e. Healing abscess
   f. Tuberculosis
   g. Emphysema

   (Metaplasia often adjoins a carcinoma or a carcinoma in situ.)
3. Viral changes and the presence of virocytes (viral inclusions may be seen) in
   a. Viral pneumonia
   b. Acute respiratory disease caused by adenovirus
   c. Herpes simplex infection
   d. Measles
   e. Cytomegalic inclusion disease
   f. Varicella
4. Degenerative changes, as seen in viral diseases of the lung
5. Fungal and parasitic diseases (in parasitic diseases, ova or parasite may be seen)
6. Tumors (benign and malignant)

Interfering Factors

1. False-negative results may be due to
   a. Delays in preparation of the specimen, causing a deterioration of tumor cells.
   b. Sampling error (diagnostic cells may not have exfoliated into the material examined).
2. The frequency of false-negative results is about 15%, in contrast with about 1% in studies for cervical cancer. This high frequency occurs even with careful examination of multiple deep cough specimens.

Patient Preparation

1. Explain the purpose and procedure of the test.
2. Emphasize that sputum is not saliva. If patient is having difficulty producing sputum, a hot shower before obtaining a specimen may improve the yield.
3. Advise the patient to brush his or her teeth and rinse his or her mouth well before obtaining the sputum specimen to avoid introduction of saliva into the specimen. The specimen should be collected before the patient eats breakfast.
4. If a bronchoscopy is performed, maintain NPO for 6 hours before procedure.
5. Manage pain with sedation as indicated.
6. Provide emotional support.
7. Instruct patient to breathe in and out of nose with mouth open during procedure; fiberoptic bronchoscope is inserted through the nose or mouth; rigid bronchoscope is inserted through mouth.
8. See Chapter 1 guidelines for safe, effective, informed *pretest* care.

Patient Aftercare

1. If specimen obtained by bronchoscopy: check blood pressure, pulse and respirations every 15 minutes, four times, then every 2 hours to 4 hours, then as ordered. Assist and teach patient to not eat or drink until gag reflex returns. Maintain bed rest and elevate head of bed 45°. Manage pain as indicated. Auscultate chest for breath sounds every 2 to 4 hours and then as ordered. Perform postural drainage and oropharyngeal suctioning as ordered. Refer to bronchoscopy care in Chapter 12.
2. Follow guidelines in Chapter 1 for safe, effective informed *posttest* care.

CYTOLOGIC STUDY OF THE GASTROINTESTINAL TRACT ●

Normal Values

Negative. Squamous epithelial cells of the esophagus may be present.

Explanation of Test

Exfoliative cytology of the gastrointestinal tract is useful in diagnosis of benign and malignant diseases. It is not, however, a specific test for these diseases. Many benign diseases, such as leukoplakia of the esophagus, esophagitis, gastritis, pernicious anemia, and granulomatous diseases, may be recognized because of their characteristic cellular changes. Response to radiation may also be noted from cytologic studies.

Procedure

1. For esophageal studies, a nasogastric Levin tube is passed approximately 40 cm (to the cardioesophageal junction) with the patient in a sitting position.

2. For stomach studies, a Levin tube is passed into the stomach (approximately 60 cm) with the patient in a sitting position.
3. For pancreatic and gallbladder drainage, a special double-lumen gastric tube is passed orally to 45 cm, with the patient in a sitting position. Then the patient is placed on his or her right side and the tube is passed slowly to 85 cm. It takes about 20 minutes for the tube to reach this distance. Tube location is confirmed by biopsy. Lavage with physiologic salt solution is done during all upper gastrointestinal cytologic procedures.
4. Specimens can also be obtained during endoscopy procedures.
5. During endoscopy, cytologic brushings may be taken of suspicious areas. The material obtained may be smeared on a slide and immediately fixed, or the brush may be placed in a specimen cup containing 50% alcohol or saline (check with the cytology laboratory for their preference) and taken to the laboratory for processing. (See Chap. 12 for endoscopic procedures.)

Clinical Implications

1. The characteristics of benign and malignant cells of the gastrointestinal tract are the same as for cells of the rest of the body.
2. Abnormal results in cytologic studies of the esophagus may be a nonspecific aid in the diagnosis of
   a. Acute esophagitis, characterized by increased exfoliation of basal cells with inflammatory cells and polymorphonuclear leukocytes in the cytoplasm of the benign squamous cells
   b. Vitamin B_{12} and folic acid deficiencies, characterized by giant epithelial cells
   c. Malignant diseases, characterized by typical cells of esophageal malignancy
3. Abnormal results in studies of the stomach may be a nonspecific aid in the diagnosis of
   a. Pernicious anemia, characterized by giant epithelial cells. An injection of vitamin B_{12} will cause these cells to disappear within 24 hours.
   b. Granulomatous inflammations seen in chronic gastritis and sarcoid of the stomach, which are characterized by granulomatous cells
   c. Gastritis, characterized by degenerative changes and an increase in the exfoliation of clusters of surface epithelial cells
   d. Malignant diseases, most of which are gastric adenocarcinomas. Lymphoma cells can be differentiated from adenocarcinoma. The Reed–Sternberg cell, a multinucleated giant cell, is the characteristic cell found along with abnormal lymphocytes in Hodgkin's disease.
4. Abnormal results in studies of the pancreas, gallbladder, and duodenum may reveal malignant cells (usually adenocarcinoma), but it is sometimes difficult to determine the exact site of the tumor.
5. Abnormal results in examination of the colon may reveal

- **a.** Ileitis, characterized by large multinucleated histocytes (bovine tuberculosis commonly manifests itself in this area)
- **b.** Ulcerative colitis, characterized by a hyperchromatic nuclei surrounded by a thin cytoplasmic rim
- **c.** Malignant cells (usually adenocarcinoma)

Interfering Factors

The barium and lubricant used in Levin tubes will interfere with good results because their presence will distort the cells and prevent accurate evaluation.

Patient Preparation

1. The patient should be told the purpose of the test, the nature of the procedure, and to anticipate some discomfort.
2. A liquid diet is usually ordered 24 hours before testing. The patient is encouraged to take fluids throughout the night and in the morning before the test.
3. No oral barium should be administered for the preceding 24 hours.
4. Laxatives and enemas are ordered for colon cytologic studies.
5. Because insertion of the nasogastric tube can cause considerable discomfort, the patient and clinician should devise a system (eg, raising a hand) to indicate discomfort. (See gastric analysis procedure in Chap. 15.)
6. The patient should be informed that panting, mouth-breathing, or swallowing can help to ease the insertion of the tube.
7. Sucking on ice chips or sipping through a straw also makes insertion of the tube easier.
8. Ballottement and massage of the abdomen are needed to release cells when a gastric wash technique is used.
9. See Chapter 1 guidelines for safe, effective *pretest* care.

Clinical Alert

Immediately remove the tube if the patient shows signs of distress: coughing, gasping, or cyanosis.

Patient Aftercare

1. Interpret test results and monitor appropriately. The patient should be given food, fluids, and rest after the tests are completed.
2. Provide rest. Patients having colon studies will be feeling quite tired.
3. Potential complications of endoscopy include respiratory distress, esophageal, gastric, or duodenal perforation. Complications of proctosigmoidoscopy include possible bowel perforation. Decreased blood pressure, pallor, diaphoresis, and bradycardia are signs of vasovagal stimulation and require immediate notification of physician.
4. Follow Chapter 1 guidelines for safe, effective, informal *posttest* care.

CYTOLOGIC STUDY OF THE FEMALE GENITAL TRACT (PAPANICOLAOU SMEAR) ●

Normal Values

Normal: no abnormal cells.

Maturation Index (MI): The MI is a ratio of parabasal to intermediate to superficial cells. The following are representative ratios:

Normal child:	80/20/0
Preovulatory adult:	0/40/60
Premenstrual adult:	0/70/30
Pregnant adult (2nd mo):	0/90/10
Postmenopausal adult (aged 60):	65/30/5

Background

Characteristic physiologic cellular changes occur in the genital tract from birth through the postmenopausal years. Hormonal evaluation by cytologic examination should be performed only on vaginal smears taken from the lateral vaginal wall or from the vaginal fornix. Smears from the ectocervix or endocervix cannot be used for hormonal evaluation because certain conditions, such as metaplasia and cervicitis, interfere with a correct assessment. There are three major cell types occurring in a characteristic pattern in normal vaginal smears.

1. Superficial squamous cells (mature squamous, usually polygonal, containing a pyknotic nucleus).
2. Intermediate squamous cells (mature squamous, usually polygonal, containing a clearly structured vesicular nucleus, which may be either well preserved or peptolytically changed as a result of bacterial cytolysis).
3. Parabasal cells (immature squamous, usually round or oval, containing one or, rarely, more than one relatively large nucleus). These cells occur either well preserved or in proteolytic clusters as a result of degeneration or necrosis.

NOTE: *Deviation from normal physiologic cell patterns may be indicative of pathologic conditions.*

A hormonal cytologic study is valuable in the assessment of many endocrine-related conditions, especially ovarian function.

Explanation of Test

The Papanicolaou (PAP) smear is used principally for diagnosis of precancerous and cancerous conditions of the genital tract, which includes the vagina, cervix, and endometrium. This test is also used for hormonal assessment and for diagnosis of inflammatory diseases. Because PAP smear is of great importance in the early detection of cervical cancer, it is recommended that all women over the age of 20 have the test at least once a year.

The value of the PAP smear depends on the fact that cells readily exfoliate (or can be easily stripped) from genital cancers. Cytologic study can also be used for assessing response to the effect of administered sex hormones. It should be noted that the microbiologic examination of cytologic samples is not as accurate as bacterial culture, but it can provide valuable information.

Specimens for cytologic examination of the genital tract are usually obtained by vaginal speculum examination or by colposcopy with biopsy. Material from the cervix, endocervix, and posterior fornix is obtained for most smears. Smears for hormonal evaluation are obtained from the vagina.

All PAP smears are usually reported on a five-point scale. The meaning of the classes varies, however, and is not universally agreed on. The following is the scale:

1: Absence of atypical or abnormal cells, negative
2: Atypical cytology, dysplastic, borderline but not neoplastic
3: Cytology suggestive of, but not inclusive of, malignancy (*suspect* is the term most often used)
4: Cytology strongly suggestive of malignancy or strongly suspect
5: Cytology conclusive of malignancy, cancer cells present

Clinical Alert

It is important to remember that cytologic findings alone do not form the basis of a diagnosis of cancer nor of other diseases. Often they are used to justify further procedures, such as biopsy.

Cells are also examined for hormonal effect and organisms. Cells examined for hormonal effect may be reported on a six-point scale.

1: Marked estrogen effect
2: Moderate estrogen effect
3: Slight estrogen effect
4: Atrophic
5: Compatible with pregnancy
6: No evaluation—specimen too bloody or inflamed or scanty

Cells also can be examined for microorganisms using routine staining techniques. These cells may be reported on a five-point scale.

1: Normal flora
2: Scanty or absent
3: *Trichomonas*
4: *Candida*
5: Other (cocci, coccobacilli, mixed bacteria)

In an effort to standardize reporting of cervical–vaginal cytologic specimens, the Bethesda System for reporting cervical–vaginal diagnoses was developed by a 1988 National Cancer Institute workshop. This reporting system is being adopted by numerous laboratories nationwide; it was slightly modified after a second workshop in 1991. The terminology of this reporting system appears in Table 11-1.

New Developments

Many new computerized technologies are being developed to aid in the manual screening of cervical–vaginal smears. Of note is the new screening system, PAPNET, which combines neural network and image processing technologies. This system may detect a few abnormal cells that may be difficult to detect when scattered among hundreds of thousands of normal cells. PAPNET is being used in some places as a quality control procedure to review smears that are classified as negative after manual screening.

Procedure

1. The patient is usually asked to remove clothing from the waist down.
2. The patient is placed in a lithotomy position on an examining table.
3. An appropriately sized bivalve speculum lubricated and warmed with only water is gently inserted into the vagina to expose the cervix.
4. The posterior fornix and external os of the cervix are scraped with a wooden spatula, and obtained material is spread on slides immediately and placed in preservative or fixative before air-drying can occur.
5. Label the specimen properly with name, date, age, reason for examination, last menstrual period, and area from which specimen is obtained and send to laboratory with a properly completed information sheet.
6. Examination takes only about 5 minutes.

NOTE: *The best time to take a PAP smear is 2 weeks after the first day of the last menstrual period and definitely not when the patient is menstruating.*

NOTE: *Cytologic specimens should be considered infectious until fixed with a germicidal fixative. Observe universal precautions when handling specimens from all patients.*

Procedure for Hormonal Smears, "Maturation Index"

Obtain a specimen by scraping the proximal portion of the lateral wall of the vagina, avoiding the cervical area. Otherwise the same as above.

Clinical Implications

1. Abnormal cytologic responses can be classified as protective, destructive, reparative (regenerative), or neoplastic.
2. Inflammatory reactions and microbes can be identified to help in the diagnosis of vaginal diseases.
3. Precancerous and cancerous lesions of the cervix can be identified. The stages of neoplastic disease can be arbitrarily classified as dysplasia (mild,

TABLE 11-1
The 1991 Bethesda System

ADEQUACY OF THE SPECIMEN

- Satisfactory for evaluation
- Satisfactory for evaluation but limited by (specify reason)
- Unsatisfactory for evaluation (specify reason)

GENERAL CATEGORIZATION (OPTIONAL)

- Within normal limits
- Benign cellular changes
- Epithelial cell abnormality

DESCRIPTIVE DIAGNOSES

Benign Cellular Changes

- Infection
  - *Trichomonas vaginalis*
  - Fungal organisms morphologically consistent with *Candida* spp.
  - Predominance of coccobacilli consistent with shift in vaginal flora
  - Bacteria morphologically consistent with *Actinomyces* spp.
  - Cellular changes associated with herpes simplex virus
  - Other
  - Reactive changes
  - Reactive cellular changes associated with
  - Inflammation (includes typical repair)
  - Atrophy with inflammation (atrophic vaginitis)
  - Radiation
  - Intrauterine contraceptive device (IUD)
  - Other

Epithelial Cell Abnormalities

- Squamous cell
  - Atypical squamous cells of undetermined significance: Qualify*
  - Low-grade squamous intraepithelial lesion encompassing: HPV mild dysplasia/CIN 1
  - High-grade squamous intraepithelial lesion encompassing:
  - Moderate and severe dysplasia, CIS/CIN 2 and CIN 3
  - Squamous cell carcinoma
- Glandular cell
  - Endometrial cells, cytologically benign, in a postmenopausal woman
  - Atypical glandular cells of undetermined significance: Qualify*
  - Endocervical adenocarcinoma
  - Endometrial adenocarcinoma
  - Extrauterine adenocarcinoma
  - Adenocarcinoma, NOS

Other Malignant Neoplasms: Specify

Hormonal Evaluation (applies to vaginal smears only)

- Hormonal pattern compatible with age and history
- Hormonal pattern incompatible with age and history: Specify
- Hormonal evaluation not possible due to: Specify reason

*Atypical squamous or glandular cells of undetermined significance should be further qualified as to whether a reactive or a premalignant process is favored.

Cellular changes of human papillomavirus (HPV) previously termed koilocytosis, koilocytotic atypia, or condylomatous atypia are included in the category of low-grade squamous cell intraepithelial lesion.

moderate, and severe), carcinoma in situ (preinvasive carcinoma), microinvasive carcinoma, and invasive carcinoma.

4. Hormonal cytologic reports will include several factors:
   a. Hormonal cell pattern: The report will state that the pattern is, or is not, compatible with the age and menstrual history of the patient. The reason for noncompatibility is given.
   b. Maturation index: Maturation index is a proportion of the major cell types (parabasal, intermediate, and superficial) in each 100 cells counted. The MI will be expressed as a ratio (eg, MI = 100/0/0). See *Normal Values* for representative MIs.
5. The following facts should be kept in mind when hormonal cytologic reports are reviewed (Table 11-2).
   a. The degree of maturity of the epithelium cannot be expressed in degrees of estrogenic effects or estrogen deficiencies because more than one hormonal stimulus is involved (estrogen, progesterone, and adrenal hormones).
   b. Surgical removal of the ovaries does not necessarily result in epithelial atrophy.
   c. Only two cell types can be identified with accuracy if the age and menstrual history of the patient are not known.
      (1) Abundant superficial squamous cells, indicative of unequivocal estrogenic effect
      (2) Parabasal cells, indicative of lack of cell maturation owing to lack of hormonal stimulation
   d. From a single specimen, it is impossible to predict whether ovulation will occur, whether it has recently occurred, or what stage of menstrual cycle the patient is in. Serial specimens must be examined to obtain the above results.
   e. An intermediate cell type is always intermediate, regardless of its size.
   f. No hormonal assessment should be made without knowing the age of the patient, her menstrual history, and her history of hormone administrations.

Clinical Alert

A cytobrush should **not** be used to obtain a cervical specimen on a pregnant patient.

Interfering Factors

1. Medications, such as tetracycline and digitalis, which affect the squamous epithelium, will alter test results.
2. The use of lubricating jelly in the vagina and recent douching will interfere with test results by distorting the cells and preventing accurate evaluation.

TABLE 11-2
Vaginal Cytologic Smear Findings in Gynecologic and Related Endocrinopathies

Condition	*Usual Smear Types*
Adrenal hyperplasia, congenital	Atrophic to atypical intermediate proliferation
Adrenogenital syndrome (hyperplasia)	Atrophic to atypical intermediate proliferation
Adrenal tumor (masculinizing)	Usually atrophic; sometimes "multihormonal" with cells from all layers
Chiari–Frommel syndrome	Markedly atrophic
Cushing's syndrome	Intermediate proliferation or atypical regressive types
Eunuchoidism, ovarian	Atrophic
Feminizing testicular syndrome	Proliferative; nuclear sex chromatin-negative
Follicular cytosis	Persistently high estrogen index (EI) and karyopyknotic index (KI)
Gonadal dysgenesis	Atrophic; nuclear sex chromatin-negative in 80%
Hirsutism, genetic	Normal cycling
Hypothalamic (psychogenic) amenorrhea	Most often atrophic to sight proliferation, but great variation from atrophic to highly proliferative
Menopausal syndrome	At first highly proliferative, some with cycling; later, intermediate proliferation or atrophic
Ovarian tumors, feminizing	Proliferative, some with high EI and KI, occasionally regressive
Ovarian tumors, masculinizing	Variation, many atrophic, some with atypical proliferation or "multihormonal"
Precocious puberty, constitutional	Proliferative, some with high EI and KI, some with cycling
Pituitary hypogonadism	Atrophic to slight proliferation
Pseudocyesis	"Progestational" types with varying regression
Stein–Leventhal syndrome	Variation; most with intermediate proliferation, occasionally highly proliferative
Uterine defect (congenital absence or irresponsiveness)	Normal cycling

(Adapted from Rakoff AI: Hormonal cytology in gynecology. Clin Obstet Gynecol 4:1045–1061, 1961.) In Keebler CM, Regan JW (eds): Manual of Cytotechnology, 7th ed, Chicago, American Society of Clinical Pathologists, 1993

3. The presence of infection will interfere with hormonal cytology.
4. Heavy menstrual flow may make the interpretation of the results difficult and may obscure atypical cells.

Patient Preparation

1. Explain the test purpose and procedure.
2. Instruct the patient not to douche for 2 to 3 days before the test because this may remove the exfoliated cells.
3. Instruct the patient not to use vaginal medication or vaginal contraceptives during the 48 hours before examination. Intercourse is not recommended the night before the examination.
4. Have the patient empty her bladder and rectum before examination.
5. Ask the patient to give the following information:
   - **a.** First day of last menstrual period
   - **b.** Use of hormone therapy or birth control pills
   - **c.** All medications taken
   - **d.** Any radiation therapy

This information must be sent to the laboratory along with specimens for cytology.

Patient Aftercare

Risks from the cervical–vaginal smear procedure are exceedingly rare. Patient should be asked to notify the doctor if any unusual pain or discharge occurs following the procedure. Give the patient a perineal pad after the procedure to absorb any bleeding.

CYTOLOGIC STUDY OF ASPIRATED BREAST CYSTS AND NIPPLE DISCHARGE ●

Normal Value

Negative for neoplasia.

Background

Nipple discharge is normal usually only during the lactation period. Any other nipple discharge is abnormal and, when it occurs, breasts should be examined for mastitis, duct papilloma, or intraductal cancer. (However, certain situations increase the possibility of finding a normal nipple discharge, such as pregnancy, perimenopause, and use of birth control pills.) About 3% of breast cancers and 10% of benign lesions of the breast are associated with abnormal nipple discharge.

The contents of all breast cysts obtained by needle biopsy are examined to detect malignant cells.

Procedure

BREAST CYST

The contents of the identified breast cyst are obtained by percutaneous aspiration. See page 746 for specific guidelines.

NIPPLE DISCHARGE

NOTE: *This procedure should be limited to patients who have no palpable masses in the breast or other evidence of breast cancer.*

1. The nipple should be washed with a cotton pledget and patted dry.
2. The nipple is gently stripped, or milked, to obtain a discharge.
3. Fluid should be expressed until a pea-sized drop appears.
4. The patient may assist by holding a bottle of fixative beneath the breast so that the slide may be dropped in immediately.
5. The discharge is spread immediately on a slide and then dropped into the fixative bottle containing 95% alcohol.
6. The specimen is identified with pertinent data, including from which breast it was obtained.
7. The specimen is sent without delay to the laboratory.

Clinical Implications

Abnormal results are helpful in identifying

1. Benign breast conditions, such as mastitis and intraductal papilloma
2. Malignant breast conditions, such as papilloma, intraductal cancer, or intracystic infiltrating cancer

Interfering Factors

Use of drugs that alter hormonal balance, such as phenothiazines, digitalis, diuretics, and steroids, often results in a clear nipple discharge.

Patient Preparation

1. Explain purpose and procedure.
2. Follow guidelines in Chapter 1 for safe, effective, informed *pretest* care.

Patient Aftercare

1. No special instructions are needed for care after nipple discharge procedure, as it is not an invasive procedure as are others in this chapter. Patient should be instructed to contact the doctor if pain or discharge occurs.
2. Follow guidelines in Chapter 1 for safe, effective, informed *posttest* care.

Clinical Alert

Any discharge, regardless of color, should be examined. A bloody or blood-tinged discharge is especially significant.

CYTOLOGIC STUDY OF URINE

Normal Value

Negative. Epithelial and squamous cells are normally present in urine. (See also Chap. 3, especially *Microscopic Examination of Sediment*.)

Explanation of Test

Cells from the epithelial lining of the urinary tract exfoliate readily into the urine. Urine cytologic evaluation is most useful in the diagnosis of cancer and inflammatory diseases of the bladder, the renal pelvis, the ureters, and the urethra. This study is also valuable in detecting cytomegalic inclusion disease and other viral diseases and in detecting bladder cancer in high-risk populations, such as workers exposed to aniline dyes, smokers, and patients previously treated for bladder cancer. A Papanicolaou stain of smears prepared from the urinary sediment, filter preparations, or cytocentrifuged smears is useful to identify abnormalities.

Procedure

1. Obtain a clean-voided urine specimen of at least 180 ml (adults) and 10 ml (children).
2. Obtain a catheterized specimen, if possible, when cancer is suspected.
3. Deliver the specimen immediately to the cytology laboratory. Urine should be as fresh as possible when it is examined. If a delay is expected, an equal volume of 50% alcohol may be added as a preservative.

Clinical Implications

1. Findings possibly indicative of *inflammatory conditions* of the *lower urinary tract* include
   a. Epithelial hyperplasia
   b. Atypical cells
   c. Abundance of red blood cells
   d. Leukocytes

   NOTE: *Inflammatory conditions could be due to any of the following: 1) benign prostatic hyperplasia; 2) adenocarcinoma of the prostate; 3) kidney stones; 4) diverticula of bladder; 5) strictures; 6) malformations.*

2. Findings indicative of viral diseases include:
   a. Cytomegalic inclusion disease: large intranuclear inclusions

   NOTE: *Cytomegalic inclusion disease is a viral infection that usually occurs in childhood but is also seen in cancer patients treated with chemotherapy and in transplant patients treated with immunosuppressives. The renal tubular epithelium is usually involved.*

      (1) Cytomegaloviruses or salivary gland viruses are related to the herpes–varicella agents.
      (2) Infected people may excrete virus in the urine or saliva for months.
      (3) About 60% to 90% of adults have experienced infection.
      (4) In closed populations, such as the mentally retarded or households, high infection rates may occur at an early age.

   b. Measles: Characteristic cytoplasmic inclusion bodies may be found in the urine preceding the appearance of Koplik's spots.

3. Findings possibly indicative of malacoplakia and granulomatous disease of the bladder or upper urinary tract
   a. Histiocytes with multiple granules in an abundant, foamy cytoplasm
   b. Michaelis–Gutmann bodies in malacoplakia
4. Cytologic findings possibly indicative of malignancy. If the specimen shows evidence of any of the changes associated with malignancy, cancer of the bladder, renal pelvis, ureters, kidney, and urethra may be suspected. Metastatic tumor should be ruled out as well.

Patient Preparation

1. Patient preparation depends on type of procedure being done. Explain the procedure, benefits, and risks to the patient.
2. If a cystoscopy is done, the patient will be given anesthesia (this may be general, spinal, or local anesthesia). Refer to Chapter 12 for cytoscopy care.
3. See Chapter 1 guidelines for safe, effective informed *pretest* care.

Patient Aftercare

1. Interpret test results and monitor appropriately. If a cystoscopy is performed, the patient should experience minimal discomfort following the procedure if it is performed gently and with adequate lubrication.
2. Complications may include mild dysuria and transient hematuria, but these should disappear within 48 hours after the procedure. The patient should be able to void normally after a routine cystoscopic examination.
3. Follow Chapter 1 guidelines for safe, effective, informed *posttest* care.

CYTOLOGIC STUDY OF CEREBROSPINAL FLUID (CSF) ●

Normal Values

1. Total cell count
   Adult: 0–10/mm^3 (all mononuclear cells)
   Infant: 0–20/mm^3
2. Negative for neoplasia.
3. A variety of normal cells may be seen. Large lymphocytes are most common. Small lymphocytes are also seen, as are elements of the monocyte–macrophage series.
4. The CSF of a healthy person should be free of all pathogens.

Explanation of Test

Spinal fluid obtained by lumbar puncture is examined for the presence of abnormal cells and for an increase or decrease in the normally present cell population. Most of the usual laboratory procedures for study of CSF involve an examination of the white cells and a white blood cell count; chemical and microbiologic studies are also done. In recent years, cell studies of the CSF have been used to identify neoplastic cells. These studies have been especially helpful in the diagnosis and treatment of the different phases of leukemia. The nature of neoplasia is such that for tumor cells to exfoliate, they must actually invade the CSF circulation and enter such areas as the ventricle wall, the choroid plexus, or the subarachnoid space.

Procedure

1. Usually, three specimens of at least 1 to 3 ml are obtained by lumbar puncture (see Chap. 5).
2. Generally, only one specimen of 1 to 3 ml goes to the cytology laboratory. Other tubes are sent to different laboratories for examination.
3. The specimen is labeled with the patient's name, date, and type of specimen.
4. The sample is immediately sent to the cytology laboratory for processing.

Clinical Alert

The laboratory should be given adequate warning that a CSF specimen will be delivered. Time is a critical factor; cells begin to disintegrate if the sample is kept at room temperature for more than 1 hour.

Clinical Implications

1. Cerebrospinal fluid abnormalities may indicate
   - **a.** Malignant gliomas that have invaded the ventricles or cortex of the brain: white blood cells (WBC)—150/mm^3 (The sample may be normal in 75% of patients.)
   - **b.** Ependymoma (neoplasm of differentiated ependymal cells) and medulloblastoma (a cerebellar tumor) in children
   - **c.** Seminoma and pineoblastoma (tumors of the pineal gland)
   - **d.** Secondary carcinomas
     - **(1)** Secondary carcinomas metastasizing to the central nervous system have multiple avenues to the subarachnoid space through the bloodstream.
     - **(2)** The breast and lung are common sources of metastatic cells exfoliated in the CSF. Infiltration of acute leukemia is also quite common.
   - **e.** Central nervous system leukemia
   - **f.** Fungal or sporozoan forms
     - **(1)** Congenital toxoplasmosis
       WBC: 50–500/mm^3 (mostly monocytes present)
     - **(2)** Coccidioidomycosis
       WBC: 200/mm^3
   - **g.** Various forms of meningitis
     - **(1)** Cryptococcal meningitis
       WBC: 800/mm^3 (lymphocytes are more abundant than polynuclear neutrophilic leukocytes)

(2) Tuberculous meningitis
WBC: 25–1000/mm^3 (mostly lymphocytes present)
(3) Acute pyogenic meningitis
WBC: 25–10,000/mm^3 (mostly polynuclear neutrophilic leukocytes present)

h. Meningoencephalitis (primary amebic meningoencephalitis)
(1) WBC: 400–21,000/mm^3
(2) Red blood cells are also found.
(3) Wright's stain may reveal amebas.

i. Hemosiderin-laden macrophages, as in subarachnoid hemorrhage

j. Lipophages from central nervous system destructive processes

2. Characteristics of neoplastic cells

a. Sometimes marked increase in size, most likely sarcoma and carcinomas

b. Exfoliated cells tend to be more polymorphic as the neoplasm becomes increasingly malignant.

Interfering Factors

The lumbar puncture can occasionally cause contamination of the specimen with squamous epithelial cells or spindly fibroblasts.

Patient Preparation

1. Explain the procedure to the patient (see Chap. 4). Instruct the patient that the procedure may be uncomfortable and immobilization is extremely important. The patient should be instructed to breathe normally; not to hold his or her breath. Provide the patient with physical and emotional support during the procedure.
2. See guidelines in Chapter 1 for safe, effective, informed *pretest* care.

Patient Aftercare

1. Patient should be placed in a supine position. Keep the head of the bed flat for 4 to 8 hours as ordered; if headache occurs, elevate feet 10° to 15° above head. Assist and teach patient to turn and deep breathe every 2 to 4 hours. Blood pressure, pulse, and respiration should be checked every 15 minutes for four times, then every hour for four times, then as ordered. Control pain as ordered and observe site of puncture for redness, swelling, or drainage, and report any symptoms to physician.
2. Interpret test outcomes and monitor appropriately.
3. Follow guidelines in Chapter 1 for safe, effective, and informed *posttest* care.

CYTOLOGIC STUDIES OF EFFUSIONS

Normal Value

Negative for abnormal cells.

Background

Effusions are accumulations of fluids. They may be *exudates*, which generally accumulate as a result of inflammation, or *transudates*, which are fluids not associated with inflammation. Below is a comparison of these two effusions.

Exudate	*Transudate*
1. Accumulates in body cavities and tissues because of malignancy or inflammation	**1.** Accumulates in body cavities from impaired circulation
2. Associated with an inflammatory process	**2.** Not associated with an inflammatory process
3. Viscous	**3.** Highly fluid
4. High content of protein, cells, and solid materials derived from cells	**4.** Low content of protein, cells, or solid material derived from cells
5. May have high WBC content	**5.** Has low WBC content
6. Clots spontaneously (because of high concentration of fibrinogen)	**6.** Will not clot
7. Malignant cells as well as bacteria may be detected	**7.** Malignant cells may be present
8. Specific gravity >1.015	**8.** Specific gravity <1.015

Fluid contained in the pleural, pericardial, and peritoneal or abdominal cavities is a serous fluid. Accumulation of fluid in the peritoneal cavity is called *ascites*.

Explanation of Test

Cytologic studies of effusions—either exudates or transudates—are helpful in determining the cause of these abnormal collections of fluids. The effusions are found in the pericardial sac, the pleural cavities, and the abdominal cavities. *The chief problem in diagnosis is in differentiating malignant cells from reactive mesothelial cells.*

Procedure

Material for cytologic examination of effusions is obtained by either thoracentesis or paracentesis. Both of these procedures involve surgical puncture of a cavity for aspiration of a fluid.

THORACENTESIS

1. Chest roentgenograms should be available at the patient's bedside so that the location of fluid may be determined.
2. The patient may be administered a sedative.

3. The chest is exposed. The physician inserts a long thoracentesis needle with a syringe attached.
4. At least 40 ml of fluid is withdrawn. It is preferable to withdraw 300 to 1000 ml of fluid.
5. The specimen is collected in a clean container and heparin may be added, particularly if the specimen is very bloody (5 to 10 units heparin per 1 ml of fluid). Alcohol should *not* be added.
6. The specimen should be labeled with the patient's name, date, source of the fluid, and diagnosis.
7. The covered specimen should be sent immediately to the laboratory. (If the specimen cannot be sent at once, it may be refrigerated.)

PARACENTESIS (ABDOMINAL)

1. The patient should be asked to void.
2. The patient is placed in the Fowler's position.
3. A local anesthetic is given.
4. A no. 20 needle is introduced into the patient's abdomen and the fluid is withdrawn, 50 ml at a time, until 300 ml to 1000 ml is withdrawn.
5. Follow the same procedure as in numbers 5, 6, and 7 of the foregoing for *Thoracentesis.*

Clinical Alert

Paracentesis may precipitate hepatic coma in a patient with chronic liver disease. The patient must be watched constantly for indications of shock: pallor, cyanosis, or dizziness. Emergency stimulants should be ready.

Clinical Implications

1. All effusions contain some mesothelial cells. (Mesothelial cells compose the squamous layer of the epithelium covering the surface of all serous membranes.) The more chronic and irritating the condition, the more numerous and atypical are the mesothelial cells. Histiocytes and lymphocytes are common.
2. Evidence of abnormalities in serous fluids is characterized by
   a. Degenerating red blood cells, granular red cell fragments, and histiocytes containing blood. Presence of these structures means that injury to a vessel or vessels is part of the condition causing fluid to accumulate.
   b. Mucin, which is suggestive of adenocarcinoma.
   c. Large numbers of polymorphonuclear leukocytes, which is indicative of an acute inflammatory process, such as peritonitis.

   d. Prevalence of plasma cells, which suggests the possibility of antibody formation.
   e. Numerous eosinophils, which suggests parasitic infestation, Hodgkin's disease, or a hypersensitive state.
   f. Presence of many reactive mesothelial cells together with hemosiderin histiocytes, which may indicate
      (1) Leaking aneurysm
      (2) Rheumatoid arthritis
      (3) Lupus erythematosus
   g. Malignant cells
3. Abnormal cells may be indicative of
   a. Malignancy: The most important criterion of cancer is the arrangement of chromatin within the nuclei.
   b. Inflammatory conditions

Interfering Factors

Vigorous shaking and stirring of specimens will cause altered results.

Patient Preparation

1. Explain the purpose of the test and the procedure. Procedure will vary depending on site of fluid accumulation. General patient preparation will include obtaining blood pressure, temperature, pulse, and respirations; administering sedation as ordered; preparing local anesthetic as ordered; providing emotional support; and obtaining a signed consent form.
2. Follow guidelines in Chapter 1 for safe, effective, informed *pretest* care.

Patient Aftercare

1. Monitor per agency protocols.
2. Check blood pressure, pulse, and respiration every 15 minutes for four times, then every 2 hours to 4 hours, and as ordered. Check temperature every 4 hours for 24 hours. Apply adhesive bandage or dressing to site of puncture. Check dressing every 15 to 30 minutes. Turn patient on unaffected side for 1 hour, then to position of comfort. Manage pain as indicated and measure and record total amount of fluid removed; note color and character.
3. See guidelines in Chapter 1 for safe, effective, informed *posttest* care.

CUTANEOUS IMMUNOFLUORESCENCE BIOPSY ●

Normal Values

A descriptive interpretative report is made.

Explanation of Test

Biopsy of the skin for direct epidermal fluorescent studies is indicated in the investigation of certain disorders, such as lupus erythematosus, blistering disease, and vasculitis. Skin biopsies are also used to confirm the histopathology of skin lesions, to rule out other diagnoses, and to follow the results of treatment.

Procedure

A 4-mm punch biopsy specimen of involved or uninvolved skin is obtained.

Clinical Implications

Biopsy of skin will show

1. The lesions of discoid lupus erythematosus as a bandlike immunofluorescence of immunoglobulins and complement components. Similar findings in a biopsy of normal skin are consistent with systemic lupus erythematosus and may be used to follow the results of treatment.
2. In blistering diseases such as pemphigus and pemphigoid; although circulating antibodies may not be present, a lesion may show intercellular epidermal antibody of pemphigus or basement membrane antibody of pemphigoid.

Patient Preparation

1. Explain purpose and procedure of skin biopsy.
2. Follow guidelines in Chapter 1 for safe, effective, informed *pretest* care.

Patient Aftercare

1. Monitor biopsy site for infection or bleeding.
2. See Chapter 1 guidelines for safe, effective, informed *posttest* care.

ESTRADIOL RECEPTOR AND PROGESTERONE RECEPTOR IN BREAST CANCER (ERA, PRA) ●

Normal Values

Estradiol: Negative; ≤3 femtomoles (fmol)/mg of protein
Progesterone: Negative; ≤10 fmol/mg of protein

Explanation of Test

Estrogen and progesterone receptors in the cells of breast cancer tissues are measured to determine whether a tumor is likely to respond to endocrine therapy or to the removal of the ovaries.

Procedure

A 1-g specimen of quickly frozen tumor is examined for saturation and expressed in a Scatchard plot. The specimen must **not** be placed in formalin. Some laboratories can perform ERA/PRA studies on paraffin-embedded tissue. Check with your laboratory for specific instructions.

Clinical Implications

1. Positive test for estrogen occurs at levels greater than 3 fmol and for progesterone binding at levels of 5 fmol and above.

2. Approximately 55% of estrogen receptor-*positive* tumors will respond to endocrine therapy.
3. Estrogen receptor-*negative* tumors rarely respond to endocrine therapy.
4. The finding of positive progesterone increases the predictive value of selecting patients for hormonal therapy. There is some evidence to suggest that progesterone receptor synthesis is estrogen dependent.

Patient Preparation

1. Explain purpose and procedure of testing to all persons being evaluated.
2. See Chapter 1 for safe, effective, informed *pretest* care.

Patient Aftercare

1. Interpret test outcomes and counsel about hormone therapy.
2. Follow Chapter 1 guidelines for safe, effective, informed *posttest* care.

STUDIES OF INHERITED DISORDERS: GENETIC STUDIES

OVERVIEW OF GENETIC STUDIES

Genetic testing determines the presence, absence, or activity of genes in cells. Genes are defined as the basic unit of heredity (Chart 11-1). Each gene has a specific place in a chromosome. With these tests, geneticists try to predict the course of a person's health state, especially if there is the possibility

CHART 11-1
Definitions

Gene: Basic unit of heredity; each gene occupies a certain location on a chromosome.

Chromosome: Linear thread in nucleus of every cell, contains DNA that transmits genetic information.

Genome: Complete set of chromosomes (entire genetic information) present in each cell.

DNA: Deoxyribonucleic acid is a complex protein consisting of adenine, guanine, thymine, and cytocine. Present in chromosomes and nuclei of all cells and is clinical basis of heredity.

RNA: Ribonucleic acid, a nucleic acid, controls protein synthesis in all cells of the body.

Ribosome: Contains ribonucleoprotein, synthesizes protein, receives genetic information and translates these instructions into protein.

of deviation from normal. Basic genetic technology counts chromosomes in a person's cells or measures the amount of specific gene-derived blood proteins. At the other end of the spectrum, cellular DNA is assayed with molecular probes to determine a specific genetic sequence among the 3 billion base pairs of genes that make up human DNA. Many disease states reflect hereditary components, even though general clinical studies usually focus on the specific disorder itself, rather than on its genetic component. This section will address those conditions that require information about genetic components to be diagnosed properly. Chromosomal studies, linkage studies, and direct detection of abnormal genes are common tests in this group.

Indications for Testing

1. *Genetic Counseling:* Specific genetic diagnostic studies of biologically related family members may be necessary to determine the risks and prognosis of disease. The test results could signal those people at special risk for genetically predisposed conditions.
2. *Prenatal care* (see Chap. 16): In some instances, psychological and medical management of a potential problem pregnancy may greatly improve outcomes. Serious fetal abnormalities may sometimes cause the parents to opt for termination of the pregnancy. Others individuals will choose to sustain pregnancy in spite of uncertain or potentially negative outcomes.
3. *Diagnosis:* Differential and presymptomatic studies may be done to diagnose certain diseases related to chromosomal or DNA studies in the unborn, in children, or in adults, and oncogene detection in the diagnosis of cancer.

Clinical Alert

1. Tests are not performed purely for information's sake; instead, they should be ordered for those conditions for which treatment is available. The best a predictive genetic test can offer is the degree of risk for acquiring the defect.
2. All tests should be linked to genetic counseling so that patients understand the results and their implications. In many cases, it is more comforting for patients to learn that they are from a high-risk family (no test done) than to try to interpret test results and have to hear "you have the gene, try not to let if affect your whole life."
3. The patient should be able to use test results to make informed decisions about issues such as childbearing and medical treatment.
4. Everyone is genetically defective to some degree. The majority of these defects, however, do not impair one's ability to function normally.
5. Family history is a major tool in identifying genetic disorders. Recognize and document dysmorphic features, growth problems, developmental delay, and adult mental retardation.

OVERVIEW OF CHROMOSOMES, GENES, AND DNA

Genetic information is coded within deoxyribonucleic acid (DNA), which is found in the chromosomes. Chromosomes are physical structures in the cell and the cell nucleus that can be directly, although not easily, observed. A chromosome is a gene holder. Each chromosome consists of many thousands of genes, which are considered to be smaller segments of DNA responsible for specific genetic traits. Genes are made up of strands of DNA.

Chromosomes and the genes they comprise are found in base pairs. Base pairs, the blueprint of coded information (genome) about how we should function, are in every single cell. This is why samples for DNA testing can come from anywhere in the body. These are the basic DNA concepts: DNA makes RNA; RNA makes ribosomes; ribosomes make protein; protein makes us what we are or tells us how to function. Proteins are of six different types: collagen, circulatory (eg, RBCs and WBCs), transport (eg, move substances in and out of cells as cholesterol), enzymes, immune system (eg, T and B cells), and hormones. There are 23 chromosomal pairs in each cell. One of each pair comes from the father and the other chromosome comes from the mother. Twenty-two of these pairs (the autosomes) are essentially identical. The twenty-third pair consists of the sex chromosomes. Women have two X chromosomes (XX) and males have one X and one Y chromosome (XY). The Y chromosome contains very few genes. These differences determine male or female development.

Single abnormal genes can generate a wide range of variations that manifest themselves in a certain way.

1. *Dominant inheritance:* A single copy of an abnormal gene can produce a disorder. An affected parent then has a 50% chance of transmitting this abnormal gene to any offspring. When the disorder is seen for the first time, it may be presumed that a new mutation has occurred in either the ovum or the sperm. For some conditions, manifestation of the disorder is not consistent. This then leads to speculation that *one* of the parents may have the abnormal gene in question. Examples of dominant inherited disorders include Huntington's chorea and neurofibromatosis.
2. *Recessive inheritance:* Both copies of the gene must be abnormal for the problem to be apparent. If both parents carry the same recessive gene, there is a 25% chance that their child will inherit two copies of the abnormal gene and will develop a problem. Cystic fibrosis and sickle cell disease are examples of recessive gene disorders.
3. *X-linked (sex-linked) inheritance:* Because males have only a single copy of the X chromosome genes, abnormalities of these genes will not be "covered up" by a second normal copy (as happens in females). When the female is a carrier, a 50% chance exists for any son to be affected by the disease or for any daughter to be a carrier of the disease. Examples of sex-linked disorders include hemophilia and Duchenne muscular dystrophy.
4. *Multifactorial inheritance:* This causes some defects through the interac-

tions of many genes with each other. Often these interactions are associated with environmental influences. Examples of multifactorial disorders are congenital dislocation of the hip and pyloric stenosis.

5. Genes are shared by members of a family. If one family member carries a gene for a disease, each of his or her parents, siblings, and offspring has a 50% chance of carrying the gene.

CHROMOSOMAL ANALYSIS ●

Normal Values

Women: 44 autosomes + 2 X chromosomes; karyotype: 46, XX

Men: 44 autosomes + 1 X chromosome and 1 Y chromosome; karyotype: 46, XY

Background

The karyotype, a study of chromosome distribution for an individual, determines chromosomal numbers and chromosomal structure. Alterations in either of these can produce problems. The standard karyotype can be a diagnostic precursor to genetic counseling. Additional or missing pieces of most chromosomal material causes developmental problems. Despite much speculation, we still do not know exactly how the abnormality translates into structural or functional anomalies. Predictions almost always depend on comparisons with clinical findings from other similar cases that present with the same evidence (Chart 11-2).

Explanation of Test

Standard chromosomal studies can be helpful in evaluation of the following clinical situations:

1. Multiple malformations of structure and function
2. Failure to thrive
3. Mental retardation
4. Ambiguous genitalia or hypogonadism
5. Recurrent miscarriages
6. Infertility
7. Primary amenorrhea or oligomenorrhea
8. Delayed onset of puberty
9. Stillbirths or miscarriages (particularly with associated malformations)
10. Prenatal diagnosis of potential or actual abnormalities related to chromosomal disorders (eg, Down syndrome, especially in mothers older than 35 years of age)
11. Detection of parents with chromosomal mosaicism or translocations who may be at high risk for transmitting genetic abnormalities to their children
12. Sex determination
13. Select cancers and leukemias in which abnormalities of the chromosomes may reveal prognosis or disease stage

CHART 11-2

Definition and Nomenclature of Karyotype

BACKGROUND

The karyotype is an arrangement of the cell chromosomes into a specific order from the largest size to the smallest size so that their number and structure can be analyzed. This is routinely done through banding, a technique that permits the appreciation of differences in structure between the different pairs. Before banding was developed, it was often impossible to group correct pairs of chromosomes; instead, they were arranged in groups according to size and structure and labeled A through G. The X chromosomes were part of group C, and the Y chromosomes belonged to group E. Now, they are usually placed with each other, apart from the other groups.

The different pairs of chromosomes are differentiated according to several of the following characteristics:

1. Their length.
2. The location of the centromere (the constriction that divides chromosomes into long {q} arms and short {p} arms.
3. Ratio of the long and short arms to each other.
4. Secondary constrictions.
5. Satellites, which are small variable pieces of DNA seen at the ends of some of the chromosomes.
6. Staining or banding patterns. A variety of different stains and techniques can be used. The most common is Giemsa banding. Most of the other methods, such as centromeric or fluorescent staining, are restricted to selected situations.

NOMENCLATURE OF THE KARYOTYPE

The standard conventions for listing karyotypes is as follows:

1. The first number denotes the total number of chromosomes.
2. Second, the sex chromosome complement follows (usually XX for normal females and XY for normal males).
3. Third, the missing, extra, or abnormal chromosomes are then identified.
4. The letter *p* refers to the short arm; *q* to the long arm.
5. Bands are numbered from the centromere out. As techniques evolved, these were further subdivided. For example, in the two-digit number 32, the first number (3) is the band and the second number (2) is the subdivision of that band (band 32). Decimal points indicate further division under the same system; for example (working backwards, 32.41 is the first subdivision (1) of the fourth subdivision (4) of the second subdivision of the third band.
6. A three-letter code at the end designates the banding technique. The first letter is the type of banding; the second letter denotes the general technique; the third letter indicates the stain. Probably the most common is GTG; band type G, by trypsin, using Giemsa stain. Special or unusual techniques are normally used only in very select circumstances.

(continued)

CHART 11-2 *(continued)*

More than 80 other abbreviations can be used to label other structural findings. Some of the more common ones are mentioned in clinical implications of chromosomal analyses.

Clinical Alert

1. Occasionally, it is possible to link a certain chromosomal pattern with specific genes and to then understand the clinical picture from analyzing these results. However, for the most part, the association between specific chromosomal abnormalities and specific sets of findings is not yet well understood. Interpretations from karyotype studies usually come from correlations with similar cases rather than from any theoretical considerations. Therefore, because many variables exist, predictions must be made cautiously and judiciously.
2. Most laboratories provide interpretations of results. However, it may be necessary to talk directly with laboratory personnel to fully understand the meaning of an unusual karyotype.

Procedure

Specimens for chromosomal analyses are generally obtained as follows:

1. Leukocytes from peripheral vascular blood samples are used most frequently because these are the most easily obtained. Preparation of the cells takes at least 3 days. Time is directly proportional to the complexity of the analytical process.
2. Bone marrow biopsies can sometimes be completed within 24 hours. However, the results are rarely as satisfactory as those obtained from leukocyte analysis. Bone marrow analysis is often done to diagnose certain categories of leukemias.
3. Fibroblasts from skin or other surgical specimens can be grown and preserved in long-term culture media for future studies. Growth of a sufficient amount of the specimen for studies usually requires at least a week. These specimens are especially helpful in detecting mosaicism (different chromosomal constitutions in different tissues).
4. Amniotic fluid obtained through amniocentesis requires at least a week to produce a sufficient amount of specimen for analysis. These studies are often done for prenatal detection of chromosomal abnormalities.
5. Chorionic villus sampling (CVS) can be done at earlier stages of preg-

nancy (about 9 weeks) than can amniocentesis. In fact, some initial CVS studies can be done almost immediately after conception. Occasional false-positive results represent mosaicism of the placenta (the presence of several cell lines, some of which may not be found in the fetus). These studies need confirmation of findings through long-term culture.

6. Cells may be grown from fetal tissue or from early-trimester products of conception to determine causes of spontaneous abortion. Cells from the fetal surface of the placenta may be the easiest to grow. However, these studies are not always successful.
7. The buccal smear, for detecting sex chromosomes, is taken from the inner cheek. However, this cell specimen is often inaccurate, especially in the newborn. However, it may be helpful to determine the presence or absence of the Y chromosome.

Clinical Implications

Many chromosomal abnormalities can be placed into one of the two following classes:

1. *Number of abnormalities*
   - **a.** Autosomes
     Trisomy 21 (Down syndrome)
     Trisomy 18
     Trisomy 13
   - **b.** Sex chromosomes
     Turner syndrome (single X)
     Klinefelter syndrome (XXY)
     XYY
     XXX
2. *Structure of abnormalities*
   - **a.** Deletions
     Cat-cry syndrome (5p–)
     18 p– (missing short arm of chromosome 18)
     Prader–Willi syndrome (15q– in some cases)
   - **b.** Duplications
     3q2 trisomy (extra material from the second band in the long arm of the third chromosome—Cornelia de Lange resemblance)
   - **c.** Translocations
     t (11;22): translocation of chromosomes 11 and 22
   - **d.** Isochromosomes
     i (Xq): a single chromosome with duplication of the long arms of the X chromosome; a variant of Turner syndrome
   - **e.** Ring chromosomes
     r (13): a chromosome 13 with the ends of the long and short arms joined together, as in a ring
   - **f.** Mosaicism
     46,XX/45,X: two cell lines, one normal female and the other for Turner syndrome

Patient Preparation

1. Some states require procurement of an informed, signed, and witnessed consent.
2. Explain purpose and procedure of the test together with known risks.
3. Provide information and referrals for appropriate genetic counseling, if necessary.
4. Follow Chapter 1 guidelines for safe, effective, informed *pretest* care.

Patient Aftercare

1. If an amniotic fluid specimen is obtained for analysis, follow same precautions as listed in Chapter 16.
2. Provide timely information and compassionate support and guidance for parents, children, and significant others.
3. See Chapter 1 for guidelines for safe, effective, informed *posttest* care.

The *Patient Preparation* and *Patient Aftercare* for chromosome testing are followed for all genetic testing in this section.

SPECIAL CHROMOSOMAL STUDIES

The fragile X syndrome is one of the most common genetic causes of mental retardation. An X-linked trait, it is most common in males. Females may carry this gene without exhibiting any of its characteristics; however, they also can be as severely affected as males. This syndrome takes its name from the small area on the long arm of the X chromosome that looks like a break in the arm (although it actually is not). The cells need to be grown in a special medium to reveal this pattern. A regular karyotype assay will miss it. Even with the special medium, not all cells will show the characteristic. In female carriers of this trait, the syndrome becomes harder to detect as the female ages.

Rare conditions, such as excess chromosomal breakage (Fanconi's anemia) or abnormal centromeres (Roberts' syndrome) merit special analytical processes and procedures.

DIRECT DETECTION OF ABNORMAL GENES BY DNA TESTING

Normal Values

Normal genes in chromosomes 1–22; X and Y normal chromosomes and genes.

Background

In the past, abnormal genes were indirectly detected by the effects they produced. These effects typically presented themselves as biochemical or physical manifestations. Now, it is possible to directly detect the specific sequence of DNA that causes an abnormality to occur. This technology relies on the ability to synthesize probes (pieces of DNA with specific sequences). Such probes hybridize with (attach to) specific complementary sequences and can be labeled for ease of detection. Probes manufactured for this purpose are called *allele specific oligonucleotides* (ASOs).

Sometimes detection of abnormal genes relies on the presence of what are termed as restriction sites. In this case, DNA can be "chopped" into pieces by the introduction of enzymes that attack specific sequences. The pieces that are formed depend on the presence of restriction sites (areas that have the requisite sequences). If only a few of these are present, the DNA pieces will usually be large. If there are only a few for a particular enzyme, they will be small.

Genes can contain several different DNA abnormalities. The bases that make up the genetic sequence may be changed. In some cases, they may be missing entirely, or in part, or may be partially duplicated. Any of these abnormalities can change the sequence at a restriction site. This means that sometimes a fragment will change in size because of a change in the DNA. When this happens, it provides a method for detecting a change in a gene. However, many changes that exist do not involve restriction sites, and so, cannot be detected by this method.

Explanation of Test

Genetic maps of the genetic traits for a variety of structural and functional abnormalities can be measured. The relation between genes and pathologic states is rarely simple. Almost all diseases are likely to have some genetic component (Chart 11-3). An international project is underway to identify and localize all of the genes in the human genome.

Procedure

Samples or specimens of body fluids or tissues are obtained.

Clinical Implications

1. Genes related to abnormal structure and function have been located in each of chromosomes; moreover, new ones are continually being discovered.

Chromosome Designation	*Known Number of Genes Related to Structural or Functional Abnormalities*
1	55
2	25
3	25
4	26
5	23
6	27
7	25
8	22
9	26
10	15

CHART 11-3
Genetic Disease: What Is It?*

Genetic disease is not a collection of syndromes.

62% of all pregnancy losses are due to genetic errors or causes; 50% of these are chromosomal errors that will not support life. First-trimester losses are due to genetic causes (often before pregnancy is known).

It is estimated that every person carries at least five genes that could cause illness with the wrong (environmental) circumstances or could adversely affect children. Spina bifida, cleft lip, congenital heart disease, pyloric stenosis, and clubfeet are common multifactoral diseases that are affected by environment.

No more than 3% of all genetic disease is caused by defects in a single gene (eg, sickle cell anemia) and none of these are major killers, such as heart disease or cancer. In cystic fibrosis (CF), more than 360 mutations have been linked to CF—yet it is not possible to firmly correlate the severity of the disease with different mutations. A positive test for CF does not foretell how severe the symptoms will be. On the other hand, a negative outcome can be misleading. All DNA tests need to be confirmed by biochemical tests and careful monitoring for signs and symptoms.

*Rules for what constitutes genetic disease are not clear-cut. Common adult-onset diseases are probably linked to multifactoral genes *and* environment (eg, hypertension, non–insulin-dependent diabetes, cancer, stroke, and major psychiatric illness).

Chromosome Designation	*Known Number of Genes Related to Structural or Functional Abnormalities*
11	46
12	23
13	13
14	19
15	17
17	26
18	9
19	25
20	14
21	8
22	17
X	112
Y	1

2. Precise DNA tests can be done for some diseases. These include phenylketonurea (PKU), hemophelia, thalessemia, polycystic kidneys, alpha-antitrypsin deficiency, paternity tests, forensic testing, and identification of microbes in infectious diseases.

NOTE: *See Chromosomal Analysis Patient Preparation and Aftercare.*

LINKAGE STUDIES

Explanation of Test

Specific genes have specific locations or loci (singular: locus) on chromosomes. It is sometimes possible to track an abnormal gene, otherwise undetectable by standard methods, by observing something located nearby that is transmitted along with the abnormal gene. Chromosomes can show harmless variations (polymorphisms) of their structure. These polymorphisms can sometimes help pinpoint the site of a certain gene on the chromosome. Similarly, other genes may be easily detected through their biochemical products, through physical findings, or by specific molecular probes.

Because chromosomes are specific physical structures, all genes present on a given chromosome should be transmitted as a single unit. Actually, because of the process of crossingover during formation of egg and sperm cells, there is some recombination between the two members of any chromosomal pair—a switching of material from one to another. Still, the more physically close any two genes are, the more likely it is that they will stay together or will be linked in transmission. Linkage studies are based on this fact. This means that, even if a gene cannot be identified directly, it may be possible to test for another gene in close proximity and to use that gene as a marker.

To illustrate this concept, this process is like trying to trace a package on a train going from coast to coast. All the baggage cars on the line may look alike; however, if it is known that there is a distinctive caboose on this train with the package, the caboose can be tracked and linked to the baggage car with the package. Of course, at each layover the cars may be switched onto other trains or tracks. If the cars right in front and right in back of the one with the package can be identified as the same as on the original train, it is unlikely that the package car would have been switched out by itself.

Basically then, flanking markers, one on each side of the gene, reduce the likelihood of undetected crossovers that might destroy the linkage. The closer the flankers are, and the more of them, the better the identification process. Calculations may be complex, but they can extrapolate the odds (in percentages) that the gene in question can be, or has been, passed on to offspring.

Again, it needs to be emphasized it is usually not enough just to know that gene A is linked to gene B. Which form of gene A is linked to which form of gene B in the individuals at risk becomes the crucial question.

Typically, this can be determined only through studies of those particular individuals.

Such studies, which may need input from extended families to clarify lines of linkage, can be laborious and time-consuming. Therefore, when necessary, the family unit should discuss their concerns with a medical geneticist or genetic counselor in an anticipation of becoming pregnant or as early in the pregnancy as possible.

Procedure

Obtain blood samples from those individuals to be studied.

Clinical Implications

1. Linkage studies are becoming more common as molecular study techniques evolve. Traditionally, these studies involved specific genes that were highly variable, such as from the blood groups or the immune response (HLA) genes. At other times, chromosomal studies were also helpful. This process has been greatly enhanced by the discovery of *restriction fragment length polymorphisms* (RFLP), a term often found in linkage reports. It has been discovered that certain areas of the DNA that constitutes the chromosomes are highly variable in structure and form (polymorphic). These variations affect the process by which that portion of DNA is separated into pieces by different types of enzymes. The length of the DNA fragments that result (longer or shorter) depends upon the sensitivity to different enzymes at different positions on the DNA strand. These can give the DNA characteristic "fingerprints" that become "markers" at different sites. Although the technology involved often differs from classic linkage studies, it is hoped that the results are the same.
2. Ideally, related testing techniques can be used to specifically detect certain gene disorders (eg, sickle cell anemia). These studies are more specific than linkage studies and may be done on one individual, if appropriate.

NOTE: *See Chromosomal Analysis Patient Preparation and Aftercare.*

BIBLIOGRAPHY

Andrews LB et al: Assessing Genetic Risks: Implications for Health and Social Policy. Washington, DC, National Academy Press, 1994

Beahrs OH, Myers MH (eds): Manual for Staging of Cancer, 4th ed. Philadelphia, JB Lippincott, 1992

Bibbo M (ed): Comprehensive Cytopathology. Philadelphia: WB Saunders, 1991

Cystic Fibrosis and DNA Tests: Implications of carrier screening. Congress of the United States, Office of Technology Assessment, Report OTA-BA 532, August 1992

Fiesor G et al: Enhancing cervical cancer detection using nucleic acid hybridization and acetic acid tests. Nurse Practitioner 7(26):29–30, July 1990

Keebler CM, Reagan JW (eds): Manual of Cytotechnology, 7th ed. Chicago, American Society of Clinical Pathologists, 1993

McCauly KM, Oi RH: Evaluating the Papanicolaou smear: Four possible colposcopic findings and corresponding management strategies, Part 2. Consultant, 29(1):36–42, January 1989

Molecular biology: Impact on human disease. Theme issue of FASEB Journal 6(10), July 1993

New Pap smear test may reduce false-negative readings. Nursing Health Care 15(2), February 1994

Rennee J: Trends in genetics. Grading the gene test. Scientific American pp. 88–97, June 1994

Rogers S: Bone biopsy in renal osteodystrophy. Journal of Pathology 171, 1993

Test-free or genetic information and insurance: Genetic information and insurance. National Institute of Health Group on Ethical, Legal, and Social Implications of Human Genome Research, 1993

The female patient: Total health care for women. Obstetrics Gynecology, March 1993

The Revised Bethesda System for Reporting Cervical/Vaginal Cytologic Diagnoses: Report of the 1991 Bethesda workshop. Acta Cytologic 36(3), May-June 1992

Watson A, Griffiths M: Cervicography: The nurse's role. Nursing Times 185(29): July 9, 1989

Wilkinson MM: Your role in needle biopsy of the liver. RN, August 1990

Wolberg WH, Tanner MA, Loh WL: Fine needle aspiration for breast mass diagnoses. Archives of Surgery 124:814–888, 1989

12

Endoscopic Studies

OVERVIEW OF ENDOSCOPIC STUDIES

Endoscopy is the general term given to the examination and inspection of body organs or cavities by means of endoscopes. These instruments can also provide access for certain kinds of surgical procedures or treatments. Endoscopes, known generally as *fiberoptic instruments,* are used for direct visual examination of certain internal body structures by means of a lighted lens system attached to either a rigid or flexible tube. Light travels through an optic fiber by means of multiple reflections. Fiberoptic instruments, composed of these fiber bundle systems, redirect and transmit light around twists and bends in cavities and hollow organs of the body. An image fiber and a light fiber allow visualization at the distal tip of the scope. A separate suction port allows instillation of drugs, lavage, and suction and insertion of brushes, forceps, or other instruments used for excision, sampling, or other diagnostic and therapeutic work. The fiberoptic scope can be inserted into orifices or other areas of the body not easily accessible or directly visualized by rigid scopes or other means. Procedures are done for diagnosis of pathologic conditions or for therapy, such as removal of tissue or of foreign objects. Local or general anesthetics may be used. Biopsy tissue is submitted to the laboratory for histologic examination.

This chapter includes discussions of the following procedures:

1. *Arthroscopy:* examination of joints
2. *Bronchoscopy:* visualization and examination of the trachea and bronchi
3. *Cervicography:* not an actual endoscopic examination but involves photography of the cervix; often done in conjunction with colposcopy
4. *Colonoscopy:* examination of the large intestine
5. *Colposcopy:* direct visualization of the vagina and cervix
6. *Cytoscopy:* visualization of the bladder, urethra, uteral orifices, and prostate (in men)
7. *Endoscopic retrograde cholangiopancreatography* (ERCP): visualization of pancreatic and bile ducts
8. *Esophageal manometry:* not an actual endoscopic examination; often done in conjunction with esophagogastroduodenoscopy; pressure readings evaluate esophageal muscle contraction
9. *Esophagogastroduodenoscopy (EGD) or gastroscopy:* visual examination of the upper gastrointestinal tract
10. *Mediastinoscopy:* examination or biopsy or both; of mediastinal lymph nodes
11. *Medical laparoscopy:* visualization of tissue of different abdominal organs, such as the liver and stomach
12. *Peritonoscopy:* visualization of uterus, fallopian tubes, and ovaries
13. *Proctoscopy, sigmoidoscopy, proctosigmoidoscopy:* visualization of the rectum and sigmoid colon
14. *Thoracoscopy:* examination of pleura, pleural spaces, mediastinum, and pericardium
15. *Urodynamic studies:* not an actual endoscopic examination; often done

in conjunction with cystoscopy; performed to study voiding patterns and to identify possible causes of incontinence

MEDIASTINOSCOPY

Normal Values

No evidence of disease; normal lymph glands.

Explanation of Test

This examination, performed under general anesthesia, requires insertion of a lighted mirror–lens instrument, similar to a bronchoscope, through an incision at the base of the anterior neck, to examine and biopsy mediastinal lymph nodes. Because these nodes receive lymphatic drainage from the lungs, mediastinal biopsies may identify such diseases as carcinoma, granulomatous infection, sarcoidosis, coccidioidomycosis, or histoplasmosis. Mediastinoscopy has virtually replaced scalene fat pad biopsy for suspicious nodes on the right side of the mediastinum. It is the routine method of establishing tissue diagnosis and of staging lung cancer and for evaluating the extent of lung tumor metastasis. Biopsies of nodes on the left side of the chest are usually taken through left anterior thoracotomy (mediastinotomy) or, occasionally, by scalene fat pad biopsy.

Procedure

1. Mediastinoscopy is considered a surgical procedure and is normally performed under general anesthesia.
2. The biopsy is done through a suprasternal incision.

Clinical Implications

1. Abnormal findings may include
   a. Sarcoidosis
   b. Tuberculosis
   c. Histoplasmosis
   d. Hodgkin's disease
   e. Granulomatous infections or inflammatory processes
   f. Carcinomatous lesions
   g. Coccidioidomycosis
   h. *Pneumocystis carinii* infection
2. Results assist in defining the extent of metastatic process.

Patient Preparation

1. Explain purpose of the test and the procedure the patient will experience.
2. A legal surgical consent form must be appropriately signed and witnessed preoperatively (see page 13, Chap. 1).
3. Preoperative care is the same as that for any patient having general anesthesia and surgery.
4. The patient must be NPO for 8 or more hours before the test.
5. See Chapter 1 guidelines for safe, effective, informed *pretest* care.

Patient Aftercare

Care is the same as for any patient who has had surgery and a general anesthetic.

1. Evaluate breathing and lung sounds; check wound for bleeding and hematoma.
2. Instruct patient to call physician if problems occur; many times this is done as an ambulatory surgical procedure.
3. Interpret test outcomes and monitor appropriately.
4. Follow Chapter 1 guidelines for safe, effective, informed *posttest* care.

> **Clinical Alert**
>
> 1. Previous mediastinoscopy contraindicates repeat examination because adhesions make satisfactory dissection of nodes extremely difficult or, sometimes, impossible.
> 2. Complications can result from the risks associated with general anesthesia or from preexisting conditions.

BRONCHOSCOPY

Normal Values

Normal trachea, bronchi, nasopharynx, pharynx, and select bronchioles (conventional bronchoscopy cannot visualize alveolar structures).

Explanation of Test

This test permits visualization of the trachea, bronchi, and select bronchioles with a flexible or, less frequently used, rigid bronchoscope. It is done to diagnose tumors, coin lesions, or granulomatous lesions; to find hemorrhage sites; to evaluate trauma or nerve paralysis; to biopsy; to take brushings for cytologic examinations; to improve drainage of secretions; to identify inflammatory infiltrates; or to lavage and remove foreign bodies. Bronchoscopy can determine resectability of a lesion as well as provide the means to diagnose bronchogenic carcinoma.

The examination is usually done under local anesthesia, combined with some form of sedation, in an outpatient setting, diagnostic center, or operating room. It also can be done in a critical care unit when the patient may be unresponsive or ventilator-dependent.

Procedure

1. A local anesthetic is sprayed and swabbed onto the back of the nose, the tongue, the pharynx, and the epiglottis. If the patient has a history of bronchospasms, steroids and aminophylline are frequently administered before the procedure.

2. The flexible or rigid bronchoscope is inserted carefully through the mouth or nose into the pharynx and the trachea. It also can be inserted through an endotracheal tube or tracheostomy. Suctioning, oxygen delivery, and biopsies are accomplished through bronchoscope ports designed for these purposes.
3. Because of sedation, usually with diazepam (Valium), midazolam (Versed), or meperidine (Demerol), the patient is normally comfortable. However, when the bronchoscope is advanced, some patients may feel they cannot breathe or are suffocating.

   NOTE: *Morphine sulfate is contraindicated in patients who have problems with bronchospasm or asthma because it can cause bronchospasm. Analgesics, barbiturates, tranquilizers–sedatives, and atropine may be ordered and administered one-half to 1 hour before bronchoscopy. The patient should be as relaxed as possible before and during the procedure but also needs to know that anxiety is normal. Therefore, the patient may need additional intravenous sedatives administered during the procedure. Refer to intravenous conscious sedation precautions in Appendix IV.*

4. An arterial blood gas measurement during and after bronchoscopy may be ordered, and arterial blood oxygen may remain altered for several hours after the procedure. Sputum specimens taken during and after bronchoscopy may be sent for cytologic examination or culture and sensitivity testing. These specimens must be handled and preserved according to institutional protocols.
5. Continuous pulse oximetry readings are routinely monitored and indicate levels of oxygen saturation before, during, and after the procedure.
6. The right lung, by convention, is normally examined before the left lung.

Clinical Implications

Abnormalities revealed through bronchoscopy include

1. Abscesses
2. Bronchitis
3. Carcinoma (right lung more than left)
4. Tumors (usually appear more often in larger bronchi)
5. Tuberculosis
6. Alveolitis
7. Evidence of surgical nonresectability (eg, involvement of tracheal wall by tumor growth, immobility of a main-stem bronchus, widening and fixation of the carina)
8. *Pneumocystis carinii* infection
9. Inflammatory processes
10. Cytomegalic inclusion virus infection
11. Aspergillosis
12. Idiopathic nonspecific pulmonary fibrosis
13. *Cryptococcus neoformans* infection
14. Coccidioidomycosis
15. Histoplasmosis
16. Blastomycosis
17. Phycomycosis

Clinical Considerations

The following data must be available before the procedure: history and physical examination, chest x-ray film (recent), recent arterial blood gas values, and electrocardiogram (ECG) if the patient is older than age 40 or has heart disease. Appropriate blood work, urinalysis, pulmonary function tests, and sputum studies (especially for acid-fast bacilli) must be done as well. Bronchoscopy is often done in the ambulatory surgical setting.

Patient Preparation

1. Reinforce information related to the purpose, procedure, benefits, and risks of the test.
2. Emphasize that pain is not usually experienced because lungs do not have pain fibers.
3. Explain that the local anesthetic may taste bitter, but numbness will occur in a few minutes. Feelings of a thickened tongue and the sensation of something in the back of the throat that cannot be coughed out or swallowed are not unusual. These sensations will pass within a few hours following the procedure as the anesthetic wears off.
4. An informed consent must be properly signed and witnessed (see p. 13, Chap. 1).
5. The patient must be NPO for at least 6 hours before the procedure to reduce the risk of aspiration. Gag, cough, and swallowing reflexes will be blocked during, and for a few hours after, surgery.
6. Wigs, nailpolish, makeup, dentures, jewelry, and contact lenses must be removed before the examination.
7. Use of relaxation techniques may help the patient relax and breathe more normally during the procedure. The more relaxed the patient, the easier it is to complete the procedure.
8. See Chapter 1 guidelines for safe, effective, informed *pretest* care.

Patient Aftercare

1. Usually the patient is NPO for at least 2 hours before the procedure. Be certain that swallow, gag, and cough reflexes are present before allowing food or liquids to be ingested orally.
2. Provide gargles to relieve mild pharyngitis. Monitor ECG, blood pressure, temperature, pulse, pulse oximeter readings, skin and nailbed color, lung sounds, and respiratory rate and patterns, according to institution protocols. Document observations.
3. Oxygen per mask or nasal cannula may be ordered. Humidified oxygen at specific concentrations up to 100% by mask may be necessary.
4. A chest x-ray film may be ordered to check for pneumothorax or to evaluate lungs.
5. Sputum specimens may be ordered. These must be preserved in the proper medium or solution.
6. The head of the bed may be elevated for comfort.

7. Interpret test outcomes and monitor appropriately.
8. See Chapter 1 guidelines for safe, effective, informed *posttest* care.
9. Provide written discharge instructions.

Contraindications to Bronchoscopy

Contraindications to bronchoscopy include

1. Severe hypoxemia
2. Severe hypocapnia (carbon dioxide retention)
3. Certain cardiac arrhythmias, cardiac states
4. History of being hepatitis B carrier
5. Bleeding or coagulation disorders
6. Severe tracheal stenosis

Clinical Alert

Observe for possible complications, which may include

1. Shock
2. Cardiac arrhythmias
3. Hypoxemia
4. Partial or complete laryngospasm (inspiratory stridor, a "crowing" sound); it may be necessary to intubate patient
5. Bronchospasm (pallor and increasing dyspnea are signs)
6. Infection or gram-negative bacterial sepsis
7. Pneumothorax
8. Respiratory failure
9. Bleeding following biopsy (rare, but can occur if there is excessive friability of airways, or massive lesions, or if patient is uremic or has hematologic disorders)
10. Anaphylactic reactions to drugs
11. Seizures
12. Febrile state
13. Hypoxia, respiratory distress
14. Empyema
15. Aspiration

Special Pediatric Considerations

Bronchoscopy instruments can decrease an already small airway lumen even more by causing inflammation and edema. Consequently, a child can rapidly become hypoxic and desaturate oxygen very quickly. Resuscitation, oxygen administration equipment, and drugs must be readily accessible. Close monitoring of respiratory and cardiac status is imperative after the procedure. The same precautions and treatment apply to the pediatric patient. Most children suffer cardiac arrest because of ***respiratory problems***—not cardiac problems.

THORACOSCOPY

Normal Values

Thoracic cavity and tissues are normal and free of disease.

Explanation of Test

Thoracoscopy is the examination of the thoracic cavity with an endoscope. This procedure is making a comeback because it can be used as a diagnostic device when other methods of diagnosis fail to present adequate and accurate findings. Moreover, many of the risks and discomfort associated with traditional diagnostic thoracotomy procedures are reduced. Thoracoscopy visualizes parietal and visceral pleura, pleural spaces, thoracic walls, the mediastinum, and the pericardium without the need for more extensive procedures. It can be used to perform biopsies; to perform laser procedures; and to assess tumor growth, pleural effusion, emphysema, inflammatory processes, and conditions predisposing to pneumothorax.

Procedure

1. Thoracoscopy is considered an operative procedure. The patient's state of health, the particular positioning needed, and the procedure itself determine the need for either local or general anesthesia.
2. Admission is frequently scheduled the morning of the procedure. Many patients are discharged the following day, provided the lung has reexpanded properly and chest tubes have been removed.

Clinical Implications

Abnormal findings can include

1. Carcinoma or metastasis of carcinoma
2. Empyema
3. Pleural effusion
4. Conditions predisposing to pneumothorax, ulcers
5. Inflammatory processes
6. Bleeding sites
7. Tuberculosis, coccidioidomycosis, histoplasmosis

Patient Preparation

1. Reinforce and explain the purpose of the examination and the procedure that the patient will experience.
2. The surgical consent form must be appropriately signed and witnessed before the procedure begins (see page 13, Chap. 1).
3. Required blood tests, urinalysis, recent chest x-ray film, and ECG (for certain individuals) must be completed and reviewed before the procedure.
4. The patient must be fasting for 8 hours before the procedure.
5. An intravenous line needs to be inserted for the administration of intraoperative intravenous fluids and intravenous medication. Refer to intravenous conscious sedation precautions in Appendix IV.
6. Skin preparation and correct positioning are done in the operating room.
7. After the actual thoracoscopy is completed, a chest tube is placed and connected to negative suction or sometimes to gravity drainage.
8. See Chapter 1 guidelines for safe, effective, informed *pretest* care.

Patient Aftercare

1. A postoperative chest x-ray film is taken to check for abnormal air or fluid in the chest cavity.
2. Monitor vital signs, amount and color of chest tube drainage, fluctuation of fluid in the chest tube, bubbling in the chest bottle, and respiratory status, including arterial blood gas values. Report abnormalities to the physician promptly.
3. Administer pain medication as necessary. Encourage relaxation exercises as a means to lessen the perception of pain. Monitor quality and rate of respirations. Be alert to possibility of respiratory depression related to narcotic administration or intrathecal narcotics.
4. Encourage frequent coughing and deep-breathing. Assist the patient to splint the incision to lessen discomfort. Promote leg exercises while in bed and assist with frequent ambulation if permitted.
5. Use open-ended questions to provide the opportunity to express concerns.
6. Document care accurately.
7. Interpret test outcomes and monitor appropriately.
8. Follow Chapter 1 guidelines for safe, effective, informed *posttest* care and provide written discharge instructions.

Clinical Alert

1. ***Do not clamp chest tubes unless specifically ordered to do so.*** Clamping them may cause a tension pneumothorax. Sudden onset of sharp pain, dyspnea, uneven chest wall movement, tachycardia, anxiety, and cyanosis may indicate pneumothorax. Notify physician STAT.
2. Possible complications include
   - **a.** Respiratory distress or hypoxia
   - **b.** Infection
   - **c.** Hemorrhage (watch for unusually large outputs of blood in a relatively short period into the chest bottle. Notify physician STAT).
   - **d.** Empyema
   - **e.** Atalectasis
   - **f.** Aspiration

ESOPHAGOGASTRODUODENOSCOPY (EGD); UGI; ENDOSCOPY; GASTROSCOPY

Normal Values

Upper gastrointestinal tract appearance is within normal limits.

Explanation of Test

Endoscopy is a general term for visual inspection of any body cavity with an endoscope. Endoscopic examination of the upper gastrointestinal tract (mouth to upper jejunum), therefore, may be referred to when the following examinations are ordered: panendoscopy, esophagoscopy, gastroscopy, duodenoscopy, esophagogastroscopy, or esophagogastroduodenoscopy.

An EGD allows visualization of the interior lumen of the upper gastrointestinal (GI) tract with a fiberoptic instrument designed for that purpose. Esophagogastroduodenoscopy is indicated for patients with dysphagia and weight loss, especially those with moderate to heavy alcohol and tobacco consumption. It can determine the cause of upper GI tract bleeding, can confirm suspicious x-ray study findings, can establish a diagnosis for a symptomatic patient with negative x-ray reports, can permit biopsy of upper GI tract lesions, and can confirm hiatal hernia or esophagitis. It can also differentiate a gastric ulcer as benign or malignant, or can be used as a follow-up examination for gastrectomy or other GI disturbances.

Procedure

1. This examination is usually performed in a gastrointestinal laboratory, in the operating room, or in critical care settings.
2. A spray anesthetizes the patient's throat.
3. An intravenous tranquilizer is often given before initiation of the procedure. The patient becomes relaxed and somewhat sleepy. A mouthpiece is inserted to prevent biting the endoscope and to prevent injury to the patient's teeth, tongue, or other oral structures.
4. The endoscope is then gently inserted through the mouthpiece into the esophagus and is advanced slowly into the stomach and duodenum. Air is insufflated through the scope to distend the area being examined so that optimal visualization of the mucosa may take place. Tissue biopsies and brushings for cytologic study may be obtained. Photographs may be taken to provide a permanent record of observations.
5. Sensations of pressure or bloating are normal, but there should be no actual pain.
6. Immediately after the examination is completed, the patient will be asked to relax and to remain lying on his or her side for a short time.

Clinical Implications

Abnormal results may indicate

1. Hemorrhagic areas or erosion of an artery or vein
2. Hiatal hernia
3. Esophagitis, gastritis
4. Neoplastic tissue
5. Gastric ulcers, either benign or malignant

Patient Preparation

1. Explain the purpose, procedure, sensations that may be experienced, and benefits and risks of the test. Refer to intravenous conscious sedation pre-

cautions in Appendix IV. Reassure the patient that the endoscope is thinner than most food swallowed. Inform the patient that they may be quite sleepy during the EGD and may not recall much of the experience.

2. Instruct the patient to be NPO for 8 hours before the examination. In the hospital, this restriction usually begins at midnight. Written instructions about fasting reinforce verbal instructions. An informed consent form must be signed and properly witnessed (see page 13, Chap 1).
3. Oral hygiene needs to be done before the procedure. Assist with oral care as necessary.
4. Encourage the patient to urinate and to defecate if possible before the examination.
5. See Chapter 1 guidelines for safe, effective, informed *pretest* care.

Patient Aftercare

1. No oral food or liquids are permitted for 2 hours (or longer if the patient cannot swallow).
2. Be certain the patient can swallow properly before offering liquids or food.
3. Check blood pressure, pulse, and respirations every 30 minutes for 2 hours.
4. A side-lying position with the side rails up and bed flat should be maintained until the sedative has worn off (usually about 2 hours). This position usually prevents aspiration in case of emesis.
5. Encourage the patient to belch so that air inserted into the stomach during the examination is expelled.
6. The patient should not experience discomfort or side effects once the sedative has worn off. Occasionally, a patient may complain of a slight sore throat. Sucking on lozenges after swallowing reflexes return may be helpful if these are permitted.
7. Interpret test outcomes and monitor appropriately.
8. Follow Chapter 1 guidelines for safe, effective, informed *posttest* care. Provide written discharge instructions.

Clinical Alert

Complications are rare. However, the following can occur

1. Perforation
2. Bleeding or hemorrhage
3. Local irritation
4. Drug reactions
5. Complications from unrelated diseases, such as myocardial infarction or cerebrovascular accident
6. Aspiration (bile aspiration can be a very serious complication)
7. Death (very rare)

ESOPHAGEAL MANOMETRY

Normal Values

Normal esophageal and stomach pressure readings.
Normal contractions; no acid reflux.

Explanation of Test

This procedure tests the esophagus for normal contractile activity and effectiveness of swallowing by measurement of pressures and acid sensors.

Indications for Testing

1. Abnormal esophageal muscle function
2. Difficulty in swallowing (dysphagia)
3. Heartburn
4. Chest pain of unknown cause
5. Regurgitation
6. Vomiting
7. Esophagitis

Other tests often done in conjunction with manometry include acid reflux tests and the Bernstein test (see later). These measurements are useful for evaluating heartburn, esophagitis, and chest pain of undetermined cause.

Procedure

1. A topical anesthetic is swabbed onto the nasal passage.
2. With the patient in a sitting position, a No. 8-lumen manometric catheter is passed through the nose and connected to an infusion pump, transducer, and recorder.
3. After the tube is passed, the patient lies supine for the remainder of the test.
4. Small amounts of water are then swallowed and pressure readings are taken.
5. *Acid reflux testing:* a second catheter is passed alongside the one already in place. This tube is actually a probe that is sensitive to acid. When the valve at the esophagogastric junction is not functioning properly, acid from the stomach backs up into the esophagus. The probe in the esophagus senses this acid.
6. *Bernstein testing:* Tests for acid reflux are by means of a nasogastric tube passed to a point 5-cm above the gastroesophageal junction. Concentrations of hydrochloric acid (0.1 N HCl) are infused for 10 minutes into the esophagus to reproduce symptoms of heartburn or chest discomfort. In the first 5 minutes of testing, 0.9% sodium chloride is infused as a control. Testing takes approximately 15 minutes. The patient may lie down or sit up.

Clinical Implications

Abnormal results reveal

1. Achalasia (failure of muscles, such as sphincters, to relax)
2. Esophageal spasm
3. Acid reflux

Patient Preparation

1. Explain the purpose, procedure, and benefits of the test.
2. The patient should be NPO for 6 hours before testing.
3. If the patient is diabetic, notify the testing department. Check with the patient's physician concerning insulin dosage, resumption of diet, or blood sugar testing.
4. See Chapter 1 guidelines for safe, effective, informed *pretest* care.

Patient Aftercare

1. Advise the patient that a sore throat and nasal passage irritation are common for 24 hours after the examination. Sensations of heartburn may also persist. Administer antacids if ordered.
2. Observe for or instruct patient to watch for nasal or GI bleeding or unusual pain.
3. Interpret test outcomes and counsel appropriately.
4. Follow Chapter 1 guidelines for safe, effective, informed *posttest* care. Provide written discharge instructions.

ENDOSCOPIC RETROGRADE CHOLANGIOPANCREATOGRAPHY (ERCP) AND MANOMETRY ●

Normal Values

Normal appearance and patent pancreatic ducts, hepatic ducts, common bile ducts, duodenal papilla (ampulla of Vater), and gallbladder (if persistent).

Manometry: normal pressure readings of bile and pancreatic ducts and sphincter of Oddi.

Explanation of Test

This examination of the hepatobiliary system is done through a side-viewing flexible fiberoptic endoscope by instillation of contrast medium into the duodenal papilla or ampulla of Vater. It is used to evaluate jaundice, pancreatitis, persistent abdominal pain, pancreatic tumors, common duct stones, or extra- and intrahepatic biliary tract disease, as well as malformation and strictures, and as a follow-up study in confirmed or suspected cases of pancreatic disease.

ERCP manometry can be done to obtain pressure readings in the bile duct, pancreatic duct, and sphincter of Oddi at the papilla. Measurements are obtained by a catheter that is inserted into the endoscope and placed within the sphincter zone.

Procedure

1. If barium x-ray films have been done before ERCP, a flat plate of the abdomen (KUB) should be done to check for barium. If barium is present, it will obscure views during ERCP. Screen for chest pain, shortness of breath, myocardial infarct, epigastric pain, bleeding, acute infections (including active hepatitis or pancreatitis). Debilitated patients may be more prone to complications. Fever or flulike symptoms may necessitate postponement of the procedure to a later date.

2. The patient gargles with, or has the throat sprayed with, a topical anesthetic.
3. An intravenous line is started and used for administration of sedatives such as meperidine, diazepam, or midazolam, as well as intravenous fluids and blood, if needed. The very ill patient often needs only a small dose of sedation. Resuscitation equipment must be available.
4. The patient assumes the left lateral position, knees flexed, while the endoscope is inserted into a mouthpiece, through the esophagus, to the duodenum. The mouthpiece also prevents the patient from biting down or injuring the mouth or lips. At this point, the patient assumes a prone position, with the left arm positioned behind.
5. Simethicone may be instilled to reduce bubbles from bile secretions. Glucagon or anticholinergics may be given intravenously to relax the duodenum so that the papilla can be cannulated. (Atropine increases the heart rate.)
6. A catheter is passed into the ampulla of Vater, and x-ray contrast dye is instilled through the cannula to outline the pancreatic and common bile ducts. Fluoroscopy and x-ray studies are done at this time.
7. Biopsies or cytologic brushings can be taken before the endoscope is removed.
8. The patient's vital signs, ECG, and oxygen saturation (pulse oximetry) should be monitored frequently throughout the procedure.
9. Side effects and drug allergic reactions (diaphoresis, pallor, restlessness, hypotension) need to be monitored.

Clinical Implications

Abnormal results reveal stones, stenoses, and other abnormalities that are indicative of

1. Biliary cirrhosis
2. Primary sclerosing cholangitis
3. Cancer of bile ducts
4. Pancreatic cysts
5. Pseudocysts
6. Pancreatic tumors
7. Cancer of the head of pancreas
8. Chronic pancreatitis
9. Pancreatic fibrosis
10. Cancer of duodenal papilla
11. Papillary stenosis

Patient Preparation

1. Explain the purpose, procedure, benefits, and risks of the test. If this is an outpatient procedure, the patient should arrange for a ride home and should leave all valuables at home. Blood work, urinalysis, x-ray films, and scans should be reviewed and charted before the procedure. Record baseline vital signs.
2. An informed consent form must be signed and properly witnessed (see page 13, Chap. 1).
3. Nothing by mouth for 12 hours before the ERCP is required.
4. Inform the patient that she or he:

   a. Should swallow when requested to do so (prevents damage to the oral pharynx)
   b. May experience a choking sensation
   c. Will have to lie quietly during the time x-ray films are taken
   d. Should breathe deeply to relieve gagging
   e. Will be suctioned to clear secretions
5. Refer to intravenous conscious sedation precautions in Appendix IV.
6. See Chapter 1 guidelines for safe, effective, informed *pretest* care.

Patient Aftercare

1. Check vital signs, including temperature, according to protocols.
2. Do not give oral food or fluids for at least 2 hours after the procedure or until the gag reflex returns, and the patient can swallow properly.
3. Observe the patient for signs of complications, such as urinary retention, cholangitis, or pancreatitis. Check for temperature elevation; may be the first sign of inflammation.
4. Monitor for respiratory and central nervous system depression from narcotics (naloxone may be used to reverse narcotic effects and romazicon is used for reversing diazepamlike drugs).
5. Explain that some abdominal discomfort may be present for several hours after the procedure.
6. Drowsiness may last up to 24 hours. The patient should not perform any tasks that require mental alertness, and legal documents should not be signed during this time.
7. A sore throat can be relieved by gargles, ice chips, fluids, or lozenges if permitted.
8. Notify physician of
   a. Prolonged, sharp abdominal pain, abnormal weakness, faintness
   b. Fever
   c. Nausea or vomiting
9. Interpret test outcomes and counsel appropriately.
10. Follow Chapter 1 guidelines for safe, effective, informed *posttest* care. Provide written discharge instructions.

COLPOSCOPY ●

Normal Values

Normal vaginal, cervical, and genital areas.

Explanation of Test

Colposcopy permits examination of the vagina and cervix with the colposcope, an instrument with a magnifying lens. The colposcope is also used to examine male genital lesions suspected in sexually transmitted diseases, condylomata, or human papillomavirus infection. Indications for this procedure include abnormal Papanicolaou (PAP) smear or other cervical lesions. This examination aids the diagnosis of benign, precancerous, leukoplakia, and other cancerous lesions. Biopsies and cell scrapings are done under direct visualization. Colposcopy is also valuable for assessing women with a history of exposure to diethylstilbestrol.

Advantages of colposcopy include

1. Lesions can be localized and their extent determined.
2. Inflammatory processes can be differentiated from neoplasia.
3. Invasive or noninvasive disease processes can be differentiated.

Colposcopy *cannot* readily detect endocervical lesions. Cervicitis and other changes can produce abnormal findings. When combined with findings from PAP smears, colposcopy can be a means of enhancing diagnostic accuracy. (See Tables 12–1 and 12–2 concerning correlation of findings and advantages and disadvantages of PAP smears and colposcopy; see Chap. 11, page 758 for PAP smear procedure.)

Whitish areas of epithelium (leukoplakia), mosaic staining patterns, irregular blood vasculature, hyperkeratosis, and other abnormal-appearing tissues show up on colposcopy. Leukoplakia vulvae is a precancerous condition characterized by white to grayish infiltrated patches on the vulvar mucosa. The colposcope has a definite advantage for detecting atypical epithelium, designated in the literature as *basal cell activity*. Atypical epithelium cannot be called benign and, yet, does not fulfill all criteria for carcinoma in situ. Its early detection promotes cancer prophylaxis.

Patients receiving colposcopy may often be spared having to undergo surgical conization (the removal of a cone of tissue from the cervix).

Procedure

1. With the patient in a lithotomy position, the vagina and cervix are exposed with a speculum after the internal and external genitalia have been carefully examined. A PAP smear is obtained at this time. No part of the colposcope is inserted into the vagina.
2. The cervix and vagina are then swabbed with 3% acetic acid as needed during the procedure to improve visibility of epithelial tissues (precipitates nuclear proteins within the cells). The cervical mucus must be completely removed. Do not use cotton-wool swabs because fibers left on the cervix may interfere with proper visualization.
3. Actual visualization with the colposcope begins with a field of white light and lower magnification to focus on sites of white epithelium or irregular cervical contours. The light is then switched to a green filter for magnification of vascular changes.
   a. Suspicious lesions are diagrammed, and photographs are taken for the permanent healthcare record.
   b. The transformation zone and squamocolumnar junction (where squamous epithelium meets columnar epithelium of the cervix) are areas where many women exhibit atypical cells. It is imperative that these zones be visualized completely, especially in older women, because of changes associated with aging.

TABLE 12-1
Correlation of Colposcopic and Histologic Findings

Colposcopic Term	*Colposcopic Appearance*	*Histologic Correlate*
Original squamous epithelium	Smooth, pink; indefinitely outlined vessels; no change after application of acetic acid	Squamous epithelium
Columnar epithelium	Grapelike structures after application of acetic acid	Columnar epithelium
Transformation zone	Tongues of squamous metaplasia; gland openings; nabothian cysts	Metaplastic squamous epithelium
White epithelium	White, sharp-bordered lesion visible only after application of acetic acid; no vessels visible	From minimal dysplasia to carcinoma in situ
Punctation	Sharp-bordered lesion; red stippling; epithelium whiter after application of acetic acid	From minimal dysplasia to carcinoma in situ
Mosaic	Sharp-bordered lesion, mosaic pattern; epithelium whiter after application of acetic acid	From minimal dysplasia to carcinoma in situ
Hyperkeratosis	White patch; rough surface; already visible before application of acetic acid	Usually hyperkeratosis or parakeratosis; seldom carcinoma in situ or invasive disease
Atypical vessel	Horizontal vessels running parallel to surface; constrictions and dilations of vessels; atypical branching, winding course	From carcinoma in situ to invasive carcinoma

4. Biopsies of the lesions are done with a fine biopsy forceps. Some patients note discomfort at this time.

a. Endocervical curettage ***must*** be performed before colposcope-directed biopsy so that epithelial fragments dislodged during colposcopy do not cause false-positive results in the endocervical curettage. Endocervical curettage biopsy samples should be placed in formalin.

TABLE 12-2
Pros and Cons of Colposcopy and Cytology

Advantages	*Disadvantages*
COLPOSCOPY	
Localizes lesion	Inadequate for detection of endocervical lesions
Evaluates extent of lesion	More intensive training is necessary
Differentiates between inflammatory atypia and neoplasia	Cervicitis and regenerative changes may produce abnormal findings
Differentiates between invasive and noninvasive cervical lesions	
Enables follow-up	
CYTOLOGY	
Ideal for mass screening	Cannot localize lesion
Economical	Inflammation, atrophic changes, or folic acid deficiency may produce suspicious changes
Specimen can be obtained by most healthcare personnel	Many steps between patient and cytopathologist allow misdiagnosis
Detects lesion in endocervical canal	Value of single smear is limited
Detects endocervical and endometrial carcinoma	False-negative rate is 5%–10%
High correlation with biopsy material (>90%)	

b. Sterile saline or sterile water should be used to rinse acetic acid from the vaginal area to prevent burning or irritation. Bleeding can be stopped by applying toughened silver nitrate cautery sticks or ferric subsulfate (Monsel's solution).

5. A small amount of vaginal bleeding or cramping for a few hours is not abnormal.

6. A paracervical block may be necessary for those patients who are extremely anxious.

Clinical Implications

Abnormal lesions or unusual epithelial patterns include the following

1. Leukoplakia
2. Abnormal blood vessels
3. Slight-to-moderate to marked dysplasia
4. Punctation (sharp borders, red stippling, epithelium whiter with acetic acid)
5. Mosaic (sharp borders, mosaic pattern, epithelium whiter after acetic acid)
6. Hyperkeratosis (white, rough, visible without acetic acid)

Patient Preparation

1. Explain purpose and test procedure.
2. See Chapter 1 guidelines regarding safe, effective, informed *pretest* care.

Clinical Alert

1. Patients may experience a vasovagal response. Watch for bradycardia and hypotension and treat accordingly. Have the patient sit for a short while before standing.
2. Anti-inflammatory agents, such as ibuprofen, may relieve cramping.
3. Cervical scars from previous events may prevent satisfactory visualization.
4. Complications may include heavy bleeding, infection, or pelvic inflammatory disease.
5. Development of cervical changes and potential cervical carcinoma pose a greater risk for these patients. An annual PAP smear is mandatory.

Patient Aftercare

1. Instruct the patient to abstain from sexual intercourse and to not insert anything into the vagina for 2 to 7 days (per the physician's orders) after the procedure.
2. Excessive bleeding, pain, fever, or abnormal vaginal discharge should be reported immediately.
3. Interpret test outcomes and counsel appropriately about follow-up treatment.
4. Follow Chapter 1 guidelines for safe, effective, informed *posttest* care. Provide written discharge instructions.

CERVICOGRAPHY

Cervicography may be done in conjunction with colposcopy or by itself. A photographic method records an image of the entire cervix. The patient assumes a lithotomy position, and the cervix is exposed with speculum. After the mucus is removed, 5% acetic acid is swabbed on the area for a few minutes. Photographs of the cervix are then taken with a specially designed 35-mm camera. Following this, aqueous iodine is swabbed on the cervix and another picture is taken. Finally, an endocervical smear is taken and transferred onto a slide for later evaluation. The patient should be told that brown vaginal discharge (from the iodine) for a few days is not unusual.

The photographs are processed into slides (cervigrams) that allow the entire cervix to be visible on one slide. It can provide evidence for colposcopic consultations. Moreover, the cervigram can be done in conjunction with a routine gynecologic examination. It is more sensitive to the early detection of cervical intraepithelial neoplasia and invasive cervical cancer than is the PAP smear.

FLEXIBLE PROCTOSCOPY; SIGMOIDOSCOPY; PROCTOSIGMOIDOSCOPY

Normal Values

Normal anal canal, rectal, and sigmoid colon mucosa.

Explanation of Test

These tests involve the examination of an approximate 25-cm area of the rectum and sigmoid with a proctosigmoidoscope. Rigid scopes are not as commonly used since the advent of flexible fiberoptic instruments. Flexible proctosigmoidoscopes are tubes usually measuring 60 cm in length. They incorporate a lighted lens system for illuminating the rectum and sigmoid. Their main use is the detection and diagnosis of cancers and other abnormalities such as diverticula in this area of the GI tract. These examinations should be routine for cancer screening of individuals older than the age of 50 (every 3 to 5 years).

These tests can also evaluate hemorrhoids, polyps, blood or mucus in the stool, unexplained anemia, and other bowel conditions.

Procedure

1. For rigid proctoscopy, the patient assumes a knee-to-chest position. When the flexible proctoscope is used, the patient must be in the left lateral position. The proctoscope or sigmoidoscope is then carefully inserted into the rectum.
2. The examination can be done with the patient in bed or positioned on a special tilt table.
3. The patient may feel a very strong urge to defecate and may experience a feeling of bloating or cramping. These sensations are normal.

Clinical Implications

1. Examination may reveal the following: edematous, red, or denuded mucosa; granularity; friability; ulcers, polyps; cysts; thickened areas; changes in vascular pattern; pseudomembranes; spontaneous bleeding; or normal mucosa. These findings may help confirm or rule out the following conditions:
   a. Inflammatory bowel disease
      (1) Chronic ulcerative colitis
      (2) Crohn's disease
      (3) Proctitis (acute and chronic)
      (4) Psuedomembranous colitis
      (5) Antibiotic-associated colitis
   b. Polyps
      (1) Adenomatou
      (2) Familial
      (3) Diminutive

c. Cancer and tumors
   (1) Adenocarcinoma
   (2) Carcinoids
   (3) Other tumors such as lipomas
d. Anal and perianal conditions
   (1) Hemorrhoids
   (2) Abscesses and fistulas
   (3) Strictures and stenoses
   (4) Rectal prolapse
   (5) Fissures
   (6) Contractures

Patient Preparation

1. Explain the test purpose and the procedure that the patient will experience.
2. No need to fast. However, a restricted diet the evening before the test may be allowed. Diabetic patients may need to check with their physician about diet and insulin regimens.
3. Laxatives and enemas may be taken the night before the examination. Enemas or a rectal laxative suppository may be administered the morning of the procedure. For all ages, one or two phosphate ("Fleet") enemas are frequently ordered to be taken about 1 to 2 hours before the examination. This is considered ample preparation by many endoscopy departments.
4. See Chapter 1 guidelines for safe, effective, informed *pretest* care.

> **Clinical Alert**
>
> 1. Patients with acute symptoms, particularly those individuals with suspected ulcerative or granulomatous colitis, should be examined *without* any preparation (without enemas, laxatives, or suppositories).
> 2. Perforation of the intestinal wall can be an infrequent complication of these tests.
> 3. Notify the patient's physician before administering laxatives or enemas to a pregnant woman.

Patient Aftercare

1. Interpret test outcomes, monitor, and counsel about anal, rectal, and sigmoid abnormalities.
2. Follow Chapter 1 guidelines for safe, effective, informed *posttest* care. Provide written discharge instructions.

COLONOSCOPY

Normal Values

Normal-appearing large-intestine mucosa.

Explanation of Test

Colonoscopy visualizes, examines, and photographs the large intestine with a flexible fiberoptic or video colonoscope inserted through the anus and advanced to the ileocecal valve. Air introduced through an accessory channel of the colonoscope distends the intestinal walls to enhance visualization. This technique can differentiate inflammatory disease from neoplastic disease or can evaluate polypoid lesions beyond the reach of the sigmoidoscope. Suture lines and anastomoses can be checked. Polyps, foreign bodies, and biopsy specimens can be removed through the colonoscope. Photographs of the large intestine lumen also can be taken. Before colonoscopy was available, major abdominal surgery was the only way to remove polyps or suspicious tissue to determine malignancy or nonmalignancy. Periodic colonoscopy is a valuable adjunct to the follow-up of persons with previous polyps, colon cancer, family history of colon cancer, or high-risk factors.

Clinical Implications

Abnormal findings may reveal

1. Polyps
2. Tumors, benign or malignant
3. Areas of ulceration
4. Inflammation
5. Colitis, diverticula
6. Bleeding sites
7. Strictures
8. Discovery and removal of foreign bodies

Procedure

1. A clear, liquid diet is usually ordered for 48 to 72 hours before the examination. The patient must fast for 8 hours before the actual procedure. Laxatives may be ordered to be taken for 1 to 3 days before the test; enemas may be ordered to be given the night before. To be effective, a purgative must produce fluid diarrhea. This shows that unaltered small intestinal contents are emerging and colonic residue has been cleared. Enemas must be repeated until solid matter is no longer expelled (white "clear"). Soapsuds enemas are contraindicated because they cause increased mucous secretion because of irritant stimulation.
2. Another common form of bowel preparation involves the ingestion of an oral saline isoosmotic and isotonic (relative to bowel contents) laxative. This washout solution may contain a number of salts, such as potassium chloride, sodium chloride, bicarbonate; an additive, such as polyethylene glycol; and distilled or deionized water. The glycol acts as an osmotic agent, so there is no net ion absorption or loss; water and electrolyte balances should not change significantly. The patient drinks 3 to 6 L of the prescribed solution over a 2- to 3 1/2-hour period. The typical volume taken is 1 gallon. It can be administered by nasogastric tube if necessary. This laxative acts quickly. Initial results can be expected in 30 minutes to 1 hour. Ingestion of the washout solution continues until feces is clear

liquid. However, the physician should be notified before administering more than 6 L of this solution. No special diet, laxative, or enemas are required with this method. However, patients with congestive heart failure or renal failure may be at great risk for fluid volume overload if this preparation is used.

3. The colonoscopy is done under analgesia by using combinations of medications such as meperidine hydrochloride (Demerol), diazepam (Valium), or midazolam (Versed). The patient should be responsive enough to inform the doctor of any subjective reactions during the examination. Refer to conscious sedation precautions in Appendix IV.
4. Occasionally, intravenous anticholinergics and glucagon may be used to relax bowel spasms.
5. The patient assumes the left side or Sim's position and is draped properly. A well-lubricated colonoscope is inserted approximately 12 cm into the bowel. The patient should take deep breaths through the mouth during this time. Air is then introduced into the bowel through the special port on the colonoscope to aid viewing. As the colonoscope advances, the patient may need to be repositioned several times to aid visualization of the colon. Sensations of pressure, mild pain, or cramping are not unusual.
6. The best views are obtained during withdrawal of the colonoscope. Therefore, a more detailed examination is usually performed during its withdrawal.

Clinical Considerations

1. Keep colon electrolyte lavage preparations refrigerated. However, the patient may drink the solution at room temperature. Use within 48 hours. Discard unused portions.
2. Before testing, a complete blood count, prothrombin time, platelet count, and thromboplastin time results should be reviewed and charted.
3. Preparation for patients with a colostomy or who are paralyzed is the same. They will usually receive at least 4 L of oral preparative solution.
4. Persons with known heart disease should receive prescribed antibiotics before testing.
5. Patients should not mix or drink anything with the washout preparation. Do not add ice or glucose to the solution.

Patient Preparation

1. Explain the purpose, procedure, benefits, and risks of the test. When ordered, one 12-ounce glass of liquid preparation is to be taken every 10 minutes. (Each gallon holds 10.7 twelve-ounce glasses.) The entire gallon should be taken in 2 hours, if possible. Timing is important. Slower drinking does not clean the colon properly.
2. Some patients will be receiving a clear liquid diet for 72 hours before the test; then NPO, except for medications, after a clear liquid supper the evening before the test.

3. Administer purgatives and cleaning enemas as ordered. Preparation is complete when fecal discharge is clear. If returns are not clear after 4 L of solution has been ingested, continue until returns are clear (up to *6 L total*). (See previous note, under "Procedure.")
4. A legal consent form must be signed and properly witnessed (see Chap. 1) after patient has received proper instruction about the test.
5. Iron preparations should be discontinued 3 or 4 days before the examination because iron residues produce an inky, black, sticky stool that interferes with visualization. Also, the stool can be viscous and difficult to clear. Aspirin and aspirin-containing products should also be discontinued 1 week before the examination because of the bleeding problems or localized hemorrhages they may cause.
6. Some protocols call for a functional intravenous line to be in place. Refer to intravenous conscious sedation precautions in Appendix IV.
7. Persons with valvular heart disease need antibiotics before the test.
8. Take baseline vital signs.
9. See Chapter 1 guidelines for safe, effective, informed *pretest* care.

Patient Aftercare

1. The patient should remain NPO for 2 hours after the examination.
2. Stools should be observed for visible bleeding. The patient should be instructed to report abdominal pain or other unusual symptoms because perforation and hemorrhage are possible complications.
3. Vital signs should be checked frequently for 2 hours after the procedure.
4. Most frequent adverse reactions to oral purgatives include nausea, vomiting, bloating, rectal irritation, chills, and feelings of weakness.
5. The patient may expel large amounts of flatus after the procedure.
6. Interpret test outcomes and counsel appropriately.
7. Follow Chapter 1 guidelines for safe, effective, informed *posttest* care. Provide written discharge instructions.

Clinical Alert

1. Solid food should never be taken less than 2 hours before the oral cleansing regimen is begun.
2. Orally administered colon lavage is contraindicated in
   - **a.** Actual or suspected ulcers
   - **b.** Gastric outlet obstruction
   - **c.** Weight less than 20 kg
   - **d.** Toxic colitis
   - **e.** Megacolon
3. Relative contraindications for colonoscopy include
   - **a.** Perforating disease for the colon

(continued)

(Clinical Alert continued)

- **b.** Peritonitis
- **c.** Radiation enteritis
- **d.** Recent abdominal or bowel surgery
- **e.** Acute conditions of the anus and rectum
- **f.** Serious cardiac or respiratory problems (such as recent myocardial infarction)
- **g.** Situations in which the bowel cannot be adequately prepared for the procedure.

4. Observe for possible complications, including
- **a.** Perforations
- **b.** Hypotensive episodes
- **c.** Cardiac or respiratory arrest, which can be provoked by the combination of oversedation and intense vagal stimulus from instrumentation
- **d.** Hemorrhage, especially if polypectomy has been performed
- **e.** Death (extremely rare)

5. If colon preparations are administered by lavage to the unconscious patient or to the patient with impaired gag reflexes, observe for aspiration or regurgitation, especially if a nasogastric tube is in place. Keep the head of the bed elevated. If this is not possible, position the patient on his or her side. Have continuous suction equipment and supplies readily available.

6. No barium studies are to be done during the preparation phase for colonoscopy.

7. Signs of bowel perforation include malaise, rectal bleeding, abdominal pain, distention, and fever.

PERITONEOSCOPY; LAPAROSCOPY; PELVISCOPY

Normal Values

Gynecologic examination: normal size, shape, and appearance of uterus, fallopian tubes, and ovaries.

Intra-abdominal examination: normal liver, gallbladder, spleen, and greater curvature of the stomach.

Explanation of Test

These examinations of the intra-abdominal and pelvic cavities are performed using a laparoscope or pelviscope inserted through a slit in the anterior abdominal wall. The pelvic organs as well as abdominal organs, such as the greater curvature of the stomach or the liver, can be viewed. The different types of examinations include peritoneoscopy, laparoscopy (intra-abdominal), and pelviscopy (gynecologic). These procedures are frequently performed under general anesthesia in a surgical setting; however, many are also done with local anesthesia.

Peritoneoscopy is most commonly done to evaluate liver disease and to obtain biopsies when the liver is too small, when previous liver biopsy proves inadequate, when contraindications to percutaneous liver biopsy exist (ascites), when there is unexplained portal hypertension or unexplained liver function abnormalities, and when the liver cannot be properly palpated for doing a conventional liver biopsy. It does away with the need to do a blind liver biopsy. Other indications for peritoneoscopy include unexplained ascites, staging of lymphomas or staging and follow-up of ovarian cancer, or the presence of abdominal masses. Sometimes patients with advanced chest, gastric, pancreatic, endometrial, or rectal tumors are evaluated by peritoneoscopy before attempting surgical intervention.

Gynecologic laparoscopy and pelviscopy are used to diagnose cysts, adhesions, fibroids, malignancies, inflammatory processes, or infections in persons with pelvic and abdominal pain. Evaluation of the fallopian tubes can be done for infertile patients. These procedures also provide a means to release adhesions, to obtain biopsies, or to do select operative procedures, such as tubal ligations. Gynecologic laparoscopy or pelviscopy is commonly performed under general anesthesia, as a same-day surgical procedure.

These techniques can frequently replace laparotomy. They are less stressful to the patient; use small incisions; can be done in shorter times; may be done with local, spinal, or general anesthetics; reduce potential for formation of adhesions; and hasten healing and recovery time.

Pelviscopy differs from laparoscopy in two major respects—*endocoagulation* as a method for controlling bleeding and *endoligation* as a technique that permits suturing using extracorporeal (outside the body) or intracorporeal (inside the body) ligating and suturing methods by means of special instruments.

The pelviscope is also angled at 30° for better visualization. A videocamera attachment offers the physician a choice of viewing the process on a videoscreen, instead of through the scope. Printouts and videotapes of the pelviscopy can be produced. Thus, pelviscopy is both a diagnostic and an operative modality.

Procedure

1. The patient is supine during all procedures, except gynecologic laparoscopy, in which the patient is placed in a lithotomy position.
2. The skin is cleansed and, if performed under local anesthesia, a local anesthetic is injected into areas where the scope will be introduced. Otherwise, the patient is prepared as for an abdominal procedure under general anesthesia. A sterile field is maintained.
3. An intravenous line is placed so that medications may be given intravenously as needed. Refer to intravenous conscious sedation precautions in Appendix IV.
4. An indwelling catheter is placed into the bladder to reduce the risk of bladder perforation.

5. A small incision is made near the umbilicus through which a trocar is introduced, followed by passage of the pelviscope or laparoscope. Sometimes, more than one puncture site will be made so that accessory instruments can be used during the procedure. Carbon dioxide introduced into the peritoneal cavity causes the omentum to rise away from the organs and allows better visualization. A few stitches or Steri-Strips are usually needed to close the incisions. Band-Aid-type bandages are applied as dressings.

Clinical Implications

Abnormal findings can reveal

1. Endometriosis
2. Ovarian cysts
3. Pelvic inflammatory disease
4. Metastatic stage of cancer
5. Uterine fibroids
6. Abscesses
7. Tumors, benign and malignant
8. Enlarged fallopian tubes (hydrosalpinx)
9. Ectopic pregnancy
10. Infection
11. Adhesions or scar tissue
12. Ascites
13. Cirrhosis
14. Liver nodules (often an indication of cancer)
15. Engorged peritoneal vasculature (correlates with portal hypertension)

Clinical Alert

These procedures may be contraindicated in persons known to have

1. Advanced abdominal wall cancer
2. Severe respiratory or cardiovascular disease
3. Intestinal obstruction
4. Palpable abdominal mass
5. Large abdominal hernia
6. Chronic tuberculosis
7. History of peritonitis

The endoscopy should be aborted in favor of a laparotomy in the event of uncontrolled bleeding or suspected malignancy.

Patient Preparation

1. Laboratory tests and other appropriate diagnostic modalities need to be completed before these endoscopies.
2. Bowel preparation may include an enema or suppository.
3. Explain the test purpose and procedure and the type of anesthesia chosen (general, spinal, or local) as well as postoperative expectations, such as activity, deep breathing, and shoulder pain.
4. A legal consent form must be properly signed and witnessed (see Chap. 1, page 13).

5. Sensitivity to cultural, sexual, and modesty issues is an important part of psychological support.
6. See Chapter 1 guidelines for safe, effective, informed *pretest* care.

Patient Aftercare

1. Check blood pressure frequently (according to institutional policies).
2. Observe for infection, hemorrhage, and bowel or bladder perforation.
3. Advise the patient that shoulder and abdominal discomfort may be present for 1 to 2 days because of residual carbon dioxide gas in the abdominal cavity. This can be controlled with mild oral analgesics. Sitting or resting in a semi-Fowler's position can also alleviate discomfort.
4. If the patient has had a general or spinal anesthetic, follow the usual cautions and protocols for the care of any person having those types of anesthesia.
5. Interpret test outcomes and counsel appropriately.
6. Follow Chapter 1 guidelines for safe, effective, informed *posttest* care. Provide written discharge instructions.

CYSTOSCOPY (CYSTOURETHROSCOPY) ●

Normal Values

Normal structure and function of the interior bladder, urethra, ureteral orifices, and male prostatic urethra.

Explanation of Test

These examinations are used to diagnose and treat disorders of the lower urinary tract. They provide views of the interior bladder, the urethra, the prostatic urethra, and the ureteral orifices through tubular, lighted, telescopic lens instruments called *cystoscopes* or *cystourethroscopes*. These scopes come in many sizes and variations as well as in flexible fiberoptic instruments. Urethroscopy is an important part of this examination because it allows visualization of the male prostate gland. (Kidney function may be studied separately through ureteral catheterization and collection of urine specimens from each kidney.)

Cystoscopy is the most common of all urologic diagnostic procedures. It may be indicated in the following conditions:

1. Unexplained hematuria (gross or microscopic)
2. Recurrent or chronic urinary tract infection
3. Infection resistant to medical treatment
4. Unexplained urinary symptoms, such as dysuria, frequency, urgency, hesitancy, intermittency, straining, incontinence, enuresis, or retention.
5. Bladder tumors (benign and malignant)

Because intravenous pyelogram (IVP) does not allow proper visualization of the area from the neck of the bladder to the end of the urethra, cystoscopy makes it possible to diagnose and to treat abnormalities in this area.

Cystoscopy may be used to perform meatotomy and to crush and retrieve small stones and other foreign bodies from the urethra, ureter, and bladder. Biopsy specimens can be obtained. Bladder tumors can be fulgurated, and strictures can be dilated through the cytoscope. In conjunction with cystoscopy, ureteroscopy can be done to determine the cause of hematuria, to detect tumors and stones, and to manipulate stones.

Procedure

1. The examination can be performed in an operating room designed for that purpose or in the urologist's office. Patient's age, state of health, and extent of surgical procedure determine setting.
2. The external genitalia are prepared with an antiseptic solution, such as povidone-iodine, after the patient is placed in the lithotomy position with legs in stirrups. Proper grounding, padding, and draping follow.
3. A local anesthetic jelly is instilled into the urethra. For males, the anesthetic is retained in the urethra by a clamp applied near the end of the penis. For best results, the local anesthetic should be applied 5 to 10 minutes before passage of the cystoscope.
4. The scope is connected to an irrigation system. Solutions used are nonconductive and retain clarity during the procedure (eg, glycine or sterile water). This solution also distends the bladder for purpose of better visualization.

   NOTE: *During transurethral resection procedures, venous sinuses may be opened and irrigation fluid may enter the circulatory system, causing "water intoxication." Therefore, isotonic solutions such as sorbitol, mannitol, or glycine must be used.*

5. Should blood or other matter be present in the bladder, the fiberoptic cystoscope will not provide as clear a view as a rigid cystoscope because it is more difficult to flush.
6. Institutional policies dictate general perioperative care and procedures.

Clinical Implications

Abnormal conditions revealed by cystoscopy include

1. Prostatic hyperplasia/hypertrophy
2. Cancer of the bladder
3. Bladder stones
4. Urethral strictures or abnormalities
5. Prostatitis
6. Ureteral reflux (shown on cystogram)
7. Vesical neck stenosis
8. Urinary fistulas
9. Ureterocele
10. Diverticula
11. Abnormally small or large bladder capacity
12. Polyps

Patient Preparation

1. Explain the purpose and procedure of the test. Special sensitivity to and concern for cultural, social, sexual, and modesty issues are an important part of psychological support. Emphasize that there is little pain or discomfort from cystoscopy. However, a strong desire to void may be experienced.

2. Bowel preparation and other laboratory and diagnostic tests may be necessary if more extensive procedures are planned.
3. If cystoscopy is performed in the hospital, a properly signed and witnessed surgical consent must be obtained. (see Chap. 1, page 13)
4. At times, the patient may take a full-liquid breakfast. Liquids may be encouraged until the time of the examination to promote urine formation if the procedure is a simple cystoscopy done under local anesthesia. NPO guidelines are followed when spinal or general anesthesia is planned.
5. Sometimes an intravenous line may be started for the administration of intravenous conscious sedative medications such as diazepam (Valium) or midazolam (Versed) to relax the patient. Amnesia may be a side effect. Younger men may experience more pain and discomfort than older men. Women usually require less sedation because the female urethra is shorter. The patient should be instructed to relax the abdominal muscles to lessen discomfort. (See Appendix IV concerning intravenous conscious sedation precautions.)
6. See Chapter 1 guidelines for safe, effective, informed *pretest* care.

Patient Aftercare

1. After cystoscopy, voiding patterns as well as bladder emptying should be monitored. Check vital signs as necessary (or instruct to monitor voiding and bladder emptying).
2. Fluids should be encouraged.
3. Clots may form and may cause the patient difficulty in voiding.
4. Report unusual bleeding or difficult urination to the physician promptly.
5. Urinary frequency, dysuria, pink to light red urine color, and urethral burning are common after cystoscopy.
6. Antibiotics may be prescribed before and after cystoscopy to prevent infection.
7. The potential for gram-negative shock is always present with urologic procedures because the urethra is such a vascular organ that any break in the tissues can allow bacteria to enter the bloodstream directly. Onset of symptoms can be rapid and may actually begin during the procedure if it is fairly lengthy. Observe for and *promptly* report chills, fever, increasing tachycardia, hypotension, and back pain to the physician. Blood cultures are usually ordered, followed by an aggressive regimen of antibiotic therapy.
8. Ureteral catheters may be left in place to facilitate urinary drainage, especially if there is concern about edema.
9. Routine catheter care is necessary for retention of ureteral catheters and follows institutional protocols. The patient may need instructions if discharged with catheter in place.
10. Interpret test outcomes and counsel appropriately.
11. Follow Chapter 1 guidelines for safe, effective, informed *posttest* care. Provide written discharge instructions.

Clinical Alert

1. If urethral dilation has been part of the procedure, the patient is advised to rest and to increase fluid intake.
2. Evaluate and instruct patient to watch for edema. Edema may cause urinary retention, hesitancy, weak urinary stream, or urinary dribbling anytime within several days postprocedure. Warm sitz baths and mild analgesics may be helpful. However, an indwelling catheter may sometimes be necessary for relief.

● URODYNAMIC STUDIES

CYSTOMETROGRAM (CMG); URETHRA PRESSURE PROFILE; RECTAL ELECTROMYOGRAM; CYSTOURETHROGRAM ●

Normal Values

Normal bladder sensations of fullness, heat, and cold. Normal adult bladder capacity of 400 to 500 ml, and residual urine less than 30 ml. First desire to void is at 175 to 250 ml. Fullness felt at 350 to 450 ml. Stream is strong and uninterrupted.

Patients will have low voiding pressure without dyssynergia (failure of muscular coordination); detrusor muscle reflex contraction intentionally suppressed on command. Detrusor muscle is the external longitudinal layer of the muscular coat of bladder. Rectal electromyographic readings are normal. Urethra pressure profile reveals normal urethral closing mechanism.

Explanation of Test

These measurements identify abnormal voiding patterns in incontinent persons by determining if a detrusor muscle and external sphincter reflex exists. The cystometrogram reflects functional level of the neuroanatomic connections between the spinal cord, the brain, and the bladder and is often done in conjunction with cystoscopy. These studies are indicated when there is evidence of neurologic disease, such as spina bifida, myelomeningocele, spinal cord injury, tumors, extensive pelvic dissection, cordotomy, neurectomy, cerebrovascular aneurysm, or specific neuropathies, such as those found in multiple sclerosis, diabetes, and tabes dorsalis. This examination can also evaluate symptoms of dysuria, scant or weak urinary stream, frequency, enuresis, overflow or stress incontinence, residual urine, or recurrent infection. Neurogenic bladder dysfunctions are grouped into five classes according to the bladder responses: autonomic, reflex, uninhibited, sensory paralytic, and motor paralytic. Frequently, crossover between categories is found.

Procedures

CYSTOMETROGRAM PROCEDURE

1. The patient voids, and urine flow rate, voiding pressure, and amount of urine voided are recorded.
2. An indwelling catheter is inserted into the bladder and residual urine is measured. The catheter is then connected to the cystometer. (A cystometer evaluates the neuromuscular mechanism of the bladder by measuring bladder capacity and pressure.) The bladder is gradually filled with sterile saline, sterile water, or carbon dioxide gas in predetermined increments, and pressure readings are taken at these increments.
3. During the cystometric examination, observations about the patient's perception of heat and cold, bladder fullness, urge to void, and ability to inhibit voiding when bladder contractions occur are recorded.
4. After the fluid or gas is instilled and measurements are completed, the catheter may be either removed or left in place. Incontinence, voiding patterns, and voided amounts are recorded. If the catheter is removed, the gas is removed before other studies are begun or before catheter removal.
5. Instruct the patient to report the following sensations:
   - **a.** Flushing
   - **b.** Sweating
   - **c.** Pain
   - **d.** Nausea
   - **e.** Bladder fullness
   - **f.** Strong urge to void
6. After the cystometric examination, cholinergic or anticholinergic drugs (eg, methantheline bromide [Banthine, atropine], or bethanechol chloride [Urecholine]) may be injected to determine their effects on bladder function. Answers to the following questions are sought:
   - **a.** Is an atonic bladder capable of being stimulated by cholinergic parasympathomimetic drugs, such as bethanechol chloride, *or* are detrusor muscle fibers so decompensated that no response can be elicited?
   - **b.** Can overactive motor stimuli be sufficiently altered with cholinergic-blocking parasympatholytic drugs, such as atropine, to allow a near-normal bladder volume that will produce an acceptable voiding pattern?

   To determine the effect of these drugs, the cystometric study may be performed as a control, followed by repeat study 20 to 30 minutes after injection of the drugs.
7. A change in posture from supine to standing or walking may be required during the examination.
8. *Sleep examination* studies may be performed in conjunction with an electroencephalogram to evaluate persons having nocturnal incontinence (see Chap. 15 for EEG study.)

RECTAL ELECTROMYOGRAPHIC PROCEDURE

1. Electrodes are applied close to the anus, and a ground is attached to the thigh.

2. A needle electrode may be introduced into the periurethral striated muscle.
3. These electrodes record electromyographic activity during voiding and produce a simultaneous recording of urine flow rate (see Chap. 15 for EMG study.)

URETHRAL PRESSURE PROFILE PROCEDURE

A special catheter, connected to a transducer, is slowly withdrawn and the pressures along the urethra are recorded.

CYSTOURETHROGRAM PROCEDURE

1. This study evaluates stress incontinence (in women), bladder wall and urethral abnormalities, and tumors. It can be used to assess reflux and to identify urine extravasation following trauma.
2. An x-ray contrast medium is instilled into the bladder through a catheter until the bladder is filled. The catheter is clamped and x-ray films are taken with the patient assuming several different positions.
3. After the catheter is removed, more x-ray films are taken as the patient voids and the contrast material passes through the urethra (voiding cystourethrogram).

Clinical Implications

1. Abnormal results reveal motor and sensory defects and abnormal patterns that point to inappropriate or absent contractions of the pelvic floor muscle and internal sphincter during voiding.
   - **a.** The most common cause of incontinence is a vesical–sphincter dyssynergia. This is a disturbance of muscular coordination between the external urethral sphincter–pelvic floor musculature and the detrusor muscle. This dyssynergia is thought to be responsible for incomplete emptying of the bladder, inappropriate voiding, perineal dampness, and predisposition to urinary tract infections.
   - **b.** Detrusor hyperreflexia is a detrusor muscle reflex that the patient cannot suppress on command owing to upper or lower motor neuron lesions, as in
     - **(1)** Cerebrovascular aneurysm
     - **(2)** Parkinson's disease
     - **(3)** Multiple sclerosis
     - **(4)** Cervical spondylosis
     - **(5)** Spinal cord injury above the conus medularis
   - **c.** Urethrovesical hyperreflexia is caused by benign prostatic hypertrophy and stress urge incontinence.
   - **d.** Detrusor areflexia occurs when the detrusor reflex cannot be evoked because the peripheral innervation of the detrusor muscle has been interrupted. This results in difficulty in initiating voiding without a residual volume being present in the bladder. If it is due to inter-

rupted peripheral innervation of the detrusor muscle, the cause may be associated with trauma to the cauda equina or conus medullaris, spinal arachnoiditis, spinal cord birth defects, diabetic neuropathy, or anticholinergic effects of phenothiazides. In postmenopausal women, the urethral pressure profile may be altered because the mucosal sphincter is deprived of estrogen.

Patient Preparation

1. Explain the purpose and procedure of the test. Be sensitive to the patient's potential anxiety and embarrassment. Tell the patient that he or she may experience slight discomfort and the urge to void.
2. Sedation is not given because patient participation is necessary to verify sensations and perceptions. However, the patient must avoid movement during the examination unless instructed otherwise.
3. See Chapter 1 guidelines for safe, effective, informed *pretest* care.

Patient Aftercare

1. Encourage the patient to increase oral fluid intake to dilute the urine and to minimize bladder sensitivity.
2. Explain that some minor discomfort or burning may be noted, especially if carbon dioxide is used, but will lessen and disappear with time.
3. Interpret test outcomes and counsel appropriately.
4. Follow Chapter 1 guidelines for safe, effective, informed *posttest* care. Provide written discharge instructions.

Clinical Alert

1. Certain patients with cervical cord lesions may exhibit an autonomic reflex that produces an elevated blood pressure, severe headache, lower pulse rate, flushing, and diaphoresis. Propantheline bromide (Pro-Banthine) alleviates these symptoms.
2. Careful use of sterile technique reduces the incidence of urinary tract infections. Preprocedural urinary tract infections can lead to sepsis as a result of bacterial spread into the blood stream.

ARTHROSCOPY

Normal Values

Normal joint: normal vasculature and color of the synovium, capsule, menisci, ligaments, and articular cartilage.

Explanation of Test

Arthroscopy is a visual examination and frequently associated surgical procedure of a joint by means of a fiberoptic endoscope system. It is most commonly done for the diagnosis of athletic injuries and for the differential diagnosis of acute or chronic joint disorders. For example, degenerative processes versus injuries can be accurately differentiated. Postoperative rehabilitation programs can be initiated to shorten recovery periods. Arthroscopy can also assess response to treatment or can identify whether other corrective procedures are indicated.

Although the knee is the joint most frequently examined, the shoulder, ankle, hip, elbow, wrist, and metacarpophalangeal joints can also be explored. Calcium deposits, biopsy specimens, bone spurs, torn meniscus or cartilage, and scar tissue can be removed during the procedure. Currently, many of these procedures are performed in an ambulatory surgical setting.

Clinical Implications

Abnormal results reveal the following:

1. Torn or displaced meniscus or cartilage. Symptoms relate to clicking, locking, or swelling of the joint.
2. Trapped synovium
3. Loose fragments of joint contents
4. Torn or ruptured ligaments
5. Necrosis
6. Nerve entrapment
7. Fractures or nonunion of fractures
8. Ganglions
9. Infections
10. Osteochondritis dissecans—inflammation of bone or cartilage occurs when cartilage fragment and underlying bone detach from the articular surface (common in the knee).
11. Chronic inflammatory arthritis
12. Secondary osteoarthritis caused by injury, metabolic disorders, and wearing away of weight-bearing joints
13. Chondromalacia of femoral condyle—wearing down of back of kneecap—grinding sensations

Procedure

1. The examination is usually performed under general anesthesia for the following reasons:
   a. The joint is very painful.
   b. Definitive treatment or surgical intervention can be done at the same time if within the realm of arthroscopic surgery.
   c. An inflated tourniquet may be used in part of the procedure to minimize bleeding at the site.
   d. Complete muscle relaxation permits a thorough examination and eliminates risk of inadvertent patient movement while the arthroscope is in the joint.
2. The surgical site is draped and prepared according to institutional protocols. Proper monitoring equipment is attached to the patient.
3. A tourniquet is applied to the appropriate area of the extremity after it is exsanguinated by the use of an elastic bandage or elevation. Some sur-

geons will choose not to inflate the tourniquet unless bleeding cannot be controlled by irrigation.

4. The joint is aspirated with a 15- or 16-gauge needle. (A specimen of aspirate may be sent to the laboratory.) The joint is then injected with 75 to 100 ml of normal saline or lactated Ringer's solution to distend the joint before inserting the arthroscope. Additional puncture sites allow manipulation of accessory instruments. The wound is irrigated with an appropriate solution throughout the procedure.
5. Joint washings are collected and examined for loose bodies or cartilage fragments.
6. All parts of the joint are carefully examined. Photographs or videotapes of the procedure may be taken. Surgical interventions may be chosen for those problems that can be corrected in this manner.
7. As the arthroscope, accessory pieces, and irrigating needles are slowly withdrawn, the joint is compressed to squeeze out excess irrigation fluid.
8. Steroids or local anesthetics may be injected into the joint for postoperative pain control and reduction of inflammation. The wound is closed with sutures or adhesive strips, and small dressings are applied to the wound. Compressive dressings and splints or immobilizers may then be applied to the extremity.

Patient Preparation

1. History and physical examination, requisite laboratory work, x-ray films, and other preoperative requirements should be completed, reviewed, and documented on the patient's record.
2. Explain the purpose and procedure of the test. The patient should be NPO from midnight before the examination unless otherwise ordered (eg, if scheduled late in the day, a liquid breakfast may be permitted).
3. A properly signed and witnessed consent form must be completed.
4. Peripheral pulses are checked. The surgical site is prepared, positioned, and draped according to institutional protocols. An intravenous line is started.
5. Crutch walking should be taught before the procedure if this is anticipated postoperatively.
6. See Chapter 1 guidelines for safe, effective, informed *pretest* care.

Patient Aftercare

1. Assess vital signs, bleeding, neurologic, and circulatory status of the affected extremity (color, pulse, temperature, capillary refill times, sensation, and motion).
2. Apply ice immediately and elevate (if ordered) to minimize swelling and pain. Dressing changes and suture removal are at the physician's discretion. Dressing is kept clean and dry. Notify physician of unusual bleeding or swelling.
3. Appropriate pain medication should be administered.

4. The patient can usually be up and about after recovery from the anesthetic. Crutches may be used. The degree of weight-bearing and joint motion is at the discretion of the physician.
5. Exercises and physical therapy may be ordered postoperatively. These are designed to strengthen and maximize use of the joint.
6. If discharged the same day, arrangements for transportation to home by another person should be arranged preoperatively. Patient should not drive for at least 24 hours.
7. Patient should consume no alcohol for 24 hours after the procedure. Progress diet from fluid to regular as tolerated.
8. Instruct patient to report altered sensation, numbness, tingling, coldness, duskiness (bluish color), swelling, bleeding, or abnormal pain to the physician immediately.
9. Interpret test outcomes and counsel appropriately.
10. Follow Chapter 1 guidelines for safe, effective, informed *posttest* care. Provide written discharge instructions.

Clinical Alert

1. Arthroscopy is usually contraindicated if ankylosis or fibrosis is present because it is very difficult to maneuver the examining instrument in this type of joint.
2. For knee arthroscopy, the posterior approach is not used because of the neurovascular structures present in that area.
3. Do not place pillows under the knee because flexion contractures can occur as a result. If the patient's *entire* leg is ordered to be elevated, make sure the knee is not flexed. Pad the pressure points (eg, the heel).
4. If there is risk of sepsis or if sepsis is present in any part of the body, the procedure should not be done.
5. Arthroscopy is usually not done less than 7 to 10 days after arthrography because chemical synovitis caused by a contrast medium can adversely affect the visual examination. However, it may be necessary to perform arthroscopy if the patient is experiencing severe pain. In this event, the joint will be thoroughly irrigated to remove contrast medium.
6. Be alert for signs of thrombophlebitis postoperatively. Instruct patient to watch for calf tenderness, pain, or heat and to report these symptoms to the physician immediately. *Warn the patient not to massage the affected area.*
7. Other complications may include hemarthrosis, adhesions, neurovascular injury, pulmonary embolus, effusion, scarring, and compartmental syndrome as a result of swelling. Compartmental syn-

(continued)

(Clinical Alert continued)

drome is a musculoskeletal complication that occurs most commonly in the forearm or leg. The compartment of fascia surrounding muscles does not expand when bleeding or edema occurs. Consequently, the neurovascular status of the extremity may be severely compromised. This prevents an emergency situation and usually requires surgical intervention to release pressure. Assess the neurovascular status of an affected extremity frequently for 24 hours after the procedure.

SINUS ENDOSCOPY

Normal Values

Normal sinuses or resolution of sinus disease.

Explanation of Test

The examination visualizes the anterior ethmoid, middle turbinate, and middle meatus sinus areas. Even though the primary purpose of sinus endoscopy is to relieve infections and other symptoms and to alter structural abnormalities from the aforementioned areas, it can also be a valuable diagnostic tool. Retained secretions may contribute to chronic recurrent sinus infections, which may lead to systemic infections, cyst formation, or mucoceles that can erode sinus walls into areas of the eyeball, eye orbit, or brain.

Those patients having recurrent episodes of acute or chronic sinusitis not responsive to antibiotic or allergy therapy are candidates for sinus endoscopy as both a diagnostic and a therapeutic modality.

Procedure

Sinus endoscopy may be an outpatient or an office procedure. Normally, the *diagnostic* procedure is performed in the office. More extensive examination and an operative procedure normally require outpatient admission to a healthcare facility or special diagnostic center.

1. A cocaine solution of select concentration is usually sprayed into the nares to produce local anesthesia. The endoscope is introduced to permit visualization of the nasal interior; the sinus cavities are *not* opened. (**Note:** some patients become very talkative and euphoric as a response to the cocaine.)
2. Sinus computed tomography (CT) scans may be a necessary adjunct to this procedure to permit visualization of these areas not accessible through endoscopy.
3. The actual treatment for underlying disease or malformations is performed with local or general anesthesia and intravenous sedation.

Diagnostic and surgical techniques will varying according to preoperative findings.

4. Endoscopes used for diagnosis and treatment are available in 0°, −30°, −70°, and 120° angles of view. These appear to be the current instruments of choice, although fiberoptic scopes are available.

Clinical Implications

Abnormalities that may be revealed include

1. Chronic sinusitis—edematous or polypoid mucosa
2. Cysts
3. Mucocele
4. Sinus erosion
5. Anatomical deformities or obstruction
6. Pathologic sinus discharge—infectious process
7. Enlarged middle turbinates

Patient Preparation

1. Explain purpose, benefits, risks, and procedure. (Steps 2 through 6 following refer to treatment modalities.) Procedure may take place in the office or outpatient hospital setting.
2. A properly signed and witnessed surgical consent form, appropriate laboratory and diagnostic test results, history and physical examination, current drug therapies, and allergies need to be reviewed and documented in the healthcare record before the procedure.
3. Preprocedure preparation may require the patient to
   - **a.** Be processed through preadmission testing if procedure will be done in a hospital surgical setting
   - **b.** Be NPO after midnight
   - **c.** Remove facial prostheses, dentures, hairpieces, and jewelry before the procedure
   - **d.** Have an intravenous line placed
   - **e.** Arrange transportation home when discharged
4. In the surgical suite, the patient assumes a supine position. The face and throat are prepared according to established protocols, and the area is properly draped. Eye pads taped in place protect the eyes from injury. Other positioning and pressure point padding are done as necessary.
5. Intravenous sedation is administered as needed. The nose is sprayed with a topical anesthetic, and a small amount of 1% lidocaine with 1:200,000 aqueous epinephrine is injected into the appropriate areas (unless contraindicated because of allergy or for other reasons) to provide anesthesia and control of bleeding. Refer to Appendix IV for intravenous conscious sedation precautions.
6. At the end of the procedure, a 10-ml syringe is filled with antibiotic ointment. A small catheter attached to the syringe tip allows ointment to be directed to the appropriate areas. A small (2 × 2) "mustache dressing" taped to the end of the nose collects secretions and blood. Usually this can be changed as needed. Nasal packing may be inserted into the nares.

7. See Chapter 1 guidelines for safe, effective, informed pretest care.

Patient Aftercare

1. Oral fluids are encouraged following nausea or vomiting (patient may experience nausea/vomiting if blood is swallowed—blood is irritating to the GI system).
2. Postprocedural instructions may include
   a. Taking prescribed medications as ordered (usually a broad-spectrum antibiotic and pain medication). Soothing gargles may be ordered.
   b. Reporting excessive bleeding or sinus discharge, unusual pain, fever, nausea or vomiting, or visual problems immediately. Include phone numbers of hospital and physician and instruct the patient to contact the physician (or the outpatient surgical department, or emergency department if unable to reach physician) in the event of an emergency. (This process may differ according to various HMO or health insurance regulations and protocols.)
   c. Patient should not drive or sign legal documents for 24 hours (because of anesthetics and sedation).
3. If the patient has received intravenous sedation, follow the usual cautions that are involved in the care of any person having this type of sedation. Refer to Appendix IV. This patient may require closer monitoring, positioning on the side to prevent aspiration, and a longer recovery time.
4. Interpret test outcomes and counsel appropriately.
5. Follow Chapter 1 guidelines for safe, effective, informed *posttest* care. Provide written discharge instructions.

Clinical Alert

1. Sinuses are poorly visualized through routine sinus x-rays films.
2. If sinus problems appear related to dental problems, the patient should see a dentist or oral surgeon before sinus endoscopy is performed.
3. Severe nasal–septal deviation needs to be corrected before endoscopy.
4. Potential complications include bleeding, cerebrospinal fluid leak, and visual disturbances.
5. Direct trauma to the nasofrontal duct is associated with increased risk of postoperative stenosis.

BIBLIOGRAPHY

Barnie DC: Care planning for the endoscopy unit: Master care plan for the post-procedure patient. Gastroenterol Nurs 11(4):266–267, Spring 1989

Barsevick AM, Louver D: Women's informational needs about colposcopy. Image 22(1):23–26, Spring 1990

Bennett JR et al: Therapeutic Endoscopy and Radiology of the Gut, 2nd ed. Baltimore, Williams & Wilkins, 1990

Brunner LS, Suddarth DS: The Lippincott Manual of Nursing Practice, 5th ed. Philadelphia, JB Lippincott, 1991

Kallacky MA, MacMillan W, Sheets EE: Should you be doing colposcopy? Patient Care, June 15, 1988

McCauly KM, Oi RH: Evaluating the Papanicolaou smear: Four possible colposcopic findings and corresponding management strategies, Part 2. Consultant 29(1):36–42, January 1989

Nichols CD: Wrist orthoscopy. AORN J 49(3):759–771, March 1989

Raufman JP et al: Endoscopic procedures in the AIDs patient: Risks, precautions, indications, and allegations. Gastroenterol Clin North Am 17(3):495–506, September 1988

Rivera ML: Pelviscoscopy: Broadening the scope of laparoscopy. Today's OR Nurse 11:16–20, November 1989

Watson A, Griffiths M: Cervicography: The nurse's role. Nurs Times 185(29), July 9, 1989

13

Ultrasound Studies

OVERVIEW OF ULTRASOUND STUDIES

Ultrasonography is a noninvasive procedure for visualizing soft-tissue structures of the body by recording the reflection of ultrasonic waves directed into the tissues. This diagnostic procedure, which requires very little patient preparation, is now used in many branches of medicine for accurate diagnosis of certain pathologic conditions (Chart 13-1). It may be used diagnosti-

CHART 13-1
Uses of Ultrasound

1. **Obstetrical ultrasound:** commonly performed to evaluate fetal health, size, number, levels of amniotic fluid, and maternal and placental anatomy.
2. **Abdominal ultrasound:** used to characterize soft-tissue organs including
   - Liver: to evaluate organ size and the presence of masses or diffuse parenchymal conditions. Doppler ultrasound is helpful in demonstrating signs of portal hypertension and other vascular problems.
   - Gallbladder (GB) and biliary tract: to detect disease as well as gallstones. Because ultrasound examination of these structures does not rely on the administration and concentration of x-ray contrast media, GB sonograms can be readily performed on patients with significant liver disease or in obstructed ducts.
   - Pancreas: to detect pathologic states such as tumor involvement, pseudocysts, and inflammatory processes.
   - Kidneys: to diagnose cysts, masses, hydronephrosis, and certain diffuse conditions. Doppler evaluation of the renal vessels and parenchyma are commonly used to evaluate transplanted kidneys and in the staging of known renal cell carcinoma.
   - Aorta and other large abdominal vessels: to detect aneurysms, the presence of clots or tumors, and other defects.
   - Spleen and lymph nodes: to evaluate organ size and pathologic states such as lymphoma and metastatic spread of known cancers.
   - Additional structures: to demonstrate suspected ascites, abscesses, retroperitoneal tumors, and signs of appendicitis.
3. **Pelvic ultrasound:** gynecologic scan is done to evaluate the urinary bladder, uterus, and ovaries. Is used to monitor follicle development during infertility treatments and is also used as a guide for oocyte retrieval.
4. **Male reproductive organs sonogram:** to evaluate scrotal masses and swelling and is combined with Doppler examination of the penis to detect physiologic causes for male impotence. Transrectal ultrasound is an accepted method of screening males for prostatic disease.

(continued)

CHART 13-1 *(continued)*

5. **Head and neck sonograms:** to evaluate pathologies in the following structures:
   - Thyroid and parathyroid for differentiating cysts from solid tumors.
   - Carotid and vertebral arteries: to demonstrate vessel patency and flow patterns.
   - Eye: to assist the ophthalmologist in the removal of foreign bodies and in the evaluation of the eye's structure.
   - Neonatal brain: to diagnose cerebral hemorrhage and other intracranial pathologies.
   - Adult cerebral blood flow: by using a method known as transcranial Doppler, the larger blood vessels within the brain may be interrogated to rule out vascular disturbances.
6. **Breast sonograms:** performed to differentiate cysts from solid lesions and to guide cyst aspirations and needle biopsies.
7. **Extremities sonograms:** used to evaluate arterial and venous blood flow and to characterize soft-tissue masses such as Baker's cysts. Sonography is often used to evaluate the pediatric hip for dislocations or other structural deformities.
8. **Invasive procedures:** serve as a **guide** for diagnostic procedures, such as amniocentesis, thoracentesis, and biopsy.
9. **Heart sonograms:** performed to evaluate the cardiac structure as well as blood flow through chambers and valves.

cally with the obstetric, gynecologic, or cardiac patient and in patients with abnormal conditions of the kidney, pancreas, gallbladder, lymph nodes, liver, spleen, thyroid, and peripheral blood vessels. Frequently, it is used in conjunction with radiography or nuclear medicine scans. The procedure is relatively quick (often requiring only a few minutes to an hour) and causes little discomfort. No harmful effects have yet been established at the low intensities that are used (under 100 mW/cm^2). However, the ultrasound technique is a relatively new procedure, and long-term effects have not been documented. As with any diagnostic procedure, ultrasound must be weighed by its benefits and risks and should not be used frivolously.

Principles and Technique

Ultrasound uses high-frequency sound waves for the characterization of the position, size, form and nature of soft-tissue organs. Its "real-time" image acquisition can readily demonstrate motion, such as seen in the fetus and the heart. Diagnostic ultrasound developed from military research in sonar—a sort of underwater radar procedure. Sonograms, which are images produced through the application of diagnostic ultrasound, are really echo-reflection maps. These "maps" represent variations in a tissue's acoustic impedance as sound passes through it. The basic physical principles involved in producing sonograms are as follows:

1. An ultrasound beam is directed into the patient's body and passes through it.
2. The body tissues, comprising structures of different acoustic impedances, reflect the sound waves with varying degrees of intensity.
3. These various echo (reflection) waves are electronically processed and displayed.
4. Recordings of these displays may be made for documentation purposes on a variety of media including x-ray film, videodisk or tape, digital media, and paper.

Evidence of a pathologic process is detectable because lesions often contain tissues with acoustic properties different from the acoustics of normal, surrounding tissues. However, ultrasound cannot be used diagnostically with the air-filled lung or the gas-filled intestine because the ultrasound beam is almost totally reflected by air-containing organs. For this reason, sonographic studies of air-filled structures are generally not diagnostic.

Most sonograms performed today produce a display that is shown in real-time on a cathode ray tube (CRT) or high-resolution videomonitor. This real-time method permits a rapid and repetitive generation of images that demonstrate the motion of the tissues visualized. The technologist chooses representative images from the display to "freeze" and save as permanent "hard-copy" records.

Doppler Method

A phenomenon known as the *Doppler effect* can be combined with diagnostic ultrasound imaging to produce detailed visualization of the **anatomy** of blood vessels as well as the **nature of blood flow** through them. Spectral maps characterize blood flow direction, velocity, and the presence of flow disturbances. Instead of a gray-scale image, **color flow Doppler** provides a color-coded depiction of selected blood flow parameters. Doppler and color flow Doppler examinations are used to establish the patency of a given blood vessel and are useful in investigating perfusion to certain organs such as the liver, placenta, kidneys, and brain. These methods are also helpful in evaluating complications in transplanted organs. It is the method of choice to evaluate potential torsion of the ovary or testes. Recently, much work has focused on the Doppler evaluation of neoplasms in an effort to demonstrate the deranged vascular patterns associated with malignant lesions.

Procedure

1. A gel or lubricant is applied to the skin over the area to be examined to conduct the sound waves.
2. An operator, known as a **sonographer,** holds a microphonelike device

called a **transducer.** The transducer is moved over a specific body part, producing a display that is viewed on the monitor.

3. Sonography of structures in the abdominal region often require the patient to control breathing patterns. Deep inspiration and exhalation may be used.
4. Selected images are recorded for documentation purposes.
5. The examination causes no physical pain. However, in certain applications, pressure may be applied to the transducer, causing some degree of discomfort. Long examinations may leave the patient feeling tired.
6. Tests usually take 20 to 45 minutes. This time refers to the actual procedure time and does not include waiting and preparation times.
7. Certain tests are best performed with a full urinary bladder.
8. Some examinations may require the patient to fast. Each individual examining department will determine its own guidelines for patient preparation.

Advances in technology have allowed the development of very small transducers that are capable of being placed within body orifices and other structures. The close proximity of these transducers to the area being examined offers better detail than examinations that require the sound to pass through skin and subcutaneous tissues. Catheter-sized transducers are used to visualize blood vessels "from the inside out" during angiographic procedures. Small transducers passed through the esophagus permit exquisite visualization of the heart during transesophageal echocardiography.

Slim transducers that are introduced into the vagina during gynecologic sonography are commonly used. Transrectal visualization of the prostate gland is an accepted method of screening for disease in that organ. Before insertion, these transducers are thoroughly cleansed and draped with condoms or other sheathing materials.

Benefits and Risks of Ultrasound Studies

1. Noninvasive procedure with no radiation risk.
2. Requires little, if any, patient preparation and aftercare
3. Procedure is safe for both patient and examiner (this is true even for the developing fetus).
4. As far as we know, examination can be repeated as many times as necessary without being injurious to the patient. No harmful cumulative effect has been seen.
5. Studies can obviate the need for extended hospitalization.
6. Because ultrasound studies demonstrate structure, rather than function, they may be useful with patients whose organ function is impaired.
7. Useful in detection and examination of moving parts, such as the heart.
8. Does not require the injection of contrast materials, isotopes, or ingestion of opaque materials.
9. Fasting is not required in many instances.

Disadvantages of Ultrasound Studies

1. An extremely skilled technician is required to operate the transducer. The scans must be read immediately and interpreted for adequacy. If the scans are not satisfactory, the examination must be repeated.
2. Air-filled structures (eg, lungs) cannot be studied by ultrasonography.
3. Certain patients (eg, restless children, extremely obese patients) cannot be studied adequately unless they are specially prepared.

Difficult-to-Study Patients

The following are general categories of patients who may provide some difficulties in ultrasound studies:

1. *Postoperative patients:* If possible, dressings should be removed and a sterile coupling agent and probe should be applied gently to the skin.
2. *Patients with abdominal scars:* The scar tissue causes attenuation of the ultrasound.
3. *Children:* Because the procedure requires the patient to remain very still, some children may need to be sedated so that their movements do not cause artifacts. However, the technician remains with the child during the entire procedure so, in most cases, there is little apprehension and little need for sedation.
4. *Obese patients:* Certain patients cannot be studied adequately in any case. For example, it may be very difficult to obtain an accurate scan on a very obese patient, owing to alteration of the sound beam by fatty tissue. There is no preparation that would help here.

Interfering Factors

1. Barium has an adverse effect on the quality of abdominal studies, so echograms should be scheduled before barium studies are done.
2. If a patient has a large amount of gas in the bowel, the examination may be rescheduled because air (bowel gas) is a very strong reflector of sound and will not permit visualization.
3. Because gel or lubricant on the skin is used as a conductor, the examination cannot be performed over an area of open wounds or dressings.

Inadequate contact between the skin and the probe may be one of the causes of unsatisfactory scans. Sufficient quantities of the coupling agent, such as oil, must be applied to the skin and frequently reapplied.

OBSTETRIC SONOGRAM ●

Normal Values

Normal image of placental position, size, and structure.

Normal fetal position and size with evidence of fetal movement, and cardiac and breathing activity.

Adequate amniotic fluid volumes.

Accuracy of Obstetric Measurements

Crown–rump length measured before 12 weeks has predictive value of ±5 days.

Biparietal diameter measured at 17 to 26 weeks has predictive value of ±11 days.

Biparietal diameter measured in third trimester has predictive value of ±3 weeks.

Gestational age is also estimated by measuring fetal extremities, particularly the femur and head, and abdominal circumferences, orbits, and numerous other anatomic structures.

Explanation of Test

Ultrasound studies of the obstetric patient are valuable in (1) confirming pregnancy; (2) facilitating amniocentesis by locating a suitable pool of amniotic fluid; (3) determining fetal age; (4) confirming multiple pregnancy; (5) ascertaining whether fetal development is normal, through sequential studies; (6) determining fetal viability; (7) localizing the placenta; (8) confirming masses associated with pregnancy; and (9) postmature pregnancy (evaluation of amount of amniotic fluid and degree of placental calcification). A pregnancy can be dated with considerable accuracy if one sonogram is done at 20 weeks and a follow-up is done at 32 weeks. There is a good reliability between those two points in fetal growth. This validation is most important when early delivery is anticipated, and prematurity is to be avoided. Conditions in which determination of pregnancy duration are useful are maternal diabetes, Rh immunization, preterm labor, and any medical condition that is worsening with the progress of labor (Table 13–1).

The pregnant uterus is ideal for echographic evaluation because the amniotic fluid–filled uterus provides strong transmitting interfaces between the fluid, placenta, and fetus. Ultrasonography has become the method of choice in evaluating the fetus, thereby eliminating the need for potentially injurious x-ray studies that were used previously. Because ultrasonography, as used in obstetrics, is about 98% accurate in detecting placental site, radionuclide studies of the pregnant patient have been abandoned.

Procedure

1. The pregnant woman lies on her back, with her abdomen exposed during the test. This may cause some shortness of breath and supine hypotensive syndrome and can be relieved by elevating the upper body or by turning the patient onto her side.
2. Transabdominal: In the second trimester, the patient is usually scanned with a full bladder. Exceptions to this requirement are made when ultrasound is used to locate the placenta before amniocentesis, in the evaluation of an incompetent cervix, or in labor and delivery. A full bladder allows the examiner to assess the true position of the placenta, repositions

TABLE 13-1
Major Uses of Obstetric Ultrasound: Levels 1 and 2§

Indications During First Trimester

- Confirm pregnancy
- Confirm viability
- Rule out ectopic pregnancy
- Confirm gestational age*
  - Birth control pill use
  - Irregular menses
  - No dates
  - Postpartum pregnancy
- Previous complicated pregnancy
  - Cesarean delivery
  - Rh incompatibility
  - Diabetes mellitus
  - Fetal growth retardation
- Clarify dates/size discrepancy
  - Large for dates—rule out
    - Leiomyomata
    - Bicornuate uterus
    - Adnexal mass
    - Multiple gestation
    - Poor dates
    - Missed abortion
    - Blighted ovum

Indications During Second Trimester

- Establish or confirm dates*
- If no fetal heart tones
- Clarify dates/size discrepancy
  - Large for dates—rule out
    - Poor estimate of dates
    - Molar pregnancy
    - Multiple gestation
    - Leiomyomata
    - Polydydramnios
    - Congenital anomalies
  - Small for dates—rule out
    - Poor estimate of dates
    - Fetal growth retardation
    - Congenital anomalies
    - Oligohydramnios
- If history of bleeding—rule out total placenta previa
- If Rh incompatibility—rule out fetal hydrops

Indications During Third Trimester

- If no fetal heart tones
- Clarify dates/size discrepancy
  - Large for dates—rule out
    - Macrosomia (diabetes mellitus)
    - Multiple gestation
    - Polyhydramnios
    - Congenital anomalies
    - Poor estimate of dates†
  - Small for dates—rule out
    - Fetal growth retardation
    - Oligohydramnios
    - Congenital anomalies
    - Poor estimate of dates‡
- Determine fetal position—rule out
  - Breech
  - Transverse lie
- If history of bleeding—rule out
  - Placenta previa
  - Abruptio placentae
- Determine fetal lung maturity
  - Amniocentesis for lecithin/sphingomyelin ratio
  - Placental maturity (grade 0–3)
- If Rh incompatibility—rule out fetal hydrops

*Accuracy +3 days
†Accuracy +1–1.5 days
‡Accuracy only +3 weeks;
§Ultrasound is a diagnostic tool for assessment of fetal age, health, and growth as well as identified as either level 1 or level 2. Level one ultrasound is performed to assess gestational age, number of fetuses, fetal viability and death, and the placenta. Level two ultrasound is used for assessment of specific congenital anomalies or abnormalities. See, also, Fetal Echocardiography on pages 837 and 853.

the uterus and cervix for better visibility, serves as a reference point, and acts as a sonic window to the pelvic organs.

3. A coupling agent, such as special transmission gel, lotion, oil, or mineral oil, is applied liberally to the skin to prevent air from absorbing sound waves. The sonographer slowly moves the transducer over the entire abdomen to obtain a picture of the uterine contents.
4. Endovaginal: During the first trimester, some laboratories use a *transvaginal* approach when performing obstetric sonograms. This method does *not* require a full bladder. A slim transducer, properly covered and lubricated, is gently introduced into the vagina. Because the sound waves do not have to transverse abdominal tissue, exquisite image detail is produced. Check with the individual laboratory to determine the approach to be used.
5. The examining time is about 30 to 60 minutes

Clinical Implications

1. In the *first trimester,* the following information can be obtained:
   - **a.** Number, size, and location of gestational sacs
   - **b.** Presence or absence of fetal cardiac and body movement
   - **c.** Presence or absence of uterine abnormalities (eg, bicornuate uterus, fibroids) or adnexal masses (eg, ovarian cysts, ectopic pregnancy)
   - **d.** Pregnancy dating (eg, biparietal diameter, crown–rump length)
   - **e.** Coexistence and location of an intrauterine device
2. In the *second* and *third trimesters,* ultrasound can be performed to obtain the following information:
   - **a.** Fetal viability, number, position, gestational age, growth pattern, and structural abnormalities
   - **b.** Amniotic fluid volume
   - **c.** Placental location and maturity, abnormalities
   - **d.** Uterine fibroids and anomalies
   - **e.** Adnexal masses

   Early diagnosis of fetal structural abnormalities makes the following choices possible: (1) intrauterine surgery or other therapy to fetus if possible; (2) discontinuation of pregnancy; and (3) preparation of family for care of child with a disorder, or plan or other options.
3. *Fetal viability:* Fetal heart activity can be demonstrated as early as **5** and **6** weeks in most cases. This information is helpful in establishing dates and in management of a woman who experiences vaginal bleeding. Incomplete, complete, and missed abortions, as well as molar pregnancies can be differentiated.
4. *Gestational age:* Indications for gestational age include uncertain dates for the last menstrual period or last normal menstrual period; recent discontinuation of oral hormonal suppression of ovulation; bleeding episode during the first trimester; amenorrhea of at least 3 months duration; uterine size that does not agree with dates; previous cesarean birth; and other high-risk conditions. The method of fetal age estimation

used depends on the stage of pregnancy: (1) determination of gestational sac size (about 4 to 5 weeks); (2) measurement of crown–rump length (between 6 and 12 weeks; (3) measurement of biparietal diameter (BPD; starting at 12 weeks to term); and (4) other parameters, such as extremity length, especially femur, abdominal, and head circumferences (12 weeks to term). The crown–rump length method is the *most* accurate age estimator. Other age predictors, such as BPD and femur length, are most accurate during the second trimester. The accuracy of all other methods suffers as the pregnancy reaches term.

5. *Fetal growth:* Some of the conditions that serve as indicators for ultrasound assessment of fetal growth include the following: poor maternal weight gain or pattern of weight gain; previous intrauterine growth retardation (IUGR); chronic infections; ingestion of drugs, such as anticonvulsants or heroin; maternal diabetes; pregnancy-induced or other hypertension; multiple pregnancy; and other medical or surgical complications. Serial evaluation of BPD and limb length can help differentiate between wrong dates and IUGR. *Doppler* evaluation of the umbilical artery, uterine artery, and fetal aorta can also assist in the detection of IUGR. Intrauterine growth retardation can be symmetric (the fetus is small in all diameters) or asymmetric (head and body growth vary). Symmetric IUGR may be due to low genetic growth potential, intrauterine infection, maternal undernutrition or heavy smoking, or chromosomal aberration. Asymmetric IUGR may reflect placental insufficiency secondary to hypertension, cardiovascular disease, or renal disease. Depending on the probable cause, the therapy varies.
6. *Fetal anatomy:* Depending on the gestational age, the following structures may be identified: head (including blood vessels and ventricles), neck, spine, heart, stomach, small bowel, liver, kidneys, bladder, and extremities. Structural defects may be identified before delivery. The following are examples of structural defects that may be diagnosed by ultrasound: Hydrocephaly, anencephaly, and myelomeningocele are often associated with polyhydramnios. Potter's syndrome (renal agenesis) is associated with oligohydramnios. These can be diagnosed before 20 weeks, as can skeletal defects (dwarfism, achondroplasia, osteogenesis imperfecta), and diaphragmatic hernias. Other structural anomalies that can be diagnosed by ultrasound are pleural effusion (after 20 weeks), intestinal atresias or obstructions (early to second trimester), hydronephrosis and bladder outlet obstruction (second trimester to term with fetal surgery available). Two-dimensional studies of the heart, together with echocardiogram, allow diagnosis of congenital cardiac lesions and prenatal treatment of cardiac arrhythmias.
7. *Detection of fetal death:* Inability to visualize the fetal heart beating and the separation of bones in the fetal head are signs of death. With real-time scanning, the absence of cardiac motion for 3 minutes is diagnostic of fetal demise.
8. *Placental position and function:* The site of implantation, such as ante-

rior, posterior, under, or in lower segment, can be described, as well as the location of the placenta on the other side of midline. The pattern of uterine and placental growth and the bladder fullness influence the apparent location of the placenta. For example, in approximately 15% to 20% of all pregnancies, when ultrasound scanning is done in the second trimester, the placenta seems to be overlying the os. At term, the evidence of placenta previa is only 0.5%; therefore, the diagnosis of placenta previa can seldom be confirmed until the third trimester. Placenta abruptio (premature separation of placenta) can also be identified.

9. *Fetal well-being:* The following physiologic measurements can be accomplished with ultrasound: heart monitor, beat-to-beat variability, fetal breathing movements (FBM), urine production (following serial measurements of bladder volume), fetal limb and head movements, and analysis of vascular waveforms from fetal circulation. Fetal breathing movements are decreased with maternal smoking and alcohol use and increased with hyperglycemia. Fetal limb and head movements serve as an index of neurologic development. Identification of amniotic fluid pockets is also used to evaluate fetal status. A pocket of amniotic fluid measuring at least 1 cm is associated with normal fetal status. The presence of one pocket measuring less than 1 cm or the absence of a pocket is abnormal. It is associated with increased risk of perinatal death.
10. *Assessment of multiple pregnancy:* Two or more gestational sacs, each containing an embryo, may be seen after 6 to 7 weeks. Of those diagnosed in the first trimester, only approximately 30% will deliver, secondary to loss or absorption of one. Of value is the assessment of the relative fetal growth of twins, where IUGR or twin-to-twin transfusion is suspected. One cannot unequivocally diagnose whether they are monozygotes or heterozygotes with ultrasound alone. Routine ultrasound cannot be totally relied on to exclude the possibility of triplets or quadruplets instead of only twins.
11. If fetal position and amniotic fluid volumes are favorable, fetal sex can be determined by visualizing genitalia. It must be cautioned, however, that sex determination is not the purpose of obstetric sonography.

Interfering Factors

1. Artifacts can be produced when the transducer is moved out of contact with the skin. This can be resolved by adding more coupling agent to the skin and repeating the scan.
2. Artifacts (reverberation) may be produced by echoes emanating from the same surface several times. This can be avoided by careful positioning of the transducer.
3. A posterior placental site may be difficult to identify because of the angulation of the reflecting surface or insufficient penetration of the sound beam because of the patient's size.

4. Schedule uterine examination before barium x-ray examination whenever possible because barium deflects the ultrasound beam.

Patient Preparation

1. A brief explanation of procedure to be performed is given, emphasizing that it is not uncomfortable or painful and that it does not involve ionizing radiation that may be harmful to the mother and fetus. The studies can be repeated without harm, but the procedure is being studied carefully to determine whether there are any long-term adverse side effects. Benefits of the procedure should be explained.
2. Most studies are performed using a transabdominal approach with a full bladder. The patient is asked to drink five or six glasses of fluid (coffee, tea, water, juice, soda) approximately 1 to 2 hours before the examination. If she is unable to do so, intravenous fluids may be administered. She is asked to refrain from voiding until the examination is completed. Tell the patient the examination will be done when she has a strong urge to void. Discomfort due to pressure applied over a full bladder may be experienced. If the bladder is not sufficiently filled, three to four 8-oz. glasses of water should be ingested, and rescanning is done 30 to 45 minutes later. The examination will not be conducted if the bladder is empty.
3. Some laboratories use a transvaginal (endovaginal) approach during the first trimester of pregnancy. No patient preparation is required for this method. Contact the laboratory performing the study to determine method to be used.
4. Explain that a liberal coating of coupling agent must be applied to the skin so that there is no air between the skin and the transducer and to permit easy movement of the transducer over the skin. A sensation of warmth or wetness may be felt. Although the acoustic couplant does not stain, the patient should be advised not to wear good clothing for the examination.
5. The woman may face the screen, and the sonographer can explain the images in basic terms. In some institutions, the father is encouraged to observe the testing. A photograph or videotape for the family to keep is often provided.
6. See Chapter 1 guidelines for safe, effective, informed *pretest* care.

Clinical Alert

1. A full bladder may not be needed or desired in patients in the late stages of pregnancy or active labor. However, if a full bladder is required, and the woman has not been instructed to report with a full bladder, at least another hour of waiting time may be required before the examination can begin.

(continued)

(Clinical Alert continued)

2. A transvaginal (endovaginal) scan does *not* require the patient to have a full bladder. Contact the laboratory to determine method to be used.
3. Fetal age determinations are most accurate during the crown–rump stage in the first trimester. The next most accurate time for age estimation is during the second trimester. Sonographic dating during the third trimester has a large margin of error (up to ±3 weeks).
4. Endovaginal studies, when indicated, typically involve the use of a latex condom to sheath the transducer before insertion into the vaginal vault. Contact the laboratory if the patient has a known or suspected latex sensitivity.

PELVIC GYNECOLOGIC SONOGRAM; PELVIC/UTERINE MASS ULTRASOUND DIAGNOSIS ●

Normal Values

Normal pattern image of bladder, uterus, fallopian tubes, and vagina.

Explanation of Test

Pelvic ultrasound examines the area from the umbilicus to the pubic bone in women. Ultrasound studies may be used in the evaluation of pelvic masses and postmenopausal bleeding and to aid in the diagnosis of cysts and tumors. Information can be provided on the size, location, and structure of the masses. These examinations cannot give definitive diagnoses of a pathologic process, but they can be used as an adjunct procedure when the diagnosis is not readily apparent. These studies are also used in treatment planning and follow-up radiation therapy of gynecologic cancer.

This test may be performed using a transvaginal (endovaginal) *or* transabdominal approach. With the transvaginal method, a slim, covered, and lubricated transducer is gently introduced into the vagina. A full bladder is *not* required. Because the sound waves do not have to traverse through abdominal tissue, exquisite image detail is produced. This approach is most advantageous for examining the obese patient, the patient with a retroverted uterus, or for those who have difficulty maintaining bladder distention. The transvaginal method is the approach of choice in monitoring follicular size during fertility workups and during the aspiration of follicles for *in vitro* fertilization.

For pelvic sonograms by the transabdominal approach, a full bladder is necessary. The distended bladder serves four purposes: (1) It acts as a "window" for transmission of the ultrasound beam; (2) it pushes the uterus away from the pubic symphysis, thereby providing a less obstructed view; (3) it pushes the bowel out of the pelvis; and (4) it may be used as a comparison in evaluating the internal characteristics of a mass under study.

Procedures

TRANSABDOMINAL METHOD

1. The patient lies on the back on the examining table during the test.
2. A coupling agent is applied to the area under study.
3. The active face of the transducer is placed in contact with patient's skin and swept across the area being studied.
4. Examination time is about 30 minutes.

TRANSVAGINAL (ENDOVAGINAL) METHOD

1. The patient lies on an examining table with hips slightly elevated in a modified lithotomy position. The patient is draped.
2. A slim vaginal transducer, protected by a condom or sterile sheath, is lubricated and introduced into the vagina. Some laboratories prefer that the patient insert the transducer herself. A depth of less than 8 cm is all that is usually required.
3. Scans are performed by using a slight rotation or movement of the handle and by varying the degree of transducer insertion. Typically, the transducer is inserted only several inches into the vaginal vault.
4. Examination time is about 15 to 30 minutes.

Clinical Implications

1. Uterine abnormalities, such as fibroids, intrauterine fluid collections, and variations in structure such as bicornuate uterus, can be detected. Uterine and cervical carcinomas may be visualized, although definitive diagnosis of cancer cannot be made by sonography alone.
2. Very small adnexal masses may not be demonstrated by ultrasound studies. Masses identified on ultrasound may be evaluated in terms of size and consistency.
3. *Cysts*
   a. Ovarian cysts (the most common ovarian mass detected by ultrasound) will appear as smoothly outlined, well-defined masses. Cysts cannot be confirmed as either malignant or benign, but ultrasound studies can increase the suspicion that a particular mass is malignant.
   b. A corpus luteum cyst is a single simple cyst commonly visualized in early pregnancy.
   c. Theca–lutein cysts are associated with hydatidiform mole, choriocarcinoma, or multiple pregnancy.
   d. Parovarian cysts are thin-walled, cystic masses that can become quite large. When the urinary bladder is not distended, these large cysts are often situated low in the pelvis and confused with the urinary bladder.
   e. Because normal ovaries often have numerous visible small cysts, the diagnosis of polycystic ovaries is difficult on the basis of ultrasound alone.

f. Dermoid cysts or benign ovarian teratomas are found in the young adult woman and have an extremely variable appearance. Because of their echogenicity, they are often missed on ultrasound. The only initial clue may be an indentation of the urinary bladder. When a dermoid is suspected on ultrasound, a pelvic x-ray film should be obtained.

4. Solid ovarian tumors, such as fibromas, fibrosarcomas, Brenner tumors, dysgerminomas, and malignant teratomas, are not distinguishable by diagnostic ultrasound. Ultrasound will document the presence of a solid lesion but can go no further in narrowing the diagnosis.

5. Metastatic tumors of the ovary are common and may be solid or cystic in ultrasonic appearance. They are quite variable in size and may be bilateral. Because ascites is often present, the pelvis and remainder of the abdomen should be scanned for fluid.

6. Pelvic inflammatory disease: Ultrasound differentiation between pelvic inflammatory disease and endometriosis is difficult. Evaluation of laboratory results plus clinical history leads to correct diagnosis. Other entities may have similar ultrasonic presentations and include (1) appendicitis with rupture into the pelvis; (2) chronic ectopic pregnancy; (3) posttrauma with hemorrhage into the pelvis; and (4) pelvic abscesses from various causes, such as Crohn's disease or diverticulitis.

7. Bladder distortion: Any distortion of the bladder raises the possibility of an adjacent mass. Tumor, infection, and hemorrhage are the major causes of increased thickness to the urinary bladder wall. Masses such as calculi and catheters may be seen within the bladder lumen. Urinary bladder calculi are highly echogenic. A urinary bladder diverticulum appears as a cystic mass adjacent to the urinary bladder. It may be mistaken for a cystic mass arising from some other pelvic structure, so attempts are made to demonstrate its communication with the bladder.

8. Ultrasound studies can help determine whether a pelvic mass is mobile.

9. Solid pelvic masses, such as fibroids and malignant tumors, may be differentiated from cystic masses, which will show sound patterns similar to the bladder.

10. Lesions may be shown to have metastasized.

11. Studies may aid in the planning of tumor radiation therapy.

12. Position of an intrauterine contraceptive device may be determined.

Interfering Factors

1. Results may be only fair, may vary with the patient's habits and preparation (see "Clinical Implications"), and can be used only in conjunction with other studies. However, masses 1 cm and smaller can be seen with high-resolution equipment.
2. The success of a transabdominal scan is dependent on full bladder distention.

Patient Preparation

1. Explain the purpose and procedure of the test. Fasting is not required.
2. For transabdominal scans, have patient drink four glasses of water or liquid 1 hour before the examination. Advise the patient not to void until the test is over.
3. If a transvaginal (endovaginal) approach is to be used, no patient preparation is required. Contact the laboratory performing the study to determine method to be used.
4. Explain that a liberal coating of coupling agent must be applied to the skin so that there is no air between the skin and the transducer and to permit easy movement of the transducer over the skin. A sensation of warmth or wetness may be felt. Although the acoustic couplant does not stain, the patient should be advised not to wear good clothing for the examination.
5. If a transvaginal (endovaginal) approach is to be used, no patient preparation is required. Determine if the patient has a latex sensitivity and communicate such sensitivities to the examining laboratory. See latex precautions in Appendix II.
6. Reassure the patient that there is no pain or discomfort involved.
7. See Chapter 1 guidelines for safe, effective, informed *pretest* care.

Clinical Alert

1. If the patient is NPO or in certain emergency situations, the patient may be catheterized and the bladder filled through the catheter.
2. Endovaginal studies, when indicated, typically involve the use of a latex condom to sheath the transducer before insertion into the vaginal vault. Contact the laboratory if the patient has a known or suspected latex sensitivity. See Appendix II concerning latex precautions.

Patient Aftercare

1. Interpret test outcomes and counsel about any gynecologic problems.
2. Follow Chapter 1 guidelines for safe, effective, informed *posttest* care.

KIDNEY (RENAL) **SONOGRAM**

Normal Values

Normal pattern image, indicating normal size and position of kidney.

Explanation of Test

This noninvasive test is used to visualize the kidney parenchyma and associated structures, including renal blood vessels. It is often performed following an intravenous pyelogram (IVP) to define and characterize mass lesions or the cause of a nonvisualized kidney. Because no contrast medium is administered, renal ultrasound is valuable in visualizing the kidneys of patients with iodine hypersensitivities. This procedure is also helpful in monitoring the status of a transplanted kidney, guiding stent and biopsy needle placement, and evaluating the progression of chronic conditions.

Procedure

1. The patient lies quietly on an examining table. Scans are often performed with the patient in the decubitus position.
2. Warm oil or gel is applied to the patient's skin.
3. For visualization of the upper ports of the kidney, the patient must inspire as deeply as possible.
4. The total study time varies from 15 to 30 minutes.

Clinical Implications

1. Abnormal pattern readings reveal
   - **a.** Cysts
   - **b.** Solid masses
   - **c.** Hydronephrosis
   - **d.** Obstruction of ureters
   - **e.** Calculi
2. Results provide information on the size, site, and internal structure of a nonfunctioning kidney.
3. Results differentiate between bilateral hydronephrosis, polycystic kidneys, and the small, end-stage kidneys of glomerulonephritis or pyelonephritis.
4. Results may be used to follow kidney development in children with congenital hydronephrosis; this approach is safer than repeated IVP studies.
5. Perirenal fluid collections, such as those associated with complications of transplantation, may be detected. These collections include abscess, hematomas, urinomas, and lymphocele.
6. Solid lesions may be differentiated from cystic lesions.
7. The spread of cancerous conditions from the kidney into the renal vein or IVC can be detected.

Interfering Factors

1. Retained barium from x-ray studies will cause poor results.
2. Obesity adversely affects tissue visualization.

Patient Preparation

1. Explain the purpose and procedure of the test.
2. Assure the patient that there is no pain involved; the only discomfort is that caused by lying quietly for a long period.
3. Explain that a liberal coating of coupling agent must be applied to the skin so that there is no air between the skin and the transducer and to

allow easy movement of the transducer over the skin. A sensation of warmth or wetness may be felt. Although the acoustic couplant does not stain, the patient should be advised not to wear good clothing for the examination.

4. Explain that the patient will be instructed to control breathing patterns while the images are being made.
5. Fasting is usually not necessary but may be required in certain laboratories. Check with your ultrasound department for guidelines.
6. See Chapter 1 guidelines for safe, effective, informed *pretest* care.

Patient Aftercare

1. Interpret test outcomes and counsel about renal disorders.
2. Follow Chapter 1 guidelines for safe, effective, informed *posttest* care.

Clinical Alert

1. Scans cannot be done over open wounds or dressings.
2. This examination must be performed before a barium x-ray study. If such scheduling is not possible, at least 24 hours must elapse between barium procedure and renal echogram.
3. Biopsies are often done using ultrasound as a guideline. If a biopsy is done, a surgical consent form must be signed by the patient.

HEPATOBILIARY SONOGRAMS; GALLBLADDER (GB)/LIVER ULTRASOUND

Normal Values

Normal size, position, and configuration of the gallbladder and bile ducts. Normal adjacent liver tissue.

Explanation of Test

These tests are helpful in differentiating hepatic disease from biliary obstruction. Unlike the oral cholecystogram, this procedure allows visualization of the gallbladder and ducts in impaired liver function. Stones and evidence of cholecystitis are readily visualized. This procedure is indicated as an initial study for persons with right upper quadrant pain. It is also useful as a guide for biopsy or other interventional procedures.

Procedure

1. The patient is asked to lie quietly on an exam table. Scans are generally performed in supine and decubitus positions.
2. The skin is covered with a layer of coupling gel, oil, or lotion.

3. The patient will be asked to regulate breathing patterns as instructed during the examination.
4. Total exam time is about 20 to 30 minutes.

Clinical Implications

1. Abnormal patterns of the gallbladder reveal
   a. Size variations
   b. Thickened wall, indicative of cholecystitis
   c. Benign and malignant lesions, such as polyps. (**Note:** results of sonograms alone cannot differentiate cancers from benign processes.)
   d. Gallstones
2. Bile duct abnormalities such as
   a. Dilation of ducts
   b. Duct obstruction by calculi or tumor
   c. Congenital abnormalities, such as choledochal cysts
3. Adjacent liver pathologic processes, including
   a. Parenchymal disease, such as cirrhosis
   b. Masses, including cysts, solid lesions, and metastatic tumors (**Note:** results of sonograms alone cannot differentiate cancers from benign processes.)

Interfering Factors

1. Intestinal gas overlying area of interest interferes with sonographic visualization.
2. Barium from recent radiographic studies will compromise the study.
3. Obesity adversely affects tissue visualization.

Patient Preparation

1. Explain the purpose and procedure of the test.
2. Instruct the patient to remain NPO for 12 hours before the examination to fully dilate the gallbladder and improve anatomic visualization.
3. Assure the patient that there is no pain involved; however, the patient may feel uncomfortable lying quietly for a long period.
4. Explain that a liberal coating of coupling agent must be applied to the skin so that there is no air between the skin and the transducer and to permit easy movement of the transducer over the skin. A sensation of warmth or wetness may be felt. Although the acoustic couplant does not stain, advise patient not to wear good clothing for the examination.
5. Explain that the patient will be instructed to control breathing patterns while the images are being made.
6. See Chapter 1 guidelines for safe, effective, informed *pretest* care.

Patient Aftercare

1. Interpret test outcomes and counsel about hepatobiliary problems.
2. Follow Chapter 1 guidelines for safe, effective, informed *posttest* care.

Clinical Alert

1. Scans cannot be done over open wounds or through dressings.
2. This examination must be performed before barium x-ray studies. If such scheduling is not possible, at least 24 hours must elapse between the barium procedure and the sonogram.
3. The gallbladder's ability to contract may be tested by administering a fatty substance and rescanning.

ABDOMINAL ULTRASOUND

Normal Values

Normal size, position and appearance of the liver, gallbladder, bile ducts, pancreas, kidneys, spleen, abdominal aorta, and inferior vena cava

Explanation of Test

This noninvasive procedure visualizes all solid organs of the upper abdomen, including the liver, gallbladder, bile ducts, pancreas, kidneys, spleen, and large abdominal blood vessels. Some diagnostic laboratories may perform organ-specific studies, such as renal or hepatobiliary ultrasound. Abdominal ultrasound is valuable in detecting a variety of pathologic processes, including fluid collections, masses, infections, and obstructions.

Procedure

1. The patient is asked to lie quietly on an exam table. Scans are generally performed in supine and decubitus positions.
2. The skin is covered with a layer of coupling gel, oil, or lotion.
3. The patient will be asked to regulate breathing patterns as instructed during the examination.
4. Total exam time is about 30 to 60 minutes.

Clinical Implications

1. Abnormal pattern liver abnormalities reveal
   - **a.** Cysts, tumors, and metastases (**Note:** the results of sonograms alone cannot differentiate malignant from benign conditions.)
   - **b.** Parenchymal disease, such as cirrhosis
   - **c.** Variations to portal venous flow
2. Gallbladder and bile duct abnormalities, including
   - **a.** Duct dilation or obstruction
   - **b.** Gallstones
   - **c.** Cholecystitis
   - **d.** Tumors (**Note:** the results of sonograms alone cannot differentiate malignant from benign conditions.)
3. Pancreas abnormalities, such as

a. Pancreatitis
b. Pseudocyst
c. Cysts and tumors including adenocarcinoma (**Note:** the results of sonograms alone cannot differentiate malignant from benign conditions.)

4. Kidney abnormalities, such as
   a. Hydronephrosis
   b. Cysts, tumors, abscesses (**Note:** the results of sonograms alone cannot differentiate malignant from benign conditions.)
   c. Abnormal size, number, location of kidneys
   d. Calculi
   e. Perirenal fluid collections
5. Spleen abnormalities, such as
   a. Splenomegaly
   b. Evidence of lymphatic disease, lymph node enlargement
   c. Evidence of trauma
6. Vascular abnormalities in the upper abdomen, including
   a. Aneurysm
   b. Thrombi
   c. Abnormal blood flow patterns
7. Miscellaneous pathologic processes, such as
   a. Ascites
   b. Mesenteric or omental cysts or tumors
   c. Congenital absence or malplacement of organs
   d. Retroperitoneal tumors

Interfering Factors

1. Intestinal gas overlying the area of interest interferes with sonographic visualization.
2. Barium from recent x-ray studies will compromise the study.
3. Obesity adversely affects tissue visualization.

Patient Preparation

1. Explain test purpose and procedure.
2. Instruct patient to remain NPO for 12 hours before the exam to fully dilate the gallbladder and improve anatomic visualization of all structures.
3. Assure the patient that there is no pain involved. However, the patient may feel uncomfortable lying quietly for a long time.
4. Explain that a liberal coating of coupling agent must be applied to the skin so that there is no air between the skin and the transducer and to allow easy movement of the transducer over the skin. A sensation of warmth or wetness may be felt. Although the acoustic couplant does not stain, the patient should be advised not to wear good clothing for the exam.

5. Explain that the patient will be instructed to control breathing patterns while the images are being made.
6. See Chapter 1 guidelines for safe, effective, informed *pretest* care.

Clinical Alert

1. Scans cannot be done over open wounds or through dressings.
2. This examination must be performed before barium x-ray studies. If such scheduling is not possible, at least 24 hours must elapse between the barium procedure and the sonogram.

Patient Aftercare

1. Normal diet and fluids are resumed.
2. Interpret test outcomes and counsel appropriately.
3. See Chapter 1 guidelines for safe, effective, informed *posttest* care.

ABDOMINAL AORTA SONOGRAM

Normal Values

Normal pattern image showing regular contour and diameter of the aorta. The walls strongly reflect echoes, whereas the blood-filled lumen is echo-free.

Explanation of Test

This noninvasive ultrasound examination is used to evaluate the abdominal aorta and its major tributaries for structural abnormalities, such as aneurysms and the presence of thrombus. Many laboratories will include Doppler evaluations to characterize blood flow through the vessels. Typically, the path of the abdominal aorta is traced from its most proximal portion to the region of the bifurcation into the iliac arteries.

Procedure

1. The patient is asked to lie quietly on an exam table. Scans are generally performed in supine and decubitus positions.
2. The skin is covered with a layer of coupling gel, oil, or lotion.
3. The patient will be asked to regulate breathing patterns as instructed during the examination.
4. Total exam time is about 30 minutes.

Clinical Implications

1. The typical abnormal pattern reveals aortic aneurysms with or without thrombus. Intimal dissections and leaks may be detected as well.
2. Para-aortic lymphadenopathy may be visualized.

Interfering Factors

1. Intestinal gas overlying the area of interest interferes with sonographic visualization.
2. Barium from recent radiographic studies will compromise the study.
3. Obesity adversely affects tissue visualization.

Patient Preparation

1. Explain the purpose and procedure of the test.
2. Instruct the patient to remain NPO for 12 hours before the examination to improve anatomic visualization of all structures.
3. Assure the patient that there is no pain involved. However, the patient may feel uncomfortable lying quietly for a long period.
4. Explain that a liberal coating of coupling agent must be applied to the skin so that there is no air between the skin and the transducer and to permit easy movement of the transducer over the skin. A sensation of warmth or wetness may be felt. Although the acoustic couplant does not stain, advise patient not to wear good clothing for the exam.
5. Explain that the patient will be instructed to control breathing patterns while the images are being made.
6. See Chapter 1 guidelines for safe, effective, informed *pretest* care.

Clinical Alert

1. Scans cannot be done over open wounds or through dressings.
2. This examination must be performed before barium x-ray studies. If such scheduling is not possible, at least 24 hours must elapse between the barium procedure and the sonogram.

Patient Aftercare

1. Resume normal diet and fluids.
2. Interpret test outcomes and counsel about follow-up care for structural abnormalities.
3. Follow Chapter 1 guidelines for safe, effective, informed *posttest* care.

THYROID SONOGRAM

Normal Values

Normal, homogenous pattern of the thyroid and adjacent structures.

Explanation of Test

This ultrasound study is used to determine the size of the thyroid, to differentiate cysts from tumors, and to reveal the depth and dimension of thyroid goiters and nodules. The response of a mass in the thyroid to suppressive therapy can be monitored by successive examinations. Theoretically, this technique offers the possibility of a good estimation of thyroid weight—information that is important in radioiodine therapy for Graves' disease.

The examination is easy to do, is done before surgery, and gives 85% accuracy. Often, these studies are done in conjunction with radioactive iodine-uptake tests. With pregnant patients, ultrasound studies are the method of choice; radioactive iodine is harmful to the developing fetus.

Procedure

1. The patient lies on the back on the examining table, with the neck hyperextended.
2. A pillow is placed under the shoulder for comfort and to bring the transducer into better contact with the thyroid.
3. An acoustic couplant such as gel, lotion, or oil is applied to the patient's neck. This affords good contact between the transducer and the patient's skin and permits the transducer to be moved easily across the neck's surface.
4. An alternative procedure involves separation of the neck surface from the transducer by a plastic bag filled with water. The water-filled bag is clipped on a stand and hung over the patient's neck. This water bath device permits proper transmission of the ultrasound waves through the thyroid.
5. Examining time is about 30 minutes.

Clinical Implications

1. An abnormal pattern reading will present a cystic, complex, or solid echo pattern.
2. Solitary cold nodules identified on radioisotope scans may appear as echo-free cysts on ultrasound. Most often, cysts are benign. Solid-appearing lesions may represent benign adenomas or malignant tumors. A biopsy is the only definitive method to differentiate the nature of such tumors.
3. Overall gland enlargement is indicative of goiter or thyroiditis.

Interfering Factors

1. Nodules smaller than 1 cm in diameter may escape detection.
2. Cysts not originating in the thyroid may show the same ultrasound characteristics as thyroid cysts.
3. Lesions larger than 4 cm in diameter frequently contain areas of cystic or hemorrhagic degeneration and give a mixed echogram that is difficult to correlate with specific disease.

Patient Preparation

1. Explain the purpose and procedure of the test.
2. Assure the patient that there is no pain involved. However, the patient

may feel uncomfortable maintaining his or her neck in position during the exam.
3. Explain that a liberal coating of coupling agent must be applied to the skin so that there is no air between the skin and the transducer and to permit easy movement of the transducer over the skin. A sensation of warmth or wetness may be felt. Although the acoustic couplant does not stain, the patient should be advised not to wear good clothing for the exam.
4. Advise the patient to refrain from wearing necklaces to the laboratory.
5. See Chapter 1 guidelines for safe, effective, informed *pretest* care.

Clinical Alert

Thyroid biopsies are often performed using ultrasound guidance. If a biopsy is performed, a witnessed informed consent must be signed by the patient in advance of the procedure.

Patient Aftercare

1. Interpret test outcomes and counsel about follow-up treatment for thyroid abnormalities.
2. Follow Chapter 1 guidelines for safe, effective, informed *posttest* care.

HEART SONOGRAM; ECHOCARDIOGRAM; DOPPLER ECHOCARDIOGRAPHY

Normal Values

Normal position, size, and movement of heart valves and chamber walls as visualized in 2-D, M-mode, and Doppler mode. Color M-mode and color Doppler assessment of the heart structures appear within normal limits.

Explanation of Test

This noninvasive technique for examining the heart can provide information about the position, size, movements of the valves and chambers, and velocity of blood flow by means of reflected ultrasound. Echoes from pulsed high-frequency sound waves are used to locate and study the movements and dimensions of cardiac structures, such as the valves and chamber walls. Because the heart is a blood-filled organ, sound can be transmitted through it readily to the opposite wall and to the heart–lung interface. This test is commonly used to determine biologic and prosthetic valve dysfunction and pericardial effusion; to evaluate velocity and direction of blood flow; to furnish direction for further diagnostic study; and to follow cardiac patients over an extended period. One of the advantages of this diagnostic technique is that it is a noninvasive procedure that can be performed at the patient's bedside using mobile equipment, or it can be done in the laboratory.

Different modes of performing echocardiograms are capable of providing a great variety of information about cardiac structure and function. These modes include

Two-dimensional (2-D): used to produce gray scale, cross-sectional images of the heart's anatomy
M-mode: used to generate depictions of rapidly moving structures, such as valves; used for standardized dimensional measurements
Continuous and pulsed-wave Doppler: used to determine velocity of blood flow
Color 2-D: useful for identifying areas of disturbed or eccentric blood flow
Color M-mode: used for evaluating movement of cardiac structures

Specialized types of echocardiograms include

Stress echocardiograms: used to provide information relative to the function of heart structures during high cardiac output states
Transesophageal echocardiograms: when a miniature ultrasound transducer is placed at the end of a tube inserted into the esophagus to provide a closer view of cardiac structures without interference from superficial chest tissues
Fetal echocardiograms: performed through the pregnant abdomen when there is a question of congenital cardiac defect

These special echocardiograms may require a signed informed consent form before performance and involve more complicated procedures. Check with the individual laboratory for specific guides and protocols.

Procedure

1. A specific diagnosis should accompany the request for the test (eg, "rule out pericardial effusion" or "determine severity of mitral stenosis").
2. The patient lies on examining table in a slight side-lying position.
3. The skin surface overlying the chest is lubricated with acoustic gel to permit maximum penetration of the ultrasound beam. The transducer is held over various regions of the chest and upper abdomen to obtain different views of the heart.
4. There is no pain or discomfort involved. Electrocardiogram (ECG) leads may be attached for a simultaneous ECG reading during the echo procedure.
5. Examination time is 30 to 45 minutes.

Clinical Implications

Abnormal values help diagnose the following:

1. Acquired cardiac disease such as

   a. Valvular disease, stenosis, and prolapse
   b. Cardiomyopathies
   c. Evidence of coronary artery disease
   d. Pericardial diseases, including effusion, tamponade, and pericarditis
   e. Endocarditis
   f. Cardiac neoplasm
   g. Intracardiac thrombi
2. Prosthetic valve function
3. Congenital heart disease

Interfering Factors

1. Dysrhythmias
2. The hyperinflation of the lungs with mechanical ventilation, especially with positive end-expiratory pressure (PEEP) of greater than 10 mm, precludes adequate ultrasound imaging of the heart.
3. False-negative and false-positive diagnoses have been identified (especially in M-mode echocardiograms), including pleural effusion, dilated descending aorta, pericardial fat pad, tumors encasing the heart, clotted blood, and loculated effusions.
4. Doppler study results can vary greatly if the transducer position does not provide satisfactory angles for the beam.

Patient Preparation

1. Explain the purpose and procedure of the test.
2. Assure patient that no pain is involved. However, the patient may feel uncomfortable lying quietly for a long period.
3. Explain that a liberal coating of coupling agent must be applied to the skin so that there is no air between the skin and the transducer and to permit easy movement of the transducer over the skin. A sensation of warmth or wetness may be felt. Although the acoustic couplant does not stain, the patient should be advised not to wear good clothing for the examination.
4. See Chapter 1 guidelines for safe, effective, informed *pretest* care.

Clinical Alert

Certain specialized echocardiographic procedures, such as stress echoes and transesophageal echocardiograms (see Chap. 15) may require individualized patient preparation. Check with the laboratory to determine specific protocols and preparation.

Patient Aftercare

1. Interpret test outcomes and counsel about cardiac disorders.
2. Follow Chapter 1 guidelines for safe, effective, informed *posttest* care.

EYE AND ORBIT SONOGRAMS

Normal Values

Pattern image indicating normal soft tissue of eye and retrobulbar orbital areas, retina, choroid, and orbital fat.

Explanation of Test

Ultrasound can be used to describe both normal and abnormal tissues of the eye when no alternative visualization is possible because of opacities. This information is of invaluable assistance in the management of eyes with large corneal leukomas or conjunctival flaps and in the evaluation of eyes for keratoprosthesis. Orbital lesions can be detected and distinguished from inflammatory and congestive causes of exophthalmos, with a high degree of reliability. An extensive preoperative evaluation before vitrectomy surgery or for vitreous hemorrhages is also done. Here, the vitreous cavity is examined to rule out retinal and choroidal detachments and to detect and localize vitreoretinal adhesions and intraocular foreign bodies. Also, persons who are to have intraocular lens implants after removal of cataracts must be measured for exact length of the eye. These exact measurements must be to the nearest 0.1 mm.

Procedure

Two techniques are used: immersion and contact. The immersion technique gives a more sophisticated evaluation because the transducer is placed away from the eye in a water bath.

1. The eye area is anesthetized by instilling eye drops.
2. If the immersion technique is used, the probe is immersed within the fluid, and sound waves are directed along the visual axis.
3. In the contact method, the probe gently touches the corneal surface.
4. If a lesion in the eye is detected, as much as 30 minutes may be required to accurately differentiate the pathologic process.
5. Orbital examination can be done in 8 to 10 minutes

Clinical Implications

1. Abnormal patterns are seen in
   - **a.** Alkali burns with corneal flattening and loss of anterior chamber
   - **b.** Detached retina
   - **c.** Keratoprosthesis
   - **d.** Extraocular thickening in thyroid eye disease
   - **e.** Pupillary membranes
   - **f.** Cyclotic membranes
   - **g.** Vitreous opacities
   - **h.** Orbital mass lesions
   - **i.** Inflammatory conditions
   - **j.** Vascular malformations
   - **k.** Foreign bodies
2. Abnormal patterns are also seen in tumors of various types based on specific ultrasonic patterns.
   - **a.** Solid, such as meningioma, glioma, and neurofibroma

b. Cystic, such as mucocele, dermoid, and cavernous hemangioma
c. Angiomatous, such as diffuse hemangioma
d. Lymphangioma
e. Infiltrative, such as metastatic lymphoma and pseudotumor

Interfering Factors

If at some time the vitreous humor in a particular patient has been replaced by a gas, no result can be obtained.

Patient Preparation

1. Explain the purpose and procedure of the test.
2. Topical anesthetic drops are instilled into the eyes before examination. This is usually done in the examining department.
3. See Chapter 1 guidelines for safe, effective, informed *pretest* care.

Patient Aftercare

1. Instruct the patient to refrain from rubbing the eyes until the effects of anesthetic have disappeared. This type of friction could cause corneal abrasions.
2. Advise the patient that minor discomfort and blurred vision may be experienced for a short time.
3. Follow Chapter 1 guidelines for safe, effective, informed *posttest* care.

URINARY BLADDER SONOGRAM

Normal Values

Normal pattern image of the exact dimensions and contour of the bladder and little residual volume.

Explanation of Test

This examination is done in the investigation of possible bladder tumor and provides a simple method of estimating postvoid residual urine volume. This test reduces the need for urinary catheterization and risk of subsequent urinary tract infection.

Procedure

1. The patient, with bladder fully distended, is instructed to lie on his or her back on an examination table.
2. A coupling agent is applied to the anterior pelvic region to permit maximum penetration of the ultrasound beam.
3. The active face of the transducer is placed in contact with the patient's skin and swept across the area being studied.
4. Typically, when the full-bladder scans are completed, the patient is in-

structed to void. Additional images are taken to check for residual volume.

5. Total exam time is about 20 to 30 minutes.

Clinical Implications

Abnormal results reveal the following:

1. Tumors of bladder
2. Cancerous extension to urinary bladder
3. Thickening of bladder wall
4. Masses posterior to bladder
5. Ureterocele

Interfering Factors

1. Residual barium from previous x-ray studies will affect test results.
2. Overlying gas or fat tissue interferes with the image.

Patient Preparation

1. Explain the purpose and procedure of the test.
2. The bladder should be full to start, then emptied to complete the examination.
3. Assure the patient that there is no pain involved. Some discomfort may be experienced from maintaining a full urinary bladder.
4. Explain that a liberal coating of coupling agent must be applied to the skin so that there is no air between the skin and the transducer and to permit easy movement of the transducer over the skin. A sensation of warmth or wetness may be felt. Although the acoustic couplant does not stain, the patient should be advised not to wear good clothing for the examination.
5. See Chapter 1 guidelines for safe, effective, informed *pretest* care.

Patient Aftercare

1. Patient may return to normal routines.
2. Interpret test outcomes and counsel about bladder abnormalities.
3. Follow Chapter 1 guidelines for safe, effective, informed *posttest* care.

INTRAUTERINE CONTRACEPTIVE DEVICE (IUCD, IUD) LOCALIZATION ●

Normal Values

An intrauterine device (IUD) can be visualized ultrasonically if it has not perforated the uterus.

Explanation of Test

Ultrasonography has been useful for confirming the presence and exact location of an IUD and for identifying the type of contraceptive device within the endometrial cavity. X-ray studies will indicate only that the device is in the pelvis. Most of these devices are sufficiently different in acoustic impedance from the normal uterus that they are easily detected. The precise appearance depends on the type of device used, the position of the device within the uterus, and the position of the device relative to the transducer.

Procedure

1. The patient lies on her back on the examining table. A full bladder is necessary.
2. A coupling gel is applied to the entire abdomen.
3. The transducer is moved across the area being studied.
4. Assure the patient that there is no pain involved. The only discomfort is the feeling of a full bladder.
5. Explain that a liberal coating of coupling agent must be applied to the skin so that there is no air between the skin and the transducer and to permit easy movement of the transducer over the skin. A sensation of warmth or wetness may be felt. Although the acoustic couplant does not stain, the patient should be advised not to wear good clothing for the examination.

Clinical Alert

Some laboratories use an endovaginal approach to assist in IUD localization. Refer to the description of pelvic sonogram on page 840.

Clinical Implications

1. A typical pattern will identify the presence of an IUD.
2. If the device has perforated the uterus, it is seldom possible to visualize it ultrasonically because it blends with the surrounding bowel echoes.

Interfering Factors

Overlying gas or obesity interferes with obtaining a satisfactory result.

Patient Preparation

1. Explain the purpose and procedure of the test.
2. Fasting is not required.
3. Instruct the patient to drink three to four glasses of liquid, preferably water, 1 hour before examination. Advise the patient not to void until the test is completed.
4. The only discomfort involved is the feeling of a full bladder.
5. See Chapter 1 guidelines for safe, effective, informed *pretest* care.

Patient Aftercare

1. Interpret test outcomes and counsel about IUD placement.
2. Follow Chapter 1 guidelines for safe, effective, informed *posttest* care.

BREAST SONOGRAM ●

Normal Values

Symmetric echo pattern in both breasts, including subcutaneous, mammary, and retromammary layers.

Explanation of Test

Ultrasound mammography is useful for differentiating cystic, solid, and complex lesions; in diagnosing disease in women with very dense breasts; and in the follow-up of women with fibrocystic disease. It is recommended as the initial method of examination in young women with palpable masses and in pregnant women with a newly palpable mass. The pregnant patient presents a dilemma because malignancies in pregnancy grow rapidly, and the increased glandular tissue causes difficulties in mammography. Ultrasound may now be used to evaluate women who have silicone prosthesis (as opposed to silicone-injected) augmented breasts. The prosthesis is readily penetrated by the ultrasound beam. Such prostheses are known to obscure masses on physical examination, and x-ray beams are absorbed by the prosthesis, thereby obscuring portions of the breast parenchyma.

Breast sonography is a valuable guide during breast biopsies and needle localization procedures. In addition, sonographic visualization of the breast is an alternative for women who absolutely refuse to have an x-ray mammogram or for those who should not be exposed to radiation.

Two types of breast sonography are performed. Most commonly, a hand-held transducer is slowly moved across the breast tissue, similar in technique to most other forms of sonography. A few institutions perform breast sonography by using a dedicated (automated) breast sonography apparatus. These units comprise a special examination table that houses an ultrasound machine within a tank of treated water. The patient lies on her abdomen, with breast suspended within the water tank, during the study. Either form of breast sonography is capable of producing detailed images of its soft-tissue contents.

Procedure

1. The patient is asked to lie on an examining table.
2. A coupling medium, generally a gel, is applied to the exposed breast to promote the transmission of sound.
3. In most laboratories, a hand-held transducer is slowly moved across the breast. On occasion, an automated breast scanner is used that will require the patient to assume a prone position with the breast immersed in a

tank of water. The tank contains transducers that are moved by remote control to image the breast.
4. Total examining time is 15 minutes.

Clinical Implications

Unusual and distinctive echo patterns will indicate the presence of

1. Cysts
2. Benign solids
3. Malignant tumors
4. Tumor metastasis to muscles and lymph nodes

Interfering Factors

1. Women with back problems or those with limited flexibility may have difficulty maintaining the positions necessary for the procedure.
2. Although the tank is built to accommodate breasts of most sizes, 1% of breasts are too large to examine by this method.

Patient Preparation

1. Explain the purpose and procedure of the examination. There is no discomfort involved. Many diagnostic departments will show the patient a videotape that explains the test.
2. On the day of examination, the patient should wear a two-piece outfit because the garments on the torso will be removed before examination.
3. Explain that a liberal coating of a coupling agent must be applied to the skin so that there is no air between the skin and transducer. This also permits easy movement of the transducer over the skin. A sensation of warmth or wetness may be felt. Although the acoustic couplant does not stain, the patient should be advised not to wear good clothing for the examination.
4. See Chapter 1 guidelines for safe, effective, informed *pretest* care.

> **Clinical Alert**
>
> If the breast sonogram is to be performed on the same day as an x-ray mammogram, advise the patient not to apply any powders, lotions, or other cosmetics to the upper body on the day of the exam.

Patient Aftercare

1. The breasts are cleansed and dried, and the patient is advised to contact her referring physician for outcomes.
2. Answer patient questions concerning follow-up procedures.
3. See Chapter 1 guidelines for safe, effective, informed *posttest* care.

SCROTAL SONOGRAM

Normal Values
Normal scrotal structure.

Explanation of Test
This noninvasive ultrasound study is useful in diagnosing testicular masses, hydroceles, spermatoceles, and diffuse processes. Doppler ultrasound or color-flow Doppler evaluation is helpful in demonstrating the presence of torsion of the testes.

Procedure
1. The patient lies on his back. The penis is gently retracted, and the scrotum is supported on a rolled towel.
2. After an acoustical gel is applied to the skin, the transducer is repeatedly passed over the scrotum. Sonographic images are generated.
3. Total examining time is about 30 minutes.

Clinical Implications
Abnormal results are associated with

1. Abscess (cystic and solid pattern)
2. Infarcted testes
3. Tumor
4. Hydrocele
5. Spermatocele
6. Adherent scrotal hernia
7. Cryptorchism
8. Chronic epididymitis

Patient Preparation
1. Explain purpose and procedure of the test.
2. Assure the patient that there is no pain involved.
3. Explain that a liberal coating of coupling media must be applied to the scrotum. A sensation of warmth or wetness will be felt. Although the acoustic couplant does not stain, the patient should be advised not to wear any good clothing for the examination.
4. See Chapter 1 guidelines for safe, effective, informed *pretest* care.

Patient Aftercare
1. Interpret test outcomes and counsel about follow-up treatment.
2. Follow Chapter 1 guidelines for safe, effective, informed *posttest* care.

PROSTATE SONOGRAM (TRANSRECTAL)

Normal Values
Normal size, contour, and consistency of prostate tissue.

Explanation of Test

This diagnostic technique is valuable in the diagnosis of prostatic cancer when used in association with rectal examination and laboratory testing of blood samples for levels of prostate-specific antigen (see page 379).

Carcinoma of the prostate is the second most common cause of cancer-related deaths in American men. Sonography can be used to evaluate prostate tissue, the seminal vesicles, and surrounding tissue. Small, subclinical tumors may be identified using this method. It is also useful in evaluating palpable nodules and as a guide to biopsy. Sonography may be used to stage a known carcinoma and to assist in radiation "seed" placement. The volume of the prostate can be determined, and transrectal sonography may also be used in the evaluation of micturition disorders.

Procedure

1. Approximately 1 hour before the study, a self-administered enema is used to eliminate fecal material from the rectum.
2. The patient lies on his left side with knees bent toward the chest.
3. A digital rectal exam usually precedes insertion of the rectal transducer.
4. A draped and lubricated rectal probe is inserted. Water may be introduced into the sheath surrounding the transducer. The patient may feel slight pressure at this time.
5. Scans are performed in various planes by using a slight rotational movement of the transducer.
6. Total exam time is approximately 30 minutes.

Clinical Implications

Abnormal results are associated with

1. Prostatitis
2. Benign prostatic hypertrophy
3. Carcinoma of the prostate

Interfering Factors

Fecal material in the rectum will interfere with results.

Patient Preparation

1. Explain the purpose and procedure of the examination.
2. Approximately 1 hour before the study, a self-administered enema is used to eliminate fecal material from the rectum.
3. Assure the patient that there is no pain involved. Anxiety and rectal pressure can be alleviated by advising the patient to breath slowly during the transducer insertion.
4. See Chapter 1 guidelines for safe, effective, informed *pretest* care.

Patient Aftercare

1. Return to normal routine at home or in the nursing unit.
2. Interpret test outcomes and counsel about prostate abnormalities.
3. Follow Chapter 1 guidelines for safe, effective, informed *posttest* care.

● DUPLEX SCANS

CAROTID/CEREBROVASCULAR SONOGRAM; LOWER EXTREMITY VENOUS (LEV) SONOGRAM; LOWER EXTREMITY ARTERIAL (LEA) SONOGRAM ●

Normal Values

Carotid: normal vascular anatomy of common carotid artery, internal and external carotids (often vertebral arteries); no stenosis or occlusion; normal blood flow patterns in major arteries.

LEV: normal venous anatomy of lower extremity; spontaneous, phasic blood flow pattern; normal venous augment (exhibit increased flow superior to site of venous compression) and possesses intact valves.

LEA: normal arterial anatomy of lower extremity; normal triphasic blood flow; no plaques or other pathologic processes; normal segmental blood pressure.

Explanation of Test

These noninvasive Doppler procedures provide anatomic and hemodynamic information. Carotid duplex scans examine the major arteries supplying the brain as an indication of cerebrovascular blood flow. Carotid scans evaluate ischemia, headache, dizziness, hemiparesis, paresthesia, speech and visual disturbances. Testing is commonly done before major cardiovascular surgery and after surgery.

LEV examines venous blood flow in the lower extremities. It is most commonly used to assess deep vein thrombosis and can also be used to "map" veins to be harvested and used for grafts. The large veins of the thigh and upper calf are well visualized by this modality, without the administration of contrast medium. In many institutions, it has replaced x-ray venography as a screen for deep venous thrombosis detection.

LEA visualizes and documents arterial blood flow in the lower extremities. It can determine the presence, amount, and location of plaques and is helpful in assessing the cause of claudication. Graft patency and condition may also be evaluated.

Procedure

1. The patient is usually asked to lie on the examining table with the neck slightly extended. For carotid tests, the head is turned to one side—for lower extremities, the head is slightly elevated and the exposed leg is turned slightly outward.
2. Acoustic coupling gel is applied to the testing area (neck or leg) to enhance sound transmission. During Doppler evaluation, an audible signal, representing blood flow, can be heard.
3. **Carotid procedure:** A hand-held transducer is gently moved up and

down neck while images of appropriate blood vessels are made. Both right and left carotid vessels are examined; time is approximately 30 to 60 minutes.

4. **LEV procedure:** A hand-held transducer is maneuvered over the blood vessels from the groin region to the calf. Both legs are examined for comparison. Examination time is approximately 30 minutes.
5. **LEA procedure:** A hand-held transducer is maneuvered over the blood vessels from the iliac region to the calf area. Both legs are examined for comparison. Following the imaging portion of the procedures, many laboratories perform segmental blood pressure assessment. A variable number of blood pressure cuffs will be placed in the extremity from high on the thigh to just superior to the ankle. Cuffs are inflated and pressure readings are obtained. Examination time is approximately 60 minutes.

Clinical Implications

1. Abnormal images and Doppler signals represent evidence of
   - **a.** Plaque
   - **b.** Stenosis
   - **c.** Occlusion
   - **d.** Dissection
   - **e.** Aneurysm
   - **f.** Carotid body tumor
2. Abnormal LEV images and Doppler signals represent evidence of
   - **a.** Deep venous thrombosis
   - **b.** Venous obstruction
   - **c.** Incompetent valves
3. Abnormal flow patterns such as spectral broadening and monophasic flow represent evidence of
   - **a.** Arterial calcification or plaques
   - **b.** Ischemia
   - **c.** Vessel occlusion
   - **d.** Graft diameter reduction
   - **e.** Pseudoaneurysm
   - **f.** Aneurysm
   - **g.** Hematoma

Interfering Factors

1. Severe obesity will compromise exam quality. Pressures may be unobtainable.
2. Cardiac arrhythmias and disease may cause changes in hemodynamic patterns.
3. In arterial wall hardening (commonly seen in diabetic persons), pressures may be extremely elevated.

Patient Preparation

1. Explain test purpose and procedure. Assure patient that no radiation is employed, no contrast media are injected, and no pain is involved. Some slight discomfort may be experienced when blood pressure cuffs are inflated for extremity test.

2. Advise that a liberal coating of coupling agent must be applied to the skin to promote sound transmission. A sensation of warmth or wetness may be felt during application. Although gel does not stain, tell patient to wear washable clothing.
3. For lower extremity testing, when legs must be examined, advise patient to wear clothing that can easily be removed from lower body. As appropriate for type of test, have patient remove necklaces, earrings, or bracelets before examination.
4. See Chapter 1 guidelines for safe, effective, informed *pretest* care.

Patient Aftercare

1. Remind patient to remove any residual gel from the skin.
2. Interpret test outcomes, provide support, and counsel appropriately concerning abnormal blood flow. Monitor and counsel for arterial or venous disease.
3. See Chapter 1 guidelines for safe, effective, informed *posttest* care.

Clinical Alert

1. An upper extremity arterial study (UEA) is essentially the same procedure performed on the arteries of the lower extremities (LEA).
2. An upper extremity venous study (UEV) is essentially the same procedure performed on the veins of the lower extremities (LEV).

BIBLIOGRAPHY

Berman MC: Diagnostic Medical Sonography, Vol. 1, Obstetrics and Gynecology. Philadelphia, JB Lippincott, 1991

Bernstein EF: Recent Advances in Noninvasive Diagnostic Techniques in Vascular Disease. St. Louis, CV Mosby, 1990

Carroll BA: Carotid sonography, Radiology 178:303–313, 1991

Craig M: Diagnostic Medical Sonography, Vol. 2, Echocardiography. Philadelphia, JB Lippincott, 1991

Hagen-Ansert SL: Textbook of Diagnostic Ultrasonography, 3rd ed. St. Louis, CV Mosby, 1989

Kawamura DM: Diagnostic Medical Sonography, Vol. 3, Abdomen. Philadelphia, JB Lippincott, 1992

Kremkau FW: Diagnostic Ultrasound: Principles and Instruments, 4th ed. Philadelphia, WB Saunders, 1993

Martin JP: Prep talks—transrectal ultrasound: A new screening tool for prostate cancer. Am J Nurs 91(2):69, February 1991

McIntyre L: A three phase ultrasound examination for deep venous thrombosis. J Diagn Med Sonogr 8:33–37, 1991

Mittelstaedt CA: General Ultrasound. Churchill Livingstone, 37, 1992

Peters BE, Kocherl GP: Diagnostic Medical Ultrasound Examination Review, 2nd ed. New Hyde Park, NY, Medical Examination Publishing, 1989

Ridgway DP: Introduction to Vascular Scanning. Appleton Davies, 1992

Rumak CM: Diagnostic Ultrasound, Vol. 1 and 2. St. Louis, CV Mosby, 1991

Sanders RC: Clinical Sonography, a Practical Guide. Boston, Little, Brown, 1991

Tempkin BB: Ultrasound Scanning: Principles and Protocols. Philadelphia, WB Saunders, 1993

14

Pulmonary Function and Blood Gas Studies

OVERVIEW OF LUNG FUNCTION TESTS

Pulmonary Physiology

There are three aspects of pulmonary function: perfusion, diffusion, and ventilation. *Perfusion* relates to blood flow through pulmonary vessels; *diffusion* refers to movement of oxygen and carbon dioxide across alveolar capillary membranes; *ventilation* relates to air exchange between alveolar spaces and the atmosphere.

During breathing, the lung–thorax system acts as a bellows to provide air to the alveoli so that adequate gas exchange can take place. Like a spring or rubber band, the lung tissue also possesses the property of elasticity. When the inspiratory muscles contract, the thorax and lungs expand; when the same muscles relax, and the force is removed, the thorax and lungs return to their resting position. Also, when the thorax and lungs expand, the alveolar pressure is lowered below atmospheric pressure. This permits air to flow into the trachea, bronchi, bronchioles, and alveoli. Expiration is mainly passive. It occurs because the thorax and lungs recoil to their resting position. Hence, alveolar pressure increases above atmospheric pressure and air flows out through the respiratory tract. The major function of the lung is to provide adequate ventilation to meet the metabolic demands of the body during rest, as well as during maximal exercise. The primary purpose of pulmonary blood flow is to conduct mixed venous blood through the capillaries of the alveoli so that oxygen (O_2) can be taken up by the blood and carbon dioxide (CO_2) can be removed from the blood.

Use of Tests

Pulmonary function tests determine the presence, nature, and extent of pulmonary dysfunction caused by obstruction or restriction, or a combination of both.

When ventilation is disturbed by an increase in airway resistance, the ventilatory defect is called an *obstructive* ventilatory impairment. When ventilation is disturbed by a limitation in chest wall excursion, the defect is referred to as a *restrictive* ventilatory impairment. When ventilation is altered by both increased airway resistance and limited chest wall excursion, the defect is termed a *combined* or *mixed* defect. (Table 14–1 summarizes conditions that affect ventilation.)

Pulmonary function studies may reveal locations of, and abnormalities in, airways, alveoli, and pulmonary vascular bed early in the course of a disease when the results of physical examination and x-ray studies still appear normal.

Indications for Tests

1. For early detection of pulmonary or cardiac pulmonary disease
2. For differential diagnosis of dyspnea
3. For presurgical assessment (eg, ability to tolerate intraoperative anesthetics, especially during thoracic procedures)

TABLE 14-1
Conditions That Affect Ventilation

CLASSIFICATION OF VENTILATORY IMPAIRMENTS

Restrictive Ventilatory Impairments

Characterized by interference with chest wall or lung movement; "stiff lung;" an actual reduction in the volume of air that can be inspired.

Examples of Restrictive Ventilatory Impairments	***Caused by***
Chest wall disease	Injury, kyphoscoliosis, spondylitis, muscular dystrophy, other neuromuscular diseases
Extrathoracic conditions	Obesity, peritonitis, ascites, pregnancy
Interstitial lung disease	Interstitial pneumonitis, fibrosis, pneumoconioses (eg, asbestosis, silicosis) granulomatosis, edema, sarcoidosis
Pleural disease	Pneumothorax, hemothorax, pleural effusion, fibrothorax
Space-occupying lesion	Tumors, cysts, abscesses

Obstructive Ventilatory Impairment

Characterized by need for increased effort to produce airflow; respiratory muscles must work harder to overcome obstructive forces during breathing. Prolonged and impaired airflow during expiration. Airway resistance increases and lungs become very compliant.

Examples of Obstructive Ventilatory Impairment	***Caused by***
Peripheral airway disease	Bronchitis, bronchiectasis, bronchiolitis, bronchial asthma, cystic fibrosis
Pulmonary parenchymal disease	Emphysema
Upper airway disease	Pharyngeal, tracheal, or laryngeal tumors; edema, infections, foreign bodies, collapsed airway, stenosis

Mixed Defect Ventilatory Impairment

Combined or mixed; exhibits components of both obstructive and restrictive ventilatory imairments.

Examples of Mixed Ventilatory Impairment	***Caused by***
Pulmonary congestion	Increases in both airway resistance and limited expansion of chest cavity and/or chest wall; obstruction caused

(continued)

TABLE 14-1 *(Continued)*

Examples of Mixed Ventilatory Impairment	***Caused by***
Pulmonary congestion	by bronchial edema; compression of respiratory airway caused by increased interstitial (and intravenous fluid) pressure; restriction caused by impaired elasticity; anatomic deformity such as kyphosis, lordosis, scoliosis

Combined or mixed, a component of both obstructive and restrictive ventilatory impairments

Examples of Mixed Ventilatory Impairment	***Caused by***
Pulmonary congestion Increases in both airway resistance and limitation in expansion of chest cavity	Obstructive caused by bronchial edema and compression of respiratory airway caused by increased interstitial and intravenous fluid pressure; restrictive caused by increase in elastic resistance of lung caused by increased interstitial and intravenous fluid pressure

4. For evaluation of risk factors for other diagnostic procedures
5. For detection of early respiratory failure
6. For monitoring progress of bronchopulmonary disease
7. For periodic evaluation of workers exposed to materials harmful to the respiratory system
8. For epidemiologic studies of select populations to determine risks for, or causes of, pulmonary diseases
9. For workers' compensation claims
10. For monitoring pharmacologic or surgical intervention

Classification of Tests

Pulmonary function tests evaluate the ventilatory system and alveoli in an indirect, overlapping way. The patient's age, height, weight, race, and sex are recorded before testing because they are the basis for calculating predicted values.

Pulmonary function tests are generally divided into three categories:

1. *Airway flow rates* typically include measurements of instantaneous or average airflow rates during a maximal forced exhalation to assess airway

patency and resistance. These also assess responses to inhaler bronchodilators or bronchial provocations.

2. *Lung volumes and capacities* measure the various "air-containing compartments" of the lung to assess air-trapping (hyperinflation, overdistention, or reduction in volume). These also differentiate obstructive versus restrictive ventilatory impairments.
3. *Gas exchange* (diffusion capacity) measures the rate of gas transfer across the alveolar–capillary membranes to assess the diffusion process. It can also monitor for side effects of drugs, such as bleomycin (neoplastic) or amiodarone (antiarrhythmic), that can cause interstitial pneumonitis or fibrosis. Diffusion capacity, in the absence of lung disease (eg, anemia), can also be evaluated.

SYMBOLS AND ABBREVIATIONS

Pulmonary function studies and blood gas analyses measure quantities of gas mixtures and their components, blood and its constituents, as well as various factors affecting these quantities. Symbols and abbreviations given here are based on standards developed by American physiologists. Familiarity with major and secondary symbols facilitate interpretation of any combination of these symbols (Charts 14–1 to 14–4).

PULMONARY FUNCTION TESTS

SPIROMETRY

Lung capacities, volumes, and flow rates are clinically measured by a spirometer. The electrical recording of the amounts of gas breathed in and out produces a spirogram. Spirometers can be grouped into two major categories: the mechanical (volume displacement) types; such as water-filled, dry-rolling seal, wedge, or bellows; and the electronic (flow-sensing) types, such as Fleisch pneumotach or hot-wire anemometer.

The water-seal spirometer has been the basic tool for many years. It consists of a bell, suspended in a sleeve of water (Fig. 14–1). The bell rises and falls in response to inhalation and exhalation through a tube connected to the spirometer. The proportional movements of the bell are recorded, either on a kymograph (a rotating drum on which a tracing is made with a stylus) or by an electrical potentiometer. Measured actual values are then compared with the predicted values by regression equations, using age, height, weight, race, and sex, and they are expressed as a percentage of predicted values. Typically a percentage of predicted value higher than 80% is considered to be within normal limits.

Spirometry determines the effectiveness of the various mechanical forces

CHART 14-1
Gas Volumes: Symbols and Abbreviations

Large capital letters denote primary symbols for gases.

V = Gas volume
$\dot{V}$ = Gas volume per unit time (the dot over the symbol indicates the factor per unit time)
P = Gas pressure or partial pressure of a gas in a gas mixture (exhaled air) or in a liquid (blood)
F = Fractional concentration of a gas

Small capital letters indicate the type of gas measured in relation to respiratory tract location or function.

A = Alveolar gas
D = Dead space gas
E = Expired gas
I = Inspired gas
T = Tidal gas

Chemical symbols for gases may be placed after the small capital letters previously listed.

O_2 = Oxygen
CO = Carbon monoxide
CO_2 = Carbon dioxide
N_2 = Nitrogen

COMBINATIONS OF SYMBOLS
The following are some examples of the ways these symbols may be combined:

V_T = Tidal volume
V_E = Volume of expired gas
P_{ACO_2} = Partial pressure of carbon dioxide in alveolar gas

BLOOD GAS SYMBOLS
Large capital letters are used as primary symbols for blood.

C = Concentration of a gas in blood
S = Percentage saturation of hemoglobin
Q = Volume of blood
$\dot{Q}$ = Volume of blood per unit time (blood flow)

To indicate whether blood is capillary, venous, or arterial, *lower case letters* are used as subscripts.

v = Venous blood
a = Arterial blood
c = Capillary blood
s = Shunted blood

CHART 14-2
Combinations of Symbols and Abbreviations

Blood gas symbols may be combined in the following ways:

Po_2	=	Oxygen tension or partial pressure of oxygen
Pao_2	=	Arterial oxygen tension or partial pressure of oxygen in arterial blood
P_{AO_2}	=	Alveolar oxygen tension or partial pressure of oxygen in the alveoli
Pco_2	=	Carbon dioxide tension or partial pressure of carbon dioxide
$Paco_2$	=	Partial pressure of carbon dioxide in arterial blood
$Pvco_2$	=	Partial pressure of carbon dioxide in venous blood
So_2	=	Oxygen saturation
pH	=	Hydronium (hydrogen) ion concentration
pH_a	=	Hydronium (hydrogen) ion concentration in arterial blood
Sao_2	=	Percentage saturation of oxygen in arterial blood as measured by hemoximetry (direct method)
Svo_2	=	Percentage saturation of oxygen in venous blood
Spo_2	=	Percentage saturation of oxygen in arterial blood as determined by pulse oximetry (indirect method)
Tco_2	=	Total carbon dioxide content

CHART 14-3
Lung Volume Symbols: Pulmonary Function Terminology

This list indicates terms used in measuring lung volumes as well as the units used in expressing these measurements.

FVC	=	*Forced vital capacity*: maximal amount of air that can be exhaled forcibly and completely following a maximal inspiration (units; L)
FEV_1	=	*Forced expiratory volume* in 1 second: volume of air expired during the first second of the FVC maneuver (units; L)
FEV_3	=	*Forced expiratory volume* in 3 seconds: volume of air expired during the first 3 seconds of the FVC maneuver (units; L)
FEV_t/FVC	=	Ratio of a timed forced expiratory volume to the forced vital capacity (eg, FEV_1/FVC) (units, percent)
$FEF_{200-1200}$	=	*Forced expiratory flow* between 200 ml and 1200 ml flow of expired air measured after the first 200 ml and during the next 1000 ml of the FVC maneuver (units; L/sec)

(continued)

CHART 14-3 *(continued)*

FEF_{25-75}	=	*Forced expiratory flow* between 25% and 75%: flow of expired air measured between 25% and 75% of the FVC maneuver (units, L/sec)
PEFR	=	*Peak expiratory flow rate*: maximum flow of expired air attained during an FVC maneuver (units; L/sec or L/min)
PIFR	=	*Peak inspiratory flow rate*: maximum flow of inspired air achieved during a forced maximal inspiration (units; L/sec or L/min)
FEF_{25}	=	Instantaneous flow rate at 25% of lung volume achieved during an FVC maneuver (units; L/sec or L/min)
FEF_{50}	=	Instantaneous flow rate at 50% of lung volume achieved during an FVC maneuver (units; L/sec or L/min)
FEF_{75}	=	Instantaneous flow rate at 75% of lung volume achieved during an FVC maneuver (units; L/sec or L/min)
FIVC	=	*Forced inspiratory vital capacity*: maximal amount of air that can be inhaled forcibly and completely following a maximal expiration (units; L)
FRC	=	*Functional residual capacity*: volume of air remaining in the lung at the end of a normal expiration (units; L)
IC	=	*Inspiratory capacity*: maximal amount of air that can be inspired from end tidal expiration (units; L)
IRV	=	*Inspiratory reserve volume*: maximal amount of air that can be inspired from end tidal inspiration (units, L)
ERV	=	*Expiratory reserve volume*: maximal amount of air that can be expired from end tidal expiration (units, L)
RV	=	*Residual volume*: volume of gas left in the lung following a maximal expiration (units, L)
VC	=	*Vital capacity*: maximal volume of air that can be expired following a maximal inspiration (units, L)
TLC	=	*Total lung capacity*: volume of gas contained in the lungs following a maximal inspiration (units, L)
DLCO	=	Carbon monoxide diffusing capacity of the lung—rate of diffusion of carbon monoxide across the alveolar–capillary membrane (ie, rate of gas transfer across the alveolar–capillary membrane (units, $ml/mm^{-1}/torr^{-1}$)
DL/VA	=	Carbon monoxide diffusing capacity per liter of alveolar volume (units, $ml/mm^{-1}/torr^{-1}$ L^{-1} of alveolar volume)
CV	=	*Closing volume*: volume at which the lower lung zones cease to ventilate, presumably as a result of airway closure (units, percentage of VC)
MVV	=	*Maximal voluntary ventilation*: maximal number of liters of air a patient can breathe per minute by a voluntary effort (units, L/min)
$V_{ISO}\dot{V}$	=	*Volume of isoflow:* volume in which flow was the same with air and with helium during an FVC maneuver

CHART 14-4
Miscellaneous Symbols

This list refers to an assortment of symbols found throughout the chapter.

A	=	Age in years
W	=	Weight in pounds
H	=	Height in inches
torr	=	A unit of pressure equal to 1/760 of normal atmospheric pressure or to the pressure necessary to support a column of mercury 1 mm high at 0°C and standard gravity
f	=	Frequency of breathing
C	=	Compliance
He	=	Helium
Hg	=	Mercury
D	=	Diffusing capacity
CO	=	Carbon monoxide
D_{LO_2}	=	Oxygen diffusing capacity of the lung (ml/mm^{-1}/torr^{-1})
$A\text{–}aD_{O_2}$	=	Alveolar-to-arterial oxygen gradient
BSA	=	Body surface area (unit, m^2)
H_2CO_3	=	Carbonic acid
HCO_3	=	Bicarbonate
TGV	=	Thoracic gas volume (also expressed as V_{TG})
Raw	=	Airway resistance
F-V	=	Flow volume
V-T	=	Volume time
pH	=	Negative logarithm of the hydrogen ion concentration, used as a positive number to indicate acidity or alkalinity
BE	=	Base excess–deficit

involved in lung and chest wall movement. The values obtained provide quantitative information about the degree of obstruction to airflow, or the restriction of the amount of inspired air (Figs. 14–2 and 14–3).

Procedure for Spirometry: Spirometry Measures PVC, FEV_1, $FEV_{1,2,3}$, $FEF_{200–1200}$, $FEF_{25–75}$

1. The patient may sit or stand.
2. The patient is fitted with a mouthpiece connected to the spirometer, and a noseclip closes the nares so that only mouth-breathing is possible.
3. The patient is then asked to inhale maximally, hold the breath momentarily, and then exhale forcibly and completely.
4. Between brief rest periods, Step 3 is repeated twice. (A minimum of three tracings are obtained. The two best ones should come within 5% of each other.)
5. The entire procedure takes about 15 to 20 minutes.

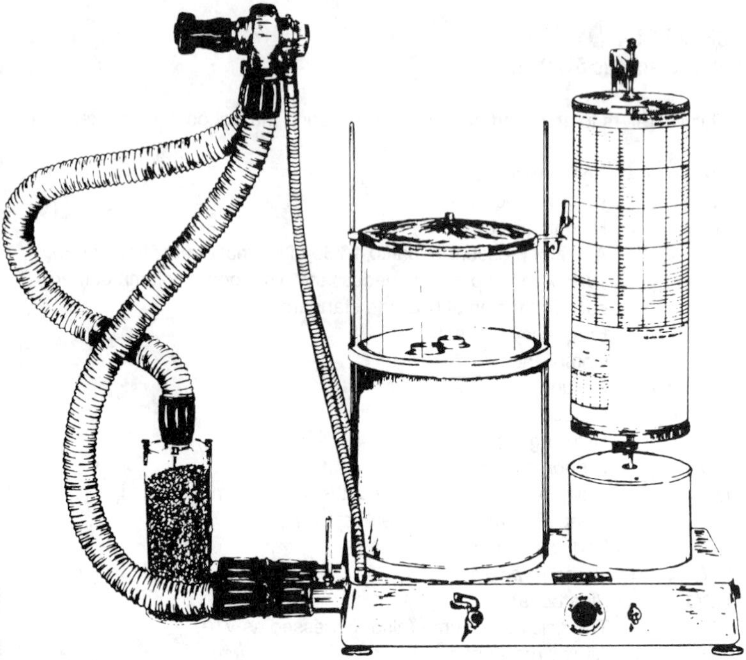

FIGURE 14-1
The Collins Stead–Wells spirometer. (Courtesy of Warren E. Collins, Inc, Braintree, MA)

Clinical Alert

1. Before testing, assess ability to comply with breathing requirements.
2. Patient may experience light-headedness, shortness of breath, or other slight discomforts. These symptoms are generally transitory. An appropriate rest period is usually all that is needed. If symptoms persist, testing is terminated.
3. Rarely, momentary loss of consciousness (caused by anoxia during forced expiration) may occur. Follow established protocols for testing this.
4. Assess for contraindications, such as pain or altered mental status.

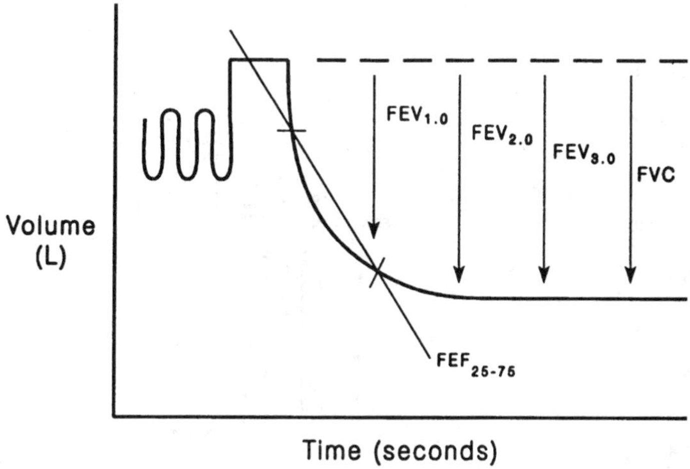

FIGURE 14-2
Typical volume–time spirogram illustrating the measurements of FVC, FEV_1, FEV_2, FEV_3, and FEF_{25-75} (see test for further explanation).

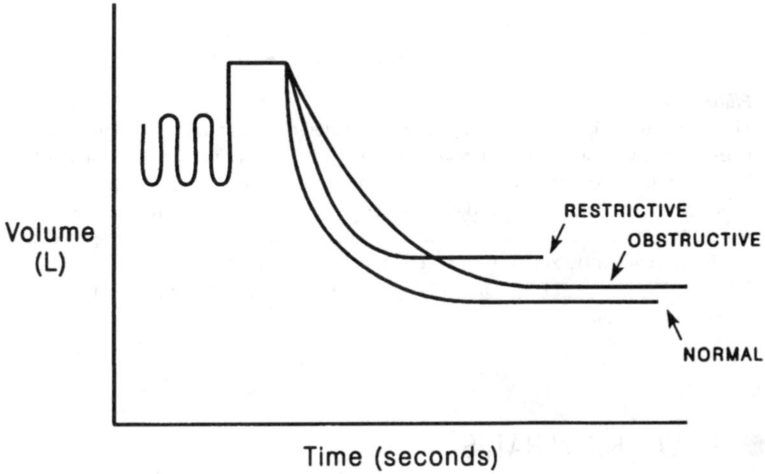

FIGURE 14-3
Examples of normal, obstructive, and restrictive volume–time spirograms.

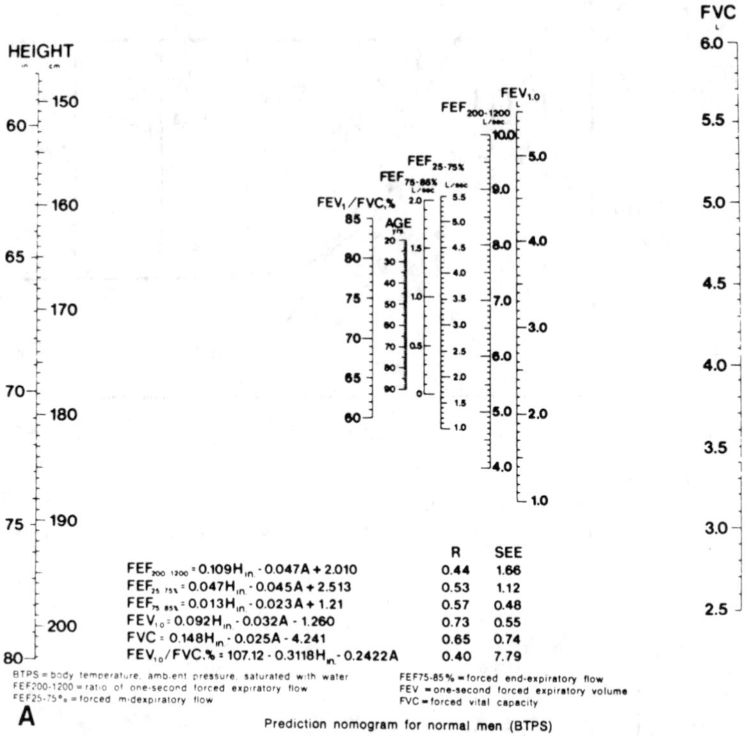

FIGURE 14-4

This is an example of a typical nomogram for determining various expiratory flow rates in normal males (*A*) and normal females (*B*). The values are determined by laying a ruler across the height scale and age scale (corresponding to the patient's height and age) and then reading the values where the ruler crosses the other scales. When the test site has computer equipment, the values are computed electronically. Values obtained in this determination include the FVC, FEV, FEF_{25-75}, PEFR, PIFR, FEF_{25}, FEF_{50}, and FEF_{75}. See Figure 14-5 for an example of a flow–volume loop.

● AIRWAY FLOW RATES

Airway flow rates provide information about the severity of airway obstruction and serve as an index of dynamic function. The lung volume at which the flow rates are measured is useful in identifying central or peripheral location of airway obstruction.

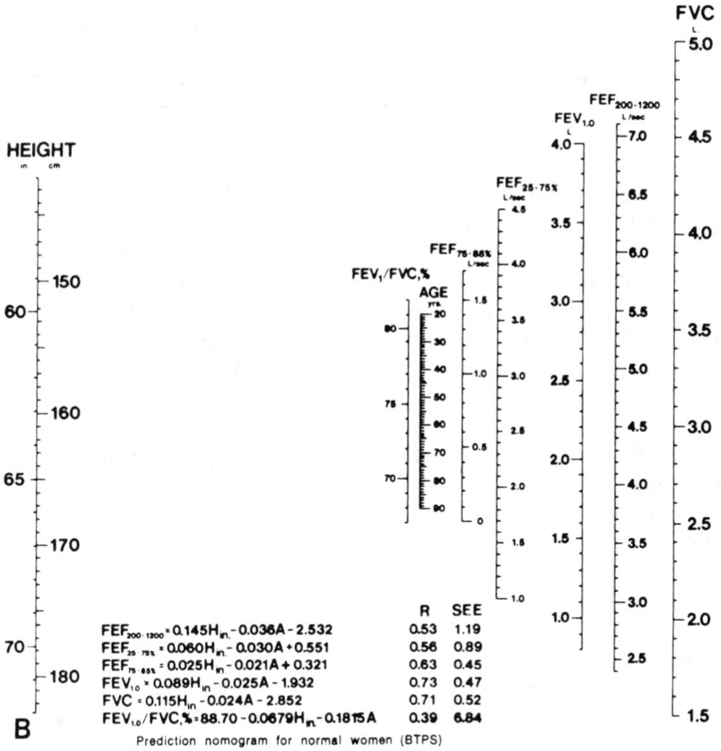

B

FIGURE 14-4
(Continued)

FORCED VITAL CAPACITY (FVC); **FORCED EXPIRATORY VOLUME** (FEV); **TIMED** (FEV_+) ●

Normal Values

FVC = approximately 3.00 to 5.00 L
FEV+ includes
FEV_1 = 80% to 85% of FVC
FEV_2 = 90% to 94% of FVC
FEV_3 = 95% to 97% of FVC

Predicted values for patients, based on age, height, race, and sex, are calculated from a nomogram (Fig. 14–4).

Explanation of Test

The forced expiratory maneuver (spirometry) is useful in quantifying the extent and severity of airway obstruction. The maximum amount of air that can be exhaled rapidly and forcibly, after a maximum deep inspiration, is recorded as the FVC, corrected for body temperature, pressure, and saturation (BTPS), and is expressed in liters.

The volumes exhaled within 1, 2, and 3 seconds are referred to as FEV_1, FEV_2, and FEV_3, or timed vital capacities. These measurements are useful for evaluating a patient's response to bronchodilators. Generally, if the FEV_1 is less than 80%, or the FEF_{25-75} is less than 60%, of their respective predicted values, a bronchodilator, such as albuterol sulfate (Proventil) or ipratropium bromide (Atrovent), is administered with a mininebulizer, and the spirometry is repeated. An increase in the FEV_1 or the FEF_{25-75} of 20% or more above the prebronchodilator level suggests a significant response to the bronchodilator and is consistent with a diagnosis of reversible obstructive airway disease, such as asthma. The person with emphysema typically does not demonstrate this type of response to bronchodilators.

Procedure

1. The patient is asked to exhale forcibly and rapidly after a maximum air inspiration.
2. These measurements are obtained from spirometry tracings (see Spirometry).
3. Brochodilators are administered with a mininebulizer, and spirometry is repeated.

Clinical Implications

1. Obstructive ventilatory impairments, such as asthma, lead to decreases in airway flow rates and, in the more severe forms, apparent loss of volume, because of airway collapse during the forced expiratory effort.
2. Decreased values occur in chronic lung diseases that cause trapping of air (emphysema), chronic bronchitis, or asthma.
3. In restrictive ventilatory impairments, the FVC is reduced, however, flow rates can be normal or elevated.

Patient Preparation

1. Explain the purpose and procedure of the spirometry test (see page 871). Emphasize that this is a noninvasive test; however, it does require cooperation and effort.
2. Withhold bronchodilators for 4 to 6 hours before study, if tolerated.
3. Assess for interfering factors and contraindications, such as pain or physical or mental impairment.
4. Follow guidelines in Chapter 1 for safe, effective, informed *pretest* care.

Patient Aftercare

1. Evaluate complaints of fatigue, shortness of breath, or chest discomfort or pain. Monitor and provide rest as necessary.
2. Assess patient and test outcomes and monitor appropriately for signs of asthma, emphysema, and other chronic lung diseases.
3. Follow guidelines for safe, effective, informed, *posttest* care in Chapter 1.

FLOW–VOLUME LOOPS (F-V LOOPS)

Normal Values

Quantitative: A "scooped-out," concave appearance of the expiratory portion of the F-V loop is characteristic of obstructive ventilatory impairment. This contrasts with the normal F-V loop, which may actually be somewhat convex on the descending portion of the expiratory limb. The restrictive F-V loop looks similar in configuration to the normal loop, except that it is smaller.

Explanation of Test

This test provides both a graphic analysis and a quantitative measurement of flow rates for any lung volume. It evaluates the dynamics of both large- and medium-sized (central) airways and is also quite helpful in ruling out small peripheral airway obstruction. Values obtained include FVC, FEV_1, FEF_{25-75}, PEFR, PIFR, FEF_{25}, FEF_{50}, and FEF_{75}. Figure 14–5 is an example of a flow–volume loop.

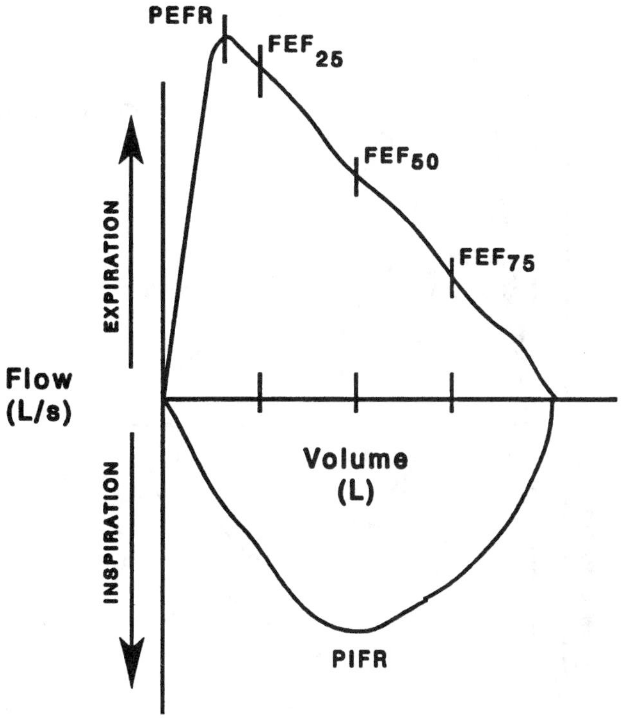

FIGURE 14-5
Typical flow–volume loop illustrating the measurements of PEFR, PIFR, FEF_{25}, FEF_{50}, and FEF_{75} (see text for further explanation).

Procedure

The procedure is the same as that for spirometry, except for the addition of a maximal, forced inspiration at the end of the forced expiratory maneuver.

Clinical Implications

Abnormal configurations of the flow–volume loops indicate (Fig. 14–6)

1. Obstructive ventilatory impairments
   a. Small-airway obstructive disease, such as bronchitis and asthma
   b. Large-airway obstructive disease, such as tumors of the trachea and bronchioles
2. Restrictive ventilatory impairments, such as interstitial pulmonary fibroses and obesity, among others

Patient Preparation

1. Explain the purpose and procedure of the spirometry test. Tell the patient that he or she will also need to perform a maximal forced inspiration.

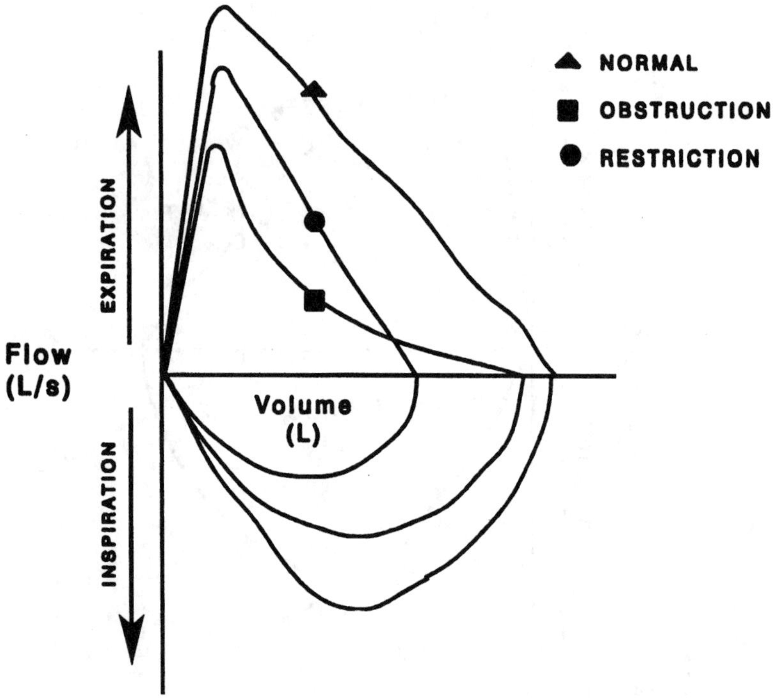

FIGURE 14-6
Examples of a normal, obstructive, and restrictive flow–volume loop.

2. A light meal may be eaten before the test. However, no caffeine should be taken before testing.
3. Follow Chapter 1 guidelines for safe, effective, informed *pretest* care, if possible.

Patient Aftercare

1. See Chapter 1 for safe, effective, informed *posttest* care guidelines.
2. See aftercare guidelines for forced vital capacity.
3. Evaluate for dizziness, shortness of breath, chest discomfort. Generally, these symptoms are transitory, and after a short rest, they will subside. If persistent, use established follow-up protocols.

PEAK INSPIRATORY FLOW RATE (PIFR) ●

Normal Values

Approximately 300 L/min.
Predicted values are based on age, sex, and height.

Explanation of Test

Peak inspiratory flow rate identifies reduced breathing on inspiration, and it is totally dependent on the effort the patient makes to inhale. The PIFR is the maximum airflow achieved during a forced maximal inspiration (see indications for tests, pages 868 and 878).

Procedure

1. The PIFR is obtained from the flow–volume loop procedure using the spirometer, with a special X-Y recorder.
2. The patient is instructed to inhale maximally, exhale forcibly and completely, and then inhale forcibly and completely (see Fig. 14–5).

Clinical Implications

1. The PIFR is reduced in neuromuscular disorders, weakness, poor effort, and extrathoracic airway obstruction (ie, substernal thyroid, tracheal stenosis, and laryngeal paralysis).
2. The PIFR will be altered in upper airway obstruction.

Interfering Factors

Poor patient effort is the major interfering factor.

Patient Preparation

1. Explain the purpose and procedure of the spirometry test. Assess patient ability to comply.
2. Follow Chapter 1 guidelines for safe, effective, informed, *pretest* care.

Patient Aftercare

1. See Chapter 1 guidelines for safe, effective, informed *posttest* care.
2. See aftercare guidelines for forced vital capacity.

PEAK EXPIRATORY FLOW RATE (PEFR)

Normal Values

Approximately 450 L/min.
Predicted values are based on age, sex, and height.

Explanation of Test

This measurement of lung volume flow rate is used as an index of large-airway function. It is the maximum flow of expired air attained during an FVC maneuver (see indications for tests, pages 868 and 878).

Procedure

1. The PEFR is obtained from the flow–volume loop procedure using the spirometer with an X-Y special recorder (see Fig. 14–5).
2. The patient is asked to inspire maximally, exhale forcibly and completely, and then to inhale forcibly and completely.

Clinical Implications

1. The value is normally decreased in an obstructive disease such as emphysema, during acute exacerbations of asthma, and in upper airway obstruction (UAO), as in tracheal stenosis.
2. The value is usually normal in restrictive lung disease, except for reduction in severe restrictive situations.

Interfering Factors

Poor patient effort is the major interfering factor.

Patient Preparation

1. Explain the purpose and procedure of the spirometry test. Assess patient ability to comply.
2. See Chapter 1 guidelines for safe, effective, informed, *pretest* care guidelines.

Patient Aftercare

1. See Chapter 1 guidelines for safe, effective, informed *posttest* care.
2. See aftercare guidelines for forced vital capacity.

LUNG VOLUMES AND CAPACITIES

Lung volumes can be considered as basic subdivisions of the lung (not actual anatomic subdivisions). They may be subdivided as follows:

1. Total lung capacity (TLC)
2. Tidal volume (VT)
3. Inspiratory capacity (IC)
4. Inspiratory reserve volume (IRV)
5. Residual volume (RV)
6. Functional residual capacity (FRC)
7. Expiratory reserve volume (ERV)
8. Vital capacity (VC)

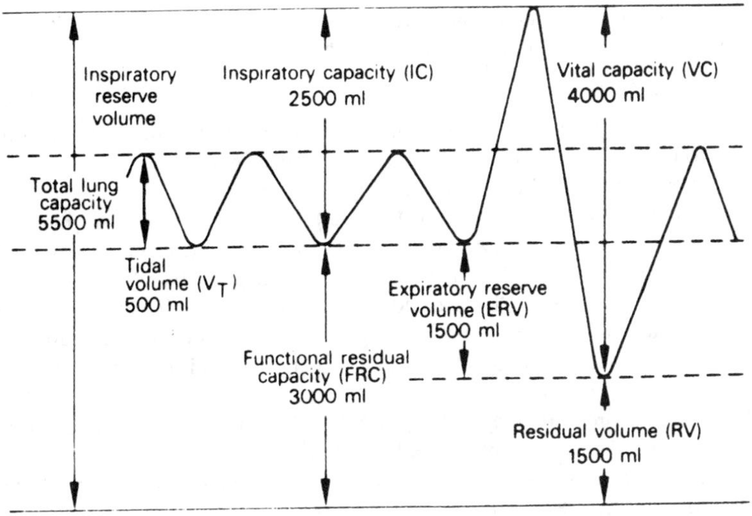

FIGURE 14-7
Subdivisions of lung volume in the normal adult. (Geschickter CF: The Lung in Health and Disease. Philadelphia, JB Lippincott, 1973)

Combinations of two or more volumes are termed *capacities*. These volumes and capacities are shown graphically in Figure 14–7. Also shown are values found in normal adult men. Measurement of these values can provide information about the degree of air-trapping or hyperinflation. There are two methods for the determination of lung volumes:

1. The multiple-breath nitrogen washout technique (open circuit)
2. The helium-dilution technique (closed circuit)

Both methods employ the use of a gas (oxygen or helium, respectively) to either wash out or dilute the air left in the lung at end tidal expiration.

FUNCTIONAL RESIDUAL CAPACITY (FRC)

Normal Values

Approximately 2.50–3.50 L.

Predicted values are based on age (A), height (H), weight (W), and sex. The observed value should be 75% to 125% of the predicted value.

Explanation of Test

Functional residual capacity is used to evaluate both restrictive and obstructive lung defects. Changes in the elastic properties of the lungs are reflected in the FRC and residual volume (RV). This test measures the volume of gas contained in the lungs at the end of a normal quiet expiration. The residual volume is expressed mathematically as the difference between the FRC and expiratory reserve volume (ERV); (RV = FRC − ERV); (see following).

Procedure

1. After being fitted with nose clips, the patient is instructed to breathe through the mouthpiece on the lung volume apparatus.
2. Depending on the instrument used, the patient
   a. Breathes 100% oxygen (O_2) until either the alveolar nitrogen (O/ON_2A) reaches 1%, or 7 minutes elapse (whichever comes first). Calculation of the FRC is based on the fact that 81% of the air in the lung is N_2. The N_2 is "washed" out of the lungs by having the patient breathe 100% O_2 and then, the volume of N_2 collected is measured.
   b. Rebreathes a 10% to 12% helium (He) and room-air mixture until equilibrium is reached
3. Results are recorded by either an X-Y recorder on semilog paper (Fig. 14–8) or by a respirometer on a kymograph drum.
4. The following values are then computed. The choice of the formula depends on the method used:

$$\text{FRC} = \frac{\%N_2 \text{ final} \times V_E}{\%N_2A}$$

(nitrogen washout or open circuit technique)
or

$$\text{FRC} = \frac{\%\text{He initial} - \%\text{He final}}{\%\text{He final}} \times \text{initial volume}$$

(helium dilution or closed circuit technique)

5. The test should be repeated a second time. Results between the FRCs should not vary more than 5% to 10%.

Clinical Implications

1. A value less than 75% is consistent with restrictive ventilatory impairment.
2. A value greater than 125% demonstrates air-trapping, consistent with obstructive airway disease. This represents hyperinflation, which is consistent with emphysema, asthma, or bronchiolar obstruction.

Patient Preparation

1. Explain the purpose and procedure of the test. Explain that this is a noninvasive test requiring patient cooperation. Assess patient's ability to comply.
2. Record the patient's age, sex, weight, and height.
3. Follow Chapter 1 guidelines for safe, effective, informed *pretest* care.

Patient Aftercare

1. Explain test outcomes; allow the patient to rest if necessary.
2. See Chapter 1 for safe, effective, informed *posttest* care.

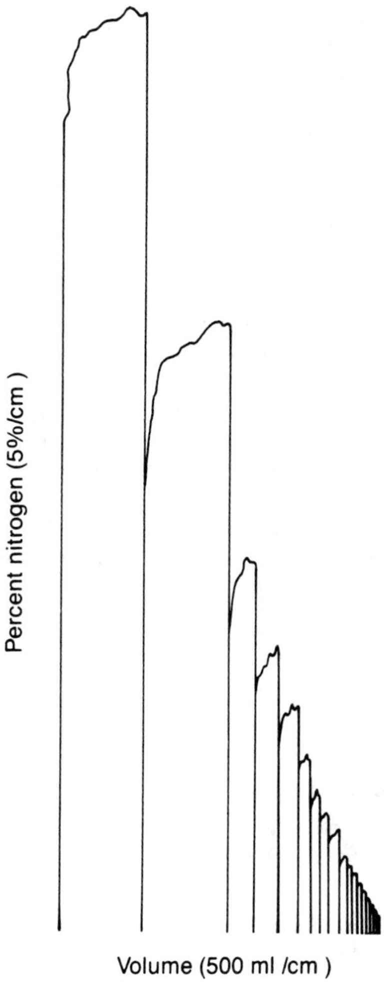

FIGURE 14-8
Typical tracing of a multiple breath nitrogen workout curve for determining FRC. The patient breathes 100% oxygen until alveolar nitrogen reaches 1%.

RESIDUAL VOLUME (RV)

Normal Values

Approximately 1200 to 1500 ml.
Predicted values are based on age, sex, and height.

Explanation of Test

Residual volume can be helpful in differentiating between restrictive or obstructive ventilatory defects. It is the volume of gas remaining in the lungs after a maximal exhalation. Because the lungs cannot be completely emptied, and because all the gas cannot be expelled by maximal expiratory effort, RV is the only lung volume that cannot be measured directly from the spirometer. It is calculated mathematically as follows: Residual volume equals the functional residual capacity minus the expiratory reserve volume (RV = FRC – ERV), (see Fig. 14–4).

Procedure

The RV is determined indirectly from other tests. There is no actual procedure.

Clinical Implications

1. An increase (greater than 125% of predicted) in the RV indicates that, in spite of a maximal expiratory effort, the lungs still contain an abnormally large amount of gas (air-trapping). This type of change occurs in young asthmatics. It is usually reversible, as in emphysema, but is permanent and indicative of air-trapping.
2. Increased RV is also characteristic of emphysema, chronic air-trapping, and chronic bronchial obstruction.
3. The RV and the FRC usually increase together, although not always.
4. The RV sometimes decreases in diseases that occlude many alveoli.
5. An RV of less than 75% of predicted value is consistent with restrictive disorders.

Interfering Factors

Residual volume normally increases with age.

Patient Preparation

1. Explain the purpose of the test and how results are calculated.
2. See Chapter 1 guidelines for safe, effective, informed *pretest* care.

Patient Aftercare

1. Interpret test results and monitor as necessary.
2. Follow Chapter 1 guidelines for safe, effective, informed *posttest* care.

EXPIRATORY RESERVE VOLUME (ERV) ●

Normal Values

Approximately 1200 to 1500 ml.
Predicted values are based on age, height, and sex.

Explanation of Test

Expiratory reserve volume measures the largest volume of gas that can be exhaled at end-tidal expiration. This measurement identifies lung or chest wall restriction. The ERV can be estimated mathematically by subtracting the inspiratory capacity (IC) from the vital capacity (VC). The ERV constitutes approximately 25% of the VC and can vary greatly in patients of comparable age and height.

Procedure

1. Record the patient's age and height.
2. Have the patient breathe normally into a spirometer for several breaths and then exhale maximally from the end-tidal expiratory level.
3. Results are recorded on a spirogram.
4. Repeat this maneuver until two values are within 5% of one another.

Clinical Implications

1. A decreased ERV indicates a chest wall restriction owing to nonpulmonary causes.
2. Decreased values are associated with elevated diaphragms, as seen in massive obesity, ascites, or pregnancy. Decreased values also occur with massive enlargement of the heart, pleural effusion, kyphoscoliosis, or thoracoplasty.
3. Decreases of ERV also seen in obstruction owing to increase in the RV impinging on the ERV.

Patient Preparation

1. Explain the purpose and procedure of the spirometry test. Inform the patient that it is noninvasive. Assess patient's ability to comply.
2. Follow Chapter 1 guidelines for safe, effective, informed, *pretest* care.

Patient Aftercare

1. Interpret test outcomes and counsel about respiratory abnormalities.
2. Follow Chapter 1 guidelines for safe, effective, informed *posttest* care.

INSPIRATORY CAPACITY (IC) ●

Normal Values

Approximately 2500 to 3600 ml.
Predicted values are based on age, height, and sex.

Explanation of Test

Inspiratory capacity measures the largest volume of air that can be inhaled from the end-tidal expiratory level. This measurement is used to identify lung or chest wall restriction. IC measurement mathematically equals the tidal volume plus the inspiratory reserve volume ($IC = IRV + V_T$).

Procedure

1. Record the age, sex, and height of the patient.
2. The patient breathes normally into a spirometer for several breaths and then inhales deeply or maximally, expanding the lungs as much as possible from end-tidal expiration. Normal breathing is then resumed.

3. Step 2 is usually repeated two or more times until the two best values are within 5%. The largest inspired volume value is selected.

Clinical Implications

1. Changes in the IC usually parallel increases or decreases in the vital capacity.
2. Decreases in IC can be related to either restrictive or obstructive ventilatory impairments.

Patient Preparation

1. Instruct the patient about the purpose, procedure for the inspiratory test, and need for patient cooperation.
2. Follow Chapter 1 guidelines for safe, effective, informed *pretest* care.

Patient Aftercare

1. Interpret test outcomes and counsel about ventilatory impairment.
2. See Chapter 1 guidelines for safe, effective, informed *posttest* care.

VITAL CAPACITY (VC) ●

Normal Values

About 3.00 to 5.00 L.
Predicted values are based on age, sex, and height.

Explanation of Test

Vital capacity identifies defects of lung or chest wall restriction. It measures the largest volume of gas that can be expelled from the lungs after the lungs are first filled to the maximum extent and then emptied to the maximum extent. The VC is the mathematical sum of the inspiratory capacity (IC) and the expiratory reserve volume (ERV) (VC = EC + ERV).

Procedure

1. With a spirometer, the patient inhales as deeply as possible and then exhales completely, with no forced or rapid effort.
2. Results are recorded on graph paper.
3. The procedure should be repeated at least twice. The VCs should compare within 5% of each other.

Clinical Implications

1. A *reduced* VC is defined as less than 80% of the predicted value.
2. The VC can be lower than expected in either a restrictive or an obstructive disorder.
3. Decreased VCs can be related to depression of the respiratory center in the brain, neuromuscular diseases, pleural effusion, pneumothorax, pregnancy, ascites, limitations of thoracic movement, scleroderma, kyphoscoliosis, or tumors.

Interfering Factors

1. The VC increases with physical fitness and greater height.
2. The VC decreases with age (after age 30).
3. The VC is generally less in women than in men of the same age and height.
4. The VC is decreased by approximately 15% in black people (African-Americans) and 20% to 25% in the Oriental populations as compared with white people (Caucasian) of the same age, height, and sex.
5. Inadequate patient effort causes lower VC values.

Patient Preparation

1. Explain the purpose and procedure of the test and the need for patient cooperation. Assess for interfering factors.
2. Follow Chapter 1 guidelines for safe, effective, informed *pretest* care.

Patient Aftercare

1. Interpret outcomes, monitor patient signs and symptoms, and follow up if necessary.
2. See Chapter 1 guidelines for safe, effective, informed *posttest* care.

TOTAL LUNG CAPACITY (TLC) ●

Normal Values

Approximately 4.00 to 6.00 L.
Predicted values are based on age, height, and sex.

Explanation of Test

Total lung capacity is used mainly to evaluate obstructive defects as well as to delineate restrictive from obstructive pulmonary disease. It measures the volume of gas contained in the lungs at the end of a maximal inspiration. Mathematically, it is the sum of the VC and the RV, or the sum of the primary lung volumes (see Fig. 14–4). This value is calculated indirectly from other tests.

Procedure

1. The patient is instructed to breath normally into a spirometer and then to inhale maximally and exhale maximally. The total amount of air exhaled is the VC (see foregoing).
2. The total lung capacity is then derived by the following formula: TLC = VC + RV

Clinical Implications

1. An obstructive impairment is characterized by an *elevated* TLC. However, a normal or *increased* TLC does not mean that ventilation or the surface

area for diffusion is normal. The TLC may be normal or *increased* in bronchiolar obstruction with hyperinflation and in emphysema.

2. The TLC is *decreased* in edema, atelectasis, neoplasms, pulmonary congestion, pneumothorax, or thoracic restriction.
3. A *decreased* TLC is the *hallmark* of a *restrictive* ventilatory impairment.

Patient Preparation

1. Explain purpose and procedure of spirometry test. Even though it is noninvasive, it does require patient effort and cooperation.
2. Follow Chapter 1 guidelines for safe, effective, informed, *pretest* care.

Patient Aftercare

1. Interpret outcomes and monitor for complaints of nausea, lightheadedness, or chest pain.
2. See Chapter 1 guidelines for safe, effective, informed *posttest* care.

● GAS EXCHANGE

Common measurements determine the rate of gas transfer across alveolar–capillary membranes to assess the diffusion process.

CARBON MONOXIDE-DIFFUSING CAPACITY OF THE LUNG (DLCO) ●

Normal Values

Approximately 25 ml/min per torr.

Predicted values are based on patient's height (H), age (A) in years, and sex.

DLCO (in men) = 0.0984 × (H) −0.1777 × (A) + 19.93

DLCO (in women) = 0.1118 × (H) −0.117 × (A) + 7.72

Background

Carbon monoxide (CO) combines with hemoglobin about 210 times more readily than does oxygen (O_2). If there is a normal amount of hemoglobin in the blood, the only other significant limiting factor to CO uptake is the state of the alveolar capillary membranes. Normally, there are insufficient amounts of CO in the blood to affect the test.

Two categories of factors determine the rate of gas (CO) transfer across the lung: physical and chemical. Physical determinants are CO-driving pressure, surface area, thickness of capillary walls, and diffusion coefficient for CO. Chemical determinants are red cell volume and reaction rate with hemoglobin.

Explanation of Test

This test is used to diagnose pulmonary vascular disease, emphysema, and pulmonary fibrosis and to evaluate the extent of functional pulmonary capillary bed in contact with functional alveoli. Alveolar volumes (VA) can also be determined. The DL measures the diffusing capacity of the lungs for CO. The DLO_2 is obtained by multiplying DLCO by 1.23 (DLO_2 = DLCO × 1.23).

Procedure

1. Record the patient's age, height, weight, and sex.
2. Two techniques are used by laboratories.
   a. *Single-breath* or *breathing-holding technique:* The patient is instructed to exhale to residual volume, then maximally inhale a diffusion gas mixture (10% helium, 0.3% carbon monoxide, and the balance room air), breath-hold for 10 to 12 seconds and then exhale. A sample of alveolar gas is collected after washout of dead space volume.

$$DLCO = \frac{VA \times 60}{(PB - PH_2O) \times t^{I}} \ln \frac{FACO_0}{FACO_t}$$

where

$FACO_0$ = initial alveolar CO concentrations
$FACO_t$ = alveolar CO concentration at end of breath-holding time
VA = alveolar volume
60 = conversion factor for seconds to 1 minute
t = breath-holding time in seconds
PB = barometric pressure in mmHg
PH_2O = water vapor pressure in mmHg
ln = natural logarithm

   b. *Steady-state technique:* The patient is asked to breathe from a bag containing 0.1% to 0.2% CO for several minutes. This method requires an arterial blood sample. During the final 2 minutes, the exhaled air is collected into a neoprene bag and then analyzed for O_2, CO_2, and CO concentrations. An arterial blood gas sample is also drawn during the final 2 minutes of the procedure.

$$DLCO = \frac{VCO(STPD)}{PACO}$$

VCO = ml of CO transferred per minute

PACO = partial pressure of CO in the alveoli

Clinical Implications

1. *Decreased values* are associated with
   a. Multiple pulmonary emboli
   b. Emphysema
   c. Lung resection
   d. Pulmonary fibroses
      (1) Sarcoidosis
      (2) Scleroderma

(3) Systemic lupus erythematosus
(4) Asbestosis
(5) Pulmonary resection
(6) Pneumonia

e. Anemia
f. Elevated carboxy-hemoglobin (COHb) levels

2. *Increased values* are observed in polycythemia, left-to-right shunts, and exercise.
3. The value is relatively normal in chronic bronchitis.

Interfering Factors

Exercise (with an increased cardiac output) and polycythemia will increase the value. Because elevated levels of COHb (as seen in smokers) and anemia will decrease the value, the DLCO is corrected for COHb levels higher than 10% and hemoglobin values less than 8%.

Patient Preparation

1. Explain the purpose and procedure. Assess for interfering factors and inform that this noninvasive test requires patient cooperation. Assess patient's ability to comply.
2. Follow Chapter 1 guidelines for safe, effective, informed *pretest* care.

Patient Aftercare

1. Explain test outcomes and possible need for follow-up testing to monitor course of therapy (eg, anti-inflammatory drugs and bronchodilators).
2. See Chapter 1 guidelines for safe, effective, informed *posttest* care.

MAXIMUM VOLUNTARY VENTILATION (MVV)

Normal Values

Approximately 160 to 180 L/min.

Based on age (A) in years, height (H) in inches, and sex; a healthy person may vary by as much as 25% to 35% of mean group values.

MVV (in men) = 3.39 × (H) − 1.26 × (A) − 21.4

MVV (in women) = 138 − 0.77 × (A)

Explanation of Test

Maximum voluntary ventilation measures several physiologic phenomena occurring at the same time (eg, thoracic cage compliance, lung compliance, airway resistance, and available muscle force). It is an indicator of the number of liters of air that a person can breathe per minute with maximum voluntary effort.

Procedure

1. The patient breathes into a spirometer as deeply and rapidly as possible

for 10 to 15 seconds. Generally, the frequency reaches 40 to 70 breaths per minute, and tidal volumes are about 50% of VC (Fig. 14–9).

2. Actual values are then extrapolated from the 10- to 15-second time interval to a 1-minute time period.
3. Typically, the maneuver is performed twice. The largest value is reported.

Interfering Factors

Poor patient effort can be ruled out by using the following formula to predict the MVV of the patient: Predicted MVV = $35 \times FEV_1$

This is a useful check to determine whether the recorded MVV is indicative of adequate patient effort. Low values can be related to patient effort and not to abnormal physiologic function.

Clinical Implications

1. Obstructive ventilatory impairments of moderate to severe degree, abnormal neuromuscular control, or poor patient effort are causes of low values.
2. In restrictive disease, the value will usually be normal; although in more severe forms, MVV may be decreased.

Patient Preparation

1. Explain the purpose and procedure of the maximum ventilation test. Explain that it is a noninvasive test which requires patient cooperation. Assess patient's ability to comply.
2. Record the patient's age, height, and sex.
3. Follow Chapter 1 guidelines for safe, effective, informed *pretest* care.

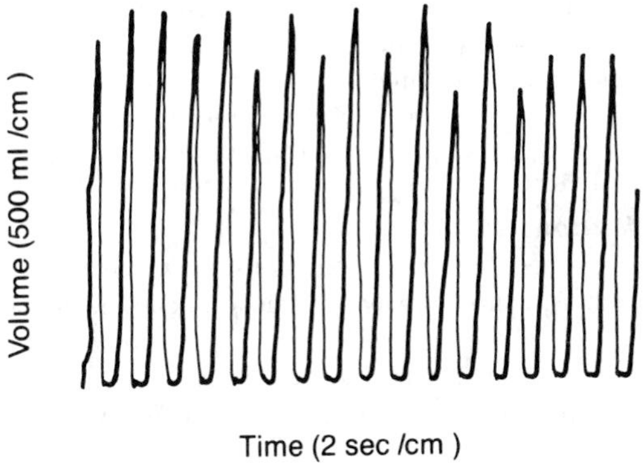

FIGURE 14-9

Maximum voluntary ventilation. Patient breathes into a spirometer as deeply and rapidly as possible for 10 to 15 seconds.

Patient Aftercare

1. Explain test outcome and possible need for follow-up testing and treatment.
2. See Chapter 1 guidelines for safe, effective, informed *posttest* care.

CLOSING VOLUME (CV) ●

Normal Values

Average is 10% to 20% of vital capacity.

Values are derived from mathematical regression equations and are based on age (A) in years and sex.

CV (in men) = 0.562 + 0.357 × (A).

CV (in women) = 2.812 + 0.293 × (A).

Explanation of Test

In the healthy person, the concentration of alveolar nitrogen previously diluted with a single breath of 100% O_2 rapidly increases near the end of expiration. This rise is due to closure of the small airways in the bases of the lung. The point at which this closure occurs is termed *closing volume.*

Closing volume is used as an index of pathologic changes occurring within the small airways (those airways smaller than 2 mm in diameter). Conventional pulmonary function tests are not sensitive enough to make this determination. The principle of determination relies on the fact that the upper lung zones contain a proportionately larger residual volume of gas than the lower lung zones and that there is a gradient of intrapleural pressure from the top of the lung to the bottom of the lung. Additionally, the uniformity of gas distribution within the lungs can be measured.

Procedure

1. The patient is asked to exhale completely, then inhale 100% oxygen, and then to exhale completely at the rate of approximately 1/2 L/sec.
2. During exhalation, both volume and percentage of alveolar nitrogen are monitored simultaneously on an X-Y recorder. A sudden increase in nitrogen represents the closing volume (Fig. 14–10).

Clinical Implications

1. Values are increased for those conditions in which the airway is narrowed (bronchitis, early airway obstruction, chronic smokers, the elderly).
2. A change in the slope of the nitrogen curve by more than 2% is indicative of maldistribution of inspired air (ie, uneven alveolar ventilation).

Interfering Factors

1. Value increases with age.
2. Patients in congestive heart failure may show increases in their closing volume.

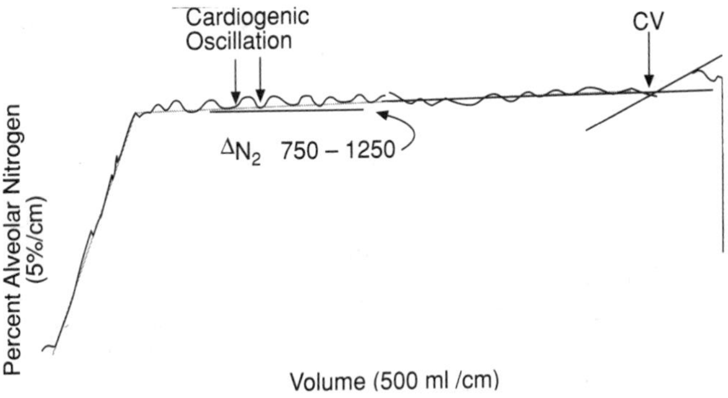

FIGURE 14-10
Typical single-breath nitrogen washout curve for determination of closing volume (CV). The patient inspires 100% oxygen to total lung capacity and then exhales slowly (0.5 LPS) until the lung is empty. The change in the slope of the curve over 1 liter (ΔN_2 750–1250) is an index of the eveness of alveolar ventilation.

Patient Preparation

1. Explain the purpose and procedure of the test. Inform the patient that this is a noninvasive test that requires patient cooperation. Assess patient's ability to comply with breathing requirements and instructions. Assess for interfering factors.
2. Follow Chapter 1 guidelines for safe, effective, informed *pretest* care.

Patient Aftercare

1. Explain meaning of test outcomes and possible need for follow-up testing and treatment for early small-airway disease. Congestive heart failure, with subsequent edema, may also contribute to decreasing patency of the small airways.
2. See Chapter 1 guidelines for safe, effective, informed *posttest* care.

VOLUME OF ISOFLOW (VISOV̇) ●

Normal Values

Average is 10% to 25% of the vital capacity.
Values cover a wide range based on age (A).

$\text{VISO}\dot{V} = 0.450 \times (A) + 4.69$

Explanation of Test

This test is designed to detect pathologic changes occurring in the small airways and may be more sensitive than conventional pulmonary function tests. Helium (He) has the unique property of lowering gas density. Therefore, after breathing a helium–oxygen gas mixture, the effects of convective acceleration and turbulence are negated. Any abnormality observed in the flow–volume loop is then due to an increase in resistance (nonturbulent) to laminar flow, which indicates small-airway abnormalities, or lung disease.

Procedure

1. The patient is fitted with nose clips and is then instructed to perform a baseline flow–volume loop maneuver into the mouthpiece of the spirometer interfaced with an X-Y recorder.
2. The patient breathes an 80% He and 20% O_2 gas mix for several breaths and then performs another flow–volume loop maneuver (HeliOx flow–volume loop).
3. The flow–volume loop tracings are superimposed on each other, and the volume of isoflow is measured at the point where the two loops intersect.

Clinical Implications

An *increased* volume of isoflow is consistent with early small-airway obstruction (ie, asthma).

Patient Preparation

1. Explain the purpose and procedure of the test.
2. Follow guidelines in Chapter 1 for safe, effective, informed *pretest* care.

Patient Aftercare

1. Interpret test outcomes and possible need for follow-up testing and treatment.
2. See Chapter 1 guidelines for safe, effective, informed *posttest* care.

BODY PLETHYSMOGRAPHY ●

Normal Values

Based on age (A) years, height (H; cm), weight (W; kg), and sex of the patient

VTG = approximately 2.50 to 3.50 L
VTG (in men) = 0.052 × (H) − 5.16 × (W)
VTG (in women) = 0.0469 × (H) − 4.85 × (W)
CL = 0.2 L/cm H_2O
Raw = 0.6 to 2.4 cm H_2OL^{-1} sec^{-1}
Gaw = 0.42 to 1.67 L sec^{-1} cmH_2O^{-1}
SGAW = 0.10 to 0.15 L sec^{-1} cmH_2O^{-1} L^{-1}

Explanation of Test

This test measures thoracic gas volume (VTG), compliance of the lung (CL), airway resistance (Raw) and airway conductance (Gaw). The VTG equals all the air contained within the thorax, whether it is in ventilatory communication with the rest of the lung. Compliance is an indication of the elasticity of the lung, and airway resistance is a measurement of resistance to airflow in the tracheobronchial tree. Airway conductance, the reciprocal of airway resistance, is the flow generated per unit of pressure. The specific airway conductance relates to conductance per liter of lung volume.

The measurement of VTG, by body plethysmography, is an application of Boyle's law, $P^1 \times V^1 = P^2 \times V^2$ as long as T is constant.

P = pressure
Patm = atmospheric pressure
V = volume
T = temperature
Palv = alveolar pressure

$$\text{Compliance (C)} = \frac{\text{change in volume}}{\text{change in pressure}} = \frac{V\,(\text{L})}{P\,(\text{cm } H_2O)}$$

$$\text{Airway resistance (Raw)} = \frac{P\text{atm} - P\text{alv}}{\text{flow}}$$

$$\text{Airway conductance} = \text{Gaw} = \frac{1}{\text{Raw}}$$

$$\text{Specific airway conductance} = \frac{\text{Gaw}}{\text{VTG}}$$

Airway resistance increases with decreased lung volumes and decreases with higher lung volumes in a nonlinear, hyperbolic fashion. Therefore, to provide a volume-standardized Raw measurement, airway conductance Gaw, and specific airway conductance (SGaw) are typically calculated.

Procedure

1. The patient sits in the plethysmograph (body box), is fitted with nose clips, and breathes through a mouthpiece connected to a transducer.
2. Once the body box door is secured, the test is not begun for a few minutes, to allow the box pressure to stabilize.
3. The patient is then instructed to perform a panting maneuver while holding the cheeks rigid and the glottis open against a closed shutter located within the transducer assembly. Box and mouth pressures are recorded on the oscilloscope to provide data for VTG.
4. Next, the patient is told to breathe rapidly and shallowly. Box pressure changes versus flow are recorded on the oscilloscope to provide data for Raw.
5. To determine CL, a balloon catheter must be passed through the nose into the patient's esophagus. The inflated balloon is connected to a transducer, and the patient is instructed to breathe normally. A recording of intraesophageal pressure changes during normal respiration (which mimics changes in intrapleural pressure), and provides data for CL.

Clinical Implications

1. An *increased* VTG demonstrates air trapping, consistent with obstructive pulmonary disease.
2. An *increased* Raw demonstrates increased resistance to airflow through the tracheobronchial tree, seen in asthma, emphysema, bronchitis, and other forms of obstruction. The Raw distinguishes between a restrictive ventilatory defect versus an obstructive ventilatory defect.
3. An *increase* in CL (ie, lung is more distensible) is seen in obstructive diseases.
4. A *decrease* in CL (ie, lung is more stiff) is seen in fibrotic diseases, restrictive diseases, pneumonia, congestion, and atelectasis.

Patient Preparation

1. The age, height, weight, and sex are recorded.
2. Explain the purpose and procedure of the test and instruct and demonstrate actual maneuvers that will be necessary. Assess for compliance with procedure.
3. Assure patients that although they are in an airtight chamber, the test takes only a few minutes. A technician will be in constant attendance to open the door should that be necessary. Assess for ability to comply with test requirements and instructions. Tactfully assess for predisposition to claustrophobia, panic attacks, or other similar responses.
4. Follow Chapter 1 guidelines for safe, effective, informed *pretest* care.

Patient Aftercare

1. Allow time to rest quietly if necessary.
2. Explain meaning of test outcomes. See Chapter 1 guidelines for safe, effective, informed *posttest* care.

BRONCHIAL PROVOCATION

Normal Values

Positive response to inhaled antigen: >20% decrease in FEV_1 from baseline.
Negative response: <20% decrease in FEV_1 from baseline.

Explanation of Test

Bronchial provocation challenge testing is performed in patients with normal pulmonary function tests, but who are suspected of having underlying bronchial hyperreactivity. Additionally, the asthmatic patient is more sensitive to bronchoconstrictive effects of cholinergic agents (methacholine chloride) than the normal person. Airway resistance tests are sensitive in monitoring responses to bronchoconstrictive agents.

Clinical Implications

A positive response to methacholine or histamine is consistent with bronchial hyperreactivity. Approximately 5% to 10% of asthmatics do not respond to the methacholine challenge test.

Procedure

1. The patient performs an FVC maneuver, and the baseline FEV_1 is measured and recorded.
2. The patient then inhales methacholine chloride (0.075–25.00 mg) by nebulizer, waits 5 minutes, and inhales increasing concentrations. The FVC maneuver is repeated after each successive concentration inhaled. A 20% reduction in the FEV_1 is considered a positive response.
3. Of note, when or if a decrease in the FEV_1 greater than 20% from baseline is reached, an inhaled bronchodilator is administered.
4. If a patient goes through all dilution ratios and a 20% reduction in the FEV is not reached, the test is considered negative.
5. If the methacholine causes no change, histamine testing may be ordered.

Patient Preparation

1. Explain the purpose, procedure, and the need for patient cooperation. Assess patient's ability to comply.
2. Withhold bronchodilators for 8 hours and antihistamines for 48 hours, if tolerated.
3. Follow Chapter 1 guidelines for safe, effective, informed *pretest* care.

Clinical Alert

1. Inhalation of methacholine can cause bronchospasm, chest pain, shortness of breath, and general discomfort.
2. These effects can be reversed with a bronchodilator.

Patient Aftercare

1. Explain meaning of test outcomes.
2. If test is positive, patient is advised to avoid antigens that may be causing hypersensitivity reaction and bronchospasms.
3. See Chapter 1 guidelines for safe, effective, informed *posttest* care.

CARBON DIOXIDE (CO_2) RESPONSE

Normal Values

The act of breathing in successively greater concentrations of CO_2 should result in an increase in minute volume (VE) when compared with VE when breathing in room air (0.03% CO_2) alone.

Normal: linear increase in VE of 3 L min^{-1} $mgHg^{-1}$ PCO_2

Explanation of Test

This test evaluates respiratory response to increasing concentrations of inspired CO_2. As alveolar levels of CO_2 increase, so does arterial CO_2. The central chemoreceptors respond by initiating impulses to the respiratory control centers. This, in turn, causes the rate and depth of breathing to increase in the healthy person.

Procedure

1. VE is determined while the patient breaths room air for several minutes into an instrument that records frequency (f) of breathing and tidal volume (VT). The minute volume is then mathematically calculated for 1 minute: VE = f × VT.
2. Next, the patient breathes a gas mixture of 2% CO_2 and room air for 5 minutes. During the last 2 minutes, f and VT are recorded and the VE calculated.
3. The patient then breathes gas mixtures of 4% CO_2 and 6% CO_2 with room air. Mixtures can be increased to 8% CO_2. The previous process is repeated with each successive concentration.
4. A graph is then constructed to plot changed VE against increased inspired CO_2 concentrations ($FICO_2$).

Clinical Implications

Lack of response to increasing inspired CO_2 concentrations suggests a disturbance in the normal physiologic pathway of ventilatory changes to hypercapnia. This may be due to central nervous system depressants (eg, anesthetics, barbiturates, or narcotics) or airflow obstruction (eg, chronic obstructive pulmonary disease).

Patient Preparation

1. Explain purpose, procedure, and need for patient cooperation. Assess patient's ability to comply.
2. Follow Chapter 1 guidelines for safe, effective, informed *pretest* care.

Patient Aftercare

1. Interpret test outcome and advise that pharmacologic intervention may be necessary to sensitize the chemoreceptors.
2. See Chapter 1 guidelines for safe, effective, informed *posttest* care.

EXERCISE STRESS TESTING ●

Normal Values

Normal response to graded exercise as an increase in ventilation and cardiac output to maintain alveolar and arterial gases at optimal levels to meet metabolic demands. The patient's ventilatory, alveolar–arterial gas responses are the primary objectives of a pulmonary exercise stress test. No significant or abnormal changes in the electrocardiographic (ECG) complex, arterial blood pressures, airflow patterns during inspiration and expiration, arterial blood gas values and chemistry, and hemodynamic pressures should occur.

Normal Ventilatory and Blood Gas Response to Graded Exercise	
Value	***Change***
O_2 consumption ($\dot{V}O_2$)	Increases
CO_2 production ($\dot{V}CO_2$)	Increases
Ventilatory equivalents for O_2 and Co_2	No change
Respiratory exchange ratio (RER)	Increases
Minute ventilation (VE)	Increases
Blood lactate	Increases
VD/$\dot{V}$T ratio	Decreases
A − aDO$_2$	No change
Arterial blood gas tensions (eg, PaO_2, $PaCO_2$)	No change
Bicarbonate concentration (HCO_3)	Decreases
Oxygen saturation (SaO_2)	No change

Background

Respiratory disease reduces the ability to perform exercise. Dynamic exercise that involves large-muscle groups produces increases in metabolic O_2 consumption and CO_2 production. This increase in metabolic demand leads to stresses on other mechanisms taking part in O_2 and CO_2 transport. Exercise testing measures the functional reserves of these mechanisms by testing underload. Analysis of bronchogenic and cardiovascular disorders includes procedures that measure respiratory outcomes and blood gas studies during exercise. Ventilation and gas exchange in healthy individuals are normally altered during exercise. However, specific abnormalities are noted in the presence of cardiovascular or respiratory impairment. Exercise tests are valuable for assessing severity and type of impairment of existing as well as undiagnosed conditions.

Explanation of Test

Exercise testing is done to evaluate fitness, functional capacity, and other limiting factors in obstructive and restrictive diseases. Efficiency of the cardiopulmonary system may be altered during exercise. Accordingly, exercise testing assesses ventilation, gas exchange, and cardiovascular function during increased demands. Dyspnea on exertion caused by cardiovascular disorders can be differentiated from that due to respiratory causes. Precise information about the mechanisms that influence O_2 and CO_2 transport during exercise can be obtained by using a staged approach.

An exercise test can detect or exclude many conditions, even though the response may be nonspecific. For example, if a person complains of severe shortness of breath in the presence of a normal exercise response, a likely cause may be psychogenic in origin. However, a few conditions exhibit diagnostic responses. Exercise-induced asthma and myocardial ischemia are two examples. These tests can also reveal the degree of impairment in conditions affecting the respiratory and circulatory systems and may uncover unsuspected abnormalities.

The majority of clinical problems can be assessed during the simple procedures included in stage 1 and should be completed before more complex tests. Abnormal results indicate that more precise information is required through more complex stage 2 protocols. If stage 3 protocols are implemented, arterial blood analysis is necessary. In 75% of patients, stage 1 is sufficient. Oxygen titration can be done during graded exercise to determine the oxygen needs for improving exercise tolerance increased functional capacity.

Clinical Alert

1. *Absolute contraindications to exercise testing include*
   - **a.** Acute febrile illness
   - **b.** Pulmonary edema
   - **c.** Systolic B/P >250 mm Hg
   - **d.** Diastolic B/P >120 mm Hg
   - **e.** Uncontrolled hypertension
   - **f.** Uncontrolled asthma
   - **g.** Unstable angina
2. *Relative contraindications to exercise testing include*
   - **a.** Recent myocardial infarction (less than 4 weeks)
   - **b.** Resting tachycardia >120 bpm
   - **c.** Epilepsy
   - **d.** Respiratory failure
   - **e.** Resting ECG abnormalities

Procedure

1. *Stage 1*
   - **a.** Blood pressure readings, ECG analysis, and ventilation are made during incremental cycle ergometry or treadmill.
   - **b.** Measurements are made at the end of each minute. The test continues until maximum allowed symptoms occur (to a symptom-limited maximum). The O_2 uptake and CO_2 output are measured if possible.
   - **c.** Total examining time is approximately 30 minutes.
2. *Stage 2*
   - **a.** Requires more complex analytical methods.
   - **b.** Exercise builds to a steady state, usually 3 to 5 minutes for each workload.
   - **c.** Stage 1 measurements plus mixed venous CO_2 tension by means of rebreathing techniques are done.
3. *Stage 3*
   - **a.** Requires blood gas sampling and analysis.
   - **b.** An indwelling catheter is inserted into the brachial or radial artery.
   - **c.** In addition to stage 2 tests, measurements for cardiac output, alveolar ventilation, ratio of dead space to tidal volume, alveolar–arterial O_2

tension difference, venous admixture ratio, and lactate levels are determined.

Clinical Implications

Altered values may reveal

1. Cardiac dysrhythmias or ischemia
2. Degree of functional impairment as a result of obstructive or restrictive ventilatory disease
3. Hypoventilation
4. Work load level at which metabolic acidosis (lactic acidosis) occurs.

Interfering Factors

1. The exercise tolerance of any person is affected by the degree of impairment related to
   a. Mechanical factors
   b. Ventilatory efficiency
   c. Gas exchange factors
   d. Cardiac status
   e. Physical condition
   f. Sensitivity of the respiratory control mechanism
2. Obese persons will have a higher than normal oxygen consumption at any given work rate, even though muscular and work efficiency values are normal.

Patient Preparation

1. Explain purpose, procedure for exercise stress testing, and assess for contraindications, interfering factors, and ability to comply.
2. Follow Chapter 1 guidelines for safe, effective, informed *pretest* care.

Patient Aftercare

1. Explain meaning of test outcomes and possible need for lifestyle changes.
2. See Chapter 1 guidelines for safe, effective, informed *posttest* care.

● BLOOD GASES; ARTERIAL BLOOD GASES (ABGs)

OVERVIEW OF ARTERIAL BLOOD GAS TESTS ●

Arterial blood gases (ABGs) are obtained to assess adequacy of oxygenation and ventilation, to evaluate the acid–base status by measuring the respiratory and nonrespiratory components, and to monitor effectiveness of therapy. The ABGs are also used to monitor critically ill patients, to establish baseline values in the perioperative and postoperative period, to detect and treat electrolyte imbalances, to titrate appropriate oxygen flow rates, to qualify a patient for home oxygen use, and in conjunction with pulmonary function testing.

Reasons for using *arterial* blood rather than *venous* blood to measure blood gases include the following:

1. Arterial blood is a better way to sample a mixture of blood from various parts of the body.
   a. Venous blood from an extremity gives information mostly about that extremity. The metabolism in the extremity can differ from the metabolism in the body as a whole. This difference is accentuated in the following instances:
      (1) In shock states, when the extremity is cold or underperfused
      (2) During local exercise of the extremity, as in opening and closing a fist
      (3) If the extremity is infected
   b. Blood from a central venous catheter is usually an incomplete mix of venous blood from various parts of the body. For a sample to be completely mixed, the blood would have to be obtained from the right ventricle or pulmonary artery.
2. Arterial blood indicates how well the lungs are oxygenating blood.
   a. If it is known that arterial oxygen (O_2) concentration is normal (indicating the lungs are functioning normally), but that the mixed venous O_2 concentration is low, it can be inferred that the heart and circulation are failing.
   b. Oxygen measurements of central venous catheter blood reveal tissue oxygenation but do not separate contributions of the heart from the lungs. If central venous catheter blood has a low O_2 concentration, it means either that the lungs have not oxygenated the arterial blood well or that the heart is not circulating the blood effectively. In this case, the body tissues must take on more than the normal amount of O_2 from each cardiac cycle because the blood is flowing slowly and permits this to occur. Consequently, this produces a low venous O_2 concentration.
3. Arterial samples provide information about the ability of the lungs to regulate acid–base balance through retention or release of CO_2. Effectiveness of the kidneys in maintaining appropriate bicarbonate levels can also be gauged.

NOTE: *Arterial puncture sites must satisfy the following three requirements:*

1. Have available collateral blood flow
2. Are superficial or easily accessible
3. Have relatively nonsensitive periarterial tissues

The radial artery is usually the site of choice, but brachial and femoral arteries can also be used. Samples can be drawn from direct arterial sticks or from indwelling arterial lines.

Clinical Alert

1. Before obtaining an arterial blood sample, assess for these contraindications to an arterial "stick" or indwelling line: absent palpable radial artery pulse, positive Allen test (in this case, only one artery supplies blood to the area [radial artery occlusion]), cellulitis or infection in the area, arteriovenous fistula or shunt, severe thrombocytopenia, or prolonged prothrombin time or partial thromboplastin time (relative contraindication). A Doppler probe or finger pulse transducer may be used to assess circulation. This may be especially helpful on dark-skinned or uncooperative patients.
2. Before obtaining an arterial blood sample, record the most recent hemoglobin value, mode and flow of oxygen therapy, and temperature. If the patient has been recently suctioned or placed on a ventilator, or if oxygen concentration has been changed, wait at least 15 minutes before drawing the sample. This waiting period allows circulating blood levels to return to baseline. Hyperthermia and hypothermia also influence oxygen release from hemoglobin at the tissue level.

Procedure for Obtaining Arterial Blood Sample

Observe universal and latex allergy precautions and follow agency protocols.

1. The patient assumes a sitting or supine position.
2. Perform the Allen's test to assess collateral circulation (use pressure to obliterate both radial and ulnar pulse; make hand ***blanch:*** release pressure over only the ulnar artery). In a positive test, flushing is immediately noted. The radial artery can then be used for puncture. If collateral circulation from the ulnar artery is inadequate (negative Allen's), another site must be chosen.
3. Elevate the wrist with a small pillow and ask the patient to extend the fingers downward (this will flex the wrist and position the radial artery closer to the surface).
4. Palpate the artery and maneuver the patient's hand back and forth until a satisfactory pulse is felt.
5. Swab the area liberally with an antiseptic agent such as one with an iodine base.
6. Optional: Inject the area with a small amount of 1% plain lidocaine (Xylocaine), 0.25 ml or less, if necessary to anesthetize site. Assess for allergy first. This allows a second attempt without undue pain.
7. Prepare a 20- or 21-gauge needle on a preheparinized self-filling syringe, puncture the artery and collect a 3- to 5-ml sample. During the procedure, if a dull or sharp pain radiating up the arm occurs, withdraw the needle slightly and reposition. If repositioning does not alleviate pain, the needle should be completely withdrawn.

8. Withdraw the needle and place a 4″ × 4″ absorbent bandage over the puncture site and maintain pressure over the site with two fingers for a minimum of 2 minutes or until there is no bleeding evident, or a pressure dressing, secured to the site with elastic tape, may be necessary for several hours.
9. Meanwhile, all air bubbles in the blood sample must be expelled as quickly as possible. Air in the sample will change values. The syringe should then be capped and gently rotated to mix heparin with blood.
10. Place the sample on ice and transfer to the laboratory. This will prevent alterations in gas tensions because metabolic processes continue after blood is drawn.
11. Label sample with patient's name, identification number, date, time, mode of O_2 therapy, and flow rate.

Patient Preparation

1. Explain purpose and procedure for obtaining arterial blood sample.
2. If patient is apprehensive reassure that a local anesthetic can be used.

Patient Aftercare

1. Evaluate color, motion, sensation, degree of warmth, capillary refill time, and quality of pulse in the affected extremity or at the puncture site.
2. Monitor puncture site and dressing for arterial bleeding for several hours. No vigorous activity (extremity) should be done for 24 hours.

Clinical Alert

1. Some patients may experience light-headedness, nausea, or vasovagal syncope during the arterial puncture. Respond according to established protocols.
2. Arterial gases will not indicate to what degree the patient is suffering from an abnormality. Therefore, the vital signs and mental function of the patient must be used as guides to determine adequacy of tissue oxygenation.
3. The arterial puncture site must have pressure applied and must be watched carefully for bleeding for several hours. Instruct the patient to report any bleeding from the site.
4. Information for the laboratory should include the fraction of inspired oxygen (FIO_2), or if on room air, note the time the sample was obtained. Do not use blood for ABGs if sample is more than 3 hours old.
5. In the clinical setting, such as the perioperative or intensive care environment, ABG studies usually include the following: pH, PCO_2, SaO_2, CO_2 content, O_2 content, PO_2, base excess/deficit, HCO_3, hemoglobin, hematocrit, CO, Na^+, K^+ (Chart 14-5).

CHART 14-5
Normal Values for Commonly Ordered AB Studies

STUDY COMPONENT	NORMAL VALUE
pHa	7.35–7.45
Paco2	35–45 torr
Saco2	95% or higher
CO2 content	23–30 mmol/L
O2 content	15–22 vol%
Pao2	80 torr or greater
Base excess deficit	Above 3 mEq/L = excess; Below 3 mEq/L = deficit
HCO3	24–28 mEq/L
(Hb)	12–16 g/dl (women); 13.5–17.5 g/dl (men)
(Hct)	37–47% (women); 40–54% (men)
CO	<7%
[Na+]	135–148 mmol/L
[K+]	3.5–5 mEq/L

ALVEOLAR TO ARTERIAL OXYGEN GRADIENT (A-aDO_2); ARTERIAL TO ALVEOLAR OXYGEN RATIO (a/A)

Normal Values

1 mm Hg = 1 torr.

$A - aDO_2$ = <10 torr if breathing room air at rest
20 to 30 mm Hg if breathing room air at maximum exercise
a/A ratio = 75% (regardless of age or FIO_2)

Normal Values

$$a/A \text{ ratio} = \frac{PaO_2}{FIO_2\,(PB - PH_2O) - (PaCO_2 \times 1.25)}$$

Explanation of Test

This test gives an approximation of the O_2 in the alveoli and arteries. It identifies the cause of hypoxemia and intrapulmonary shunting that are caused by (1) ventilated alveoli, but no perfusion; (2) unventilated alveoli, with perfusion; or (3) collapse of both alveoli and capillaries.

Procedure

After an arterial blood sample is obtained and analyzed, the following mathematical formula is solved:

$A = aDO_2 = PAO_2 - PaO_2$
$PAO_2 = FIO_2\,(PB - PH2O) - (PaO_2 \times 1.25)$

P_B = barometric pressure (mm Hg or torr)
P_{H_2O} = water vapor pressure (mm Hg or torr)
F_{IO_2} = fractional concentration of inspired oxygen (eg, 0.21 for room air, 0.40 for 40% oxygen and so forth)
Pa_{CO_2} = partial pressure of arterial carbon dioxide (mm Hg or torr)
1.25 = conversion factor for respiratory quotient
Pa_{O_2} = partial pressure of arterial oxygen (mm Hg or torr)
P_{AO_2} = alveolar oxygen tension (mm Hg or torr)
D = difference

Clinical Implications

1. *Increased* values may be due to
   - **a.** Mucus plugs
   - **b.** Bronchospasm
   - **c.** Airway collapse as seen in
     - **(1)** Asthma
     - **(2)** Bronchitis
     - **(3)** Emphysema
2. Hypoxemia, due to an increased $A - aD_{O_2}$ difference is caused by
   - **a.** Atrial septal defects
   - **b.** Pneumothorax
   - **c.** Atelectasis
   - **d.** Emboli
   - **e.** Edema

Interfering Factors

Values increase with age and increasing O_2 concentration.

Patient Preparation

1. Explain purpose, benefits, and risks of arterial blood sampling (see page 906).
2. Follow Chapter 1 guidelines for safe, effective, informed *pretest* care.

Patient Aftercare

1. Interpret test outcome and assess, monitor, and intervene appropriately for hypoxemia and ventilatory disturbances.
2. Frequently observe puncture site for bleeding (see page 908).
3. See Chapter 1 guidelines for safe, effective, informed *posttest* care.

PARTIAL PRESSURE FOR CARBON DIOXIDE (P_{CO_2}) ●

Normal Values

Pa_{CO_2} (arterial blood): 35 to 45 torr
Pv_{CO_2} (venous blood): 41 to 51 torr
Carried in blood in two ways: 10% carried in plasma, 90% carried in red blood cells.

Explanation of Test

This test measures the pressure or tension exerted by dissolved CO_2 in the blood and is proportional to the partial pressure of CO_2 in the alveolar air. The test is commonly used to detect a respiratory abnormality and to determine the alkalinity or acidity of the blood. To maintain CO_2 within normal limits, the rate and depth of respiration vary automatically with changes in metabolism. This test is an index of the effectiveness of alveolar ventilation and is the most physiologically reflective blood gas measurement. An arterial sample directly reflects how well air is exchanged with blood in the lungs.

The CO_2 tension in the blood and in cerebrospinal fluid (CSF) is the major chemical factor regulating alveolar ventilation. When the CO_2 of arterial blood rises from 40 torr to 45 torr, it causes a threefold increase in alveolar ventilation. A CO_2 of 63 torr in arterial blood increases alveolar ventilation tenfold. When the F_{ICO_2} >0.05 concentration of inspired air exceeds 5%, the lungs can no longer be ventilated fast enough to prevent a dangerous rise of CO_2 concentration in tissue fluids. Any further increase in CO_2 begins to depress the respiratory center, causing a progressive decline in respiratory activity, rather than an increase.

Procedure

1. Obtain an arterial blood sample according to protocols. See pages 906 and 907 for specimen collection.
2. A small amount of this blood is introduced into a blood gas analyzing machine and the CO_2 tension is measured by a silver–silver chloride electrode (Severinghaus electrode).

Clinical Implications

1. A *rise* in Pa_{CO_2} (hypercapnia) is usually associated with hypoventilation (CO_2 retention); a *decrease,* with hyperventilation ("blowing off" CO_2). Reduction in Pa_{CO_2}, through its effect on plasma bicarbonate concentration, decreases renal bicarbonate reabsorption. For each milliequivalent per liter fall in HCO_3, the Pa_{CO_2} falls by 1 to 1.3 mm Hg. Because HCO_3 and P_{CO_2} bear this close mathematical relationship, and this ratio, in turn, defends the hydrogen ion concentration, the outcome is that the steady-state P_{CO_2} in simple metabolic acidosis is equal to the last two digits of the pH_a. Also, addition of 15 to the bicarbonate level equals the last two digits of the pH_a. Failure of the Pa_{CO_2} to achieve predicted levels defines the presence of superimposed respiratory acidosis on alkalosis.
2. The causes of *decreased* Pa_{CO_2} include
   - **a.** Hypoxia
   - **b.** Nervousness
   - **c.** Anxiety
   - **d.** Pulmonary emboli
   - **e.** Pregnancy
   - **f.** Pain
   - **g.** Other cause of hyperventilation
3. The causes of *increased* Pa_{CO_2} include
   - **a.** Obstructive lung disease
     - **(1)** Chronic bronchitis
     - **(2)** Emphysema

b. Reduced function of respiratory center
  (1) Overreaction
  (2) Head trauma
  (3) Anesthesia
c. Other less common causes of hypoventilation, such as pickwickian syndrome

Clinical Alert

Increased $Paco_2$ may occur, even with normal lungs, if the respiratory center is depressed. Always check laboratory reports for abnormal values. When interpreting laboratory reports, remember that $Paco_2$ is a gas and is regulated by the lungs not the kidneys.

Patient Preparation

1. Explain purpose, benefits, and risks of invasive arterial blood sampling procedure. Assess ability to cooperate.
2. Follow Chapter 1 guidelines for safe, effective, informed *pretest* care.

Patient Aftercare

1. Interpret test outcome. Assess, monitor, and intervene appropriately for hypoxemia and ventilatory disturbances.
2. See Chapter 1 guidelines for safe, effective, informed *posttest* care.

OXYGEN SATURATION (So_2)

Normal Values

Arterial blood oxygen saturation (Sao_2) = 95% or higher
Mixed venous blood oxygen saturation (Svo_2) = 75%
Newborn: 40 to 90%
Values decrease with age.

Explanation of Test

This measurement is a ratio between the actual oxygen (O_2) content of the hemoglobin (Hb) compared with the potential maximum O_2- carrying capacity of the hemoglobin. The percentage of So_2 is a measure of the relation between O_2 and hemoglobin. It does not indicate O_2 content of arterial blood. The maximum amount of O_2 that can be combined with hemoglobin is called the O_2 capacity. The combined measurements of O_2 saturation, partial pressure of O_2, and of hemoglobin will indicate the amount of O_2 available to tissue (tissue oxygenation). Pulse oximetry (Spo_2) is a noninvasive technique that permits continuous real-time monitoring and trending of arterial oxygen saturation. However, it cannot differentiate carboxyhemoglobin (COHb). As a result, the Spo_2 is generally higher than the Sao_2 by the amount of COHb.

Procedure

1. Obtain arterial blood sample. Two methods are used for determining oxygen saturation: direct method and calculated method.
   - **a.** The blood sample is introduced into hemoximeter, a spectrophotometric device for direct determination of oxygen saturation.
   - **b.** Oxygen saturation is calculated from oxygen content and oxygen capacity by following formula:

$$\text{Percentage saturation} = \frac{100 \times O_2 \text{ content volume \%}}{O_2 \text{ capacity volume \%}}$$

   that is

$$\text{Percentage saturation} = 100 \times \frac{\text{volume of } O_2 \text{ actually combined with Hb}}{\text{volume of } O_2 \text{ to which Hb can combine}}$$

   The O_2 content of the blood sample is measured both before and after exposure to the atmosphere.
2. Pulse oximetry: A small cliplike sensor is placed on a digit over the fingernail (or toenail, if necessary). The instrument, using transmitted light waves and sensors, determines oxygen saturation noninvasively.

Limitations

1. Oxygen saturation measures only the percentage of oxygen being carried by hemoglobin. It does not reveal the actual amount of oxygen available to the tissues (oxygen content).
2. Pulse oximetry equipment evaluates pulsatile blood flow. Many factors can interfere with the ability to measure flow:
   - **a.** Digit motion
   - **b.** A decrease in blood flow to the digit (cool extremity, decreased peripheral pulses, vasoconstriction, nailbed thickening, ambient light, digit malformation, vasoconstrictive drugs, or localized obstruction)
   - **c.** Decrease in hemoglobin (anemia) or abnormal hemoglobin (carboxyhemoglobin)

Interfering Factors

Recent smoking or exposure to close second-hand smoke or carbon monoxide can increase the carboxyhemoglobin levels, as can use of certain paint and varnish-type stripping agents, especially when applied in closed and poorly ventilated areas, thereby decreasing arterial blood oxygen saturation with little or no effect in the arterial blood partial pressure of oxygen ($PaCO_2$).

Clinical Implications

1. Abnormal results occur in pulmonary diseases with cyanosis and erythrocytosis.
2. Venous to arterial shunts.
3. Rh incompatibility caused by blocking antibodies.

4. Values are usually normal in polycythemic vera.
5. Values are decreased in ventilation/perfusion mismatching.

Patient Preparation

1. Explain purpose, benefits, and risks of invasive arterial blood sampling. Assess compliance with procedure.
2. Follow Chapter 1 guidelines for safe, effective, informed *pretest* care.

Patient Aftercare

1. Interpret test outcomes. Assess, monitor, and intervene appropriately for bleeding at puncture site, for hypoxemia, and for other respiratory dysfunctions.
2. See Chapter 1 guidelines for safe, effective, informed *posttest* care.

OXYGEN (O_2) CONTENT ●

Normal Values

Arterial blood: 15 to 22 vol%
Venous blood: 11 to 16 vol%
(Vol % = volume percentage = ml/dl of blood)

Explanation of Test

The actual amount of O_2 in the blood is termed the *oxygen content.* Blood can contain less O_2 than it is capable of carrying. About 98% of all O_2 delivered to the tissues is transported in chemical combination with hemoglobin: 1 g of hemoglobin can carry or is capable of combining with 1.34 ml of O_2, whereas 100 ml of blood plasma can carry up to only 0.3 ml of O_2. This measurement is determined mathematically (see later).

Procedure

1. An arterial or venous blood sample is obtained.
2. The oxygen saturation, Po_2, and hemoglobin concentration are measured.
3. The mathematical formula for calculating O_2 content is:

$$Cao_2 \text{ content} = Sao_2 \times Hb \times 1.34 + Pao_2 \times 0.003$$
$$Cvo_2 = Svo_2 \times Hb \times 1.34 + Pvo_2 \times 0.003$$

Clinical Implications

Decreased arterial blood O_2 content is associated with

1. Chronic obstructive lung disease
2. Postoperative respiratory complications
3. Flail chest
4. Kyphoscoliosis
5. Neuromuscular impairment
6. Obesity-caused hypoventilation
7. Anemia

Patient Preparation

1. Explain purpose, benefits, and risks of invasive arterial blood sampling.
2. Follow Chapter 1 guidelines for safe, effective, informed *pretest* care.

Patient Aftercare

1. Interpret test outcome. Assess, monitor, and intervene appropriately for bleeding at puncture site, hypoxemia, and ventilatory disturbances.
2. See Chapter 1 guidelines for safe, effective, informed *posttest* care.

PARTIAL PRESSURE OF OXYGEN (PO_2)

Normal Values

PaO_2, arterial blood = 80 torr or greater
PvO_2, venous blood = 30 to 40 torr

Background

Oxygen (O_2) is carried in the blood in two forms: dissolved and in combination with hemoglobin. Most of the O_2 in the blood is carried by hemoglobin. It is the partial pressure of a gas that determines the force it exerts in attempting to diffuse through the pulmonary membrane. The partial pressure reflects the amount of O_2 passing from the pulmonary alveoli into the blood and is directly influenced by the FIO_2.

Explanation of Test

This test measures the pressure exerted by the amount of O_2 dissolved in the plasma. It evaluates the ability of the lungs to oxygenate the blood and is used to assess the effectiveness of oxygen therapy. Partial pressure of oxygen indicates the ability of the lungs to diffuse O_2 across the alveolar membrane into the circulating blood.

Procedure

1. An arterial blood sample is obtained (see page 907).
2. A sample of blood is introduced into a blood gas analyzing machine, and the O_2 tension is measured by the Clark electrode.

Clinical Implications

1. *Increased levels* are associated with
   - **a.** Polycythemia
   - **b.** Increased FIO_2
   - **c.** Hyperventilation
2. *Decreased levels* are associated with
   - **a.** Anemias
   - **b.** Cardiac decompensation
   - **c.** Insufficient atmospheric O_2
   - **d.** Intracardiac shunts
   - **e.** Chronic obstructive pulmonary disease (COPD)
   - **f.** Restrictive pulmonary disease
   - **g.** Hypoventilation due to neuromuscular disease

3. *Decreased* arterial PO_2 with normal or decreased arterial blood PCO_2 tension is associated with
   a. Diffuse interstitial pulmonary infiltration
   b. Pulmonary edema
   c. Pulmonary embolism
   d. Postoperative extracorporeal circulation

Clinical Alert

Supplemental oxygen will increase the $PaCO_2$. However, it can also alter CO_2 retention in COPD patients because ventilatory efforts, normally stimulated by *hypoxic states in these patients,* are no longer stimulated. The normal COPD hypoxic state has been altered by the administration of oxygen, and the patient breathes less effectively because their "hypoxic drive is knocked out." (The respiratory stimulus for a healthy person relates to the "building up" of CO_2—it is not a situation of hypoxia.)

Patient Preparation

1. Explain purpose, benefits, and risks of arterial blood sampling. Assess level of cooperation and understanding.
2. Follow guidelines in Chapter 1 for safe, effective, informed *pretest* care.

Patient Aftercare

1. Interpret test outcome. Assess, monitor, and intervene appropriately for bleeding at puncture site or for respiratory and ventilatory disturbances.
2. See Chapter 1 guidelines in Chapter 1 for safe, effective, informed *posttest* care.

CARBON DIOXIDE (CO_2) CONTENT; TOTAL CARBON DIOXIDE (TCO_2) ●

Normal Values

23 to 30 mmol/L

Background

In normal blood plasma, more than 95% of the total CO_2 content is contributed by bicarbonate (HCO_3^-), *which is regulated by the kidneys.* The other 5% of CO_2 is contributed by the dissolved CO_2 gas and carbonic acid (H_2CO_3). Dissolved CO_2 gas, which is regulated by the lungs, therefore contributes little to the total CO_2 content. Total CO_2 content gives little information about the lungs.

The HCO_3^- in the extracellular spaces exists first as CO_2, then as H_2CO_3, and thereafter, much of it is changed to sodium bicarbonate ($NaHCO_3$) by the buffers of the plasma and red cells.

Explanation of Test

This test is a general measure of the alkalinity or acidity of the venous, arterial, or capillary blood. It measures CO_2 from

1. Dissolved CO_2
2. Total H_2CO_3
3. HCO_3^-
4. Carbaminohemoglobin (CO_2HHb)

Procedure

1. A 6-ml venous or arterial blood sample is collected in a heparinized syringe.
2. If the collected blood sample cannot be studied immediately, the syringe should be placed in an iced container.
3. CO_2 content = $HCO_3 + H_2 CO_3$.

Clinical Implications

(see also Table 14–2)

1. *Elevated* CO_2 content levels occur in
   - **a.** Severe vomiting
   - **b.** Emphysema
   - **c.** Aldosteronism
   - **d.** Use of mercurial diuretics
2. *Decreased* CO_2 content levels occur in
   - **a.** Severe diarrhea
   - **b.** Starvation
   - **c.** Acute renal failure
   - **d.** Salicylate toxicity
   - **e.** Diabetic acidosis
   - **f.** Use of chlorothiazide diuretics

NOTE: *In diabetic acidosis the supply of ketoacids exceeds the demands of the cell. Blood plasma acids rise. Blood plasma HCO_3^- decreases because it is used in neutralizing these excess acids.*

Clinical Alert

1. A double use of the term CO_2 is one of the main reasons why understanding acid–base problems may be difficult. Use the terms *CO_2 content* and *CO_2 gas* to avoid confusion. Remember the following:
   - **a.** *CO_2 content* is mainly bicarbonate and a base. It is a solution and is regulated by the kidneys.
   - **b.** *CO_2 gas* is mainly acid. It is regulated by the lungs.
2. Panic value is 6.0 or less and is usually associated with severe metabolic acidosis, with the pH often less than 7.1. *This is a life-threatening situation.*

TABLE 14-2
Summary of Changes in Two Primary Disturbances (Ventilatory and Acid–Base Disturbances) and Four Underlying Disturbances of Acid–Base Imbalance

Ventilatory Disturbance Form	*pH*	*Bicarbonate (HCO_3^-)*	*pao_2*	*Occurrence*
1. Respiratory acidosis (acute) caused by decreased alveolar ventilation and retention of CO_2	Decrease	Normal	Increase	*Depression of respiratory centers* Drug overdose Barbiturate toxicity Use of anesthetics *Interference with mechanical function of thoracic cage* Deformity of thoracic cage Kyphoscoliosis *Airway Obstruction* Extrathoracic tumors Asthma Bronchitis Emphysema *Circulatory Disorders* Congestive heart failure Shock
Respiratory acidosis, compensated (chronic); compensatory mechanism is by the disturbance not involved. Renal reabsorption of the bicabonate ion	Normal	Increase	Increase	

2. Respiratory alkalosis (acute) caused by increased alveolar ventilation and excessive blowing off of CO_2 and water	Increase	Normal	Decrease	*Hyperventilation* *Hysteria* *Lack of oxygen* *Toxic stimulation of the respiratory centers* High fever Cerebral hemorrhage Excessive artificial respiration Salicylates
Respiratory alkalosis compensated (chronic); compensatory mechanism is by the disturbance not involved: glomerular filtration of the bicarbonate ion	Normal	Decrease	Decrease	
3. Nonrespiratory metabolic (acute) acidosis caused by accumulation of fixed body acids or loss of HCO_3 (bicarbonate) from the extracellular fluid	Decrease	Decrease	Normal	*Acid gain* Renal failure Diabetic ketoacidosis Lactic acidosis Anaerobic metabolism *Hypoxia* Base loss Diarrhea Renal tubular acidosis
Nonrespiratory, metabolic acidosis compensated (chronic); compensatory mechanism is by the disturbance not involved: *Hyperventilation* through stimulation of central chemoreceptors.	Normal	Decrease	Decrease	

(continued)

TABLE 14-2 *(Continued)*

Ventilatory Disturbance Form	***pH***	***Bicarbonate (HCO_3^-)***	***pao_2***	***Occurrence***
4. Nonrespiratory or metabolic alkalosis (acute) cause by loss of fixed body acids or gain in bicarbonate (HCO_3) in extracellular fluid	Increase	Increase	Normal	*Acid loss* Loss of gastric juice Vomiting *Potassium or chloride depletion* *Base gain* Excessive bicarbonate or lactate administration
Nonrespiratory or metabolic alkaloses, compensated (chronic); compensatory mechanism is by disturbance not involved: *hypoventilation*	Normal	Increase	Increase	

Note: 1. Although these four basic imbalances occur individually, a combination of two or more is observed more frequently. These disturbances may have an antagonistic or a synergistic effect on each other.

2. Compensation is most efficient in respiratory acidoses. Uncompensated disturbances are referred to as acute, and compensated as chronic.
3. The degree of hypoventilation is precisely related to the degree of hypobicarbonatemia. For each milliequivalent per liter (mEq/L) fall in bicarbonate, Pco2 falls by 1 to 1.3 torr. A close mathematical relationship prevails between bicarbonate and Pco2. Their ration (HCO_3 and Pco_2) defines the prevailing hydrogen ion concentration. For this reason, the steady-state Pco_2 in simple metabolic acidosis is equal to the last two digits of the pH. Failure of the Pco_2 to reach predicted levels defines the presence of superimposed respiratory acidosis or alkalosis.
4. Decreases in Pao2 are interpreted separately and referred to as hypoxemia.
5. Acid–base disturbances force kidney and lungs to compensate for changes in pH. Hyper- or hypoventilation can restrict pH to normal within 15 minutes; the kidney, however, can take up to 2 to 3 days to compensate.

Interfering Factors
A number of drugs may cause increased or decreased CO_2 levels.

Patient Preparation
1. Explain purpose, benefits, and risks of arterial blood sampling. Assess ability to comply.
2. Follow guidelines in Chapter 1 for safe, effective, informed *pretest* care.

Patient Aftercare
1. Interpret test outcomes. Assess, monitor, and intervene appropriately for acid–base imbalances.
2. Monitor and intervene for bleeding at puncture site or for respiratory/ventilatory disturbances.
3. See Chapter 1 guidelines for safe, effective, informed *posttest* care.

BLOOD pH

Normal Values
pH_a = arterial blood: 7.35 to 7.45
pH_v = venous blood: 7.31 to 7.41

Background
The pH is the negative logarithm of the hydrogen ion concentration in the blood. The sources of hydrogen ions are (1) volatile acids, which can vary between a liquid and a gaseous state; and (2) nonvolatile acids, which cannot be volatilized but remain fixed (eg, dietary acids, lactic acids, and ketoacids).

> **NOTE:** *Values from 1 to 7 represent an acid state; 7 is neutral; and 7 to 14 represents an alkaline state. Limits of pH compatible with life fall within the 6.9 to 7.8 range.*

Explanation of Test
Blood pH measures the body's chemical balance and represents a ratio of acids to bases. It is also an indicator of the degree to which the body adjusts to dysfunctions by means of its buffering systems. It is one of the best ways to determine if the body is too acid or too alkaline and is an indicator of the patient's metabolic and respiratory status. Lower pH numbers (<7.35) indicate an acid state; higher pH numbers (>7.45) indicate an alkaline state. This extracellular fluid balance is extremely delicate and intricate and must be kept within the very narrow margin of 7.35 to 7.45 pH (slightly alkaline).

Procedure
1. An arterial blood sample is obtained.
2. The pH can be determined by direct method or indirect method.

a. *Direct method:* A small amount of blood is analyzed by a blood gas machine in which the pH is measured by a modified Severinghaus electrode.

b. *Indirect method:* The Henderson–Hasselbalch equation is solved: pH = pK + log *A*; pK refers to pH at which the associated and unassociated forms of an acid will exist in equal concentrations.

$$\text{pH} = \text{pK}' + \log \frac{(HCO_3) \text{ major blood base}}{(H_2CO_3) \text{ major blood acid}}$$

Clinical Implications

1. Generally speaking, the pH is *decreased* in acidemia or acidosis because of increased formation of acids. The pH is *increased* in alkalemia or alkalosis because of a loss of acids.

2. When interpreting an acid–base abnormality, certain steps should be followed:

a. Check the pH to determine whether an alkalotic or acidotic state exists.

b. Check P_{CO_2} to determine whether a respiratory acidosis or alkalosis is present. (**Remember:** P_{CO_2} is **the breathing component.**)

c. Check HCO_3 to determine a metabolic acidosis or alkalosis. (This is the "renal" component.)

3. See Table 14–2 for a more complete explanation of the changes occurring in acute and chronic respiratory and metabolic acidosis and alkalosis.

4. Metabolic acidemia (acidosis)

a. Renal failure

b. Ketoacidosis in diabetes and starvation

c. Lactic acidosis

d. Strenuous exercise

e. Severe diarrhea

5. Metabolic alkalemia (alkalosis)

a. Hypokalemia

b. Hypochloremia

c. Gastric suction or vomiting

d. Massive doses of steroids

e. Sodium bicarbonate administration

f. Aspirin intoxication

6. Respiratory alkalemia (alkalosis)

a. Acute pulmonary disease

b. Myocardial infarction

c. Chronic and acute heart failure

d. Adult cystic fibrosis

e. Third trimester of pregnancy and process of labor and delivery

f. Anxiety, neuroses, psychoses

g. Pain

h. Central nervous system diseases

i. Anemia

j. Carbon monoxide poisoning

k. Acute pulmonary embolus

l. Shock

7. Respiratory acidemia (acidosis)

a. Acute and chronic respiratory failure

b. Ventilatory failure

c. Neuromuscular depression

d. Obesity
e. Pulmonary edema
f. Cardiopulmonary arrest

Clinical Alert

1. *Ventilatory failure is a medical emergency. Aggressive and supportive measures must be taken immediately.*
2. Rate and depth of respirations may give a clue to blood pH.
   a. Acidosis usually *increases* respirations.*
   b. Alkalosis usually *decreases* respirations.*
3. Respiratory alkalosis may reflect hyperventilation in response to treatment for hypoxemia. However, correction of hypoxemia is essential.
4. Metabolic alkalosis, which is compensated through hypoventilation, may produce hypoxemia.

*This is the body's way of adjusting once the state is established.

Interfering Factors

A number of drugs may alter these acid–base components.

Patient Preparation

1. Explain purpose, benefits, and risks of invasive blood sampling for pH determination.
2. Follow guidelines in Chapter 1 for safe, effective, informed *pretest* care.

Patient Aftercare

1. Interpret test outcome. Assess, monitor, and intervene appropriately for metabolic and respiratory acidosis and alkalosis (see Table 14–2).
2. Frequently observe the arterial puncture site for bleeding (see page 908). Be prepared to initiate proper interventions in the event of life-threatening situations.
3. See Chapter 1 guidelines for safe, effective, informed *posttest* care.

BASE EXCESS/DEFICIT

Normal Values (plus or minus 3 mEq/L)

Positive value indicates a base excess (ie, nonvolatile acid deficit).
Negative value indicates a base deficit (ie, nonvolatile acid excess).

Explanation of Test

This test quantifies the patient's total base excess or deficit so that clinical treatment of acid–base disturbances (specifically those that are nonrespiratory) can be initiated. It is also referred to as the whole-blood buffer base and is the sum of the concentration of buffer anions (in mEq/L) contained in whole blood. These buffer anions are the bicarbonate (HCO_3^-) ion present in plasma red blood cells, and hemoglobin, plasma proteins, as well as phosphates in plasma and red blood cells.

The total quantity of buffer anions is 45 to 50 mEq/L or about twice that of HCO_3^-, (24 to 28 mEq/L). Thus, the quantity of HCO_3^- ions accounts for only about half of the total buffering capacity of the blood. Therefore, the base excess/deficit measurement provides a more complete picture of the buffering taking place and is a critical index of nonrespiratory changes in acid–base balance versus respiratory changes in acid–base balance.

Procedure

Calculation is made from the measurement of pH, $PaCO_2$, and hematocrit. These values are plotted on a nomogram, and the base excess/deficit is read.

Clinical Implications

1. A negative value (lower than 3 mEq/L) reflects a nonrespiratory or metabolic disturbance, a true base deficit, or a nonvolatile acid accumulation caused by
   a. Dietary intake of organic and inorganic acids
   b. Lactic acid
   c. Ketoacidosis
2. A positive value (higher than +3 mEq/L) reflects a nonvolatile acid deficit or true base excess.

ANION GAP (AG) OR R FACTOR ●

Normal Values

< ±12 mEq/L
< 16 mEq/L if potassium concentration is used to calculate the anion gap

Explanation of Test

This test is a measurement of the difference between sodium (Na^+) and potassium (K^+) ion concentrations (the measured cations) and the sum of chloride (Cl^-) and bicarbonate (HCO_3^-) concentrations (the measured anions). This difference reflects the concentrations of anions that are present in the extracellular fluid, including phosphates, sulfates, ketone bodies, lactic acid, and proteins. Increased amounts of these unmeasured anions are produced in the acidotic state.

Primary hypobicarbonatemia is brought about by any combination of these three mechanisms: (1) overproduction of acids, which causes replacement of $NaHCO_3^-$ by the Na^+ salt of the offending acid (eg, Na^+ lactate replaces HCO_3^- in lactic acidosis); (2) loss of $NaHCO_3^-$ through diarrhea along with renal retention of dietary NaCl, which causes hyperchloremic metabolic acidosis; (3) generalized renal failure or specific forms of renal tubular acidosis, which causes retention of acids that are normally produced by intermediary metabolism or by urinary excretion of alkali (Table 14-3).

Hyperbicarbonatemia with sustained increases of HCO_3^- levels is brought about by a source of *new* alkali and the presence of factors that stimulate renal retention of excess HCO_3^- (Table 14-4). These mechanisms include excessive gastrointestinal loss of acid, exogenous alkali in persons whose kidneys avidly retain $NaHCO_3^-$, and renal synthesis of HCO_3^- in excess of daily consumption. Other pathophysiologic factors that affect renal reabsorption of more than 25 mEq of HCO_3^- and contribute to sustained hyperbicarbonatemia include extracellular fluid volume contraction, hypercapnia, hypokalemia, hyperaldosteronemia, and hypoparathyroidism.

Procedure

This measurement is obtained by determining the difference between the sum of the serum cations and the sum of the serum anions.

$$AG = (Na^+ + K^+) - (Cl^- + HCO_3^-) \quad \text{or} \quad AG = Na^+ - (Cl^- + HCO_3^-)$$

Clinical Implications

1. An anion gap occurs in acidosis because of the excess metabolic acids and excess serum chloride levels. If there is no change in sodium content, anions, such as phosphates, sulfates, and organic acids, will increase the anion gap because these components replace bicarbonate.
2. *Increased* anion gap is associated with an increase in metabolic acid when there is an excessive production of metabolic acids as in
   - **a.** Alcoholic ketoacidosis
   - **b.** Diabetic ketoacidosis
   - **c.** Fasting and starvation
   - **d.** Ketogenic diets
   - **e.** Lactic acidosis
   - **f.** Salicylate, ethylene glycol (antifreeze), and methanol or propyl alcohol poisoning

TABLE 14-3
Subclassification of Anion Gap Metabolic Acidosis (Hypobicarbonatemia) into High- and Low-Potassium Forms*

High-Potassium Form	*Low-Potassium Form*
Acidifying agents	Diarrhea
Mineralocorticoid deficiency	Ureteral sigmoidostomy and malfunctioning
Renal diseases, such as systemic lupus erythematosus, interstitial nephritis, amyloidosis, hydronephrosis, sickle cell nephropathy	Ileostomy
Early nonspecific renal failure	Renal tubular acidosis, both proximal and distal

*All metabolic acidoses can be classified on the basis of how they affect the anion gap.

TABLE 14-4
Classification of Anion Gap Metabolic Alkalosis (Hyperbicarbonatemia) on the Basis of Urinary Excretion

Saline-**Responsive** *Urinary Chloride Excretion of Less Than 10 mEq/day*	*Saline*-**Unresponsive** *Urinary Chloride Excretion of Less Than 10 mEq/day*
1. Excess body bicarbonate content (a) Renal alkalosis Diuretic therapy Poorly reabsorbable anion therapy, such as carbenicillin, penicillin, sulfate, phosphate (b) Gastrointestinal alkalosis Gastric alkalosis Intestinal alkalosis, such as chloride diarrhea (c) Exogenous alkali Baking soda Sodium citrate, lactate, gluconate, acetate Transfusions Antacids **2.** Normal body bicarbonate content Contraction alkalosis—This means that the urinary loss of sodium chloride and water without bicarbonate loss will cause extracellular fluid contraction around an unchanged body content of alkali, resulting in hyperbicarbonatemia. This is especially important in persons with edema and persons who have excess body stores of water, sodium, bicarbonate, and chloride.	**1.** Excess body bicarbonate content (a) Renal alkalosis—normotensive conditions Bartter's syndrome Severe potassium depletion Refeeding alkalosis Hypercalcemia and hypoparathyroidism (b) Hypertensive conditions—endogenous mineralocorticoids Primary aldosteronism Hyperreninism Adrenal enzyme deficiency: 11- and 17-hydroxylase Liddle syndrome (c) Exogenous mineralocorticoids Licorice Carbenoxolone Chewing tobacco

3. *Increased anion* gap is also associated with decreased loss of metabolic acids, as in renal failure. In the absence of renal failure or intoxication with drugs or toxins, an increase in anion gap is assumed to be due to ketoacidosis or lactate accumulation.
4. *Increased* bicarbonate loss, with resulting normal anion gap, is associated with
   - **a.** *Decreased* renal losses as in
     - **(1)** Renal tubular acidosis
     - **(2)** Use of acetazolamide
   - **b.** *Increased* chloride levels as in

(1) Altered chloride reabsorption by the kidney
(2) Parenteral hyperalimentation
(3) Administration of sodium chloride or ammonium chloride

c. Loss of intestinal secretions as in
(1) Diarrhea
(2) Intestinal suction or fistula
(3) Biliary fistula

5. *Low* anion gap is associated with
   a. Multiple myeloma
   b. Hyponatremia owing to viscous serum
   c. Bromide ingestion (hyperchloremia)

Clinical Alert

1. Interpret test outcomes and assess and monitor appropriately for acid–base disturbances.
2. AG may provide evidence of a mixed, rather than a simple, acid–base disturbance.
3. Lactic acidosis should be considered in any metabolic acidosis with increased AG of >15 mEq/L.

LACTIC ACID

Normal Values

0.5 to 2.2 mEq/L venous blood
0.5 to 1.6 mEq/L arterial blood

Background

Lactate is a product of carbohydrate metabolism. Lactic acid is produced during periods of anaerobic metabolism when cells do not receive adequate oxygen to allow conversion of fuel sources to carbon dioxide and water. Lactic acid will accumulate because of excess production of lactate and decreased removal of lactic acid from blood by liver.

Explanation of Test

This measurement contributes to the knowledge of acid–base volume and is used to detect lactic acidosis in persons with underlying risk factors, such as cardiovascular and renal disease, which predispose them to this imbalance. Lactate will be elevated in a variety of conditions in which hypoxia occurs, as well as in liver disease. Lactic acidosis can occur both in diabetics and nondiabetics. It is often fatal.

Procedure

A venous or arterial blood sample of at least 4 ml is obtained. *The specimen must be brought to the laboratory immediately.*

Clinical Implications

1. Values will be *increased* in
   a. Lactic acidosis
   b. Cardiac failure
   c. Pulmonary failure
   d. Hemorrhage
   e. Diabetes
   f. Shock
   g. Liver disease
2. Lactic acidosis can be distinguished from ketoacidosis by the absence of severe ketosis and hyperglycemia in this state.

Interfering Factors

Lactic acid levels normally rise during strenuous exercise when blood flow and oxygen cannot keep pace with increased needs of exercising muscle.

Clinical Alert

An unexplained decrease in pH associated with a hypoxia-producing condition is reason to suspect lactic acidosis.

Patient Preparation

1. Explain purpose and procedure of arterial blood sampling for lactic acid determination. Assess patient cooperation.
2. Follow guidelines in Chapter 1 for safe, effective, informed *pretest* care.

Patient Aftercare

1. Frequently observe the puncture site for bleeding. Manual pressure and a pressure dressing should be applied to the puncture site if necessary.
2. Base *posttest* assessments on patient outcomes; monitor and intervene appropriately for ventilatory and acid–base disturbances and hypoxemia.
3. See guidelines in Chapter 1 for safe, effective, informed *posttest* care.

BIBLIOGRAPHY

American Thoracic Society: Single breath carbon monoxide diffusing capacity (transfer factor): Recommendations for a standard technique. Am Rev Respir Dis 136:1299–1307, 1987

American Thoracic Society: Standardization of spirometry—1987 update. Am Rev Respir Dis 139:1285–1298, 1987

American Thoracic Society: Lung function testing: Selection of reference values and interpretive strategies. Am Rev Respir Dis 144:1202–1218, 1991

Anderson S: Six easy steps to interpreting blood gases. Am J Nurs 42–45, August 1991

Cherniack RM: Pulmonary Function Testing, 2nd ed. Philadelphia, WB Saunders, 1992

Kryger MH, Roth T, Dement WC: Principles and Practice of Sleep Medicine. Philadelphia, WB Saunders, 1989

Leff AR, Schumacker PT: Respiratory Physiology–Basics and Applications. Philadelphia, WB Saunders, 1993

Madama VC: Pulmonary Function Testing and Cardiopulmonary Stress Testing. Albany, Delmar Publishers, 1993

Ruppel G: Manual of Pulmonary Function Testing, 6th ed. St. Louis, CV Mosby, 1994

Shapiro BA, Harrison RA, Cane RD, et al: Clinical Application of Blood Gases. Chicago, Year Book Medical, 1989

Snow MG: Determination of functional residual capacity. Respir Care 34:586–594, 1989

Spyr J, Preach M: Pulse oximetry—understanding the concept and knowing the limits. RN 53 (5):38–45, May 1990

Stiesmeyer JK: A four-step approach to pulmonary assessment. Am J Nurs 22–28, August 1993

Zavala DC: Manual on Exercise Testing: A Training Handbook, 3rd ed. Iowa City, University of Iowa Press, 1993

15

Special System and Organ Function Studies

OVERVIEW OF SPECIAL STUDIES

These special studies have been selected for discussion because of their great value in aiding diagnosis of diseases in certain organs and systems. Tests after death serve to identify previously undiagnosed disease; evaluate accuracy of predeath diagnosis; provide information about sudden, suspicious, or unexplained deaths; assist postmortem legal investigations; and control quality in healthcare settings.

ELECTROENCEPHALOGRAPHY (EEG)

Normal Values

Normal, symmetric patterns of electrical brain activity; range of alpha, 8 to 11 Hertz (Hz; cycles per second).

Explanation of Test

The EEG measures and records electrical impulses from the brain cortex. This test is used to diagnose epilepsy and to evaluate brain tumors, abscesses, subdural hematomas, cerebral infarcts, and intracranial hemorrhages. It can also assist in diagnosing narcolepsy and Alzheimer's disease. It is common practice to use the EEG pattern along with other clinical procedures, drug levels, patient body temperature, and a thorough neurologic examination to determine electrocerebral silence or "brain death." Recordings are obtained using guidelines set by the American Electroneurodiagnostic Society. When this electrocerebral silence pattern is recorded and there is no chance of neurologic recovery, the patient may be declared brain dead, despite assisted cardiovascular and respiratory support.

Procedure

1. An EEG can be done any time.
2. Electrodes with conduction gel are fastened to the scalp with skin glue or paste. Nineteen to 25 electrodes are attached according to an internationally accepted measurement named the *10–20 System*. This system correlates electrode placement with anatomic structure of the brain.
3. The patient may lie on a bed or couch.
4. The patient is instructed to keep the eyes closed and to relax as much as possible.
5. Before beginning the examination, the patient may be asked to breathe deeply through the mouth 20 times a minute for 3 minutes. This hyperventilation may cause dizziness or numbness in hands or feet but is not a cause for alarm. Rapid, shallow breathing causes alkalosis, which causes vasoconstriction, which may activate a seizure pattern.
6. A flashing light at frequencies of 1 to 30 times per second may be placed close to the face. This technique, called *photic stimulation*, may cause an abnormal pattern not otherwise recorded on the EEG.
7. Some patients may be ordered to be sleep-deprived before the test to

promote rest and sleep during the test. Sleep is especially helpful in bringing out abnormalities, especially different forms of epilepsy.

8. Electrodes, glue, and paste are removed from the scalp after the test.

Clinical Implications

1. Abnormal EEG pattern readings will reveal generalized seizures (eg, grand mal and petit mal epilepsy), if the EEG is recorded during the seizure. If a patient suspected of having epilepsy shows a normal EEG, the test may have to be repeated using sleep deprivation or special electrodes.
   a. Also abnormal during other types of seizure activity (eg, focal [psychomotor], infantile myoclonic, or jacksonian seizures).
   b. Between seizures, 20% of patients with petit mal epilepsy and 40% with grand mal epilepsy show a normal EEG pattern.
   c. The diagnosis of epilepsy can be made only by correlating the clinical history with the EEG abnormality, if one exists.
2. An EEG may often be normal in the presence of cerebral disease. However, most brain abscesses and glioblastomas cause EEG abnormalities.
   a. Electroencephalographic changes caused by cerebrovascular accidents depend on the size and location of the infarcts or hemorrhages.
   b. Following a head injury, a series of EEGs may be helpful in predicting the likelihood of epilepsy as a result of the trauma if a previous EEG is available for comparison.
   c. In dementia, the EEG may be either normal or abnormal.
   d. In early stages of metabolic disease, the EEG will be normal; in the later stages, it will be abnormal.
3. The EEG is abnormal in most diseases or injuries that alter the level of consciousness. The more profound the change in consciousness, the more abnormal the EEG pattern.

Interfering Factors

1. Sedative drugs or a state of mild hypoglycemia alter a normal EEG.
2. Oily hair, hair spray, and other hair care products interfere with the placement of EEG patches and with accurately represented EEG tracings.
3. Artifacts may even appear in technically well-done EEGs. Eye and body movements cause changes in wave patterns and must be noted so that they will not be misinterpreted for brain waves.

Patient Preparation

1. Explain test purpose and procedure. Some persons are very fearful, even though it is neither painful nor uncomfortable. Emphasize that the EEG is not a test of thinking or intelligence, that no electrical impulses pass through the body, and that the test bears no relation to any type of shock treatment.
2. Food may be taken if the patient is sleep-deprived. ***No coffee, tea,*** or

cola is permitted within 8 hours before the test. Emphasize that food should be eaten to prevent hypoglycemia.

3. Smoking is usually allowed before the test.
4. Hair should be shampooed the evening before the EEG so that EEG patches will remain firmly in place during the test.
5. If a sleep study is ordered, an adult patient should sleep as little as possible the night before (up past midnight) so that sleep occurs during the test.
6. If a sleep-deprivation study is ordered for a child, call the EEG department for special instructions.
7. See Chapter 1 guidelines for safe, effective, informed *pretest* care.

Patient Aftercare

1. The hair should be shampooed after the test. Oil applied to the adhesive before shampooing may promote easier removal of this substance.
2. If the patient received a sedative during the test, allow him or her to rest. Put bedside rails in raised position for safety reasons.
3. Skin irritation from the electrodes usually resolves within a few hours.
4. Interpret test results and monitor appropriately. Explain that repeat testing may be necessary.
5. Follow Chapter 1 guidelines for safe, effective, informed *posttest* care.

TESTS OF EVOKED RESPONSES OR POTENTIALS (AUDITORY BRAIN STEM RESPONSE [ABR]; VISUAL-EVOKED RESPONSE [VER]; SOMATOSENSORY-EVOKED RESPONSE [SER]) ●

These tests use conventional EEG recording techniques, with specific electrode placement for each procedure, along with computer data-processing to evaluate electrophysiologic integrity of the auditory, visual, and sensory pathways.

Normal Values

AUDITORY BRAIN STEM–EVOKED POTENTIALS (ABR)

Absolute latency, measured in milliseconds (msec), of the first five waveforms at a sound stimulation rate of 11 clicks/second.

Wave	*Mean*	*Standard deviation (SD)*
I	1.7	0.15
II	2.8	0.17
III	3.9	0.19
IV	5.1	0.24
V	5.7	0.25

VISUAL-EVOKED RESPONSE (VER)

Absolute latency, measured in milliseconds of the first major positive peak (P_{100})

Wave	*Mean*	*Range*	*SD*
P_{100}	102.3	89–114	5.1

SOMATOSENSORY–EVOKED RESPONSE (SER)

Absolute latency of major waveforms, measured in milliseconds at a stimulation rate of 5 impulses per second

Wave	*Mean*	*SD*
EP	9.7	0.7
A	11.8	0.7
B	13.7	0.8
II	11.3	0.8
III	13.9	0.9
N_2	19.1	0.8
P_2	22	1.2

Explanation of Test

AUDITORY BRAIN STEM RESPONSE

This study evaluates suspected peripheral hearing loss, cerebellopontine angle lesions, brain stem tumors, infarcts, multiple sclerosis, or comatose states.

Special stimulating techniques permit recording the signals generated by subcortical structures in the auditory pathway. Stimulation of either ear evokes potentials that can reveal lesions in the *brain stem* involving the auditory pathway, without affecting hearing. Evoked potentials of this type are also used to evaluate hearing in infants, children, and adults through *electrical response audiometry.*

VISUAL-EVOKED RESPONSE

This test of visual pathway function is valuable in diagnosing lesions involving the optic nerves and optic tracts, multiple sclerosis, and other disorders. Visual stimulation excites retinal pathways and initiates impulses that are conducted through the central visual path to the primary visual cortex. Fibers from this area project to the secondary visual cortical areas on the occipital convexity. Through this path, a visual stimulus to the eyes causes an electrical response in the occipital regions that can be recorded with electrodes placed along the vertex and the occipital lobes.

SOMATOSENSORY-EVOKED RESPONSE

This test assesses patients with spinal cord lesions, stroke, and complaints of numbness and weakness of the extremities. It studies the conduction of impulses through the somatosensory pathway. Electrical stimuli are applied to the median or peroneal nerve at an intensity near that which produces thumb or foot twitches. It is possible to measure in milliseconds the time it takes for the current to travel along the nerve to the cortex of the brain. SERs are also used to monitor the sensory pathway conduction during surgery for spinal cord decompression or ischemia, or for scoliosis repair. A loss of the sensory potential can signal impending cord damage.

Procedures

1. *Auditory brain stem responses* are obtained through scalp electrodes placed on the vertex and on each earlobe. Stimuli, consisting of clicking noises or tone bursts, are delivered to one ear through earphones. Because sound waves delivered to one ear can be heard by the opposite ear, a continuous masking noise is simultaneously delivered to the opposite ear.
2. Electrodes used in *visually evoked* response are placed on the scalp along the vertex and occipital lobes. The patient is then asked to watch a checkerboard pattern flash for several minutes, first with one eye, then with the other, while brain waves are recorded.
3. *Somatosensory-evoked responses* are recorded through several pairs of electrodes. Electrical stimuli are applied to the median nerve at the wrist or to the peroneal nerve at the knee. Electrodes placed over the sensory cortex of the opposite hemisphere in the scalp pick up the signals. This procedure measures, in milliseconds, the time it takes for the current to travel along the nerve to the cortex of the brain.

Clinical Implications

1. Abnormal **ABRs** are associated with
   - **a.** Acoustic neuroma
   - **b.** Cerebrovascular accidents
   - **c.** Multiple sclerosis
   - **d.** Lesions affecting any part of the auditory nerve or brain stem area
2. Abnormal **VERs** are associated with
   - **a.** Demyelinating disorders, such as multiple sclerosis
   - **b.** Lesions of the optic nerves and eye (prechiasmal defects)
   - **c.** Lesions of the optic tract and visual cortex (postchiasmal defects)
   - **d.** Abnormal visual-evoked potentials may also be found in persons without a history of retrobulbar neuritis, optic atrophy, or visual field defects. However, many patients with proved damage to the postchiasmal visual path and known visual-field defects may have normal visual-evoked potentials.
3. Abnormal **SERs** are associated with
   - **a.** Spinal cord lesions
   - **b.** Cerebrovascular accident
   - **c.** Multiple sclerosis
   - **d.** Cervical myelopathy

Interfering Factors

Some difficulty with interpreting brain stem–evoked potentials may arise in persons with peripheral hearing defects that alter evoked potential results.

Patient Preparation

1. Explain the test purpose and procedure.
2. Hair should be shampooed and rinsed well before testing. Instruct patient **not** to apply any other hair preparations.
3. See Chapter 1 for guidelines for safe, effective, informed *pretest* care.

Patient Aftercare

1. Assist the patient to shampoo the hair (if necessary). Remove gel from other skin areas.
2. Interpret test results, counsel, and monitor appropriately for neurologic problems.
3. Follow Chapter 1 guidelines for safe, effective, informed *posttest* care.

COGNITIVE TESTS (EVENT-RELATED POTENTIALS [ERPS]) ●

Normal Values

No shift of P_3 components to longer latencies

ERP: absolute latency of P_3 waveform

Wave	*Mean*	*SD*
P_3	294	21

Explanation of Test

Event-related potentials are being used more frequently as objective measures of mental function in neurologic diseases that produce cognitive defects. These measurements use the method of auditory-evoked response testing (see page 934) in which sound stimuli are transmitted through earphones. A rare tone is associated with a prominent endogenous P_3 component that reflects the differential cognitive processing of that tone. Although a systematic neurologic increase in P_3 component latency occurs as a function of increasing age in normal persons, in many instances of neurologic diseases producing dementia, the latency of the P_3 component has been reported to substantially exceed the normal age-matched value.

This test is useful in evaluating persons with dementia or decreased mental functioning. It is also helpful in differentiating persons with real organic defects in cognitive function from those who are unable to interact with the examiner because of motor or language defects and those who are unwilling to cooperate because of problems such as depression or schizophrenia.

Procedure

1. The procedure is the same as that for auditory brain stem responses (see page 935).
2. Patients are asked to count the occurrences of audible rare tones.

Interfering Factors

The latency of P_3 component normally increases with age.

Clinical Implications

An increased or abnormal P_3 latency is associated with neurologic diseases producing dementia such as

1. Alzheimer's disease
2. Metabolic encephalopathy associated with hypothyroidism, or alcoholism with severe electrolyte disturbances
3. Brain tumor
4. Hydrocephalus

Patient Preparation

1. Explain the purpose and procedure of the test.
2. See Chapter 1 guidelines for safe, effective, informed *pretest* care.

Patient Aftercare

1. Interpret test results, counsel, and monitor appropriately for neurologic disease.
2. Follow Chapter 1 guidelines for safe, effective, informed *posttest* care.

BRAIN MAPPING (COMPUTED TOPOGRAPHY) ●

Normal Values

Normal frequency signals and evoked responses presented as a color-coded map of electrical brain activity.

Explanation of Test

Brain mapping uses traditional EEG data and specialized computer digitization to display the diagnostic information as a topographic map of the brain. The computer analyzes EEG signals for amplitude and distribution of alpha, beta, theta, and delta frequencies and displays the analysis as a color map. Specific or *minute* abnormalities are enhanced, allowing comparison with normal data. This methodology is used in the assessment of cognitive function and in patients with migraine headaches, episodes of vertigo or dizziness, persons who lose pieces of time, and select patients with generalized seizures, dementia of organic origin, ischemic abnormalities, or certain psychiatric disorders. With this procedure, it is possible to localize a specific area of the brain that may otherwise show a generalized area of deficit in the conventional EEG. It is helpful in evaluating children and adults to demonstrate areas of the brain possibly related to hyperactivity, dyslexia, dementia, or Alzheimer's disease.

Procedure

1. The patient should be rested, but awake, for the test so that no sleep signals appear (as indicators of beta activity).
2. The procedure is similar to the conventional EEG. Forty-two electrodes are placed on the scalp.

3. Before electrode placement, the skin is cleansed with an abrasive solution, and the electrodes are applied with a paste or adhesive.
4. The patient sits comfortably and is instructed to keep the eyes closed and to remain as still as possible.

Clinical Implications

Abnormal brain maps can pinpoint the following areas:

1. Focal seizure discharge in persons who experience generalized seizures
2. Focal irritation in persons with migraine
3. Ischemia
4. Dysfunction in states of dementia
5. Possible brain abnormalities as the cause for schizophrenic or other psychotic states

Interfering Factors

1. Tranquilizers may affect results.
2. Oily hair or other hair preparations interfere with electrode placement.
3. Eye and body movements cause change in the signals and wave patterns.

Patient Preparation

1. Explain the test purpose and procedure. There are no known risks. Emphasize that electrical impulses pass only from the *patient* to the machine not from the machine to the patient.
2. Food and fluids are permitted before testing. However, no coffee, tea, or caffeinated drinks are permitted for 8 hours before the test.
3. Hair should be recently shampooed.
4. Tranquilizers should not be taken before testing (check with physician). Other prescribed medications, such as antihypertensives and insulin, do not have to be discontinued. Notify the testing laboratory about drugs the patient has taken.
5. See Chapter 1 guidelines for safe, effective, informed *pretest* care.

Patient Aftercare

1. The conduction gel is removed, and the patient is advised to shampoo the hair.
2. Interpret test results, counsel, and monitor appropriately for seizure activity.
3. Follow Chapter 1 guidelines for safe, effective, informed *posttest* care.

ELECTROMYOGRAPHY; ELECTROMYONEUROGRAM (EMG) ●

Normal Values

Nerve conduction: Normal
Muscle action potential: Normal

1. On insertion
2. At rest
3. During minimum voluntary muscle contraction
4. During maximum voluntary muscle contraction

Explanation of Test

Electromyoneurography combines electromyography and electroneurography. These studies, done to detect neuromuscular abnormalities, measure nerve conduction and electrical properties of skeletal muscles. These tests, together with evaluation of range of motion, motor power, sensory defects, and reflexes can differentiate between neuropathy and myopathy. The EMG can define the site and cause of muscle disorders, such as myasthenia gravis, muscular dystrophy, and myotonia, as well as lesions involving the motor neurons in the anterior horn of the spinal cord. An EMG can localize the site of peripheral nerve disorders, such as radiculopathy and axonopathy. Skin and needle electrodes measure and record electrical activity. Electrical sound equivalents are amplified and recorded on tape for later studies.

Procedure

1. The test is done in a copper-lined room to screen out interference.
2. The patient lies or sits during the test.
3. A surface disk is applied to the skin to ground the patient. The muscles and nerves examined depend on the patient's signs and symptoms, history, and physical condition (special nerves innervate specific muscles).
4. The patient is told to relax (the examiner may massage certain muscles to get the patient to relax) or to contract certain muscles (eg, to point toes) at specific times during the test.
5. The test consists of two parts. The first test determines *nerve conduction.*
   a. Metal surface electrodes are coated with electrode paste and firmly placed over a specific nerve area. Electrical current is then passed through the area. This causes sensations directly proportional to the time the current is applied.
   b. The amplitude wave is read on an oscilloscope and recorded on tape for later studies.
   c. Electrical current leaves no mark but can cause unusual sensations, not usually considered unpleasant. Measurement can be taken of how fast and how well a nerve transmits messages. Nerves in the face, arms, or legs can be tested in this way.
6. The second test determines *muscle potential.*
   a. A monopolar electrode (1/2 to 3-in. very small gauge needle) is inserted, and advanced into the muscle by increments. The examiner may move the needle around without actually removing it to see if readings change, or may reinsert the needle in another muscle area.
   b. The electrode causes no pain unless the end of the needle is near a terminal nerve; then it can cause considerable pain. Ten or more in-

sertions may need to be made. No shocks are necessary because the needle detects the electricity normally present in muscle.

c. The examiner observes the oscilloscope for normal waveforms and listens for normal quiet sounds at rest. A machine-gun popping sound or rattling sound like hail on a tin roof is normally heard when the patient contracts the muscles.

d. If the patient complains of pain, the examiner removes the needle because pain yields false results.

e. Total examining time is 45 to 60 minutes if testing is confined to a single extremity, and up to 3 hours for more than one extremity. There is no completely "routine" EMG. The length of the test depends on the clinical problem.

Clinical Implications

1. Abnormal neuromuscular activity occurs in diseases or disturbances of striated muscle fibers or cell membranes.
- **a.** Muscle fiber disorders such as muscular dystrophy
- **b.** Cell membrane hyperirritability, such as myotonia, and myotic disorders, such as polymyositis, hypocalcemia, thyrotoxicosis, tetanus, and rabies
- **c.** Myasthenia (muscle weakness states)
  - **(1)** Myasthenia gravis
  - **(2)** Cancer caused by nonpituitary ACTH secretion by the tumor
    - **(a)** Bronchial cancer
    - **(b)** Sarcoid
  - **(3)** Deficiencies
    - **(a)** Familial hypokalemia
    - **(b)** McArdle's phosphorylase
  - **(4)** Hyperadrenocorticism
  - **(5)** Acetylcholine blockers
    - **(a)** Curare
    - **(b)** Botulism
    - **(c)** Kanamycin
    - **(d)** Snake venom

2. Disorders or diseases of lower motor neuron
- **a.** Lesions involving motor neuron on anterior horn of spinal cord (myelopathy)
  - **(1)** Tumor
  - **(2)** Trauma
  - **(3)** Syringomyelia
  - **(4)** Juvenile muscular dystrophy
  - **(5)** Congenital amyotonia
  - **(6)** Anterior poliomyelitis
  - **(7)** Amyotrophic lateral sclerosis
  - **(8)** Peroneal muscular atrophy
- **b.** Lesions involving nerve root (radiculopathy)

   - **(1)** Guillain–Barre syndrome
   - **(2)** Entrapment of the nerve root
     - **(a)** Tumor
     - **(b)** Trauma
     - **(c)** Herniated disk
     - **(d)** Hypertrophic spurs
     - **(e)** Spinal stenosis
 - **c.** Damage or disease to peripheral or axial nerves
   - **(1)** Entrapment of the nerve
     - **(a)** Carpal or tarsal tunnel
     - **(b)** Facial, ulnar, radial, and peroneal palsy
     - **(c)** Neuralgia paresthetica
   - **(2)** Endocrine
     - **(a)** Hypothyroidism
     - **(b)** Diabetes
   - **(3)** Toxic
     - **(a)** Heavy metals
     - **(b)** Solvents
     - **(c)** Antiamebicides
     - **(d)** Chemotherapy
     - **(e)** Antibiotics
 - **d.** Early peripheral nerve degeneration and regeneration

Interfering Factors

1. Conduction can vary with age but normally decreases with the aging process.
2. Pain can yield false results.
3. Electrical activity from extraneous persons and objects can produce false results.
4. The test is ineffective in the presence of edema, hemorrhage, or thick subcutaneous fat.

Patient Preparation

1. Explain the test purpose and procedure. There is a risk of hematoma if the patient is receiving anticoagulant therapy.
2. Sedation or analgesia may be ordered.
3. See Chapter 1 guidelines for safe, effective, informed *pretest* care.

Patient Aftercare

1. If the patient experiences pain, provide relief from the pain through appropriate interventions.
2. Provide rest or relaxing activities.
3. Interpret test results and monitor appropriately for nerve and muscle disease.
4. Follow Chapter 1 guidelines for safe, effective, informed *posttest* care.

Clinical Alert

1. When ordering the test, the more pertinent data given, the more precise will be the interpretation of findings.
2. Enzyme levels that reflect muscle activity (AST, LDH, CPK) must be determined before testing because EMG will cause elevation of these enzymes for up to 10 days after the procedure.
3. Although rare, hematomas may form at needle insertion sites. Take measures, such as application of pressure to the site, to control bleeding. Notify the physician. Ascertain whether the patient is taking anticoagulants or aspirinlike drugs.

ELECTRONYSTAGMOGRAM (ENG)

Normal Values

Vestibular–ocular reflex: Normal.
Nystagmus accompanying head turning: Expected.

Explanation of Test

This study aids in the differential diagnoses of lesions in the brain stem and cerebellum. It can diagnose the causes of unilateral hearing loss of unknown origin, vertigo, or ringing in the ears. Evaluation of the vestibular system and the muscles controlling eye movement is based on measurements of the nystagmus cycle. In health, the vestibular system maintains visual fixation during head movements by means of *nystagmus*, the involuntary back and forth eye movement caused by initiation of the vestibular–ocular reflex.

Procedure

1. The test is usually done in a darkened room with the patient in a sitting or lying position.
2. If ear wax is present, it should be removed before testing.
3. Five electrodes are taped at certain positions around the eye.
4. During the study, the patient is asked to look at different objects, to open and close the eyes, and to change position.
5. Toward the end of the test, air is gently blown into each external ear canal, first on the affected side. Water may also be used to irrigate the ears during the test.

Clinical Implications

Prolonged nystagmus following a head turn is abnormal and can be caused by lesions of the vestibular or ocular system as in

1. Cerebellum disease
2. Brain stem lesion

3. Peripheral lesion occurring in the elderly; head trauma; middle ear disorders
4. Congenital disorders

Interfering Factors

1. Test results are altered by the inability of the patient to cooperate, by poor eyesight, blinking of the eyes, or poorly applied electrodes.
2. Anxiety of the patient or medications, such as central nervous system depressants, stimulants, or antivertigo agents, can cause false-positive test results.

Patient Preparation

1. Explain the test purpose and procedure. No discomfort or known risks are associated with the test.
2. Face makeup should be removed.
3. No caffeine nor alcoholic beverages should be taken for at least 48 hours. Avoid heavy meals before testing.
4. In most cases, medications, such as tranquilizers, stimulants, or antivertigo agents, are withheld for 5 days before the test. If in doubt, consult the attending physician.
5. See Chapter 1 guidelines for safe, effective, and informed *pretest* care.

Clinical Alert

1. The test is contraindicated in persons who have pacemakers.
2. Water irrigation should not be done in the presence of a perforated eardrum. Instead, a fingercot may be inserted into the ear canal to protect the middle ear.

Patient Aftercare

1. Allow the patient to rest as necessary.
2. Nausea, vertigo, and weakness may be present and may require treatment and administration of medication.
3. Interpret test results and monitor appropriately for brain or middle ear disease.
4. Follow Chapter 1 guidelines for safe, effective, informed *posttest* care.

ELECTROCARDIOGRAPHY (ECG OR EKG) (WITH BRIEF DESCRIPTION OF VECTOR CARDIOGRAM) ●

Normal Values

Normal positive and negative deflections in an ECG record (Figure 15-1); normal cardiac cycle components. One cardiac cycle is represented by the P wave, QRS complex, and T wave. Additionally, a Y wave may be observed.

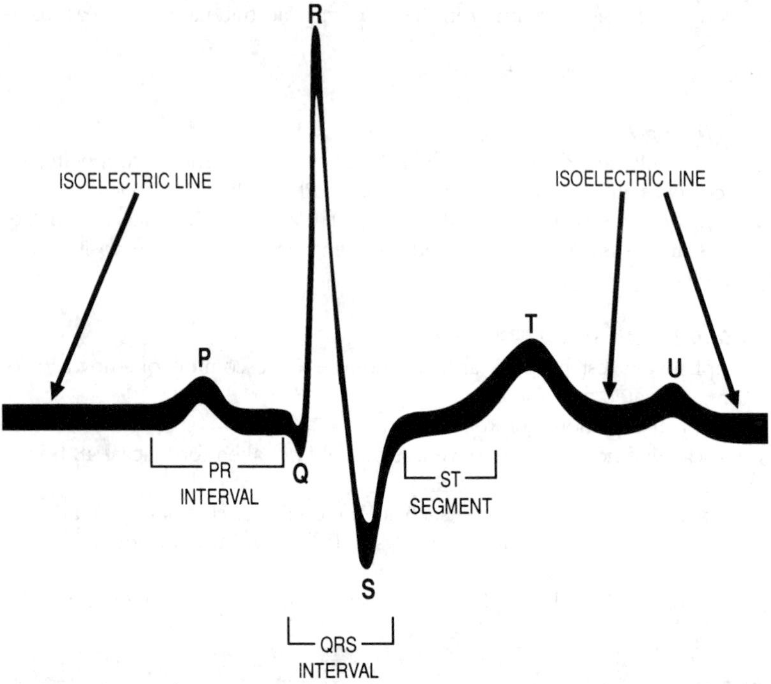

FIGURE 15-1
Electrocardiographic components of the cardiac cycle. (After Phillips RE, Feeney MK: The Cardiac Rhythms, 3rd ed. Philadelphia, WB Saunders, 1990)

This cycle is repeated continuously. P = atrial depolarization; QRS = ventricular depolarization; T = ventricular repolarization/resting stage between beats; U wave = nonspecific recovery afterpotentials.

Waves

Capital letters refer to relatively large waves (over 5 mm), and small letters refer to relatively small waves (less than 5 mm).

1. The *P wave* is upright and represents *atrial* depolarization and the electrical activity associated with the original impulse from the sinus node and its subsequent spread through the atrial sinus.
   If P waves are present; are of normal size, shape, and deflection; have normal conduction intervals to the ventricular complex; and demonstrate rhythmic timing variances between cycles, it can be assumed that the stimulus began in the sinoatrial node.
2. The T_a wave is a deflection produced by atrial repolarization and is usually not seen in the 12-lead ECG.

3. The Q(q) wave is the first downward, negative deflection resulting from ventricular depolarization.
4. The R(r′) wave is an upright, positive deflection resulting from ventricular depolarization.
5. The S(s′) wave is the first downward, negative deflection that follows the first positive deflection.
6. The QS wave is a negative deflection that does not rise above the baseline.
7. The R^1(r′) wave is the second upward, positive deflection or the first positive, upward deflection during ventricular depolarization that follows the S wave. The negative deflection following the r′ is termed the s′.
8. The T wave is a deflection produced by ventricular repolarization. There is a pause after the QRS complex, then a T wave appears. The T wave is a period of no cardiac activity, before the ventricles are again stimulated. It represents the recovery phase after contraction.
9. The U wave is a deflection (usually positive) following the T wave. It is thought to be caused by repolarization of the Purkinjes' (intraventricular) conduction system.

Intervals

1. The R–R interval is the distance between two successive R waves. In normal rhythms, the interval in seconds (or fractions of seconds) between two successive R waves, then divided into 60 seconds, will give the heart rate per minute.
2. The P–P interval will be the same as the R–R interval in normal sinus rhythm. The responsiveness of the sinus node to physiologic activity (exercise, rest, respiratory cycling) results in a rhythmic variance of P–P intervals.
3. The P–R interval measures conduction tone and includes time for atrial depolarization and normal conduction delay in the atrioventricular node; it terminates with the onset of ventricular depolarization. It is the period from the start of the P wave to the beginning of the QRS complex. This interval represents the time taken for the impulse to traverse the atria and atrioventricular node and reach the ventricles and initiate ventricular depolarization.
4. The QRS interval is ventricular depolarization time and represents the electrical impulse as it travels from the atrioventricular node through the bundle branches to the Purkinje fibers and into the myocardial cells. Normal waves consist of an initial downward deflection (Q wave), a large upward deflection (R wave), and a second downward wave (S wave). It is measured from the onset of the Q wave (or R if no Q is visible) to the termination of the S wave.

Segments and Junctions

1. The PR segment is normally isoelectric and is that portion of the ECG tracing from the end of the P wave to the onset of the QRS complex.

2. The J junction is the point at which the QRS complex ends and the ST segment begins.
3. The ST segment is that part of the ECG from the J point to the onset of the T wave. Elevation or depression is determined by comparing its location with that portion of the baseline between the end of the T wave and the beginning of the P wave or when related to the PR segment. This segment represents the period between the completion of depolarization and onset of repolarization (recovery) of the ventricular muscles.
4. The TP segment is that portion of the ECG record between the end of the T wave and the beginning of the next P wave. It is usually isoelectric.

Voltage Measurements

1. Upright deflection voltage is measured from the upper part of the baseline to the peak of the wave.
2. Negative deflection voltage is measured from the lower portion of the baseline to the nadir of the wave.

Explanation of Test

An ECG is a recording of the electrical impulses that stimulate the heart to contract and can indicate dysfunctions that influence the conduction ability of the myocardium. The ECG is helpful in diagnosing and monitoring the following: origins of pathologic rhythms; myocardial ischemia; myocardial infarction; atrial and ventricular hypertrophy; conduction delay of atrial, atrioventricular, and ventricular electrical impulses; and pericarditis. It is also helpful in the diagnosis of systemic diseases that affect the heart; determination of cardiac drug effects, especially digitalis and antiarrhythmic agents; disturbances in electrolyte balance, especially potassium and calcium; and evaluation of cardiac pacemaker or implanted defibrillator functions.

The ECG provides a continuous picture of the electrical activity during a cycle. Heart cells are charged or polarized in the resting state, but when electrically stimulated, they depolarize the contract. The body fluid is an excellent conductor of electrical current. When the depolarization (stimulation) process sweeps in a wave across the cells of the myocardium, the electrical current generated is conducted to the body's surface where it is detected by special electrodes placed on the patient's limbs and chest. An ECG tracing shows the voltage of the waves and the time duration of both waves and intervals. By studying the amplitude and time duration of the waves and intervals, disorders of impulse formation and conduction can be diagnosed.

Recording the Electrical Impulses

1. Because the electrical forces extend in several directions at the same time, a comprehensive view of heart activity can be obtained only if the flow of current in several different planes is recorded.
2. Twelve leads are simultaneously used to present this comprehensive picture.

   a. Limb leads—I, II, III, aVL, aVF, aVR—record events in the frontal plane of the heart.
   b. Chest leads—V_1, V_2, V_3, V_4, V_5, and V_6—record a horizontal view of the heart's electrical activity.
3. Occasionally, an esophageal lead, which is swallowed, is used to supply additional information. These are frequently used during surgical procedures.

ECG Versus Vectorcardiogram

The vectorcardiogram, like the ECG, records the electrical forces of the heart. The major difference between these two methods is the way in which these forces are displayed. A vectorcardiogram records a *three-dimensional* display of the heart's electrical activity, whereas the ECG shows activity in a *single plane.*

The three planes of the vectorcardiogram are

1. Frontal plane (combines the Y and X axes)
2. Sagittal plane (combines the Y and Z axes)
3. Horizontal plane (combines the X and Z axes)

The following chart compares ECG and vectorcardiograms:

ECG	*Vectorcardiogram*
Records electrical forces as deflections on a scale	Depicts electrical forces as vector loops, thereby showing the *direction* of electrical activity
Records in the frontal and horizontal planes of the body	Records on the frontal, horizontal, and sagittal planes of the body. The term *vector* indicates the direction of electrical activity

Procedures

The following steps apply to both the ECG and the vectorcardiogram:

1. The patient is usually placed in a supine position. However, recording can also be done during exercise.
2. The skin is prepared (shaving if necessary), and electrodes are placed anywhere on the four extremities and at specific sites on the chest. The right leg is the ground.
3. Twelve leads can be recorded simultaneously on newer ECG machines.
4. If a rhythm strip is ordered, a 2-minute recording of a single lead (usually lead II) is run.

Clinical Implications of ECG

1. The ECG *does not* depict the actual mechanical state of the heart or function of the valves.

2. An ECG may be quite normal in the presence of heart disease unless the pathologic process disturbs the electrical forces. It ***cannot*** predict future events.
3. An ECG should be interpreted and treatment instituted within the context of the comprehensive clinical picture.
4. ECG abnormalities are categorized into five general areas:
   - **a.** Heart rate
   - **b.** Heart rhythm
   - **c.** Axis or position of the heart
   - **d.** Hypertrophy
   - **e.** Infarction or ischemia

   Typical abnormalities in these areas include:
   - **(1)** Pathologic rhythms
   - **(2)** Conduction system diseases
   - **(3)** Myocardial ischemia
   - **(4)** Myocardial infarction
   - **(5)** Hypertrophy of the heart
   - **(6)** Pulmonary infarction
   - **(7)** Altered potassium, calcium, and magnesium levels
   - **(8)** Pericarditis
   - **(9)** Effects of drugs

Clinical Implications of Vectorcardiogram

1. The vectorcardiogram is more sensitive than the ECG in diagnosing myocardial infarction but is probably not more specific.
2. Vectorcardiography is more specific than the ECG in assessing hypertrophy or dilation of the ventricles.
3. Intraventricular conduction abnormalities can possibly be differentiated.

Clinical Considerations

1. Chest pain, if present, should be noted on the ECG strip.
2. The presence of a pacemaker and whether a magnet was used in testing should be documented in the record.
3. Reproducibility of precordial lead placement can be ensured by marking the position on the chest wall in ink when necessary.

Interfering Factors

1. Race: ST elevation with T-wave inversion is more common in black persons but disappears with maximal exercise effort.
2. Food intake: High-carbohydrate content is especially associated with an intracellular shift of potassium in association with intracellular glucose metabolism. Nondiagnostic ST depression and T-wave inversion may occur.
3. Anxiety: Episodic anxiety and hyperventilation are associated with prolonged PR interval, sinus tachycardia, and ST depression, with or without T-wave inversion. This may be due to autonomic nervous system imbalances.
4. Deep respiration: Position of the heart in the chest shifts more vertically with deep inspiration and more horizontally with deep expiration.
5. Exercise and movement: Strenuous exercise before the test can produce misleading results. Muscle twitching can also alter the tracing.

6. Position of heart within thoracic cage: There may be an anatomic cardiac rotation in both horizontal and frontal planes.
7. Position of precordial leads: Inaccurate placement of the bipolar chest leads and the transposition of right and left arm and left leg electrodes will affect test results. In normal persons, lead reversal will produce the typical ECG findings of dextrocardia in frontal plane leads and can mimic a myocardial infarction pattern.
8. A leftward shift in the QRS axis occurs with excess body weight, ascites, and pregnancy.
9. Age: At birth and infancy, there is hypertrophy of the right ventricle because, in the fetus, the right ventricle performs more work than the left ventricle. T-wave inversion in leads V_{1-3} persists into the second decade of life and into the third decade in black persons.
10. Sex: Slight ST segment depression is present in women.
11. Chest configuration and dextrocardia: In this congenital anomaly, the precordial leads must be placed over the right side of the chest.
12. Severe drug overdose, especially with barbiturates, as well as many other medications can influence ECG configuration.
13. The serious effects of electrolyte imbalance shown on the ECG can be seen as follows:
    - **a.** Increased Ca^{2+}: prolonged PR shortened QT
    - **b.** Decreased Ca^{2+}: prolonged QT

Patient Preparation

1. Explain the test purpose and procedure and the factors that interfere with accurate test results, emphasizing that ECG is painless and there is no current flow to the body. A resting ECG (without stressing the heart) is no more than a 1-minute record of the heart's electrical activity.
2. The patient must be completely relaxed to ensure a satisfactory tracing.
3. Ideally, the person should rest for 15 minutes before ECG recording. Heavy meals and smoking should be delayed for at least 30 minutes before the ECG—longer if possible.
4. See Chapter 1 guidelines for safe, effective, informed *pretest* care.

Patient Aftercare

1. It is important to recognize the limitations of an ECG. A normal ECG does not rule out coronary artery disease or areas of ischemia in the heart. On the other hand, an abnormal ECG in and of itself does not signify heart disease.
2. Interpret test results, counsel, and monitor appropriately. The resting ECG is usually normal for patients who experience only angina and no other heart problems. It can also provide evidence of prior heart damage. The ECG is one diagnostic tool in a whole repertoire of diagnostic modalities and should be viewed as such. The presence or absence of heart disease should not be presumed or decided on the basis of the ECG alone.
3. Follow Chapter 1 guidelines for safe, effective, informed *posttest* care.

Clinical Alert

1. When an ECG shows changes that indicate ischemia, injury, or infarction, these changes must be reported and acted on immediately. The goal is to increase myocardial blood supply and reduce oxygen demand.
   a. When ECG changes represent stages of ischemia, injury, or necrosis and symptoms of possible myocardial infarction appear, the first concern is to balance myocardial oxygen supply and demand as follows:
      (1) Give ordered nitroglycerin to dilate blood vessels.
      (2) Sedate with narcotics to relieve pain and anxiety.
      (3) Administer calcium channel blockers to relieve coronary spasm.
      (4) Administer oxygen to increase supply available to the myocardium.
      (5) Give β-adrenergic blocking drugs to slow rapid heart rate.
      (6) Give antiarrhythmics to correct abnormal rhythms.
      (7) Give frequent reassurance to alleviate anxiety.
   b. Monitoring for cardiac rhythm disturbances is essential. Potentially lethal dysrhythmias and ventricular tachyarrhythmias require immediate intervention and possible cardiopulmonary resuscitation.
2. Serious diagnostic error can be made if the ECG is not interpreted in the light of patient's history, signs, and symptoms.
3. The electrical axis is not synonymous with the anatomic position of the heart.

SIGNAL-AVERAGED ELECTROCARDIOGRAM (SAE)

Normal Values

Normal QRS complexes and ST segments.

Explanation of Test

The signal-averaged ECG (SAE) is a noninvasive tool for the identification of patients at risk for malignant ventricular dysrhythmias, particularly after a myocardial infarction.

During the later phase of the QRS complex and ST segment, the myocardium produces high-frequency, low-amplitude signals, termed *late potentials*. These late potentials correlate delayed activation areas within the myocardium, a condition that produces reentrant forms of ventricular tachycardia.

Indications

SAEs are performed to evaluate the etiology of ventricular dysrhythmias as a precursor to electrophysiology studies. Myocardial disorders that may result in regions of delayed conduction include myocardial infarction, nonischemic dilated cardiomyopathy, left ventricular aneurysm, and some forms of healed ventricular incisions (eg, from tetralogy of Fallot surgical intervention).

Procedure

A modification of body-surface ECG, the SAE uses computerized techniques to provide signal averaging, amplification, and filtering of electrical potentials. Electrodes are placed on the abdomen and anterior and posterior thorax. The signals received are converted to a digital signal. A typical QRS complex is used as a template against which subsequent cycles are compared. Typically, several hundred beats are averaged to analyze the late potential. Collection of data usually takes about 20 minutes. Optimal recordings are obtained if the patient is placed in a comfortable position, is quiet during recording, electrodes are properly applied, and interference from other electrical equipment is eliminated.

Clinical Implications

1. SAE provides predictive values for ventricular tachycardia in patients who have a history of myocardial infarction or chronic coronary artery disease.
2. Late potentials are a stronger predictor of sudden death or sustained ventricular tachycardia than ventricular dysrhythmias from a Holter monitor recording.
3. Evidence shows that late potentials associated with ventricular tachycardia are abolished following successful surgical intervention.
4. Patients with late potentials have a 17% incidence of sustained ventricular tachycardia or sudden death (versus 1% incidence in patients without late potentials). The incidence is even greater in the presence of decreased ejection fractions.
5. SAE may explain unexplained syncope, subsequently identified as ventricular tachycardia during EP study.

Interfering Factors

1. Increased time is required for collection of beats in the presence of slow heart rates or frequent ventricular ectopics. Additionally, patient movement, talking, and restlessness delay procurement of relevant data.
2. Bundle-branch block can interfere with averaging of impulses.
3. SAE does not provide information on the efficacy of antiarrhythmic drug therapy.
4. Late potentials are not present in every patient with ventricular tachycardia.
5. Ventricular pacing prolongs ventricular activation time and obscures late

potentials. On the other hand, atrial pacing, even at rapid rates, does not alter late potentials.

Patient Preparation

1. Explain test purpose, procedure, benefits, and risks. Caution patient to rest quietly during testing.
2. See Chapter 1 guidelines for safe, effective, informed *pretest* care.

Patient Aftercare

1. Interpret test results, counsel, and monitor appropriately when late potentials are identified.
2. Follow Chapter 1 guidelines for safe, effective, informed *posttest* care.

HOLTER CONTINUOUS ECG MONITORING ●

Normal Values

Normal sinus rhythm.

Explanation of Test

Holter monitoring is a method of continuously recording the ECG on magnetic tape for prolonged (24-hour) time periods. The tape recorder is a battery-powered device with very slow (3 3/4-in./min) tape speeds and is small enough to be carried on a strap over the shoulder or around the waist, similar to a small purse. Two ECG channels recorded simultaneously present graphic records of the electrical conduction activities. The Holter recorder is equipped with a digital clock, synchronized to the tape recorder; this allows accurate time marking. The patient carries a diary in which he or she enters any symptoms experienced during the monitoring period, the activity status, and the time at which the symptoms occurred. When a symptom occurs, the patient pushes an event-marker button on the recorder. This marks one of the channels for easy recognition during playback and evaluation.

A 24-hour recording contains over 100,000 cardiac cycles. Playback and tape analysis are done at 60, 120, or 180 times real-time. The tape may be rapidly analyzed by computers that provide summaries of heart rates, frequency, and type of arrhythmias, coupling intervals, and other variations. Another method of tape scanning superimposes each QRS complex on the preceding QRS complex. This makes variations in the QRS contours apparent. In either method of scanning, segments of the tape recording can be reproduced on ECG paper. The patient diary is also used to analyze correlations between symptoms and ECG findings.

Indications for Holter Monitoring

1. Documentation of suspected rhythm disturbances: The recording, along with the patient diary, permits correlation of rhythm disturbances with patient symptoms of such things as syncope, palpitations, chest pain, light-headedness, or unexplained dyspnea. If these symptoms have no

obvious cause, a Holter recording can detect unsuspected arrhythmias, such as supraventricular and ventricular tachycardias, bradycardia–tachycardia in patients with sick sinus syndrome, and other ventricular and supraventricular arrhythmias.

2. To record the onset and termination of a rhythmic disturbance may provide insights into the electrophysiologic mechanisms responsible for the arrhythmia.
3. To check pacemaker and automatic implantable defibrillator device functions.
4. To track effectiveness of drugs and other treatments.

Procedure

1. The patient assumes a supine position.
2. The skin is prepared and shaved, if necessary, cleansed with alcohol, and rubbed with gauze or similar rough material to assure proper electrode contact.
3. Two electrodes for each channel and one ground electrode are positioned over bony prominences. The two negative electrodes are placed on the manubrium, and their corresponding positive electrodes are placed in the V_1 and V_5 positions.
4. Leads and cables are secured. The recorder is activated and calibrated. The patient is then free to pursue normal activities except for bathing in a tub or showering.
5. After the predetermined (24 to 48 hours) time, the recorder is stopped and the electrodes are removed.
6. The tape is scanned and interpreted, and a written summary of findings is completed.

Interfering Factors

1. Incomplete diary or event: Marker not pushed during symptoms.

   NOTE: *The patient may not be aware of cardiac events, such as certain arrhythmias.*

2. Mechanical interferences (eg, scratching the electrode sites) can alter the recording.

Clinical Implications

1. Abnormal results include rhythm disturbances such as
   - **a.** Tachycardias—atrial and ventricular
   - **b.** Bradycardia
   - **c.** Premature atrial or ventricular beats
   - **d.** Heart blocks
   - **e.** Junctional rhythms
   - **f.** Atrial flutter or fibrillation
   - **g.** Other ventricular and supraventricular rhythm disturbances
2. Hypoxic/ischemic changes

Clinical Alert

Advise the patient to take a "sponge bath" while wearing the Holter monitor.

Patient Preparation

1. Explain test purpose, benefits, and procedure for keeping diary of events.
2. See Chapter 1 guidelines for safe, effective, informed *pretest* care.

Patient Aftercare

1. Interpret test results, counsel, and monitor appropriately for cardiac arrhythmias.
2. Follow Chapter 1 guidelines for safe, effective, informed *posttest* care.

STRESS/EXERCISE TESTING (GRADED EXERCISE TOLERANCE TEST)

Normal Values

Negative when the patient does not exhibit significant symptoms, arrhythmias, or other ECG abnormalities at 85% of maximum heart rate predicted for age and sex.

Explanation of Test

This test measures the efficiency of the heart during a dynamic exercise stress period on a motor-driven treadmill or ergometer, It is valuable for diagnosing ischemic heart disease and in investigating physiologic mechanisms underlying cardiac symptoms, such as angina, dysrhythmias, inordinate rises in blood pressure, and functional valve incompetence. Exercise testing also measures functional capacity for work, sport, or participation in a rehabilitation program and estimates response to medical or surgical treatment. Additionally, the function of physiologic responsive pacemakers (testing for upper rate limits) can be evaluated.

The systolic blood pressure normally increases with exercise, and the diastolic normally remains essentially unchanged. Stress exercise testing takes place in a controlled environment under controlled conditions; it requires a lower temperature (68°C) and low humidity.

Procedure

There are many different types of stress tests. Most of them include the following steps:

1. Recording electrodes are placed on patient's chest (see description of ECG) and attached to a monitor. A blood pressure–recording device is also placed.

2. As the patient walks on a motor-driven treadmill or pedals an ergometer (if walking is not possible), a computerized ECG and heart-monitoring device records the performance. The patient walks at progressively greater speeds and elevations to increase heart rate and workload.
3. The ECG, heart rate, and blood pressure are recorded at rest. The patient is asked to report any symptoms, such as chest pain or shortness of breath experienced during the test. Normal persons are symptom-free at submaximal efforts. At peak or maximal efforts, symptoms expected in normal persons include exhaustion, fatigue, and sometimes nausea or dizziness.
4. The patient is stressed in stages. Each stage consists of a predetermined treadmill speed (in miles per hour) and a treadmill grade elevation (in percentage grade).
5. The ECG, heart rate, and blood pressure are continually monitored for signs of abnormalities and any unusual symptoms, such as intolerable dyspnea, chest pain, or severe cramping (claudication) in the legs.
6. Usually, vital signs and other abnormalities are recorded at the 3- and 10-minute posttest interval as the patient rests. The test is terminated if ECG abnormalities, fatigue, weakness, abnormal blood pressure changes, or intolerable symptoms occur during the test.
7. Common criteria for stopping a test include
   - **a.** Maximum possible performance achievement
   - **b.** Emergence of signs or symptoms that indicate the presence of disease process
   - **c.** Predetermined endpoint, such as 85% of age-related maximal heart rate, arbitrary work load (one that raises heart rate to 150), or diagnostic ECG change
8. Total examination time is about 30 minutes; however, the patient should plan to be in the laboratory for 1 to 1 1/2 hours.

Clinical Implications

Abnormal responses to exercise testing include

1. Alterations in blood pressure, such as
   - **a.** Failure of systolic pressure to rise
   - **b.** Progressive fall in systolic pressure
   - **c.** Elevation of diastolic blood pressure
2. Alterations in heart rate, such as
   - **a.** Elevated rate of tachycardia
   - **b.** Bradycardia
3. Change in ECG, such as
   - **a.** Deviation of ST segments caused by ischemia; can be depression or elevation
   - **b.** Dysrhythmias, ventricular tachycardia, multifocal ventricular premature contractions, atrial tachycardia, atrioventricular block other than first-degree block

   c. Failure of physiologic pacemaker to function within established rate limits
4. Ectopic rhythms, either ventricular or supraventricular, must be considered abnormal responses, but not necessarily ischemic responses.
5. Ischemic ST segment displacement greater than 0.1 mm of 80-msec duration or longer is the most common abnormality found. Men aged 40 to 59 who develop ST depression during exercise, which is not present at rest, have five times the risk of developing overt coronary heart disease than do men who do not develop ST depression.
6. Unusual symptoms, such as
   a. Anginal pain
   b. Severe breathlessness
   c. Faintness, dizziness, light-headedness, confusion
   d. Claudication, leg pain
7. Unusual signs, such as
   a. Cyanosis, pallor, mottling of skin
   b. Cold sweat, piloerection
   c. Ataxia, glassy stare
   d. Gallop heart sounds
   e. Valvular regurgitation

Interfering Factors

Common causes of false-positive exercise ECG responses include

1. Left ventricular hypertrophy
2. Digitalis toxicity
3. ST segment abnormality at rest
4. Hypertension
5. Valvular heart disease
6. Left bundle-branch block
7. Anemia
8. Hypoxia
9. Vasoregulatory asthenia
10. Lown–Ganong–Levine syndrome
11. "Panic" or anxiety attack

Patient Preparation

1. Explain the test purpose and procedure. No food, coffee, or cigarettes are allowed before testing. Water may be taken.
2. A legal consent form must be signed.
3. The patient should wear flat walking shoes or tennis shoes; bedroom slippers are not suitable. Men should wear gym shorts or loose-fitting light trousers. Women should wear a bra, a short-sleeved blouse that buttons in front, and slacks, shorts, or pajama pants (no one-piece undergarments or panty hose).
4. Some medications should be discontinued before testing. Doses of β-

adrenergic blocking agents, such as propranolol, should be reduced or tapered off gradually before stopping. Check with the exercise laboratory for specific protocols for taking digoxin, isosorbide (Isordil), and other drugs before this test.

5. See Chapter 1 guidelines for safe, effective, informed *pretest* care.

Patient Aftercare

1. Interpret test results and monitor appropriately for abnormal responses to exercise.
2. The patient should not leave the premises until the examiner is satisfied that pretest baseline levels for heart rate, blood pressure, and ECG waveform have been met.
3. Follow Chapter 1 guidelines for safe, effective, informed *posttest* care.

Clinical Alert

Stress/exercise testing can be risky for patients with recent onset of chest pain, with significantly elevated blood pressure, or with frequent attacks of angina. The test may be rescheduled in 4 to 6 weeks if these situations occur.

CARDIAC CATHETERIZATION AND ANGIOGRAPHY (ANGIOCARDIOGRAPHY, CORONARY ARTERIOGRAPHY)

Normal Values

Heart and coronary arteries: Normal
Hemodynamic pressures and cardiac output: Normal
Percentage of oxygen saturation: Normal

Explanation of Test

This is a method to study and diagnose defects in the chambers of the heart, valves, and certain blood vessels by inserting arterial and venous catheters, which then carry contrast material into the right and left sides of the heart. As the catheters are advanced, fluoroscopy and rapidly taken x-ray pictures projected on videomonitors show the action of the heart under study. The injected contrast medium provides definition of the cardiac structures. Coronary artery circulation is filmed as well. An oscilloscope near the videomonitor shows the patient's heart rate, heart rhythm, and pressures.

Coronary arteriograms are highly useful for diagnosing heart disease, determining the extent of myocardial damage, diagnosing congenital abnormalities, identifying cardiac structure and function before surgery, and measuring hemodynamic pressures within heart chambers and great vessels. They are also useful for determining cardiac output (using contrast dilution, thermodilution, or the Fick method), and for obtaining blood samples directly from the heart to measure oxygen content of blood and oxygen saturation.

Cardiac catheterization combined with angiography is indicated in patients who exhibit angina, incapacitating chest pain, syncope, valvular and ischemic diseases; in patients with cholesteremia and familial heart disease who are experiencing chest pain; in patients with abnormal resting or exercise ECGs; in patients who have had past cardiac revascularization and now present with recurring symptoms; in young patients with a history of coronary insufficiency or ventricular aneurysm; and in patients with coronary neurosis who need assurance that their arteries are normal. This test can be done during the acute stage of myocardial infarction; if necessary, the patient can be sent to surgery immediately.

Although it is an examination with some risks, it is highly accurate as a diagnostic technique.

Procedure

1. The test is usually done in a darkened, special procedure room.
2. To decrease anxiety, inform the patient about what is being done.
3. The patient lies on a special x-ray table; after preparation, ECG leads are attached to the chest. During the procedure, the patient will be turned from side to side and may be asked to exercise (optional) to evaluate heart changes that occur during activity. Atrial pacing also can be done as part of a cardiac catheterization in persons who cannot walk (paraplegics) or cannot use a treadmill. In these instances, there is a sequence of events at which time the heart is stressed; a rest period follows, measurements are taken, the heart is paced again, and another rest period follows.
4. The catheterization procedure is done under sterile surgical conditions. The skin is prepared with an antiseptic solution. A local anesthetic is injected before making small incisions for the insertion of the catheter into an artery and vein. (Incisions are not always made.) Catheters are gently pushed into the heart and great vessels.
5. The patient may be able to watch the procedure on a videoscreen monitor if the screen is placed so that the examiner can see it.
6. After x-ray films have been taken from all angles, the catheters are removed and skin incisions (if any) are closed with a few stitches. A sterile pressure bandage is applied.
7. IV sedation may be administered if necessary.

Clinical Implications

1. Abnormal results include the following:
   - **a.** As the catheters are advanced, they will reveal altered hemodynamic pressures.
   - **b.** Injected contrast reveals altered ventricular dynamics and occluded coronary arteries.
   - **c.** An analysis of blood oxygen confirms cardiac, circulatory, or pulmonary problems.

2. Abnormal hemodynamic pressures indicate
   a. Valve stenosis or insufficiency
   b. Left and/or right ventricular failure
   c. Idiopathic hypertrophic subaortic stenosis (IHHS)
   d. Rheumatic fever sequelae
   e. Cardiomyopathies
3. Abnormal blood oxygen results indicate
   a. Congenital or acquired shunting circulation
   b. Septal defects
   c. Other cardiac and pulmonary defects or pathological processes
4. When contrast is injected into the ventricles, abnormalities of size, function, structure, ejection fractions, aneurysms, leaks, stenosis, and altered contractility can be detected.
5. When contrast is injected into coronary arteries, abnormal circulation through coronary vessels can be detected.

Patient Preparation

1. Explain the test purpose, procedure, benefits, and risks. A legal consent form must be signed before the examination. Ascertain allergies, especially the potential for a reaction to contrast components.
2. The patient should fast for at least 3 hours before testing. Check with the physician about administration of routine, scheduled medications, such as cardiac drugs or insulin.
3. Analgesics, sedatives, or tranquilizers are administered before the examination begins.
4. The patient should void before the catheterization begins.
5. The patient may wear dentures; jewelry and other accessories must be removed.
6. Instruct the patient that he or she will need to breathe deeply and to cough during the test and that certain sensations are common to the procedure.
   a. Catheter insertion, through antecubital or groin sites, may produce significant pressure sensations with introduction of the "sheath" through which the catheter is advanced.
   b. A slight shock (like hitting the "funny bone") might be felt if the nerve adjacent to the artery is touched; a tiny "bump" in the neck may be experienced as the catheter is inserted and advanced through the artery into the heart. Neither of these sensations is usually painful.
   c. When contrast is injected into the catheter, a pumping sensation (with palpitations and warm flushes) may last 30 to 60 seconds. The injection causes skin vessels to vasodilate and blood to rise to the skin surface for a short time.
   d. Nausea, vomiting, headache, and cough are side effects that some patients experience.
   e. Angina may occur with exercise or with contrast injection. This can be relieved with nitroglycerin or narcotics.
7. See Chapter 1 guidelines for safe, effective, informed *pretest* care.

Patient Aftercare

1. Bed rest is usually maintained for 2 to 12 hours after the test. Time limits are based on the exact procedure used, the physician's protocols, and the patient status. Elevation of the head may be restricted during this time because elevation puts strain on a femoral insertion site. The patient may be allowed to turn from side to side if the affected extremity is maintained in a straight position. Encourage movement of **uninvolved** extremities.
2. Check vital signs frequently. Check dressing for swelling or bleeding. Pressure to the catheter insertion site may be necessary if bleeding or hematoma develops. Notify physician immediately. Neurovascular checks should be done on bilateral extremities to compare them. This includes assessing color, motion, sensation, capillary refill times, temperature, and pulse quality. Report significant changes immediately.
3. Antibiotics may be administered to prevent infection.
4. Encourage fluids after testing unless contraindicated.
5. Keep the affected extremity extended (not elevated) and immobilized with sandbags if necessary. Apply ice or a sandbag to the site, if ordered, Analgesics, if ordered, can be administered for pain or discomfort.
6. Sutures, if used, are removed per the physician's protocols.
7. Interpret test results and monitor appropriately for cardiac, circulatory, and pulmonary problems.
8. Follow Chapter 1 guidelines for safe, effective, informed *posttest* care.

Clinical Alert

1. This procedure is contraindicated in patients with gross cardiomegaly.
2. Complications include
   a. Dysrhythmias
   b. Allergic contrast reactions (evidenced by urticaria, pruritus, conjunctivitis, anaphylaxis)
   c. Thrombophlebitis
   d. Infection at insertion site
   e. Pneumothorax
   f. Hemopericardium
   g. Embolism
   h. Liver lacerations, especially in infants and children (from poor technique)
   i. Excessive bleeding at the site
3. Notify attending physician immediately of any increased bleeding or hematoma formation, dramatic fall or elevation in blood pressure, or decreased peripheral circulation.
4. When angiography is performed, the following equipment should always be available to treat complications:
   a. Resuscitation equipment
   b. DC defibrillator
   c. External pacemaker
   d. Electrocardiographic monitor
   e. Drugs used for resuscitation

ELECTROPHYSIOLOGY STUDIES
(EP; HIS BUNDLE PROCEDURE)

Normal Values
Normal conduction intervals, refractory periods and recovery times.
Normal arrhythmias induced.

Explanation of Test
EP is an invasive test used to diagnose and treat ventricular arrhythmias; it is similar to cardiac catheterization. The difference lies in the fact that an EP study measures the activity of the electrical conduction system of the heart through solid electrode catheters instead of through the open-lumen catheters used to measure pressures. The electrode catheters are almost always inserted into *veins* because of the greater risk they pose in the arterial system. With fluoroscopy as a guide, the catheters are advanced into the right atrium and right ventricle. Besides an x-ray monitor that tracks the location of the catheter, there is also a physiologic monitor that shows the patient's ECG rhythms as well as intracardiac electrograms from the catheters themselves (Fig. 15-2).

An EP study is highly useful for diagnosing diseases of the cardiac conduction system and to point the direction toward optimal treatment. Besides measuring control resting values for the patient, the electrode catheters are also used to pace the heart in an attempt to induce the same arrhythmia that may be giving the patient problems. If the patient is taking medication to control dysrhythmias, the EP study can determine how well the medication is working by how easily the arrhythmia can be induced. This is in contrast with the trial-and-error method in which there is no way to know that a particular drug is ineffective until that drug has actually failed to resolve the problem.

An EP procedure is indicated to differentiate disorders of impulse formations (supraventricular versus ventricular rhythms). Electrophysiologic studies also provide diagnostic insight into the etiology and mechanism of conduction disorders. These studies are often part of the workup for syncope, sick sinus syndrome, or tachyarrhythmias. Finally, EP studies are indicated for testing the effectiveness of antiarrhythmic drugs.

Procedure
1. The room is usually darkened.
2. To decrease anxiety, the patient is kept informed of what is being done as the procedure evolves.
3. The patient is positioned on an x-ray table, and ECG leads are attached to exact locations on the body.
4. The procedure is done under sterile, aseptic surgical conditions. The skin is prepared. Usually one or two sites are chosen for catheter insertion (right or left antecubital area or both; right or left groin, or both). These depend on where in the heart the catheters will have to be placed and

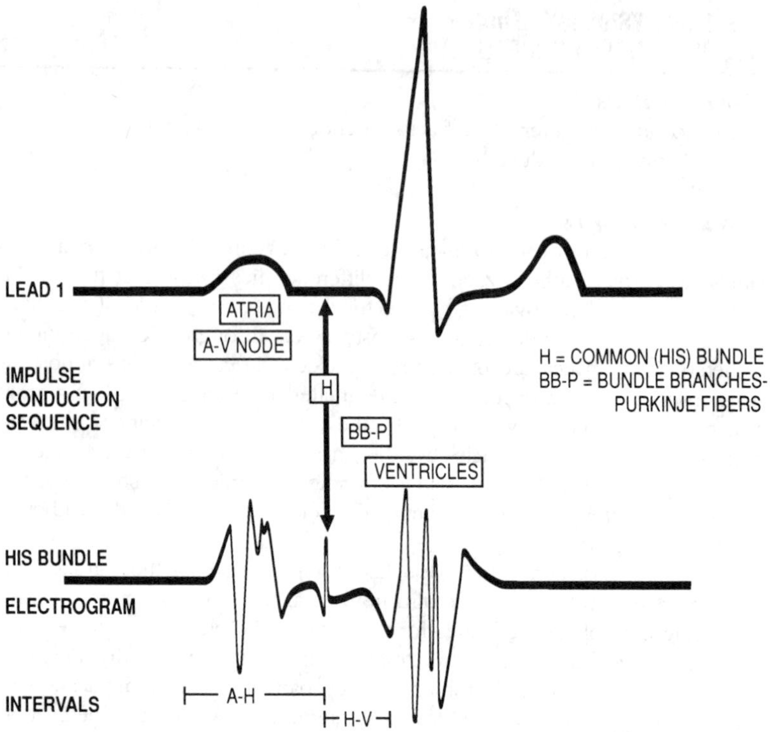

FIGURE 15-2

His bundle electrogram. Note electrophysiologic events are presented in relation to the surface electrocardiogram. (After Phillips RE, Feeney MK: The Cardiac Rhythms, 3rd ed. Philadelphia, WB Saunders, 1990)

what the patency and size of the patient's veins are. The insertion site is injected with local anesthetic before the catheter insertion takes place.

5. As the catheters are advanced toward the desired location, baseline information is recorded. Sometimes pacing may be necessary. (For example, measuring sinus node recovery times requires pacing the atrium until the sinus is fatigued and then measuring the time the sinus takes to recover.)
6. After baseline values have been determined, pacing can be used to induce arrhythmias. If a sustained arrhythmia is induced, an attempt may be made to terminate the arrhythmia through pacing. Should the patient lose consciousness, an external cardioverter/defibrillator can be used to terminate the arrhythmia.
7. A quiet conversation is continuously held with the patient to assess the level of consciousness.
8. After the procedure, the catheters are removed and a sterile pressure bandage is applied to the catheter entrance site (no stitches).

9. Each antiarrhythmic drug has certain effects that must be anticipated during the loading phase—for example, hypotension with quinidine and procainamide, abdominal cramping with quinidine, and venous pain for phenytoin. A state of "happy drunkenness" may occur. Intravenous saline is normally used to support blood pressure in the event hypotension occurs.

Clinical Implications

1. Abnormal EP results will reveal
   a. Conduction intervals longer or shorter than normal
   b. Refractory periods longer than normal
   c. Prolonged recovery times
   d. The induction of an arrhythmia in a normal subject
2. Abnormal results indicate
   a. Long AH intervals indicate disease in the atrioventricular node if sympathetic and vagal influences have been eliminated.
   b. Long HV intervals indicate disease in the His–Purkinje system.
   c. Prolonged sinus node recovery times indicate sinus node dysfunction, such as sick sinus syndrome.
   d. Prolonged sinoatrial conduction times can indicate sinus exit block.
   e. A wide or split His bundle deflection indicates that a His bundle lesion is present.
   f. The induction of sustained ventricular tachycardia by using one or two premature stimuli confirms the diagnosis of recurrent ventricular tachycardia.

Patient Preparation

1. Explain the test purpose, procedure, benefits, and risks. A description of the possible sensations that may be experienced and the procedural steps helps reduce anxiety.
   a. A peculiar sensation in the arm and neck as the catheter is advanced. The sensation feels like a "bug crawling."
   b. Palpitations or racing heart may be felt when the heart is paced.
   c. Light-headedness or dizziness may be experienced. The patient must inform the nurse or doctor any time he or she feels light-headed or dizzy.
2. Obtain a legal, signed consent form before the procedure.
3. Blood samples for potassium levels (and other drug levels if the effectiveness of a drug is to be determined) are drawn.
4. A standard 12-lead ECG should be taken before testing.
5. *Nothing* can be consumed for at least 3 hours before testing.
6. Analgesics, sedatives, or tranquilizers are not usually given before the procedure.
7. Have the patient void.

8. The patient may wear dentures.
9. Follow Chapter 1 guidelines for safe, effective, informed *pretest* care.

Patient Aftercare

1. Bed rest for 6 to 8 hours after the procedure. Instruct the patient not to flex or bend the extremity used for the catheter insertion because this may lead to bleeding or vascular occlusion.
2. Check vital signs and insertion site for swelling or bleeding every 15 minutes four times, every 30 minutes twice, and every 1 hour twice or according to institutional protocols. Neurovascular checks include assessing for pulses, color, motion, sensation, temperature, and capillary refill times of affected extremity.
3. Keep the affected extremity extended (not elevated) to decrease discomfort and risk of bleeding. Analgesics, if ordered, can be administered.
4. Normally, the patient must remain flat with a pillow permitted under the head.
5. Permit side-to-side turning and range of motion of uninvolved limbs. Maintain the affected extremity in a straight position during bed rest.
6. If an electrode catheter is left in place for sequential studies, it is sutured in place and covered with a sterile dressing. Care for site as ordered. Use sterile, aseptic technique.
7. Interpret test results and monitor appropriately. Instruct the patient concerning the importance of compliance with prescribed therapy. Should an adverse reaction to a drug occur, ECG monitoring may be necessary until the drug is metabolized.
8. Follow Chapter 1 guidelines for safe, effective, informed *posttest* care.

Clinical Alert

1. Relative contraindications: Although an acute myocardial infarction may limit detailed and prolonged EP procedures, brief but clinically useful procedures can be performed.
2. Observe the patient for complications; these include
   a. Hemorrhage at the catheter insertion site. This can be rapid and dramatic. Apply pressure to the site and notify the physician immediately.
   b. Thrombosis at the puncture site; thromboembolism
   c. Phlebitis
   d. Hemopericardium
   e. Atrial fibrillation (usually transient)
   f. Ventricular fibrillation or ventricular ectopy
3. Notify the attending physician for bleeding, hypotension, altered neurovascular status, decrease in distal perfusion, or life-threatening arrhythmias. Be aware of drug studies carried out and monitor for effects of that drug.

TRANSESOPHAGEAL ECHOCARDIOGRAPHY (TEE)

Normal Values
Normal position, size, and function of heart valves and heart chambers.

Explanation of Test
This test permits optimal ultrasonic visualization of the heart when traditional transthoracic (noninvasive) echocardiography fails or proves inconclusive. A miniaturized high-frequency ultrasound transducer is mounted on an endoscope and coupled with an ultrasound instrument to display and record ultrasound images from the heart. Endoscope controls allow remote manipulation of the transducer tip. Various images of heart anatomy can be displayed by rotating the top of the instrument and by varying the depth of insertion into the esophagus. Indications for TEE include

1. Situations in which a transthoracic echocardiogram has not been satisfactory, such as in the presence of obesity, trauma to the chest wall, and chronic obstructive pulmonary disease.
2. When results of traditional transthoracic echocardiography do not agree or correlate with other clinical findings.

Procedure
1. A topical anesthetic is applied to the pharynx. A bite block is inserted into the mouth. This reduces the risk of damage to the patient's teeth and oral structures as well as accidental damage to the endoscope.
2. The patient assumes a left lateral decubitus position while the lubricated endoscopic instrument is inserted to a depth of 30 to 50 cm. The patient is asked to swallow to facilitate advancement of the device.
3. Manipulation of the ultrasound transducer provides a number of image planes.

Clinical Implications
Abnormal TEE findings include

1. Heart valve diseases
2. Pericardial effusion
3. Congenital heart disease
4. Left ventricular dysfunction
5. Endocarditis
6. Intracardiac tumors or thrombi

Patient Preparation
1. Explain purpose and procedure, benefits, and risks.
2. The patient must be NPO status for at least 8 hours before the procedure to reduce the risk of aspiration. Premedications such as analgesics or sedatives may be ordered. Check with laboratory or physician for specific instructions.
3. See Chapter 1 guidelines for safe, effective, informed *pretest* care.

Patient Aftercare
1. Interpret test results; monitor vital signs and level of consciousness (if sedated). Ensure patent airway.

2. Position on side is sedated to prevent risk of aspiration.
3. Ascertain return of swallowing, coughing, and gag reflexes before allowing patient to take oral food or fluids.
4. Follow Chapter 1 guidelines for safe, effective, informed *posttest* care.

Clinical Alert

Swallowing reflexes may be diminished for several hours because of the effects from the topical anesthetic.

MAGNETIC RESONANCE IMAGING (MRI, MRF, MRA)

Normal Values

Soft-tissue structures: Normal brain, spinal cord, subarachnoid spaces, fat, muscles, tendons, ligaments, nerves, blood vessels, marrow of limbs and joints, heart, abdomen, and pelvis.

Blood vessels: Normal size, anatomy, and hemodynamics.

Explanation of Test

Magnetic resonance testing comprises several methodologies: MR imaging (MRI); MR blood flow scanning (MRF); magnetic resonance angiography (MRA). The most common uses include the following:

MRI OF THE BRAIN. Provides exquisite visualization of the soft tissue structures of the brain. Although bony anatomy is seen using MRI, CT is the test of choice to evaluate bone lesions and fractures.

MRI OF THE SPINE. Provides excellent demonstration of the spinal cord and subarachnoid space ***without intrathecal*** contrast injection.

MRI OF THE LIMBS AND JOINTS. Accurately demonstrates fat, muscles, tendons, ligaments, nerves, blood vessels, and bone marrow. If the region of interest is small, a ***surface coil*** (which produces the RF signal) is placed directly onto the skin overlying the part to be examined.

MRI OF THE HEART (CARDIAC MRI). Provides anatomic demonstration of the heart's structure, including the valves and coronary vessels. Image acquisition is synchronized to the ECG—a process known as "gating" to help eliminate motion artifacts.

MRI OF THE ABDOMEN AND PELVIS. Visualizes soft tissue organs, particularly the liver, pancreas, spleen, adrenals, kidneys, blood vessels, and reproductive organs.

MRI ANGIOGRAPHY. Provides both anatomic and hemodynamic information (likened to noninvasive angiography). MRI angiography is becoming a more common procedure to evaluate known vascular lesions.

Procedures

HEAD AND BODY IMAGING

1. The patient lies down on a movable examination couch ***after*** a thorough medical history is obtained.
2. Sedation may be required if the patient is claustrophobic or otherwise unable to hold still during the procedure. Ear protection aids in eliminating the "knocking" sound emanating from the scanner. Some facilities provide earphones so that patient can listen to music during the procedure. The patient is assured that a two-way communication system between the patient and the operator will allow for continual monitoring and vocal feedback.
3. The patient is positioned and asked to remain still during the procedure. The couch is moved into the tunnel-shaped gantry. The gantry is narrow and may frighten some individuals. Reassure the patient that there is sufficient air to breathe and that they will be monitored during the entire procedure. In some instances, a noniodinated contrast will be injected into a vein for better visualization of anatomy. The most commonly used contrast agent is *Gadolinium DPTA* which has very low toxicity and much fewer side effects than x-ray contrast agents. Gadolinium is generally used in examinations of the central nervous system (brain and spine).
4. There is no pain or discomfort associated with the MR exam. Throughout the procedure, the patient will hear a rhythmic knocking sound. Exam time varies between 60 and 90 minutes.

BLOOD FLOW SCANNING OF THE EXTREMITIES

1. The patient lies down during the test and remains as motionless as possible.
2. The limb to be examined is extended and rests on the system's examining table. Before testing, a finger plethysmograph is applied. Reference points on the leg are identified by a light marker: ankle, knee, and hip. The fingertips, wrist, and elbow are selected on the arm. These landmarks are stored by the computer system.
3. The examination table rotates to accommodate upper and lower extremities. The patient's limb is moved into and out of the flow cylinder during each extremity study.
4. If complete extremity studies (leg, arm, finger) are to be performed, usually the leg study will be done first.
5. Flow data are computed and projected on a graphics monitor and recorded on a computer-generated printout. Information is stored digitally for record-keeping purposes and evaluation. Data can be recorded

for a single vessel or for limb as a whole. To normalize for variations in limb size, limb circumference is measured every 5 cm, and blood flow is measured in terms of milliliters per minute per 100 cm^3 of distal tissue.

6. Flow-monitoring data are acquired in 25 seconds for a single cross-section of an extremity. A multiple cross-sectional study of both limbs requires about 30 minutes.

Interfering Factors

1. Respiratory motion causes severe artifacts in abdominal and thoracic imaging. Severely obese persons may not fit into the gantry opening.
2. Unusually large legs or bulky casts may prevent access into the blood flow scanner.

Clinical Implications

1. MRI of the brain demonstrates
   a. White matter disease (eg, multiple sclerosis)
   b. Infectious disorders affecting the brain (AIDS)
   c. Neoplasms
   d. Ischemias, CVA
   e. Aneurysms and hemorrhage
2. MRI of the spine demonstrates
   a. Disk herniation/degeneration
   b. Neoplasm (primary and metastatic)
   c. Inflammatory disease
   d. Demyelinating disease
   e. Congenital abnormalities
3. MRI of the heart demonstrates
   a. Abnormal chamber size and myocardial thickness
   b. Cardiac tumors
   c. Congenital heart disorders
   d. Pericarditis
   e. Graft patency
   f. Thrombic disorders
   g. Aortic dissection/aneurysm
4. MRI of the limbs and joints demonstrates
   a. Neoplasms of soft tissue and bone
   b. Ligament or tendon damage
   c. Osteonecrosis
   d. Bone marrow disorders
   e. Changes in blood flow
      (1) Atherosclerosis
      (2) Aneurysm
      (3) Thrombus
      (4) Embolism
      (5) Bypass grafts
      (6) Endocarditis
      (7) Shunt placement
5. MRI of the abdomen and pelvis demonstrates
   a. Neoplasms: especially useful in staging tumors
   b. Retroperitoneal structures
   c. Evaluation of renal transplants
6. MRI angiography demonstrates
   a. Aneurysms
   b. Stenosis or occlusions
   c. Graft patency
   d. Vascular malformations

Clinical Alert

Although there are no special dietary restrictions or special preparations before an MRI, there are numerous safety factors that must be considered:

1. Absolute contraindications to MRI include
   a. Implanted devices: pacemakers, cochlear implants, some prosthetic devices (consult with MR laboratory for specific information), implanted drug infusion pumps, neurostimulators, bone growth stimulators, and certain IUCD (intrauterine contraceptive devices).
   b. Internal metallic objects: metallic fragments, bullets, shrapnel; and surgical clips, pins, plates, screws, metal sutures, or wire mesh
2. In addition, MRI is generally not advised for the pregnant patient or individuals with epilepsy. All patients should be advised to remove the following materials before entering the MRI suite: hearing aids, dentures, jewelry, hair pins, and wigs and hairpieces.
3. Patients unable to hold still or who are claustrophobic may require conscious sedation before MRI procedures.

Patient Preparation

1. Explain the purpose, procedure, benefits, and risks. Safety concerns for the patient and staff during MRI procedures are based on interaction of strong magnetic fields with body tissues and metallic objects. These potential hazards are mainly due to (1) **projectiles**—metallic objects can be displaced, giving rise to potentially dangerous projectiles; (2) **torquing of metallic objects**—implanted surgical clips and other metallic structures can be torqued or twisted within the body when exposed to strong magnetic fields; (3) **local heating**—exposure to RF pulses can cause heating of tissues or metallic objects within the patient's body. For this reason, pregnant women are not routinely scanned because an increase in amniotic fluid or fetal temperature may be harmful; and (4) **interference with electromechanical implants**—electronic implants are at risk for damage from both magnetic fields and the RF pulses. Consequently, patients fitted with cardiac pacemakers, implanted drug infusion pumps, cochlear implants, and similar devices should not be exposed to MR procedures.

Clinical Alert

In the event of respiratory or cardiac arrest, the patient must be removed from the scan room before resuscitation. Most general hospital equipment (oxygen tanks, wheelchairs, IV pumps, and monitors) are not permitted in the MR suite.

2. Assess for contraindications to testing and obtain a relevant history concerning implanted heart valves, surgical and aneurysm clips, and internal orthopedic screws and rods.
3. Help the patient remove the following materials before entering the MR room: dental bridges and appliances, credit cards, keys, hairclips, shoes, belts, jewelry, or clothing with metal fasteners, wigs and hairpieces.
4. Those who are to have body imaging may experience a closed-in feeling that can be avoided if the patient keeps eyes closed during the entire test. Explain that it is better not to eat a large meal at least 1 hour before testing to reduce physiologic demands in the body and possible emesis that could occur in claustrophobic persons.
5. The patient should be helped to relax and remain as motionless as possible during testing. No pain is involved in testing.
6. Patients who are having blood flow testing should abstain from alcohol, nicotine, caffeine, and iron prescription drugs, and testing should be done 2 hours after meals to avoid unexpected vasoconstrictions or dilation. No smoking should be permitted before the test. The patient is asked to rest supine 10 minutes before the test.
7. Fasting or drinking clear liquids several hours before examination for abdominal pelvic MR may be necessary.
8. See Chapter 1 guidelines for safe, effective, informed *pretest* care.

Patient Aftercare

1. Interpret test results, counsel, and monitor appropriately.
2. Assess contrast injection site for signs of infection, inflammation, bruising, or irritation.
3. Follow Chapter 1 guidelines for safe, effective, informed *posttest* care.

Special Pediatric Considerations for MR Testing

Pediatric cautions of MR testing are as follows

1. Age: Ability to understand and cooperate, physical condition, and reasons for testing must be considered.
2. Body imaging: Most adult information applies. Tranquilizers and modified restraints may be employed in selected cases.
3. Blood flow in extremities: Simple restraints may be used to restrict motion of arms or legs. No tranquilizers or sedatives may be given because blood flow will be affected.

SLEEP STUDIES, POLYSOMNOGRAPHY (PSG) ●

Normal Values

Respiratory disturbance index (RDI): fewer than five to ten episodes per study period. The apnea/hypopnea index (AHI) is another name for RDI. The following values are normal during sleep.

ECG: Cardiac rate and rhythm
Impedance: Chest and abdominal wall movement
Airflow: nasal and oral airflow
Arterial oxygen saturation: By pulse oximetry
Leg electromyogram (EMG): Muscle activity
Electrooculogram (EOG): Retinal function
Electroencephalogram (EEG): Brain activity

Explanation of Test

These tests are used in the differential diagnosis of sleep-disordered breathing. They are indicated in persons with a history of excessive snoring, narcolepsy, excessive daytime sleepiness, insomnia, cardiac rhythm disorders, and restless leg spasms.

Procedure

1. Polysomnography (PSG) is usually scheduled for evening and night hours (for example, from 10 PM until 6 AM), within a specially designed sleep laboratory. PSG recording equipment and videomonitors record sleep events as they occur.
2. Electrodes are secured to the patient's skin. The number of electrodes used depends on the type of PSG being done. For example, a four-channel PSG will use ECG, impedance, airflow, and arterial O_2 saturation monitoring.
3. The patient is made comfortable and assured that normal body movements will not interfere with electrodes.
4. After the lights are turned off, the EEG is monitored before the patient actually falls asleep. Monitoring of sleep events continues until the test is completed.

Clinical Implications

1. Abnormal PSG recordings reveal obstructive sleep apnea syndrome (OSA). A respiratory disturbance index (RDI) of greater than five to 10 episodes of apnea/hypopnea indicates sleep apnea. *Apnea* refers to complete airway obstruction for a least 10 seconds; *hypopnea* refers to partial airway obstruction with oxygen desaturation for at least 10 seconds. Abnormal readings also occur in the presence of seizure disorders, movement disorders (restless leg syndrome), and parasomnia. During the apneic episode, the patient ceases to breathe while asleep. This response is marked by bradycardia together with decreased oxygen saturation. Often these events end with a spontaneous arousal, which then causes a sleep disturbance. The patient then exhibits tiredness when awake because sleep has been so interrupted.
2. OSA may be associated with cardiovascular conditions, especially hypertension or myocardial infarction.

3. OSA is also linked to strokes, neuromuscular diseases and, possibly, to dementia. It may be related to hypothyroidism, obesity, and type II diabetes.
4. Central sleep apnea occurs with cessation of chest wall movement and respiratory system airflow.

Interfering Factors

Electrophysiologic artifacts, defective electrodes, diaphoresis, environmental noises, or inability of the patient to fall asleep will affect sleep study results.

Patient Preparation

1. Explain test purpose and procedure. Instruct the patient to adhere to normal sleep patterns before PSG testing so that the patient comes to the test neither sleep-deprived nor overrested. No caffeine-containing products or naps should be taken for 2 to 3 days before the test.
2. Reassure patient that PSG lead wires and transducers will not interfere with changes of position during sleep. *Alleviate fears about equipment and videotaping.*
3. Instruct patient to prepare for sleep at the normal time; a shower or bath should be taken before testing.
4. See Chapter 1 guidelines for safe, effective, informed *pretest* care.

Patient Aftercare

1. Patient may resume usual activities and routines.
2. Interpret test outcome and monitor appropriately. If test results are indicative of obstructive sleep apnea syndrome (OSA), explain possible need for further treatment.
3. Follow Chapter 1 guidelines for safe, effective, informed *posttest* care.

Clinical Alert

Split-night studies may be ordered. These include monitoring a patient for half the night to document obstructive sleep apnea. Then, during the second half of the night, sleep apnea is actually treated by means of continuous positive airway pressure (CPAP) or nasal ventilation to open the obstructed airway.

GASTRIC ANALYSIS (TUBE GASTRIC ANALYSIS); **GASTRIC FLUIDS**

Normal Values

Fluid: clear or opalescent; no food, blood, drugs, or bile present
pH: 1.5 to 3.5
Culture: negative for mycobacterial organisms

Fasting specimen total acidity: 15 to 50 mmol/L; Basal acid output (BAO)—without stimulation; 0 to 5 mmol/hr; Maximal acid output (MAC) or normal secretory ability using a gastric stimulant, such as histamine—10 to 20 mmol/hr

Explanation of Test

This test examines stomach contents for the presence of abnormal substances and measures gastric acidity. It aids in diagnosing ulcers, obstruction, pernicious anemia, or carcinoma of the stomach. It can determine the cause of GI bleeding as well as the effectiveness of medical or surgical therapies. Cytologic exams of gastric washings (TB studies) can identify mycobacterial infection when previous sputum tests have been negative.

Procedure

1. Fasting gastric analysis specimens are collected either during endoscopy or by insertion of a nasogastric (NG) tube.
2. A NG tube is introduced into the stomach and checked for placement according to routine NG tube insertion protocols. Observe for signs of respiratory distress, such as coughing or cyanosis.
3. Initial gastric acid is aspirated with a syringe, tested for acid pH, and then discarded. If no acid is present, reposition tube and obtain another specimen if possible.
4. Specimens are normally collected by low suction over a period of 1 to 2 hours at 15-minute intervals (depends on type of gastric stimulant given). These are put in separate specimen cups and labeled "BAO" or "MAO" along with patient's name, date, and time.
5. The tube is removed after all specimens are collected.
6. Documentation includes date, time, and type of procedure; type and size of tubes used; number of specimens collected; appearance, consistency, and volumes of gastric fluid obtained; patient's response to testing; complications; interventions; and other pertinent information.

Clinical Implications

1. *Decreased levels* of gastric acid (hyposecretion and hypochlorhydria) occur in
   - **a.** Pernicious anemia
   - **b.** Gastric malignancy
   - **c.** Atrophic gastritis
   - **d.** Adrenal insufficiency
   - **e.** Vitiligo
   - **f.** Rheumatoid arthritis
   - **g.** Thyroid toxicosis
   - **h.** Chronic renal failure
   - **i.** Postvagotomy
2. *Increased levels* of gastric acid (hypersecretion and hyperchlorhydria) occur in
   - **a.** Peptic or duodenal ulcer
   - **b.** Zollinger-Ellison syndrome
   - **c.** Hyperplasia and hyperfunction of antral gastric cells
   - **d.** Following massive small-intestinal resection

Interfering Factors

1. Barium present from previous tests or lubricants can alter the sample.
2. Medications (antacids, histamine blockers), food, and smoking alter gastric secretions.
3. Gastric secretions are altered in patients with diabetes who use insulin, or in those who have had a surgical vagotomy.
4. Elderly patients have lower levels of gastric hydrochloric acid.

Patient Preparation

1. Assess for contraindications to the procedure. These categories include patients with carcinoid syndrome, congestive heart failure, or hypertension. The use of histamine may exacerbate these conditions.
2. Explain test purpose, procedure; inform patient that there may be some discomfort when the NG tube is inserted and that histamine may be injected.
3. Record baseline vital signs. Remove dentures before test.
4. Food, fluids, smoking, and gum chewing must be abstained from for at least 8 to 12 hours before testing.
5. Restrict ingestion of anticholinergics, cholinergics, adrenergic blockers, antacids, steroids, alcohol, and coffee for at least 24 hours before testing. Check with physician.
6. See Chapter 1 guidelines for safe, effective, informed *pretest* care.

Clinical Alert

1. If histamine is injected, flushing, dizziness, headache, faintness, and numbness of extremities and abdomen may occur during or immediately after testing. Advise patient to report these symptoms immediately. Have epinephrine immediately available.
2. Specimens for acid-fast bacillus (AFB) cultures for tuberculosis detection need to be warm when taken to the laboratory. The specimen should be taken to the laboratory immediately and laboratory personnel alerted concerning this specimen.

Patient Aftercare

1. Monitor vital signs; observe for possible drug side effects or for GI or respiratory bleeding or distress (may be sign of perforation).
2. Provide nasal and oral care after tube removal. Allow patient to rest. Provide food or fluids as tolerated or ordered. If local anesthetic was used on the throat, assess for return of gag and swallow reflexes before allowing patient to drink or eat.
3. Interpret test outcomes. Counsel patient concerning possible lifestyle al-

terations, such as cessation of smoking, restricted alcohol intake, dietary changes, stress reduction, and medication or surgical intervention.

4. Follow Chapter 1 guidelines for safe, effective, informed *posttest* care.

● TESTS AFTER DEATH

Overview of Postmortem Tests

It is the basic civil right of deceased human beings to have competent medical investigations of their deaths. This is particularly true in today's environment of social ills, drug use, crime, and violence among all sociocultural and political classes. Any death has potential civil, legal, criminal, or economic implications for the deceased, the family, and significant others and for society as a whole.

As with establishing a medical diagnosis for a living person, the medical process is similarly executed in developing a postmortem diagnosis. A history is taken (past medical history, risk factors and death interpretation); physical examination is performed (autopsy); and laboratory tests are interpreted (postmortem blood, tissue, organ, and other body fluids, vitreous, urine, bile, gastric contents).

Death Investigation

All deaths, whether from natural sequence of events, during medical treatment, in unexplained circumstances, or that are criminally related, need to be investigated for "cause" and "manner" of death so that the legal death certificate may be accurately completed, signed, and recorded. Deaths can be defined as *natural* or *medical/legal:*

Natural Death	*Medical/Legal Death*
Cessation of cardiorespiratory function due to a medical disease process (eg, metastatic cancer, cerebrovascular accident) or natural progression of life events ("old age")	Results from some "unnatural' or unexpected, unusual or suspicious event, such as homicide, suicide, or accident; specifically governed by legal statutes and require that a coroner, medical examiner, and law enforcement officials be involved

Death Interpretation

The process of postmortem interpretation follows a certain sequence. First the "history" portion of the investigation is obtained. In natural death without autopsy, the medical history, diagnostic tests before death, clinical record, and knowledge about lifestyle can provide reasonably sufficient information to arrive at conclusions about cause and manner of death. Only autopsy, however, can definitely confirm this.

Clinical Alert

Postmortem examination falls under the domain of the physician pathologist; in criminal cases, forensic pathologists, who have specialized knowledge, skills, and the latest investigative techniques at their disposal, should perform the autopsy.

Medical/legal death focuses first on the death scene investigation. Interviews "lay the groundwork" for the investigation. Evaluation of the actual site involves a detailed examination: blood stains, disrupted environment, position of body, signs of struggle or injury (manifested by fluids leaking from body orifices, eyes, ears, nose, or mouth). Color change and rigidity can be beneficial in establishing time frames for events (Chart 15-1).

The second part of the process involves the autopsy itself. It consists of a detailed examination of both external and internal body features.

Clinical Alert

In the case of medical/legal autopsy, samples of organs and specimen sections (slides) should be retained for 3 to 5 years pending outcomes of litigation and legal system appeals. Photographs should be included with reports and should be archived.

The third step of a routine death interpretation includes blood, bile, urine, and ocular fluids collection (if available) and analysis. Blood sample toxicology studies need to be performed at a state-certified laboratory. Blood samples are the *only* life/death determinants; urine samples provide information about levels of substances excreted, they do not indicate blood levels. Typical toxicology screens include

No. 1. Alcohol screens determine levels of various alcohols.
No. 2. Acid neutral screens detect barbiturates and salicylates.
No. 3. Basic screens detect tranquilizers, synthetic narcotics, local anesthetics, antihistamines, antidepressants, and alkaloids.
No. 4. Higher volatile screens use gas chromatography to detect such substances as toluene, benzene, trichloroethane, and trichloroethylene.
No. 5. Cannibis screens detect the presence of cannabis (marijuana).

All of these screens find their purpose in cases involving accidents and work-related deaths.

CHART 15-1
Time of Death

Although time of death is usually not a major issue, determination of this time is important in both natural deaths (insurance and other death benefits) and unnatural deaths (unwitnessed or when body parts have been intentionally altered to conceal an individual's distinguishing features). Time of death estimate is based on presence of

Rigor mortis: Stiffening of body as pH changes and lack of adenosine triphosphate in muscles: rigidity appears anywhere from instantly to 6–12 hr after death.

Livor mortis: Reddish-purple color (settling of blood for dependent body parts owing to gravity): onset is immediate, sometimes beginning before death, maximum or fixed in 8–12 hr.

Algor mortis: Cooling of body: body temperature interpretation is based on cocaine use, presence of infections or fever before death; death scene, heat absorption, amount and type of clothing, size of body, activity just before death, decomposition.

Decomposition: Processes occur because of chemical breakdown of cells and organs caused by intracellular enzymes and putrefaction from bacterial action.

Gastric emptying: Food in stomach: Digestion and stomach emptying varies in both life and death.

Chemical changes: Potassium in vitreous fluid of the eye. As the time since death becomes greater, so does the concentrate of potassium increase.

Insect activity: Flies and other insects are associated with decomposed bodies. Any attempt to determine time of death using insect evidence should be done only with the aid of an entomologist.

Clinical Alert

1. Time of death is expressed as an estimate of the time range during which a death could have occurred.
2. There is no single accurate marker of time of death.
3. When the time interval since death and the initial death investigation is a matter of months or years, body changes may be quite variable. Saponification: subcutaneous tissue changes owing to prolonged exposure to moisture (several months); mummification; drying process (lack of moisture), occurs quickly in hot, dry climate, exposure to air, dying of thirst; skeletization takes months to years. Examination of bones may yield general knowledge of deceased, estimate of age, stature, race, and sex.

Once the life events and scene investigation, autopsy, and laboratory tests are done, data from all sources are scrutinized and analyzed. Findings are then documented and certified on the death certificate, where it becomes a matter of public record. From there, it may be shared with the decedent's immediate family or become part of a court deposition process, or both.

> **Clinical Alert**
>
> Some examiners may be reluctant to include HIV-positive information in public record autopsy reports out of compassion for the decedent's family. Be that as it may, certain states require that every autopsy done through the medical examiner's office include an HIV test. As with other issues of confidentiality, the law needs to be obeyed. However, one must make every effort to protect the patient's/family's right to privacy to the degree that the law will allow. (**Note:** If HIV status of decedent is ***not*** directly related to the cause of death, the decedent's HIV status need not be recorded.)

AUTOPSY

Normal Values

External and internal findings: within normal limits.

Explanation of Test

An autopsy is an investigation into the cause and manner of death by direct examination. *Cause of death* is the disease or injury that through its physiologic effects, results in the actual death of the individual. *Manner of death* is the type of event(s) that lead to death (categorized as natural, homicidal, suicidal, accidental, pending, or undetermined). Interpretation of physical findings results in setting forth an opinion about probable cause of death. Before autopsy, as much pertinent information as possible is gathered about the deceased. Available medical records are reviewed thoroughly. In cases of medical/legal death investigation, not only the medical and social background but also the terminal events and circumstances of death, including the environment, presence of drugs and alcohol, and the exact condition and position of the body are thoroughly investigated.

General Procedure

1. The body is identified and "tagged" (on the great toe) with a name (if available) sex, age, and a number, then weighed and measured.
2. Next, the head and chest are photographed and marked with identification number.
3. Information about clothing and valuables is described and recorded.

These items are then removed and given to family or the law enforcement agency.

4. Fingerprints are made (fingertips in children).

5. The body is cleansed. If blood, dirt, and other materials were present initially, the face is again photographed.

7. An external examination is then performed on the entire body. The location and description of all identifying marks, scars, tattoos, incisions, injuries, and other significant findings are recorded on a body diagram.

8. All injuries are photographed in at least two views—one shows the location of the injury on the body, and the other provides a closer view of the injury itself.

9. In some instances, x-ray studies may be necessary to verify gross anatomic deformities, injuries, or pathologies (may provide clues to the cause of death). Radiography tracks bullet and other weapon trajectories through the entire body or just through a specific area, and also may be performed on exhumed organs. The x-ray studies can determine age and can establish a victim's identity by comparing bone and dental detail with previously taken films of the victim.

10. The autopsy then proceeds in an orderly manner. Observe universal precautions. Descriptions of color and distinguishing features of the hair, eyes, nose, ears, mouth, teeth, face, head, neck, genitalia, torso, and extremities are made front, side, and back in detail. Injuries, wounds, bruises, contusions, and lacerations are described, mapped, and detailed. Descriptions of size, depth, location, presence of foreign objects or materials at or near the injured areas, as well as fluids draining from body orifices and wounds are entered into the report. Internal examination includes a complete head and pelvic dissection with removal of all organs from the skull, neck, abdomen, and pelvis, Specific organs are then subjected to gross examination, including measuring size and weight. Once this is done, organ sections are prepared for microscopic slides and then examined later. The slides are saved for evidence. Virtually any part of the body can be microscopically examined. The brain and the neck organs are always removed and examined. As part of this examination, the dura matter is removed to permit visualization of the skull and calvarium.

11. Blood specimens are withdrawn by syringe from the heart or the aorta and vitreous fluid from the eyes, bile from the gallbladder, urine from the bladder. Refrigerate until examined and save for an indefinite period. In the instance of trauma, the blood sample can be retrieved from the pulmonary trunk or the chest. If clots are present and syringe sampling cannot be done, pericardial tapping is an alternative method to procure a blood sample.

12. Sometimes it is necessary to collect specimens for cultures. Most internal organs of previously uninfected persons remain sterile for about 20 hours after death.

a. Follow universal precautions; use sterile instruments and gloves when obtaining specimens for culture; scrub the body with a povidone iodine 5-minute scrub, followed by a 70% alcohol 5-minute scrub. For collection, either aspirate body fluid samples and transfer them to a sterile tube or swab.

b. Obtain blood culture specimens from the right ventricle of the heart; collect peritoneal fluid immediately after entering the peritoneal cavity; collect bladder urine directly from the bladder with a syringe and needle; sample pericardial or pleural cavity fluid on a swab or with a syringe and needle. Sear the exernal surface of an abscess to dryness with a red-hot spatula; collect pus by syringe and needle (if possible) or else on a swab.

13. The organs are returned to the body after examination is completed.

Clinical Alert

1. If an autopsy is not done, but just an external examination, collect blood from the subclavian vessel and vitreous from the eyes.
2. Do not use plastic envelopes for storing biologic samples, such as tissue or hair or foreign objects, such as bullets. Plastic captures moisture and promotes fungal growth. Instead, place objects in clean paper envelopes. Label each item properly (Chart 15-2).

Clinical Implications

CAUSES OF DEATH

1. The most common *cardiovascular* disease causes of natural sudden death are myocardial infarction, hypertensive cardiovascular disease, strenuous activity during extreme heat or cold weather, congenital drug use, anorexia nervosa.
2. The most common *brain* disease or injury causes of natural sudden death are poorly controlled epilepsy (noncompliance with treatment); absence of brain lesion in the presence of seizure disorders is cardiac arrest, related to lack of oxygen; hemorrhage, primary brain tumors, and aneurysm.
3. The most common *respiratory* causes of sudden death are epiglottitis, pulmonary thrombosis/embolus, status asthmaticus, aspiration of gastric contents/blood, cavernous TB, premature birth, fulminating pneumonia.
4. The most common *gastrointestinal* causes of natural sudden death are trauma, peritonitis, massive splenic enlargement/rupture, caustic substances, liver/pancreatic diseases, diabetes mellitus in the presence of diabetic coma (diagnosed by elevated glucose in vitreous of eye).
5. Other causes of natural sudden death are rupture of tubal pregnancy; chronically ill, bed-ridden persons with sepsis associated with decubitus ulcers; malnutrition; dehydration; environmental causes (eg, Legionnaires' disease or other diseases spread by rodent droppings).

CHART 15-2
Special Criminological Postmortem Procedures

GUNSHOT WOUND PROCEDURE

X-ray studies of all gunshot wounds incuding entrance/exit, locate bullets, fragments; **Note:** copper and aluminum jackets remain in the body; aluminum jackets are difficult to visualize on x-ray film, especially in bone. Photograph entry/exit, cleanse wound; repeat photograph.

BLUNT FORCE INJURY PROCEDURE

X-ray studies of affected areas: X-ray films of hands and forearms for "defense wounds." Photograph the wounds in original condition and after cleansing. Use rape kit if possible rape is suspected (both male and female) or when the nature of the injury suggests uncontrolled rage (hammer, axe, stab wounds).

SHARP WOUND PROCEDURE

X-ray film of wound sites. Photograph wounds in original condition, after cleansing, and after approximating wound margins. Check for defense wounds on hands and arms. Trace wounds on clear plastic sheet (optional). Save and photograph severed cartilage.

DRUG OVERDOSE PROCEDURE

Photograph evidence suggesting drug abuse; injection sites on body, drug paraphernalia/drugs; drug residue on lips, face, teeth, oral cavity, tongue, nose, hands. Assess mouth area and body for bite marks and "fall" injuries (suggests seizure activity associated with drug ingestion). Check lymph nodes, spleen, liver (abnormal in IV drug abuser).

SPECIAL BATTERY PROCEDURE

If sexual assault is suspected, the following should be done *in order:* Body supine (on back), obtain scalp and pubic hair, oral samples, semen from inner thighs. Body prone (face down), obtain anal specimen first—then vaginal specimen. Fingernail evidence. Collect 25 pubic hairs from entire vulvar area. Collect 25 head hairs from affected area. Obtain oral, anal, vaginal, cervical, and other body area specimens suspected of containing semen.

CHILD ABUSE/SIDS PROCEDURE

X-ray studies and photograph entire body. External examination of conjunctival petechiae, fingertip bruises, torso and shoulders (front and back), frenulum, back, posterior thighs and buttocks may be incised (from buckles or other sharp objects). Internal examination for

(continued)

CHART 15-2 *(continued)*

CHILD ABUSE/SIDS PROCEDURE

hematomas (due to direct injury); if present and *no* evidence of head trauma, remove eyes and examine retina (shows characteristic signs in presence of sudden infant death syndrome). Document whether recent or healed fractures and estimated time of injury. Reexamine and rephotograph following day to delineate bruises not previously evident.

Clinical Alert

1. Observe universal precautions during these procedures. Risk of disease transmission, hepatitis, and HIV exposure is high.
2. Sketch, measure, and mark wounds on diagram (both inches and centimeters) (U.S. residents relate to inches more accurately)
3. Projectile (bullet) caliber is estimated as small, medium, or large. Procure toxicologic specimens if indicated. Specimens for toxicologic analysis include all ocular fluid from both eyes; 50 ml blood in sodium fluoride preservative, 10 ml blood in sodium fluoride preservative (retainer tube); liver—3 g, bile—10 ml, urine—50 ml, stomach and small bowel contents.
4. Store specimens and fragments in paper envelopes or bags—never plastic, which allows mold, fungus to grow.
5. Route specimens and reports to appropriate department or individual.

6. The most common *unnatural* causes of sudden death are trauma to body, wounds, cuts, lacerations, traumatic amputations, self-inflicted and self-defense wounds, asphyxia, motor vehicle deaths, and airplane crashes.
7. Other *unnatural* causes of sudden death are sudden infant death syndrome (SIDS; unexpected death of apparently healthy infant. Post mortem examination may not reveal the cause of death); neonaticide (deliberate killing of infant within 24 hours of birth); infanticide, and child murder. Deaths by fire, drowning, electrical deaths, deaths by hyperthermia (heat) or hypothermia (cold), and embolism; homicide associated with rape; deaths caused by criminal abortion; and drug abuse and drug-related deaths.

Family Preparation

1. Explain rationale for postdeath procedures. (Chart 15-3 outlines information for families concerning biopsy.) Concern and respect for the deceased and significant others can reduce anxiety and objections to or misinterpretations of after-death testing. Obtain signed, witnessed consent form for autopsy.
2. Consider cultural habits and practices. Human response to the death of a loved one varies among different societies, religions, cultures, and races. In this light, postmortem examination may be offensive to some groups.

CHART 15-3
Information for Families Concerning an Autopsy

Autopsies are frequently mandatory or routine procedures, especially in sudden, suspicious, or unexplained deaths. They serve as quality control indicators to confirm pre-death diagnoses; to assess effectiveness of drug therapy, diagnostic procedures, surgical techniques, gene therapy, and other diagnostic and treatment modality. They make it possible to identify, track, and monitor disease for prevalence, incidence, trends, or association with certain lifestyle, environmental, or occupational influences. Information gathered from autopsy findings provides a framework for developing better and more sophisticated treatments for disease and illness control or eradication.

Should family members be undecided concerning an autopsy, they may wish to consider it as an option when no firm medical diagnosis has been established; on the event of unexpected or mysterious death of apparent natural causes or suspected exposure to environmental or other hazards; for presence of hereditary, genetic, or contagious disease. The cause of death could affect insurance settlements and other legal matters, if death occurs in the presence of unexpected medical or obstetric complications, during the use of experimental drugs, or as the result of certain dental, invasive, surgical, or diagnostic procedures.

3. Assure the family that nothing will be done without their permission except as required by law.
4. If fear of mutilation or delay in release of body for burial are concerns, provide clear and concise information to help with decision-making. In case of religious dilemmas, facilitate counsel and communication with clergy.
5. Conflict may occur when statutory authority is at odds with family wishes. Explanations may help.

Family Aftercare
Interpret postmortem test results and counsel appropriately.

DNA TYPING OR FINGERPRINTING ●

Normal Values
Characteristic and unique to each person.

Background
DNA is a complex protein of high molecular weight composed of deoxyribose, phosphoric acid, and four bases (adenine, guanine, thymine, and cytocine). These six substances are arranged in two long chains that twist around each other to form a "double-helix." The complementary components on each of these two chains link together between the two chains. The nucleic acid component is present in the cell nuclei chromosomes and forms the chemical foundation for heredity. It carries the genetic material for every living organism except RNA viruses. DNA provides the actual code for individual genetic characteristics through a specific sequence "blueprint" that is unique to that person alone.

Explanation
DNA testing is used during criminal investigations and tracking of parentage by a technique termed *restriction fragment length polymorphism (RFLP).* This technique allows evaluation of different DNA tissue samples from several sources to determine matching patterns (similar to comparing "bar codes").

Procedure
1. DNA can be extracted from any tissue that contains *nucleated cells* (eg, skin, saliva, hair shafts, semen).
2. The DNA samples are enzymatically digested until DNA fragments can be visually represented on x-ray film. These films are called *autorads* or *autoradiographs.* At this point, the fragments appear to resemble bar codes.
3. The autorads are compared for matching or nonmatching characteristics among several samples. If a match between two or more different au-

torads is found, there exists a high probability that the different samples come from the same source or person.

Clinical Implications

1. Even though each person has a unique DNA profile, matching characteristics in certain areas of the autorads that come from two different individuals can indicate a parent-child connection.
2. Matching DNA characteristics associated with tissue samples retrieved from both victim and suspect *may* establish presence at the scene of a crime. A nonmatch disproves that the different samples come from the same source or person.

Interfering Factors

1. Insufficient amount of DNA.
2. Sample deterioration or degradation.
3. Lack of material database to conduct effective sample comparison.

BIBLIOGRAPHY

Aher H, Rue K: How do you measure gastric pH 1. Am J Nurs p. 70, May 1991.

Bandyk D: Postoperative surveillance of infrainguinal bypass. Surg Clin North Am 70: 71–85, 1990

Bankanash MJ et al. Post mortem recording of human immunodeficiency virus type I from plasma and non-nucleic cells. Arch Pathol Lab Med 116: 1124–1127, November 1992

Berk, JL, Sampliner JE (eds): Handbook of Critical Care, 3rd ed. Boston, Little, Brown & Co, 1990

Baldridge ED: Clinical significance of free floating venous thrombi. J Vasc Surg 11: 62–69, 1990

Cheney AM, Mquinding MR: Patient teaching for x-ray and other diagnostics; transesophageal echocardiogram (TEE). RN April: 54–56, 1993

DiMaio DJ, DiMaio VJM: Forensic Pathology. New York, Elsevier Science, 1990

Farley MA, Harrington JJ: Forensic DNA Technology. Chelsea, MI, Lewis Publishers, 1990

Froede RC: Handbook of Forensic Pathology. Northfield, IL, American College of Pathologists, 1993

Greenspon AJ: Effects of atrial pacing on signal averaged ECG. Am Heart J 1: 29–34, January 1990

Hibner CS, Mosely M: What is transesophageal echocardiography? Am J Nurs, April: 74–76 1993

Howland WA: MRI madness. Am J Nurs, February 14 1994

March K: Transcranial Doppler sonography—noninvasive monitoring of intracranial vasculature. J Neurosci 22 (2): 113–116, April 1990

Milnor W: Hemodynamics. Baltimore, Williams & Wilkins, 1989

Moser DK, Woo MA, Stevenson WG: Noninvasive identification of patients at risk for ventricular tachycardia with the signal-averaged electrocardiogram. AACN Clin Issues Crit Care Nurs 1(1): 79–86, May 1990

Phillips RE, Feeney MK: The Cardiac Rhythms: A Systemic Approach to Interpretation, 3rd ed. Philadelphia, WB Saunders, 1990

Plankey ED, Knohf J: Prep talk: What patients need to know about magnetic resonance imaging. Am J Nurs 90(1): 27–28, January 1990

Rudolphi DM: Duplex scanning. Am J Nurs April: 123–124, 1990

Wong W: Brain mapping leads to better life. Med Coll Wisconsin Health News Fall: 6–7, 1992

16

Prenatal Diagnosis and Tests of Fetal Well-Being

Frances Fischbach: A MANUAL OF LABORATORY & DIAGNOSTIC TESTS, Fifth Edition.

OVERVIEW OF PRENATAL DIAGNOSIS

Tests included in this chapter monitor changes in the status of the maternal–fetal unit, identify the fetus at risk for intrauterine asphyxia, aid in the early diagnosis of infection, and identify genetic and biochemical disorders and major anomalies. Tests to predict normal fetal outcome or to identify the fetus at risk for asphyxia during labor are outlined in Table 16–1. Other commonly used diagnostics include ultrasound and magnetic resonance imaging (MRI), and testing of the mother's blood screens for presence of fetal neural tube defects. Ultrasound testing, introduced in the 1950s as a method of assessing fetal well-being, has now become a diagnostic tool for assessment of fetal age, health, growth, and identification of anomalies. (See ultrasound, Chap. 13 for complete discussion.) Level I ultrasound assesses gestational age, number of fetuses, fetal death, and the condition of the placenta. Level II ultrasound assesses specific congenital anomalies or abnormalities. In some diagnostic centers, fetal echocardiography is available (see page 853).

Although MRI is used at some prenatal centers, it is still under investigation for diagnostic evaluation in pregnancy (see Chap. 15 for a full discussion of MRI). Advantages of MRI during pregnancy include that it is a noninvasive technique, permits easy differentiation between fat and soft tissue, does not require a full bladder, and can show the entire fetus in one scan. Currently, MRI can confirm fetal abnormalities found by ultrasound and can be used for pelvimetry, placental localization, and determination of size. Future uses for MRI may include assessment of fetal blood flow, evaluation of nutritional status in intrauterine growth retardation (IUGR), and intracranial studies.

MATERNAL SERUM ALPHA-FETOPROTEIN (MSAFP)

Normal Value

25 ng/ml

Explanation of Test

Maternal serum screening of alpha-fetoprotein (AFP) for neural tube defects (NTD) is routinely offered to all pregnant women because only 5% to 10% of NTDs occur in families with previous NTD.

Procedure

1. Obtain a 10-ml venous blood sample.
2. Plan first screening at 16 to 18 weeks. If normal, no further screening is necessary. If low, consider ultrasound studies. Do a second screening after an initial elevated MSAFP. If normal, no further screening is necessary. Ultrasound may be ordered as a second screening procedure.

TABLE 16-1
Tests to Predict Fetal Outcome and Identify the Fetus at Risk for Intrauterine Asphyxia

Name of Test, Normal Values, and Clinical Implications	Test Procedure and Purpose
CONTRACTION STRESS TESTS (CST) (NIPPLE STIMULATION CONTRACTION STRESS TEST [NSCST]; BREAST STIMULATION TEST [BST])	
Normal Values Reactive; negative implies that placental support is adequate and that the fetus is probably able to tolerate the stress of labor, should it begin within a week. There should be a low risk of intrauterine death due to hypoxia.	After 26 weeks gestation, the nipples are stimulated to release oxytocin that causes uterine contractions similar to labor contractions. Test is to assess fetal heart rate in response to uterine contractions while using electronic fetal monitoring.
Clinical Alert **1.** There is a risk of hyperstimulation with all methods of CST that could result in extended fetal heart rate decelerations which could be hypoxic for fetus. **2.** Contraindications for CST include: third-trimester bleeding; presence of classic uterine incision; at risk for premature labor.	
OXYTOXIC CHALLENGE TEST (OCT)	
Normal Values Negative. Implies placental reserve is sufficient should labor begin within 1 week.	Contractions may occur spontaneously, or intravenous oxytocin is administrered to produce three good quality contractions of at least 45 seconds each in 10 minutes. The fetal heart rate is monitored for reaction to this stress. It is performed when a nonstress test is nonreactive or a BST is either positive or unsatisfactory. This is done after 28 weeks gestation.

(continued)

TABLE 16-1 *(Continued)*

Name of Test, Normal Values, and Clinical Implications	*Test Procedure and Purpose*
NONSTRESS TEST (NST)	
Normal Values	
Reactive; at least two episodes of fetal movement associated with a rise in fetal heart rate. Provides a baseline status and implies intact central and autonomic nervous systems that are not being affected by intrauterine hypoxia.	After 27 weeks gestation, it determines fetus ability to respond to fetal environment by an increase in fetal heart rate associated with fetal movement when not under the stress of labor by using electronic fetal monitoring. The mother should eat a light snack or drink orange juice before the test if she has not eaten recently.
FETAL ACOUSTICAL STIMULATION TEST (FAST)	
Normal Values	
Reactive implies intact central and autonomic nervous systems not stressed by hypoxia.	This is done after 28 weeks gestation. Often used when NST is nonreactive. Using an electronic fetal monitor and sound source or vibroacoustic source (vibration and sound) on the maternal abdomen, an evaluation of fetal movement in response to stimulation is done. Intended to induce fetal heart rate acceleration by stimulation of fetal movement.

Clinical Implications

1. Elevated MSAFP levels can indicate
   a. Neural tube defects of spina bifida (a vertebral gap) or anencephaly
   b. Underestimation of gestational age
   c. Multiple gestation
   d. Threatened abortion
   e. Rh incompatibility disease
   f. Other congenital abnormalities
2. Elevated MSAFP levels early in pregnancy are associated with other fetal defects:
   a. Congenital nephrosis
   b. Duodenal atresia
   c. Umbilical hernia or protrusion
   d. Sacrococcygeal teratoma
3. Elevated MSAFP levels in the third trimester are associated with other fetal defects:
   a. Esophageal atresia
   b. Tetralogy of Fallot
   c. Hydroencephaly
   d. Rh isoimmunization (severe)
4. Low MSAFP levels may indicate an increase in second-trimester fetal wastage, Down syndrome, and other chromosomal abnormalities (eg, trisomy 13, 18, 21). Ultrasound and then amniocentesis are indicated for follow-through.

Clinical Alert

The incidence of NTD is 1:1000 births in the United States; 1:5000 births in England.

Patient Preparation

1. Explain reason for testing mother's blood.
2. See Chapter 1 guidelines for safe, effective, informed *pretest* care.

Patient Aftercare

1. Interpret test outcomes and counsel appropriately. Explain possible need for further testing.
2. Follow Chapter 1 guidelines for safe, effective, informed *posttest* care.

HORMONAL TESTING

Normally, the amounts of all steroid hormones increase as pregnancy progresses. The maternal unit responds to altered hormonal levels even before the growing uterus is apparent. Serial testing is done to monitor rising levels of a particular hormone over a time period. Decreasing levels indicate that the maternal–placental–fetal unit is not functioning normally. A decrease in steroids does not adversely affect the mother because the hormonal level already exceeds her nonpregnant levels. For the fetus it is a different story. Maintained in a closed environment, the fetus can be quite susceptible to maternal system variations. Biochemical analyses of several hormones can monitor changes in the status of the maternal–fetal unit (see Chaps. 3 and 6).

1. In early pregnancy, human chorionic gonadotropin (hCG) provides evidence of a viable pregnancy (mother's blood).
2. The hCG, together with prolactin and luteinizing hormone (LH), prolongs the life of the corpus luteum once the ovum is fertilized. The hCG stimulates the ovary for the first 6 to 8 weeks of pregnancy, before the placental synthesis of progesterone. Its function later in pregnancy is unknown.
3. Late in pregnancy, estriol and human placental lactogen (hPL) reflect fetal homeostasis (mother's blood). hPL is a protein hormone produced by the placenta. Testing of hPL evaluates only placental functioning. Blood testing of the mother usually begins after the 30th week and may be done weekly thereafter. An hPL level of 1 μg/ml may be detected at 6 to 8 weeks of gestation. The level of hPL slowly increases throughout pregnancy and reaches a level of 7 μg/ml at term, before abruptly dropping to zero after delivery. An hPL value of 4 μg/ml after 30 weeks of gestation indicates probable fetal distress; however, falsely high values are common. Low hPL values indicate the need for further assessment by nonstress testing and amniocentesis to corroborate results (see Chap. 6, Blood Chemistry).

FETAL BIOPHYSICAL PROFILE (FBP OR BPP) ●

Normal Values

Fetal well-being of 8 points or above based on normal nonstress test, normal fetal muscle tone, movement, breathing, and volume of amniotic fluid.

Explanation of Test

This test, used in the later stages of pregnancy, assesses fetal well-being. The biophysical profile is more accurate and provides more information than the nonstress test. It can identify the fetus suffering the effects of hypoxia who is at risk of in utero distress or death. Testing of high-risk pregnancies usually begins by 32 to 34 weeks gestation, whereas those with severe complications may require earlier testing at 26 to 28 weeks.

The biophysical profile uses ultrasound imaging to evaluate five distinct parameters: (1) Evidence of cardiac rate acceleration with fetal movement (nonstress test); (2) muscle tone; (3) fetal movement; (4) fetal breathing; and (5) volume of amniotic fluid. From the sonographic evidence during a typical 20- to 30-minute survey, each parameter is assigned a value of 0 to 2 points (2 is optimal). The maximum number of points obtainable is 10 points, which indicates a normal test without evidence of fetal distress. Generally, a score of 8 or above indicates fetal well-being.

The biophysical profile also provides the clinician with valuable information concerning fetal size, position, and number of fetuses; the placental location and grade; and evidence of specific fetal activities, such as micturition and eye movements. In some laboratories, Doppler examinations of the umbilical vessels assess uterofetal blood flow. Abnormal Doppler blood flow studies (umbilical artery velocimetry) may be detected before changes are apparent from the nonstress test (NST), contraction stress test (CST), and fetal biophysical profiles (FBP). Abnormal Doppler umbilical artery waveforms become indicative of acidosis, hypoxia, or intrauterine growth retardation (IUGR), which may result in a poor outcome.

Procedure

1. Explain the test purpose and procedure.
2. Position the patient on her back (as for an obstetric sonogram). Apply a gel (coupling agent) to the skin of the lower abdomen. Then, move the ultrasound transducer across the lower abdominal area to visualize the fetus and surrounding structures.
3. Examining time is generally 30 minutes but may be variable because of fetal age or state.

Clinical Implications

1. Variables that influence FBP include fetal age, fetal behavioral states, maternal or fetal infection, hypoglycemia, hyperglycemia, and postmaturity.
2. If a fetus less than 36 weeks gestation does not have stable behaviors, a longer test may be needed. Infection may cause absence of fetal heart rate reactivity and fetal breathing movements. Frequency of fetal breathing increases during maternal hyperglycemia and decreases with maternal hypoglycemia. Other variables that influence FBP results include both therapeutic and nontherapeutic chemicals. Magnesium sulfate may decrease or eliminate fetal breathing movements and decrease fetal heart rate variability. Nicotine can decrease the profile parameters, and cocaine may also decrease the FBP score.
3. When the five major biophysical profile parameters can be observed, the fetus is considered to be free of distress. Generally a score of 8 or more points out of a possible 10 points indicates fetal well-being.
4. A score lower than 8 indicates the potential for, or the existence of, fetal distress.

Clinical Alert

A fetus that appears to lack respiratory activity may simply be sleeping. The presence of rapid eye movements must be determined sonographically to assess the fetal state properly. If no eye movement and no respirations are evident, the fetus is most likely asleep. On the other hand, if rapid eye movement is evident, but breathing is absent, the fetus is probably in distress.

Patient Preparation

1. Explain the test purpose and procedure and include information concerning each part of the test and how it relates to fetal well-being.
2. See Chapter 1 guidelines for safe, effective, informed *pretest* care.

Patient Aftercare

1. Interpret test outcomes and counsel appropriately.
2. Follow Chapter 1 guidelines for safe, effective, informed *posttest* care.

FETOSCOPY

Normal Values: Normal Fetal Development

No evidence of fetal developmental defects; negative for hemophilia types A and B and sickle cell anemia.

Explanation of Test

Fetoscopy allows direct observation of the fetus and facilitates fetal blood or skin sampling. It provides direct visualization of the fetus in 2- to 4-cm segments so that developmental defects can be more accurately identified. The fetal blood sample allows early diagnosis of disorders, such as hemophilia A and B, that are not amenable to detection within the fetus through other means. Fetoscopy can also be used for therapeutic interventions, such as shunt placement.

Procedure

1. Obtain properly signed and witnessed consent form.
2. Apply a local anesthetic to the mother's abdominal wall. Meperidine (Demerol), which crosses the placenta, may be given to the mother to quiet the fetus.
3. Real-time ultrasound locates the proper maternal abdominal area through which a small incision is made. A cannula and the trocar are then inserted into the uterus.
4. Following cannulation into the uterus, an endoscope (fetoscope), consisting of a fiberoptic light source and self-focusing lens, is inserted and then manipulated for optimal views and fetal tissue sampling that can include skin, blood samples, and amniotic fluid.

Clinical Implications

Abnormal results reveal

1. Fetal malformation
2. Neural tube defects
3. Sickle cell anemia
4. Hemophilia

Clinical Alert

1. Fetoscopy presents increased risk of spontaneous abortions (5% to 10%) and of preterm delivery (10%); amniotic fluid leakage (1%); and intrauterine fetal death.
2. Fetoscopy is offered only to those women who present a significant risk for producing a child with a major birth defect that can be diagnosed only by this method.

Patient Preparation

1. The woman (or couple) should receive genetic counseling and a thorough explanation of the procedure and its risks and limitations.
2. Antibiotics may be ordered to be administered before the procedure to prevent amnionitis. Assess for possible allergies to the drug.
3. See Chapter 1 guidelines for safe, effective, informed *pretest* care.

Patient Aftercare

1. Monitor mother and fetus for several hours after the procedure. Institute proper protocols for dealing with maternal blood pressure and pulse changes, fetal heart rate abnormalities, uterine activity, vaginal bleeding, or amniotic fluid leakage. Rh-negative mothers should receive Rh_o (D) immune globulin (RhoGAM) unless the fetus is also known to be Rh-negative. Repeat ultrasound studies should be done to check amniotic fluid volume and fetal viability.
2. Instruct patient to report pain, bleeding, infected cannulation site, amniotic fluid leakage, or fever (amnionitis).
3. Interpret test outcomes and counsel appropriately.
4. Follow Chapter 1 guidelines for safe, effective, informed *posttest care.*

PERCUTANEOUS UMBILICAL BLOOD SAMPLING (PUBS) OR CORDOCENTESIS

Normal Values

Normal fetal values.

Explanation of Test

This procedure has somewhat replaced fetoscopy because of fetoscopy risk factors. This test samples blood from the umbilical cord of the fetus in utero, and is probably a safer and easier method for obtaining fetal blood. Research on this procedure is ongoing. Fetal blood can be studied for hemophilias, hemoglobinopathies, fetal infections, chromosomal abnormalities, fetal distress, fetal drug levels, as well as other blood studies.

Procedure

Scanning is done with a linear-array ultrasound device (placed into a sterile glove) to provide landmarks as a 25-gauge spinal needle is first inserted into the maternal abdomen and then guided into the fetal umbilical vein 1 to 2 cm from the cord insertion site on the placenta. The fetal blood sample is aspirated into a syringe containing anticoagulant to prevent clotting of the sample.

> **Clinical Alert**
>
> Risks include transient fetal bradycardia, maternal infection, premature labor, and a 1% to 2% incidence of fetal loss.

Clinical Implications

1. Abnormal blood results reveal
   a. Hemoglobinopathies
   b. Hemophilia
   c. Infection
   d. Chromosomal abnormalities
2. Evidence of fetal distress correlates with abnormal blood levels obtained by this method.

Patient Preparation

1. Explain the procedure, meaning of results, benefits, and risks. Obtain properly signed and witnessed consent form.
2. Assist with relaxation exercises during procedure. Antibiotics may be given pretest to prevent infection.
3. See Chapter 1 for safe, effective *pretest* care.

Patient Aftercare

1. Monitor maternal vital signs and perform external fetal monitoring or nonstress test. Observe for signs of fetal distress.
2. Interpret test outcomes and counsel appropriately.
3. Refer to Chapter 1 guidelines for safe, effective, informed *posttest* care.

CHORIONIC VILLUS SAMPLING (CVS)

Normal Values

Negative for chromosomal and DNA abnormalities; no fetal metabolic enzyme or blood disorders.

Explanation of Test

Chorionic villus sampling (CVS) is a more recently developed procedure that can provide very early diagnosis of fetal genetic or biochemical disorders. CVS involves extracting a small amount of tissue from the villi of the chorion frondosum. This tissue is composed of rapidly proliferating trophoblastic cells that ultimately form the placenta. Although not a part of the fetus, these villi cells are genetically identical with those of the fetus and are considered fetal, rather than maternal, in origin.

Chorionic villus sampling differs from amniocentesis in several respects. In amniocentesis, the cells examined are composed of desquamated fetal cells; on the other hand, CVS cells are viable and easier to culture. Consequently, karyotyping (see Chap. 11 on genetic studies) can be performed on CVS cells much more rapidly. Normally, this provides diagnostic information within 24 hours, much more quickly than that obtained from amniotic fluid cells. Also, CVS can be performed much earlier in pregnancy, typically at 7 to 11 menstrual weeks. Because amniocentesis is generally performed after 16 weeks gestation with results available several weeks later, CVS has the advantage of providing first-trimester diagnosis. This can be of particular value if the choice is made to abort an affected fetus because first-trimester terminations of pregnancy are medically safer.

Chorionic villus sampling reveals chromosomal abnormalities and fetal metabolic or blood disorders. However, because CVS cannot measure alpha$_1$-fetoprotein (AFP) levels, it cannot detect neural tube defects or other disorders associated with elevated AFP levels.

Indications for CVS

1. Advanced maternal age (older than 35 years)
2. Fetus at risk for detectable mendelian disorders
3. Birth of previous child with evidence of chromosomal abnormality
4. Parent with known structural chromosomal rearrangement

Procedure

1. The mother is positioned on her back to permit ultrasound documentation of fetal viability, the number of fetuses in utero, and the localization of trophoblastic tissue. The patient may be asked to either maintain a full bladder or to empty the bladder to optimize the sampling path. A bimanual pelvic exam is often performed concurrently with this preliminary ultrasound examination.
2. The patient then assumes a lithotomy position. A sterile speculum is inserted, after the vagina is cleansed with an iodine-based antiseptic.
3. A sterile flexible catheter with a stainless steel obturator is introduced into the vaginal canal and advanced through the cervical canal into the trophoblastic tissue. The catheter is visually tracked by the ultrasound device.
4. Once the catheter is in place, a syringe is attached to the end of the catheter to extract approximately 5 cm^3 of tissue. The tissue sample is immediately examined under a low-power microscope to determine if both quantity and tissue quality are acceptable.
5. Up to three passes of the catheter may be made. A new, sterile catheter is used each time. After sufficient tissue has been gathered, ultrasound is

again used to monitor fetal viability. The tissue sample is used for chromosomal and enzymatic analysis as well as other tests.

Clinical Implications

Abnormal CVS results indicate

1. Abnormal fetal tissue
2. Chromosomal abnormalities
3. Fetal metabolic and blood disorders

Patient Preparation

1. Genetic counseling typically precedes any CVS procedure.
2. Explain the purpose, procedure, and risks of the test.
3. A legal consent form must be signed by the mother and the father of the baby and must be properly witnessed.
4. The patient must drink four 8-oz. glasses of water about 1 hour before the exam. The patient should not void until instructed to do so.
5. Obtain baseline maternal vital signs and fetal heart rate.
6. Advise the patient that she may experience cramping as the catheter passes through the cervical canal.
7. Help the patient relax.
8. See Chapter 1 guidelines for safe, effective, informed *pretest* care.

Patient Aftercare

1. Monitor maternal vital signs and fetal heart rate every 15 minutes for the first hour after test completion.
2. Instruct the patient to notify her physician if she experiences abdominal pain, vaginal bleeding, or abnormal discharge, elevated temperature, chills, or amniotic fluid leakage.
3. Interpret test outcomes and counsel appropriately. Rh-negative women usually receive RhoGAM.
4. Support the mother and significant others during decision-making. Provide opportunity for questions and discussion.
5. Follow Chapter 1 guidelines for safe, effective, informed *posttest* care.

Clinical Alert

1. At this time, CVS is not considered a routine alternative to amniocentesis. The safety of the CVS procedure is related to the experience and skill of the examiner. In experienced hands, the complication rate and fetal loss are only slightly greater than that for amniocentesis. Risks include leakage of amniotic fluid, bleeding, intrauterine infection, spontaneous abortion, maternal tissue contamination of specimen, Rh isoimmunization, or fetal death (5%).

(continued)

(Clinical Alert continued)

2. Transcervical CVS (as described previously) is difficult in those patients with a fundal placental implantation site or an extremely retroflexed or anteflexed uterus. In these patients, a transabdominal approach similar to that used for amniocentesis is employed.
3. CVS cannot detect neural tube defects or other disorders associated with abnormal maternal serum.
4. Some specialists advise that this procedure be reserved for those conditions that present relatively high genetic risks (such as hemoglobinopathies).

● AMNIOTIC FLUID STUDIES

Amniotic Fluid

The origin of amniotic fluid is not completely understood. It is believed to be primarily a by-product of fetal pulmonary secretions, urine, and metabolic products from the intestinal tract.

Initially, amniotic fluid is produced from the amniotic membrane cells. Later, most of it is derived from the maternal blood. The volume increases from about 30 ml at 2 weeks gestation to 350 ml at 20 weeks gestation. After 20 weeks, the volume ranges from 500 to 1000 ml. There is continuous change in volume of amniotic fluid because of fluid movement in both directions through the placental membrane. Later in pregnancy, the fetus contributes to amniotic fluid volumes through excretion of urine and the swallowing of amniotic fluid. The fetus also absorbs up to 400 ml of amniotic fluid every 24 hours through its gastrointestinal tract, bloodstream, and umbilical artery exchanges across the placenta. Probably, some fluid is also absorbed by direct contact with the fetal surface of the placenta. Amniotic fluid contains cast-off cells from the fetus and resembles extracellular fluid with suspended, undissolved material. It is slightly alkaline and contains albumin, urea, uric acid, creatinine, lecithin, sphingomyelin, bilirubin, fat, fructose, epithelial cells, leukocytic enzymes, and lanugo hair.

AMNIOTIC FLUID ANALYSIS

When amniocentesis is advised early in pregnancy (15 to 18 weeks), it is to study the fetal genetic makeup and to determine developmental abnormalities. Fetal cells are separated from the amniotic fluid by centrifugation and are then placed in a tissue culture medium so that they can be grown and harvested for subsequent karyotyping to identify chromosomal disorders. Testing in the third trimester is done to determine fetal age and well-being, to study blood groups, or to detect amnionitis.

ANMIOCENTESIS

Normal Values

Normal amniotic fluid constituents and properties vary according to age of fetus and laboratory methods. The pH is slightly alkaline. See individual tests.

Explanation of Test

Amniotic fluid is aspirated be means of a needle guided through the mother's abdominal and uterine wall into the amniotic sac. Amniocentesis is preferable done after the 15th week of pregnancy. By this time, amniotic fluid levels have expanded to 150 ml; hence, a 10-ml specimen can safely be aspirated. If amniocentesis is done to ascertain fetal maturity, it should be done after the 35th week of gestation.

Amniocentesis provides a method to detect fetal abnormalities in situations for which the risk of this may be high. The test can evaluate fetal hematologic disorders, fetal infections, inborn errors of metabolism, and can determine potential sex-linked disorders. It is not done to determine the sex of the fetus simply out of curiosity (also, see amniotic fluid analysis description on page 999).

Chromosomal abnormalities and neural tube defects, such as anencephaly, encephalocele, spina bifida, and myelomeningocele, can be determined, as can fetal age estimates, fetal well-being, and pulmonary maturity.

The development of significant maternal Rh antibody titers or a history of previous erythroblastosis can be an indication for amniocentesis.

High-Risk Parents Who Should Be Offered Prenatal Diagnosis

1. Women of advanced maternal age (35 or older) who are at risk for children with chromosomal abnormality, especially trisomy 21 (at maternal age 35 to 40, the risk for Down syndrome is 1% to 3%; at maternal age 40 to 45, there is a 4% to 12% risk; for a maternal age older than 45, the risk is 12% or greater).
2. Women who have previously borne a trisomic child or a child with another kind of chromosomal abnormality.
3. Parents of a child with spina bifida or anencephaly or who have a family history of neural tube disorders.
4. Couples in whom either parent is a known carrier of a balanced translocation chromosome for Down syndrome.
5. Couples in whom both partners are carriers for a diagnosable metabolic or structural autosomal recessive disorder. Presently, over 70 inherited metabolic disorders can be diagnosed by amniotic fluid analysis.
6. Couples in whom either partner or a previous child is affected with a diagnosable metabolic or structural dominant disorder.
7. Women who are presumed carriers of a serious X-linked genetic disorder.

8. Couples from families whose medical history reveals mental retardation, ambiguous genitalia, or parental exposure to toxic environmental agents (drugs, irradiation, infections).
9. Couples whose personal and family medical history reveals multiple miscarriages, stillbirths, or infertility.
10. Anxiety about the health status of potential offspring.
11. Abnormal ultrasound results.

Clinical Implications

1. *Elevated* levels of alpha-fetoprotein (AFP) can indicate possible neural tube defects as well as multiple gestation, fetal death, abdominal wall defects, teratomas, Rh-sensitization, fetal distress, or a normal fetus.
2. New evidence indicates that *decreased* AFP levels are associated with fetal trisomy 21.
3. Creatinine levels are reduced in fetal prematurity. Creatinine levels should be 2 mg/dl of amniotic fluid—at 37 weeks gestation—or greater.
4. Increased or decreased total amniotic fluid volumes are associated with certain types of arrested fetal development.
5. Increased bilirubin levels are associated with impending fetal death (see page 1015 for normal values).
6. Amniotic fluid color changes are associated with fetal distress and other disorders, such as chromosomal abnormalities.
7. Sickle cell anemia and thalassemia can be detected through amniotic fibroblast DNA.
8. X-linked disorders are not routinely diagnosed in utero. However, because these disorders affect only men, the fetal sex may need to be determined when the mother is a known carrier of the X-linked gene in question, as in hemophilia or Duchenne muscular dystrophy.
9. Screening for carrier state or affected fetus is done through chromosomal testing.
10. The presence of some of the over 100 detectable metabolic disorders can be detected in the amniotic fluid sample. Examples of these disorders are Tay-Sachs disease, Lesch-Nyhan syndrome, Hunter's syndrome, Hurler's syndrome, and various hemoglobinopathies. Hereditary metabolic disorders are caused by the absence of an enzyme owing to a gene deletion, by the alteration of an enzyme structure owing to a gene mutation, or through a mutation of the gene that regulates the synthesis of the enzyme. If the enzyme in question is expressed in amniotic fluid cells, it can potentially be used during prenatal diagnosis. Thus, an unaffected fetus would have normal enzyme levels, a clinically normal "carrier" of the mutant gene defect would have approximately half the normal enzyme level, and an *affected* fetus would have very small amounts of or no normal enzyme.
11. For these disorders in which an abnormal protein is not expressed in amniotic fluid cells, other test procedures are necessary, such as *DNA restriction endonuclease analysis*.

Clinical Alert

The in utero diagnosis of many genetic disorders may lead the mother or parents to consider abortion as a viable option to dealing with an unfavorable situation. Because this may be a very difficult choice in light of the controversy surrounding the issue, communication between the patients and the healthcare team needs to take place in a nonjudgmental, nonthreatening manner.

Interfering Factors

1. Fetal blood contamination can cause false-positive levels of AFP.
2. False-negative and false-positive errors in karyotyping can occur.
3. Polyhydramnios may falsely lower bilirubin values by the process of dilution.
4. Hemolysis of the specimen can alter test results.
5. Oligohydramnios may falsely increase some amniotic fluid analytic values, especially bilirubin; this can lead to errors in predicting the clinical status of the fetus.

Procedure (in Combination With Ultrasound)

1. The patient is positioned on her back with arms behind her head to prevent touching the abdomen and the sterile field during the procedure (see Obstetric Ultrasound in Chap. 13).
2. Pretap ultrasound scanning is performed to assess fetal number, viability, and position, An appropriate pocket of amniotic fluid is localized on scan. The tap site should be away from the fetus, the site of umbilical cord insertion, and any thick placental segments.
3. The skin is thoroughly cleansed with an appropriate antiseptic solution and then properly draped with sterile drapes. A local anesthetic is slowly injected at the puncture site.
4. A 3.5-in. spinal needle (20–22 gauge) with stylet is then advanced through the abdominal and uterine walls into the amniotic sac but away from the fetus and, when possible, the placenta. Continuous ultrasound surveillance tracks the position of the fetus. Should the fetus move close to the needle, the needle is withdrawn.
5. Once properly positioned, the stylet is removed from the needle, and a syringe is attached to the needle to permit aspiration of a 20- to 30-ml specimen. The first 0.5 ml of aspirated fluid is discarded to prevent contamination by maternal cells or blood.
6. Once the needle is withdrawn, an adhesive bandage is placed over the puncture site. Posttap ultrasound scanning confirms fetal viability.
7. The amniotic fluid specimen should be placed in a sterile brown or foil-

covered silicone container to protect the fluid from light and to prevent breakdown of bilirubin. Label the container properly. Include estimated weeks of gestation and expected delivery date. Deliver the sample to the laboratory immediately.

8. The laboratory workup for genetic diagnoses usually takes 2 to 4 weeks to complete. However, specimens done for fetal age, such as creatinine, take 1 to 2 hours; L/S ratio and phosphatidyl glycerol take 3 to 4 hours; Gram stain to rule out infection takes 1/2 hour, and cultures take 24 to 48 hours.
9. The procedure may have to be repeated if no amniotic fluid is obtained or if there is failure of cell growth or negative culture results.
10. Record the type of procedure done, date, time, name of physician performing the test, mother–fetal response, and disposition of specimen.

Patient Preparation

1. Elective genetic counseling should include a discussion of the risk of having a genetically defective infant, the risk of a positive test result, and problems (depression and guilt) associated with selective abortion. The father should be present and should be a partner in the decision-making process. In genetic counseling, persons must not be coerced into undergoing abortion or sterilization; this should be an individual choice.
2. Explain the test purpose, procedure, and risks; assess for contraindications to the test.
3. A properly signed and witnessed legal consent form must be obtained.
4. Instruct the patient to empty her bladder just before the test.
5. Obtain baseline fetal and maternal vital signs. Monitor fetal signs for 15 minutes.
6. Alert the patient to short-lived feelings of nausea, vertigo, and mild cramps that may occur during the procedure. Help the patient relax.
7. See Chapter 1 guidelines for safe, effective, informed *pretest* care.

Patient Aftercare

1. Check maternal blood pressure, pulse, respiration, and fetal heart tone every 15 minutes for the first half hour after test completion. Palpate the uterine fundus to assess fetal and uterine activity; monitor with external fetal monitor, if one is available, for 20 to 30 minutes.
2. Position the mother on her left side to counteract supine hypotension and to increase venous return and cardiac output.
3. Instruct the patient to notify her physician if she experiences amniotic fluid loss, signs of onset of labor, redness and inflammation at the insertion site, abdominal pain, bleeding, elevated temperature, chills, unusual fetal activity, or lack of fetal movement.
4. Follow Chapter 1 guidelines for safe, effective, informed *posttest* care.

Clinical Alert

1. Fetal loss attributable to the procedure is less than 0.5%. Repeat amniocentesis is necessary in 0.1% of all amniocentesis procedures.
2. Fetal complications include
   a. Spontaneous abortion
   b. Injury to fetus (fetal puncture)
   c. Hemorrhage
   d. Infection
   e. Rh sensitization if fetal blood enters the mother's circulation
3. Maternal complications include
   a. Hemorrhage
   b. Hematomas
4. This test is contraindicated in women with a history of premature labor or incompetent cervix, or in the presence of *placenta previa* and *abruptio placentae.* If the amniotic fluid is bloody (blood is usually of maternal origin), and if a significant number of fetal cells (Kleihauer Betke positive smear) are present in the amniotic fluid of an Rh-negative mother, the injection of human anti-D globulin (RhoGAM) should be considered. Some doctors prefer to administer RhoGAM to all Rh-negative mothers following amniocentesis, provided they are not already sensitized at that time.
5. Families need to know that prenatal diagnoses based on amniotic fluid assay are not infallible; sometimes, results may not reflect the true fetal status. Findings from amniocentesis cannot guarantee a normal or abnormal child. They can only determine the relative likelihood of specific disorders within the limits of laboratory measurements. Some conditions cannot be predicted by this method (eg, nonspecific mental retardation, cleft lip and palate, and phenylketonuria [PKU]).
6. Accurate and optimally safe results from amniocentesis are possible only if the following protocols are followed:
   a. 15 weeks or longer gestation
   b. Ultrasound monitoring to landmark suitable pools of amniotic fluid, to outline the placenta, to exclude the presence of a multiple pregnancy, and to accurately estimate fetal maturity. These considerations are necessary to correctly interpret AFP levels in amniotic fluid and maternal blood.
   c. Precise and meticulous amniocentesis technique, including use of No. 22 or No. 20 needle.
   d. Maximum of two needle insertion attempts for a single tap.
   e. Administration of anti-D immunoglobulin for the Rh-negative woman.

(continued)

(Clinical Alert continued)

7. Cytogenetic analysis can produce results that are 99.8% accurate.
8. Techniques have been developed for performing amniocentesis in the presence of multiple fetuses. Amniotic fluid must be aspirated from each individual amniotic sac followed by the injection of a small amount of contrast material into one of the sacs. When the adjacent sac is tapped and produces clear amniotic fluid, the clinician is assured that each sac has been tapped. Thus, each fetus will be accurately assessed.
9. An anteriorly located placenta does not preclude amniocentesis. A thin portion of placenta can be traversed during amniocentesis with no apparent increase in postamniocentesis complications.

● ANALYSIS OF AMNIOTIC FLUID

AMNIOTIC FLUID; ALPHA$_1$-FETOPROTEIN (AFP) ●

Normal Values

Values vary considerably according to age of fetus and laboratory methods used. Peak values are reached at 13 to 15 gestational weeks and gradually decline to term.

Background

Alpha$_1$-Fetoprotein (AFP) is synthesized by the embryonic liver and is the major protein (glycoprotein) found in fetal serum. It resembles albumin in molecular weight, amino acid sequence, and immunologic characteristics. However, it is not normally detectable after birth. Ordinarily, high levels of fetoproteins are found in the developing fetus, whereas low levels exist in maternal serum and amniotic fluid.

Explanation of Test

This prenatal amniotic fluid measurement is used to diagnose neural tube defects (malformation of the central nervous system). During those pregnancies in which the fetus has a neural tube defect, fetoprotein leaks into the amniotic fluid and causes elevated levels to be found there. Neural tube defect etiologies are not known; however, a genetic component is assumed because an increased risk of recurrence exists. Neural tube defects usually exhibit polygenic (multifactional) traits. In cases of anencephaly and open spina bifida, both maternal blood and amniotic fluid AFP levels are abnormal by the 18th week of gestation. Additionally, AFP measurements have been used as indicators of fetal distress when it can be increased in both amniotic fluid and maternal serum. However, final confirmation must come from further studies.

Procedure

In the laboratory, amniotic fluid is analyzed for level of alpha$_1$-fetoprotein. Maximum fetal serum concentrations of 2 to 3 mg/ml occur at about 16 weeks gestation and decline steadily to about 0.07 mg/ml by term.

Clinical Implications

Increased amniotic AFP levels are associated with

1. Neural tube defects, such as anencephaly (100% reliable), encephalocele, spina bifida, and myelomeningocele (90% reliable).
2. Congenital Finnish nephrosis
3. Omphalocele
4. Turner's syndrome with cystic hydromas
5. Gastrointestinal tract obstruction
6. Missed abortion
7. Fetal distress
8. Imminent or actual fetal death
9. Severe Rh immunization
10. Esophageal and duodenal atresia
11. Fetal liver necrosis secondary to herpesvirus infection
12. Sacrococcygeal feratoma
13. Spontaneous abortion
14. Trisomy 13
15. Urinary obstruction

Interfering Factors

1. Fetal blood contamination will cause increased AFP levels.
2. Increased AFP levels are associated with multiple pregnancies.
3. Some false-positives (0.1% to 0.2%) are associated with fetal death, twins, or genetic anomalies. Sometimes, no explanation can be given.

Clinical Alert

1. Any couple who has delivered a child with a neural tube defect should be offered antenatal studies in anticipation of future pregnancies. If one parent has spina bifida, the pregnancy should be closely monitored.
2. High-resolution ultrasound studies must confirm elevated AFP levels.

Patient Preparation

1. Explain test purpose and meaning of positive and negative test results.
2. Provide for genetic counseling.
3. See Chapter 1 guidelines for safe, effective, informed *pretest* care.

Patient Aftercare

1. Interpret test outcomes, counsel, and monitor appropriately.
2. Follow Chapter 1 guidelines for safe, effective, informed *posttest* care.

AMNIOTIC FLUID TOTAL VOLUME ●

Normal Values

Average amniotic fluid volumes measure approximately 350 ml at 15 weeks, 450 ml at 20 weeks, 750 ml at 25 weeks, and 1500 ml at 30 to 35 weeks; volume then decreases to 1250 ml at term.

Explanation of Test

Measurement of amniotic fluid total volumes is helpful for estimating the changes in total amounts of certain substances that circulate in the amniotic fluid, including bilirubin pigment, creatinine, and surface-active agents. Knowledge of total amniotic fluid volumes is important because marked changes in amounts of amniotic fluid can decrease the predictive value of serial concentration measurements of specific substances. This measurement is most important when test results do not agree with the clinical picture.

Procedure

1. A sample of amniotic fluid is studied using a solution of *para*-aminohippuric acid (PAH) for absorbency and dilution to calculate probable amniotic fluid volume in milliliters.
2. Corrected levels of amniotic fluid equal measured levels of specific substance times actual volume divided by average volume.

Clinical Implications

1. Polyhydramnios, or increased amniotic fluid (greater than 2000 ml), is suggested by a total intrauterine volume greater than standard deviations above the mean for a given gestational age. It is estimated that 18% to 20% of fetuses in the presence of polyhydramnios will have congenital anomalies; esophageal atresia and anencephaly are the two most common. The remainder of fetuses will have involvement secondary to Rh disease, diabetes, and other unknown causes. Polyhydramnios is also associated with multiple births (eg, twins).
2. Oligohydramnios, or reduced volume of amniotic fluid (less 300 ml), is suggested by a total intrauterine volume value of 2 standard deviations below the mean that is seen before the 25th week of gestation. A distur-

bance of kidney function caused by renal agenesis or kidney atresia may cause oligohydramnios. After this time, premature rupture of membranes, intrauterine growth retardation, and postterm pregnancies are suspected causes of decreased amniotic fluid levels.

Clinical Alert

If either polyhydramnios or oligohydramnios is suspected, the fetus should be screened with ultrasound to detect physical anomalies.

Patient Preparation

1. Explain reason for amniotic fluid testing and meaning of values.
2. See Chapter 1 guidelines for safe, effective, informed *pretest* care.

Patient Aftercare

1. Interpret amniotic fluid test results, counsel, and monitor appropriately.
2. Follow Chapter 1 guidelines for safe, effective, informed *posttest* care.

AMNIOTIC FLUID CREATININE

Normal Values

Values of 1.5 to 2 mg/dl or higher indicate fetal maturity. Values are laboratory dependent.

Background

Creatinine, a by-product of muscle metabolism found in amniotic fluid, reflects increased fetal muscle mass and the ability of the mature kidney (glomerular filtrating system) to excrete creatinine into the amniotic fluid. Amniotic creatinine progressively increases as pregnancy advances. The mother's blood creatinine level should be known before the amniotic fluid creatinine value is interpreted.

Explanation of Test

Creatinine indicates fetal physical maturity and correlates reasonably well with the level of pulmonary maturity. As pregnancy progresses, creatinine levels increase. A value of 2 mg/dl is accepted as an indicator that gestation is at 37 weeks or more. However, the use of this value alone to assess maturity is not advised for several reasons. A high creatinine value may reflect fetal muscle mass but may not necessarily reflect kidney maturity. For example, a macrosmatic fetus of a diabetic mother may have high creatinine levels because of increased muscle mass. Conversely, a small, growth-retarded infant of a hypertensive mother may have low creatinine levels owing to decreased muscle mass. Creatinine levels can be misleading if used without other supporting data. As long as maternal blood creatinine levels are not elevated, amniotic creatinine measurements have a certain degree of reliability if interpreted in conjunction with other maturity studies.

Procedure

1. A 0.5-ml amniotic fluid sample is necessary.
2. Protect the specimen from direct light.

Clinical Implications

1. Decreased creatinine values because of decreased muscle mass are associated with prematurity and small, growth-retarded infants delivered of hypertensive mothers.
2. Creatinine levels lower than expected may be due to
   a. Early gestational cycle
   b. Fetus smaller than normal
   c. Fetal kidney abnormalities

Interfering Factors

1. A chance of falling within the 5% false-positive result area.
2. Causes of elevated amniotic fluid creatinine levels that are not consistent with gestational age include abnormal maternal creatinine, diabetes, and preeclampsia.

Patient Preparation

1. Explain creatinine test purpose.
2. See Chapter 1 guidelines for safe, effective, informed *pretest* care.

Patient Aftercare

1. Interpret creatinine test outcomes and counsel about fetal maturity.
2. Follow Chapter 1 guidelines for safe, effective, informed *posttest* care.

AMNIOTIC FLUID LECITHIN/SPHINGOMYELIN RATIO (L/S) (SURFACTANT COMPONENTS) ●

Normal Values

A ratio of 2:1 or greater indicates pulmonary maturity: 1:2 dilution on shake test indicates lung maturity.

Background

Lecithin and sphingomyelin have detergent activity. These substances, produced by lung tissue, stabilize the neonatal alveoli to prevent their collapse on expiration, and thereby, to prevent consequential atelectasis. The amount of lecithin in amniotic fluid will be less than the amount of sphingomyelin until 26 weeks gestation; at 30 to 32 weeks gestation, the two lipid values are about equal. At 35 weeks, lecithin levels rise abruptly, but sphingomyelin levels stay constant or decrease slightly. Saturated phosphatidylcholine, a subfraction of total lecithins, is a major surface-active component of lung surfactant.

Explanation of Test

The relation between the phospholipids and the surface-active agents, lecithin and sphingomyelin, is used as an index of fetal lung maturity. If early delivery is anticipated because of conditions such as diabetes, premature rupture of membranes, maternal hypertension, placental insufficiency, or erythroblastosis, the L/S ratio value can be used to predict whether a mature fetal lung might function properly at birth. Unfortunately, early delivery may be necessary for fetal viability. Consequently, the birth may result in prematurity, pulmonary immaturity, or perinatal mortality. The L/S ratio should be performed on all repeat cesarean sections before delivery to determine when fetal lungs are functionally mature. Sphiromyelin exhibits surface-active properties in the lung but plays no role in the surfactant system, except to be used as a convenient marker.

Procedure

At least 3 ml of amniotic fluid is withdrawn. The fluid is then centrifuged, prepared for analysis, and the results are read in a reflectance spectrodensitometer. The ratio of lecithin and sphingomyelin is then calculated.

Clinical Implications

1. Decreased L/S ratios are often associated with pulmonary immaturity and respiratory distress syndrome (RDS).
2. An L/S ratio greater than 2:1 signifies fetal lung maturity; occurrence of RDS is extremely unlikely.
3. An L/S ratio of 1.5 to 1.9:1 indicates possible mild to moderate RDS.
4. An L/S ratio of 1 to 1.49:1 indicates immaturity of the fetal lungs with moderate to severe RDS.
5. An L/S ratio of less than 1 indicates severe RDS.

Clinical Alert

1. If the L/S ratio is less than 1.2:1, it is preferable to delay induced delivery until the fetal lung becomes more mature.
2. Fetal lung maturity appears to be regulated by hormonal factors, some stimulatory and others possibly inhibitory. Consequently, hormones such as betamethasone (Celestone) are given in 12-mg dosages for two doses, administered 12 to 18 hours apart, if premature labor occurs.
3. Under certain stressful conditions, premature fetal lung maturation may be seen. These include

(continued)

(Clinical Alert continued)

   a. Premature rupture of the membranes. (Prolonged rupture of the membranes [after 72 hours] has an acute effect on lung maturation.)
   b. Acute placental infarction
   c. Placental insufficiency
   d. Chronic *abruptio placentae*
   e. Renal hypertensive disease caused by degenerative forms of diabetes
   f. Cardiovascular hypertensive disease associated with drug abuse
   g. Severe pregnancy-induced hypertension

   This accelerated fetal lung maturation is thought to be a protective mechanism for preterm fetus should delivery actually occur.

4. Delayed fetal lung maturation may be seen in
   a. Infants born to mothers having class A, B, and C diabetes
   b. Infants born to mothers having nonhypertensive glomerulonephritis
   c. Hydrops fetalis

   In these instances, no higher L/S ratio (3:1) may be necessary to ensure adequate fetal lung maturity.

5. A lung profile of amniotic fluid to evaluate lung maturity looks not only for lecithin but also for two other phospholipids—phosphatidylglycerol (PG) and phosphatidylinositol (PI). Phosphatidylinositol increases in the amniotic fluid after 26 to 30 weeks gestation, peaks at 35 to 36 weeks, and then decreases gradually. Phosphatidylglycerol appears after 35 weeks and continues to increase until term. Results are classified as positive PG or negative PG. The lung profile is a useful adjunct to evaluating L/S ratio. It appears that lung maturity can be confirmed in most pregnancies if the PG is present in conjunction with an L/S ratio of 2:1. The PG may provide stability that makes the infant less susceptible to respiratory distress syndrome when experiencing hypoglycemia, hypoxia, or hypothermia. Research using PI in the same manner as PG is being carried out. The PG measurement is especially useful in borderline cases and in class A, B, and C diabetes in which pulmonary maturation is delayed.

Interfering Factors

1. High false-negative rates
2. Unpredictability or borderline values
3. Unpredictability of contaminated blood specimens
4. Occasional false-positive values associated with conditions such as Rh diseases, diabetes, or severe birth asphyxia

Patient Preparation

1. Explain reason for testing and meaning of values.
2. See Chapter 1 guidelines for safe, effective, informed *pretest* care.

Patient Aftercare

1. Interpret test results and counsel appropriately.
2. Follow Chapter 1 guidelines for safe, effective, informed *posttest* care.

AMNIOTIC FLUID SHAKE TEST ●

Normal Values

A 1:2 dilution on shake test indicates lung maturity.

The shake test is a qualitative measurement of the amount of pulmonary surfactant contained in the amniotic fluid. It is quick and inexpensive. It is a "bedside test" of lung maturity. In an obstetric emergency, an immediate decision about delivery can be made. The advantage of this test over the L/S ratio is that a physician, technician, or nurse can perform it, and results are highly reliable. The L/S ratio is normally not done when the shake test is positive because the shake test also indicates fetal maturity. A table of dilutions is used to determine stages of lung maturity.

Procedure

The test is based on the ability of amniotic fluid surfactant to form a complete ring of bubbles on the surface of the amniotic fluid in the presence of 95% ethanol. Exact amounts of 95% ethanol, isotonic saline, and amniotic fluid are placed in an appropriate container and shaken together for 15 seconds.

Clinical Implications

1. A complete ring of bubble formation indicates a positive test.
2. No ring of bubble formation indicates a negative test.
3. The test produces a high false-negative rate but a low false-positive rate.

Interfering Factors

Blood or meconium contamination can alter results.

AMNIOTIC FLUID FOAM STABILITY INDEX (FSI) ●

The foam stability index (FSI) is similar to the shake test. In this test, 0.5 ml of amniotic fluid is added to various amounts of 95% ethanol. The sample is then shaken and observed for foam, which indicates maturity. This test seems as reliable as the L/S ratio in normal pregnancy and seems to have a lower false-positive rate than the shake test.

Procedure

A fixed amount of undiluted amniotic fluid is mixed with increasing volumes of ethanol, and the largest volume of ethanol in which the amniotic fluid can foam and support foam is documented.

Clinical Implications
An FSI of 0.48 or greater is termed *mature;* 0.46 or less is *immature.*

Interfering Factors
Blood or meconium contamination can produce a false "mature" result.

AMNIOTIC FLUID FERN TEST

Normal Value
Positive test for amniotic fluid.

Background
Fern production is the result of electrolyte activity in the cervical glands and is under the control of estrogen. Close to term, amniotic fluid shows a typical fern pattern, similar to that seen in cervical mucus, that indicates a predominantly estrogen effect; urine will not produce a fern pattern.

Explanation of Test
This study differentiates urine from amniotic fluid. It is done to determine whether the fluid passed is urine or prematurely leaked amniotic fluid.

Procedure
1. A vaginal examination is done using a sterile speculum.
2. A few drops of fluid are placed on a slide.

Clinical Implications
1. A positive test shows the fern pattern, indicative of amniotic fluid.
2. A negative test shows no ferning or crystallization; this indicates little or no estrogen effect.
3. No fern pattern is seen if the specimen is urine.

Interfering Factors
Blood contaminating the specimen inhibits fern formation.

> **Clinical Alert**
>
> Urine can also be differentiated from amniotic fluid when the fluid is tested for urea, potassium, absence of AFP, and by odor and appearance.

Patient Preparation
1. Explain test purpose and procedure.
2. See Chapter 1 guidelines for safe, effective, informed *pretest* care.

Patient Aftercare

1. Interpret test results and counsel appropriately.
2. Follow Chapter 1 guidelines for safe, effective, informed *posttest* care.

AMNIOTIC FLUID COLOR

Normal Values

Amniotic fluid is colorless or a pale, straw yellow.

Explanation of Test

Amniotic fluid specimens may vary from no color to a pale straw yellow. White particles of vernix caseosa from fetal skin and lanugo hair may be present. Certain disorders, such as missed abortion, chromosomally abnormal fetus, and fetal anencephaly will alter amniotic fluid color.

Procedure

Every amniotic fluid specimen should be visually inspected for color.

Clinical Implications

1. *Yellow* amniotic fluid indicates blood incompatibility, erythroblastosis fetalis, or presence of bile pigment released from red blood cell hemolysis (fetal bilirubin).
2. *Dark yellow* aspirate indicates probable fetal involvement.
3. *Red* indicates blood. In this instance, it must be determined whether the blood is from the mother or the fetus. If fetal, there is cause for grave concern.
4. *Green opaque* fluid indicates meconium contamination. The fetus passes meconium because of hyperperistalsis in response to a stressor that may be very transient or may be more serious and protracted, such as hypoxia. A very good correlation states that the more meconium present, the more severe and immediate the stressor. Additional assessments, such as amnioscopy and amniography, must be made to determine if the fetus is suffering ongoing episodes of hypoxia or other stressors. A green color can also indicate erythroblastosis but is not necessarily indicative of it.
5. *Yellow-brown opaque* fluid may indicate intrauterine death and fetal maceration (although not necessarily from erythroblastosis), oxidized hemoglobin, or maternal trauma.

Clinical Alert

1. Before the amniotic membranes have ruptured, color changes and staining can be observed through amnioscopy. During this procedure, an amnioscope is placed into the vagina and against the fetal presenting part. The amniotic fluid is then visualized through the

(continued)

(Clinical Alert continued)
amniotic membranes. Problems with amnioscopy include inadvertent rupturing of membranes, insufficient dilation of the cervix and difficulty with inserting the amnioscope, intrauterine infection, and occasional difficulty in interpreting amniotic fluid color. The test may also be difficult to perform if the patient is in active labor.

2. Meconium staining also may be observed when an amniocentesis is done. After the membranes have ruptured, meconium staining may be observed in the vaginal discharge. Once meconium staining is identified, more assessments (such as fetal heart rate patterns) must be made before delivery is contemplated to determine if the fetus is suffering ongoing episodes of hypoxia.
3. The presence of meconium in the amniotic fluid is normal in breech presentations.

Patient Preparation

1. Explain test purpose and procedure if amnioscopy is done.
2. See Chapter 1 guidelines for safe, effective, informed *pretest* care.

Patient Aftercare

1. Interpret color changes, monitor, and counsel appropriately.
2. Follow Chapter 1 guidelines for safe, effective, informed *posttest* care.

AMNIOTIC FLUID BILIRUBIN OPTICAL DENSITY (OD) ●

Normal Values

An OD of 0.02 or less indicates maturity; less than 0.28 mg/dl or a 1+ is normal to slightly affected.

Background

Bilirubin is a pigment acquired by the amniotic fluid during its circulation through the gastrointestinal tract. It is not excreted by the mother, as is fetal serum bilirubin. Bilirubin may be found in amniotic fluid as early as the 12th week of gestation. It reaches its highest concentration between 16 and 30 weeks. As the pregnancy continues, the amount of bilirubin progressively decreases and finally disappears near term. Bilirubin levels increase in the presence of erythroblastotic fetuses and fetuses with anencephaly or intestinal obstruction.

Explanation of Test

This measurement is used to monitor the fetal state in an Rh_0-negative pregnant woman who has a rising anti-Rh_0 antibody titer. The rising titer is synonymous with Rh erythroblastosis fetalis, or hemolytic disease of the newborn (HDN). This determination is usually not made before 20 to 24 weeks gestation because no therapy is available for the fetus before that time. Close to term, amniotic fluid bilirubin pigment concentration will normally decrease in the absence of Rh sensitization.

Optical density is a laboratory method of measuring bilirubin. It is reported as the deviation ([t404]D[rt]) or difference between the expected and plotted curves on a spectrophotometer. Optical density levels can be interpreted by realizing that a value of 0.1 [t404]D[rt]OD (deviation of optical density) corrected will correspond to approximately 0.14 mg/dl of bilirubin. The degree of hemolytic disease falls into three zones:

1. If the optical density falls into zone 1 (low zone) at 28 to 31 weeks, the fetus will not be affected or will have very mild hemolytic disease.
2. If the optical density falls into zone 2 (midzone), there is moderate effect on the fetus. The fetal age and the trend in optical density indicate the need for intrauterine transfusion and premature delivery.
3. If the optical density falls into zone 3 (high zone), the fetus is severely affected, and fetal death is a possibility. In this case, a decision concerning delivery or intrauterine transfusion, dependent on fetal age should be made. After 32 to 33 weeks of gestation, early delivery and extrauterine treatment are preferred methods of treatment.

Procedure

1. A 2- to 10-ml sample of amniotic fluid should be collected in a lightproof container.
2. The fluid should be sent to the laboratory immediately.
3. The specimen may be refrigerated for up to 24 hours. It can be frozen if a longer time will elapse before analysis.
4. Avoid blood in the specimen. If initial aspiration produces a bloody fluid, the needle should be repositioned to obtain a specimen free of red cells. If unable to obtain a blood-free specimen, the specimen must be examined at once before hemolysis occurs.

Clinical Implications

1. A Δ OD greater than 0.04 indicates prematurity.
2. A value of 0.28 to 0.46 is 2+, zone 1; the fetus is affected by hemolytic disease but is not in danger. Amniocentesis should be repeated in 2 to 3 weeks.
3. A value of 0.47 is 3+, zone 2; the fetus is moderately affected and in danger. Amniocentesis is repeated frequently so trends can be determined.
4. A value of 0.95 is 4+, zone 3; it indicates impending fetal death.

Interfering Factors

Blood or meconium in the specimen can produce inaccurate results.

Clinical Alert

1. Difficulty in interpretation occurs if the measurement is between 0.03 and 0.04 or if the bilirubin concentration unexpectedly decreases early in pregnancy.
2. If the bilirubin level fails to decline as expected or the level increases, the fetal status is deteriorating.

Patient Preparation

1. Explain test purpose and meaning of test results.
2. See Chapter 1 guidelines for safe, effective, informed *pretest* care.

Patient Aftercare

1. Interpret test outcomes, monitor, and counsel appropriately.
2. Follow Chapter 1 guidelines for safe, effective, informed *posttest* care.

CYTOLOGIC EXAMINATION OF FETAL CELLS FOR MATURITY (LIPIDS)

Normal Values

Interpretive reports: The percentage of fat cells increases as the fetus matures.

Explanation of Test

This determination of fetal maturity is done by staining fetal fat cells from the amniotic fluid with Nile blue sulfate. The fetus sheds cells during its intrauterine life. In the last weeks of pregnancy, the sebaceous glands begin to function. These cells, with their lipid globules, slough into the amniotic fluid. The numbers of these fat cells increases as the fetus matures; thus, the percentage of these cells present in the amniotic fluid gives an indication of gestational age.

Procedure

An amniotic fluid specimen is obtained and examined.

Clinical Implications

1. When the number of sebaceous cells is fewer than 2%, the prematurity rate is 85%.
2. If more than 20% of cells in the fluid stain orange, the infant should weigh at lease 2500 g and have a gestational age of 35 weeks or greater.
3. If fewer than 10% of cells in the fluid stain orange, the gestational age is less than 35 weeks.

Patient Preparation

1. Explain test purpose and amniotic fluid sampling procedure.
2. See Chapter 1 guidelines for safe, effective, informed *pretest* care.

Patient Aftercare

1. Interpret test outcomes, monitor, and counsel appropriately.
2. Follow Chapter 1 guidelines for safe, effective, informed *posttest* care.

BIBLIOGRAPHY

Cohen S, Kenner CA, Hollingsworth A: Maternal, Neonatal, and Women's Health Nursing. Springhouse Corporation, 1991

Cunningham G, MacDonald P, Gant N, Gilstrap W III: Obstetrics, 19th ed. Norwalk, CT, Appleton & Lange, 1993

Elias S, Simpson JL (eds): alpha-Fetoprotein and Other Maternal Serum Markers for Detecting Fetal Genetic Disorders. New York, Churchill Livingstone, 1992

Fletcher MA, MacDonald MG (eds): Atlas of Procedures in Neonatology. Philadelphia, JB Lippincott, 1993

Gebauer C, Lowe N: The biophysical profile: Antepartal assessment of fetal well-being. JOGNN, Mar-Apr: 115–124, 1993

May KA, Mahlmeister LR: Maternal and Neonatal Nursing. Family-Centered Care, 3rd ed. JB Lippincott, Philadelphia, 1994

Olds S, London M, Ladewig P: Maternal–Newborn Nursing, A Family Centered Approach, 4th ed. Benjamin/Cummings Publishing, 1992

Tietz NW: Fundamentals of Clinical Chemistry, 4th ed. WB Saunders, 1992

Tyrell O, Lilford: Umbilical artery doppler velocimetry as a predictor of fetal hypoxia and acidosis at birth. *Obstet Gynecol* Sept: 332–336, 1989

APPENDICES

APPENDIX I

Examples of Conversions to Systéme International (SI) Units

Component	*System*	*Present Reference Intervals*	*Present Unit*	*Conversion Factor*	*SI Reference Intervals*	*SI Unit Symbol*
Alanine aminotransferase (ALT)	Serum	5–40	U/L	1.00	5–40	U/L
Albumin	Serum	3.9–5.0	mg/dl	10	39–50	g/L
Alkaline phosphatase	Serum	35–110	U/L	1.00	35–110	U/L
Aspartate aminotransferase (AST)	Serum	5–40	U/L	1.00	5–40	U/L
Bilirubin	Serum					
Direct		0–0.2	mg/dL	17.10	0–4	μmol/L
Total		0.1–1.2	mg/dL	17.10	2–20	μmol/L
Calcium	Serum	8.6–10.3	mg/dL	0.2495	2.15–2.57	mmol/L
Carbon dioxide, total	Serum	22–30	mEq/L	1.00	22–30	mmol/L
Chloride	Serum	98–108	mEq/L	1.00	98–108	mmol/L
Cholesterol	Serum					
Age <29 yr		<200	mg/dl	0.02586	<5.15	mmol/L
30–39 yr		<225	mg/dl	0.02586	<5.80	mmol/L
40–49 yr		<245	mg/dl	0.02586	<6.35	mmol/L
>50 yr		<265	mg/dl	0.02586	<6.85	mmol/L
Complete blood count	Blood					
Hematocrit						
Men		42–52	%	0.01	0.42–0.52	1
Women		37–47	%	0.01	0.37–0.47	1

Red cell count Men		$4.6–6.2 \times 10^6$	$/mm^3$	10^6	$4.6–6.2 \times 10^{12}/L$	
Women		$4.2–5.4 \times 10^6$	$/mm^3$	10^6	$4.2–5.4 \times 10^{12}/L$	
White cell count		$4.5–11.0 \times 10^3$	$/mm^3$	10^6	$4.5–11.0 \times 10^9/L$	
Platelet count		$150–300 \times 10^3$	$/mm^3$	10^6	$150–300 \times 10^9/L$	
Cortisol 8AM	Serum	5–25	μg/dl	27.59	140–690	nmol/L
8PM		3–13	μg/dl	27.59	80–360	nmol/L
Cortisol	Urine	20–90	μg/24 hr	2.759	55–250	nmol/24 hr
Creatine kinase High CK group (black men)	Serum	50–250	U/L	1.00	50–520	U/L
Intermediate CK group (nonblack men, black women)		35–345	U/L	1.00	35–345	U/L
Low CK group (nonblack women)		25–145	U/L	1.00	25–145	U/L
Creatinine kinase isoenzyme, MB fraction	Serum	>5	%	0.01	>0.05	1
Creatinine Men	Serum	0.4–1.3 0.7–1.3	mg/dl mg/dl	88.40 88.40	35–115	μmol/L
Women		0.4–1.1	mg/dl	88.40		
Digoxin, therapeutic	Serum	0.5–2.0	ng/ml	1.281	0.6–2.6	nmol/L
Erythrocyte indices Mean corpuscular volume (MCV)	Blood	80–100	$microns^3$	1.00	80–100	fL
Mean corpuscular hemoglobin (MCH)		27–31	pg	1.00	27–31	pg
Mean corpuscular hemoglobin concentration (MCHC)		32–36	%	0.01	0.32–0.36	1

(continued)

Examples of Conversions to Systéme International (SI) Units (*Continued*)

Component	*System*	*Present Reference Intervals*	*Present Unit*	*Conversion Factor*	*SI Reference Intervals*	*SI Unit Symbol*
Ferritin	Serum					
Men		29–438	ng/ml	1.00	29–438	μg/L
Women		9–219	ng/ml	1.00	9–219	μg/L
Folate	Serum	2.5–20.0	ng/ml	2.266	6–46	nmol/L
Follicle-stimulating hormone (FSH)	Serum					
Children		12 or <	mIU/ml	1.00	12 or <	IU/L
Men		2.0–10.0	mIU/ml	1.00	2.0–10.0	IU/L
Women, follicular		3.2–9.0	mIU/ml	1.00	3.2–9.0	IU/L
Women, midcycle		3.2–9.0	mIU/ml	1.00	3.2–9.0	IU/L
Women, luteal		2.0–6.2	mIU/ml	1.00	2.0–6.2	IU/L
Gases, arterial	Blood					
Po_2		80–95	mm Hg	0.1333	10.7–12.7	kPa
Pco_2		37–43	mm Hg	0.1333	4.9–5.7	kPa
Glucose	Serum	62–110	mg/dl	0.05551	3.4–6.1	mmol/L
Iron	Serum	50–160	μg/dl	0.1791	9–29	μmol/L
Iron-binding capacity	Serum					
TIBC		230–410	μg/dl	0.1791	41–73	μmol/L
Saturation		15–55	%	0.01	0.15–0.55	1
Lactic dehydrogenase	Serum	120–300	U/L	1.00	120–300	U/L
Luteinizing hormone	Serum					
Men		4.9–15.0	mIU/ml	1.00	4.9–15.0	IU/L
Women, follicular		5.0–25	mIU/ml	1.00	5.0–25	IU/L

Women, luteal		3.1–13	mIU/ml	1.00	3.1–31	IU/L
Magnesium	Serum	1.2–1.9	mEq/L	0.4114	0.50–0.78	mmol/L
Osmolality	Serum	278–300	mOsm/kg	1.00	278–300	mmol/kg
Osmolality	Urine	None defined	mOsm/kg	1.00	None defined	mmol/kg
Phenobarbital, therapeutic	Serum	15–40	μg/ml	4.306	65–175	μmol/L
Phenytoin, therapeutic	Serum	10–20	μg/ml	3.964	40–80	μmol/L
Phosphate (phosphorus, inorganic)	Serum	2.3–4.1	mg/dl	0.3229	0.75–1.35	mmol/L
Potassium	Serum	3.7–5.1	mEq/L g/ml	1.00	3.7–5.1	mmol/L
Protein, total	Serum	6.5–8.3	g/dl	10.0	65–83	g/L
Sodium	Serum	134–142	mEq/L	1.00	134–142	mmol/L
Theophylline, therapeutic	Serum	5–20	μg/ml	5.550	28–110	μmol/L
Thyroid-stimulating hormone (TSH)	Serum	0–5	μIU/ml	1.00	0–5	mIU/L
Thyroxine	Serum	4.5–13.2	μg/dl	12.87	58–170	nmol/L
T_3-uptake ratio	Serum	0.88–1.19	1	1.00	0.88–1.19	1
Triiodothyronine (T_3)	Serum	70–235	ng/ml	0.01536	1.1–3.6	nmol/L
Triglycerides	Serum	50–200	mg/dl	0.01129	0.55–2.25	mmol/L
Urate (uric acid)	Serum					
Men		2.9–8.5	mg/dl	59.48	170–510	μmol/L
Women		2.2–6.5	mg/dl	59.48	130–390	μmol/L
Urea nitrogen	Serum	6–25	mg/dl	0.3570	2.1–8.9	mmol/L
Vitamin B_{12}	Serum	250–1000	pg/ml	0.7378	180–740	pmol/L

(Blair ER et al (eds): Damon Clinical Laboratories Handbook. Lexi-Comp, Inc., Stow OH, 1989).

APPENDIX II

Latex/Rubber Allergy Precautions

Allergies to latex and rubber products are becoming more common in patients and healthcare workers. Therefore, measures to maximize a latex-free environment and minimize risk for susceptible individuals are mandatory. Patients with a history of spina bifida and repeated exposure to latex products, such as catheters, gloves or balloons, appear to exhibit more sensitivity and reactivity. Additionally, some healthcare workers have developed such severe sensitivity that they are no longer able to practice in a traditional healthcare setting in which latex products are used. The following list addresses some basic precautions that should be taken when dealing with a known or suspected latex allergy.

1. Question the patient about latex allergy history. Assess for signs and symptoms, such as rash, red and swollen areas on the skin, welts, eye irritation, dyspnea, itching, and chest pain. Severe allergic reactions can progress to anaphylactic shock quite rapidly. Other individuals exhibit symptoms different from what one might expect, such as hypertension and tachycardia.
2. Post **"Latex Allergy Precautions"** signs that are readily visible to all healthcare workers. "Flag" the chart. Schedule invasive procedures early in the day, if possible, when environmental latex allergen exposure should pose less risk.
3. Avoid use of latex or rubber supplies or equipment. If unsure of product, verify with manufacturer, supplier, or central supply of the institution.
4. Latex-free products include items made of clear plastic, vinyl, silicone, and silk. Use Velcro tourniquets. Transfer enema contents from Fleet kit to soap suds plastic enema bag.
5. Put on double vinyl gloves during invasive procedures. Persons caring for latex-allergic patients need to wear freshly laundered uniforms or scrubs that have not yet been exposed to other patients' latex products.
6. Use nonlatex gloves, endotracheal tubes, suction equipment and supplies, drainage tubes, adhesive tape, wound drains, tourniquets, temperature probe covers, and catheters for all procedures. Use latex-free blood pressure cuffs. If not available, put stockinette over patient's arm before applying cuff. Sphygmometer tubing can be shielded with adhesive tape if necessary. Remove rubber stoppers from vials before reconstituting medication or using diluent such as sterile water for injection or normal saline for injection. Do not draw medication through rubber stoppers.
7. Rinse syringes with sterile water or sterile saline before use. Remove latex

Frances Fischbach: A MANUAL OF LABORATORY & DIAGNOSTIC TESTS, Fifth Edition.

ports from IV tubing and replace with stopcocks or nonlatex plugs if latex-free tubing is not available.

8. Keep resuscitation equipment and emergency supplies accessible at all times in the event of severe allergic reaction or anaphylaxis.

9. In the acute care setting, all latex-containing products should be removed from the patient's environment. If possible, the patient should be assigned to a private room.

APPENDIX III

Example of Consent for Human Immunodeficiency Virus (HIV) Antibody Testing

I have asked or been asked to have my blood tested for antibodies to the HIV (human immunodeficiency virus), the virus that causes AIDS. It has been explained to me that the test is for HIV infection. It is not a test for AIDS. If I do have antibodies to the virus (a POSITIVE test), this means that I have been infected with the virus. If I do not have antibodies (a NEGATIVE test), but am in a group of persons who are at high risk for AIDS (persons who have had multiple sex partners or who share needles when using drugs), this does not mean that I will not become infected in the future. In fact, I may already be infected, but have not yet had time to develop antibodies.

I have been told that the blood tests for antibodies to the virus are not foolproof. In a small number of persons, other things such as another virus or disease may wrongly cause a positive test. This is called a false-positive test. It is also possible to have a false-negative test. In this case, I do have the antibodies to the virus, but the test did not show this. If the first test on my blood is positive, the test will be repeated. If positive again, a different test will be conducted. These tests will all be done on the blood taken after I sign this consent.

I have been told that HIV is spread through the blood from an infected person. It is also spread by having sex with an infected person. I understand that if my test is positive, I can spread the infection to others. I must not give blood or plasma or donate my organs or sperm if I am positive.

If I have a positive test, I should explain this to any sexual partner. If I am unable to tell my spouse or any other sexual partner whom I have identified, my doctor or counselor may do so but only to protect their health.

If I have a positive test, my case may be reported to public health agencies. However, the public health staff may use or give out only that information for the public health purpose for which it was given. Otherwise, information about my HIV testing cannot be revealed to anyone outside the VA without my written permission, or, a court order, a medical emergency, for research, Congressional oversight, or audit purposes, or for medical treatment provided to me by the Armed Forces.

Frances Fischbach: A MANUAL OF LABORATORY & DIAGNOSTIC TESTS, Fifth Edition.

I have been told that the results of my test (positive or negative) will be in my medical record. I understand that any VA employee who improperly releases information about my HIV testing is subject to a fine. Even though I understand every effort will be made to protect the results of my test, I also understand that disclosure of a positive test result can lead to discrimination in housing, jobs, and other areas in some communities.

I have been counseled abut the HIV test and have been given a chance to ask questions. I understand that the test is voluntary and that I will still receive care from the VA if I refuse to have the test done.

Therefore, I give my permission for my blood to be tested for HIV antibodies.

______________________________________ _______________
PATIENT OR LEGAL GUARDIAN DATE

______________________________________ _______________
WITNESS DATE

(Veterans Administration, Form 10-0121, Dec 1988)

APPENDIX IV

Intravenous Conscious Sedation Precautions

Increasing numbers of patients in ambulatory and hospital settings are receiving short-term intravenous conscious sedation for diagnostic procedures. Keep in mind the following guidelines when caring for these patients:

1. Provide a safe and caring environment.
2. Assess total patient care requirements during IV conscious sedation and recovery (age, health status, disease states, history, and physical diagnostic test results). Screen and identify patients at high risk for developing complications.
3. Recognize physiologic effects of agents used for IV conscious sedation. These include: meperidine (Demerol), diazepam (Valium), midazolam (Versed), droperidol (Inapsine), fentanyl; other combinations of medications. Be especially watchful of respiratory status because many of these drugs are respiratory depressants. If oxygen saturation drops below 90%, sedatives may need to be held or reversed. Have IV reversal agents, naloxone (Narcan) and Flumazenil (Romazicon) readily available. Oxygen therapy may be necessary until SaO_2 levels, vital signs, and cardiac rhythms are acceptable.
4. Anticipate and monitor for potential complications of IV conscious sedation. Arrhythmias should be promptly reported and treated if necessary. Monitor IV site as well as the general effects of medications given.
5. Rapidly and appropriately respond to emergencies during administration of, or recovery from, IV conscious sedation. Have resuscitative equipment, drugs, and supplies immediately available.
6. Ongoing assessment parameters during the procedures and recovery include pulse oximetry, cardiac monitoring, vital signs, and neurologic checks, if indicated. Evaluate readiness for discharge.
7. Provide both verbal and written *pretest* and relevant *posttest* instructions.

APPENDIX V

Table of Trace Minerals

Substance Tested (Specimen Needed, Reference Range [RR], and Critical Range [CR])	Clinical Significance of Values
ALUMINUM	
(Serum) RR: 0.4 μg/dl or 0.15 μmol/L	*Increase:* excessive occupational exposure, lung diseases, Shaver's disease (abrasives from aluminum oxide) *Toxicity not seen* normally, except in renal failure, when aluminum-containing antacids are used; long-term intermittent dialysis
ANTIMONY	
(Urine [24 hr/dl]) RR: <50 μg/L CR: >1 mg/L	*Increase:* excessive occupational exposure (ore mining, bronze, ceramic)
ARSENIC	
(Blood [20 ml]) (Urine [24 hr/50 ml]) (Hair [0.5 g]) (Nails) RR Blood: <3 μg/dl RR Urine: <100 μg/L/d CR Urine: <850 μg/L/d RR Hair: <65 μg/dl CR Hair: >100 μg/dl RR Nails: 90–180 μg/100 g	*Increase:* accidental or intentional poisoning. Excessive occupational exposure (ceramics, agriculture)
BERYLLIUM	
(Urine [24 hr]) RR: 0.05 μg/d CR: >20 μg/L or >2.22 μmol/L	*Increase:* excessive occupational exposure (metal extraction, refinery, rocket base, nuclear plants, extensive coal burning). Acute lung irritation, pneumonitis, berylliosis, secondary polycythemia
TRACE MINERALS	
CHROMIUM (CR)	
(plasma) 0.3 μg/L	*Decrease:* insulin resistance; impaired glucose RR: zero tolerance; increased risk CHD, hypercholesterolemia

(continued)

Substance Tested (Specimen Needed, Reference Range [RR], and Critical Range [CR])	***Clinical Significance of Values***
	Increase: excessive industrial exposure (carcinogenic); renal damage
COBALT (CO) (part of the vitamin B_{12} molecule) (plasma) RR: 0.007–6 μg/dl 0.1–0.4 ng/ml	*Decrease:* cobalamin (vitamin B12) deficiency *Increase*: cardiomyopathy after industrial exposure, during maintenance dialysis, and after drinking beer contaminated with cobalt during processing
COPPER (CU) (serum, 3 ml) RR: Total 100–200 μg/dl 16–31 μmol/L (urine, 24 hr) RR: 0–100 μg/d 0–1.6 μmol/d (plasma)	*Decrease:* rheumatoid arthritis; Menke's steely hair disease: lack of pigmentation of skin and hair; collagen abnormalities, osteoporosis; ataxia; hypochromic anemia unresponsive to iron therapy; hypercholesterolemia; impaired cardiovascular system; altered interleukin-2 production *Increase:* T-cell proliferation; hepatic GSH (glutathione); Wilson's disease (hepatolenticular degeneration); ingestion of solutions of copper salts; contaminated water or dialysis fluids; Indian childhood cirrhosis; female rheumatoid arthritis; oral contraceptive use; inflammatory conditions, cancer at injection sites or muscles *Toxicity:* hepatic or renal failure *Lethal dose:* 50–500 mg/kg body weight
FLUORINE (F) (fluoride) (plasma) RR: 20–100 μg/dl 200–1000 ng/ml	*Decrease:* marginal to deficient dietary intake from deficiencies in geochemical environments; dental caries; skeletal changes, especially in long bones *Increase:* fluorosis (excess fluorine use: >4 million ppm in water, treatment of osteoporosis, multiple myeloma, or Paget's disease); osteosclerosis; exostoses of spine and genuvalgum; excess ingestion from swallowing fluoridated toothpaste *Toxicity:* peculiar taste with salivation and thirst (salty-soapy), hemorrhagic gastroenteritis; hypoglycemia; CNS depression; renal failure *Lethal dose:* 50–500 mg/kg body weight
IODINE (I) (plasma) RR: 2–4 μg/dl	*Decrease:* simple, edemic, colloid, or euthyroid goiter; endemic cretinism (neurologic and/or

Substance Tested (Specimen Needed, Reference Range [RR], and Critical Range [CR])	***Clinical Significance of Values***
60–ng/ml Deficiency: IDD (iodine deficiency disorders)	myxedematous); (fetus) abortions, stillbirths, congenital anomalies; (child/teen) impaired mental function, retarded physical development; (adult) hypo- or hyperthyroidism, impaired mental function

IDD Severity	***(daily urine)***	***(median urine)***
RR: mild	50—100 μg/d	3.5–5 μg/dl
moderate	25–49 μg/d	2–3.4 μg/dl
severe	<25 μg/d	0–1.9 μg/dl

	Increase: prolonged excessive intake of iodine leading to iodide-goiter and myxedema (common with preexisting Hashimoto's thyroiditis); excessive consumption of seaweed, kelp supplements; high dietary intake of known goitrogens (rutabagas, turnips, cabbages); hypothyroidism in autoimmune thyroid diseases, inhibition of thionamide drugs; dysgeusias; acnelike skin lesions *Toxicity:* mucous membranes stained brown; burning pain in mouth and esophagus, laryngeal edema; shock, nephritis, circulatory collapse *Lethal dose:* 5–50 mg/kg body weight
IRON (FE) (serum, 5 ml, shows diurnal) variation—higher in AM) RR: 50–150 μg/dl (higher in males) 9.0–26.9 μmol/L CR: >400–500 mg/dl at 3–6 hr (urine, 24 hr) RR: 100–300 μg/dl Iron deficiency anemia (IDA) Transferrin <16 μg/L Ferritin <12 μg/L Red cell distribution width >15 Mean corpuscular value (MCV) <100 Concern: Ingestion of elemental iron >40–70 mg/kg body weight	*Decrease:* iron deficiency anemia: inadequate diet, (grossly iron deficient, high in cereals, low in animal protein and vitamin C); koilonychia (spoon-shaped nails); excessive menstrual loss; pregnancy, lactation; blood donors; premature infants; intestinal helmenthiasis (esp. hookworm disease); malabsorption syndromes, chronic diarrhea, gastrectomy, patients with atrophic gastritis and achlorhydia, occult GI bleeds; hereditary hemorrhagic telangiectasia; Turner's syndrome; angiodysplasia (vascular ectasis or arteriovenous anomaly; blue rubber bleb nevi (hereditary cutaneous hemangiomas); Menetrier's disease; Zollinger-Ellison syndrome, pseudo Zollinger-Ellison syndrome, (hypersecretion of gastric HCl); drugs (aspirin; aspirin and ethanol), adrenocorticosteroids or nonsteroidal anti-inflammatory agents; sports anemia; Patterson-Kelly (Plummer-Vinson) syndrome

(continued)

Substance Tested (Specimen Needed, Reference Range [RR], and Critical Range [CR])	***Clinical Significance of Values***
	Factitial iron deficiency anemia (aka, Lasthenie de Ferjol syndrome—self-induced blood letting) (Transferrin) severe protein–energy malnutrition—PEM; iron sequestration (idiopathic pulmonary hemosiderosis, paroxysmal nocturnal hemoglobinuria, chronic disease with inability to metabolize iron from reticuloendothelial cell deposits, congenital atransferrinemia [rare]) Vitamin A deficiency—lack in developmental periods causes deficits in neural functioning and behavior *Increase:* diets: high in heme iron or high in promoters of nonheme iron absorption Excessive iron absorption: hereditary hemochromatosis (African or "Bantu" siderosis); prolonged therapeutic administration of iron to subjects not iron deficient; chronic alcoholism or liver disease, pancreatic insufficiency potential; "shunt hemochromatosis"; severe anemia with ineffective erythropoiesis and increased hemolysis; diabetes in 80% of patients Transfusional hemosiderosis: β-Thalassemia major, some chronic sideroblastic anemias, hypoplastic or other refractory anemias Other: cancers (primary hepatic carcinoma, acute leukemia, early breast cancer); demyelinating disease, Alzheimer's disease; increased risk of CHD; listeriosis
MANGANESE (MN) (plasma) RR: 0.6–2 ng/ml 1–2 μg/dl (urine) RR: 0–0.3 μg/dl	*Decrease:* high in nonheme iron; certain types of epilepsy; impaired bone metabolism, weak boned in association with low concentrations of copper and zinc; possibly in alcohol abuse *Increase:* chronic inhalation of airborne manganese (mines, steel mills, chemical industries), "manganic madness," permanent crippling neurologic disorder of the extrapyramidal system (similar to lesions in Parkinson's disease)
MOLYBDENUM (MO) (plasma) RR: 1.3 μg/dl (blood—mainly within red cells) RR: 2–6 ng/ml	*Decrease:* sulfite oxidase deficiency (lethal inborn error of metabolism deranges cysteine metabolism; TPN prolonged ("acquired molybdenum deficiency"); interference with copper metabolism

Substance Tested (Specimen Needed, Reference Range [RR], and Critical Range [CR])	***Clinical Significance of Values***
	Increase: massive ingestion of tungsten (W); occupational and high dietary intake (elevated uric acid blood concentration, gout); sulfur amino acid toxicity; growth depression and anemia similar to copper deficiency
SELENIUM (SE) (component of the enzyme glutathione peroxidase, isolated from human red blood cells) (plasma) RR: 100–300 ng/ml	*Decrease:* Keshan disease (endemic cardiomyopathy); Kashin-Beck disease (endemic osteoarthritis); parenteral nutrition; decreased dietary intake owing to low soil concentrations (New Zealand, China) aspermatogenesis, TPN (cardiomyopathy), Duchenne muscular dystrophy, cataracts, tumor development *Increase:* endemic selenosis; nail and hair loss; increased dietary intake owing to high soil concentrations (North Dakota, USA, China, Venezuela), excessive intake from "health store" tablets (skin lesions, polyneuritis)
ZINC (ZN) (plasma) RR: 1000 ng/ml, 0.7–1.25 μg/ml (serum) RR: 55–150 μg/ml (decreases with aging), 11–18 μ*M* (urine, 24 hr) RR: 6–9 μ*M*	*Decrease:* decreased intake (chronic alcholics and vegetarians, young women with anorexia nervosa); decreased circulatory and splenic T lymphocytes; prolonged bed rest; decrease in absorption of tetracycline; rheumatic diseases; infection; growth retardation; male hypogonadism and hypospermism; nyctalopia (night blindness); hypogeusia; impaired wound healing, TPN without zinc supplement; acrodermatitis enteropathica (AE); dwarfism (Iran); parasitism (Egypt); compromised immune function; low facteur thymique serique (FTS); impaired embryogenesis; behavioral disturbances (impaired hedonic tone) *Increase:* zinc therapy for Wilson's disease; ingestion of food or beverage contaminated by storage in a galvanized container; long-term ingestion of excessive zinc supplements >150 mg/day (secondary copper deficiency), low serum HDL, gastric erosion, depressed immune system; lethargy in dialysis patients; hyperzincuria increasing with the severity of diabetes; inhalation of zinc oxide fumes causing neurologic damage (metal fume fever, brass-founders' ague, zinc shakes)

(continued)

Substance Tested (Specimen Needed, Reference Range [RR], and Critical Range [CR])	***Clinical Significance of Values***
	Lethal dose: IV administration of 1.5 g over a 3-day period; zinc salts 50–500 mg/kg body weight.
ULTRATRACE ELEMENTS	
ARSENIC (AS)	
(whole blood) RR: 10–64 μg/dl (plasma) RR: 4–6 μg/ml	*Increase:* dermatoses (hyperpigmentation, hyperkeratosis, desquamation and hair loss), hematopoeitic depression, liver damage characterized by jaundice, peripheral neuropathy *Toxicity:* metallic taste and odor of garlic on breath, burning pain in GI tract, shock syndrome, bloody diarrhea *Lethal dose:* 5–50 mg/kg body weight arsenic trioxide (As/kg body weight) 0.35–0.91 μmol 70–180 mg 10.2–26 nmol 0.76–1.95 mg
BORON (BO)	
(blood, 4 ml serum) RR: 1 mg/dl CR: 10–20 mg/dl (plasma) RR: 200 ng/ml (urine, 24 hr/5 ml) RR: 0.3/dl	*Decrease:* increase in total plasma calcium concentrations and urinary excretions of calcium and magnesium; decreased serum concentrations of 17β-estradiol, testosterone and iodized calcium, depressed mental alertness *Increase:* ingestion of boric acid, borate salts (antiseptic, detergent, water softener); unexpected absorption of boric acid from diapers *Toxicity:* riboflavinuria; lethargy; GI symptoms, bright, red rash *NOTE:* infant pacifiers dipped in a borax preparation and honey; reports of scanty hair; patchy, dry erythema; anemia; seizure disorders *Lethal dose (adults):* boric acid or borate salts 50–500 mg/kg body weight
BROMINE (BR) BROMIDE	
(serum) RR: 1000–2000 μg/ml (plasma) RR: 3500 ng/dl	*Decrease:* recent findings support incidence of depressed growth, conception rate, milk fat production and hemoglobin; CNS depressants *Increase:* prolonged use/exposure to bromides in medicine/photography; bromide acne; neurologic disturbances; increased spinal fluid pressure *Toxicity:* bromism or brominism *Lethal dose:* 500–5000 mg/kg body weight

Substance Tested (Specimen Needed, Reference Range [RR], and Critical Range [CR])	Clinical Significance of Values
CADMIUM (CD)	
(blood) RR: 0–5 ng/ml (plasma) RR: 0.1–0.7 μg/dl	*Increase:* (tissue) in prostatic and renal cancer; (urine) in hypertension, industrial exposure: (electroplating, atomic reactors, zinc ores, cadmium solder); (blood) poisoning from foods prepared in cadmium-lined vessels, inhaling of cadmium dust and fumes, softened drinking water, foods grown in soil heavily fertilized with superphosphate *Toxicity:* severe gastroenteritis, mild liver damage, acute renal failure; pulmonary edema; cough; ducklike gait; brown urine *Lethal dose:* several hundred mg/kg body weight
LEAD (PB)	
(blood, 2 ml, collect with oxalate-fluoride mixture) RR: 50 μg/dl or less up to 2.4 μmol/L RR: (children) <10 μg/dl (plasma) RR: 1–8 ng/ml (urine, 24 hr) RR: 0.08 μg/ml 120 μg or less per day	*Decrease:* depressed growth, altered iron metabolism *Increase:* (children) irreversible cognitive deficits, acute encephalopathy; (adults) progressive, irreversible renal disease; toxic psychosis from inhalation of tetraethyl or tetramethyllead (children and adults) hypochromic-microcytic anemia *Lead sources:* ingested or inhaled leaded paint (chips, renovation dust); contaminated soil; contaminated water (lead pipes, lead solder on copper pipes, softened water); retention of a lead object in the stomach or joint (shot, curtain weight, fishing weight, bauble); contaminated acidic foods and beverages (storage in lead-glazed ceramics, leaded crystal, galvanized or nonstainless steel pots); inhalation (burning leadpainted wood or battery casings in home fireplaces/stoves); leaded gas fumes; occupational exposure *Lethal dose:* 30 g/kg body weight

Classification System of Poisoning (Plumbism)*

Class	*Risk*	*(whole, blood, PbB)*
1	Mild	PbB 10–19 μg/dl; FEP <35 μg/dl PbB 20–24 μg/dl; FEP 35–220 μg/dl iron deficiency
2	Moderate	PbB 25–44 μg/dl; FEP <35 μg/dl minimal PbB burden; FEP 35–220 μg/dl; excess PbB burden

(continued)

Classification System of Poisoning (Plumbism)*

3	High	PbB 45–69 µg/dl; FEP <35 µg/dl; never seen; FEP 35–220 µg/dl; marked PbB burden
4	Urgent	Asymptomatic; PbB 70–100 µg/dl and/or FEP >250 µg/dl; PbB toxicity
5	Encephalopathy or impending encephalopathy	Any symptomatic patient or PbB >100 µg/dl

*Adapted from *The Merck Manual*, 16th ed.

Substance Tested (Specimen Needed, Reference Range [RR], and Critical Range [CR])	***Clinical Significance of Values***
LITHIUM (LI)	
(serum)` RR: 0.0055 µg/ml (plasma) RR: 11 ng/ml Therapeutic range (serum) RR: 1 ml or 5.5 µg/ml (plasma) RR; 0.7–2.0 mEq/L (serum) ÇR: >2 mEq/L >2 mmol/L	*Decrease:* high dietary caffeine and/or sodium intake *Increase:* therapy for bipolar disorder; diabetes insipidus; renal failure, weight gain; diminished taste perception; high "hard water" levels
NICKEL (NI)	
(plasma) RR: 2–4 µg/dl 0.2–2 ng/ml (sweat) RR: High nickel content	*Decrease:* lack in diet, depressed iron absorption *Increase:* consistent in alcoholic liver disease; nickel dermatitis; inhalation of nickel carbonyl (promotes lung cancer)
SILICON (SI)	
silicic acid (H_2SiO_3) (plasma) RR: 500 µg/dl	*Decrease:* proposed detrimental effects on brain and bone defects in connective tissue metabolism, diet low in liver (atherosclerosis development) *Increase:* long-term antacid therapy (magnesium trisilicate); siliceous renal calculi
TIN (SN)	
(plasma) RR: 23 ng/ml	*Increase:* diets high in canned fruits and juices; zinc balance negatively affected at 50 mg intakes, industrial exposure to organic tin compounds and dust

Substance Tested (Specimen Needed, Reference Range [RR], and Critical Range [CR])	***Clinical Significance of Values***
VANADIUM (V) (plasma) RR: 0.5–2.3 μg/dl 5 ng/ml	*Increase:* occupational inhalation (fuel combustion for electricity) hemorrhagic endotheliotoxic with leukocytotactic and hematotoxic components *Toxicity:* industrial processes (sore eyes and bronchi), dermatitis, depletion of ascorbic acid (lowers vanadium toxicity); daily intake of 196 mmol (10 mg) vanadium
MINERAL ELEMENTS FOUND IN THE BODY WITHOUT AN ASSIGNED METABOLIC ROLE	
ALUMINUM (AL) (serum) RR: 0–6 ng/ml <40 ng/ml dialysis patients (24 hr urine) RR: 0–32 ng/d	*Increase:* aluminum absorption with citrate-containing drugs (effervescent or dispersible analgesics), use of aluminum-containing astringents, hydroxide gels (antacids), or aluminum-containing phosphate binders; excessive occupational exposure *Toxicity:* aluminosis (lung disease), aluminum-induced encephalopathy, hypophosphatemia, dialysis dementia, iron-resistant microcytic anemia, aluminum-related osteomalacia *NOTE:* Aluminum is a neurotoxin. The primary symptom is motor dysfunction leading to dysarthria, myoclonus, or epilepsy. Aluminum toxicity is not related to Alzheimer's disease. Aluminum can be found in laboratory solutions used with tissue samples and in laboratory dust. New testing methods are being adopted to rule out contamination.
ANTIMONY (SB) (stibium) (urine: 24 hr/dl RR: <50 μ/L CR: >1 mg/L (plasma)	*Increase:* excessive occupational exposure (ore mining, bronze, ceramics), ingested compounds (stibophen, tartar enemic) *Toxicity:* acrid metallic taste, burning GI pain (as in arsenic poisoning), throat constriction, dysphagia, pulmonary edema, liver and renal failure *Lethal dose:* 5–50 mg/kg body weight
BERYLLIUM (BE) (urine, 24 hr) RR: 0.05 μg/d CR: >20 μg/L or 2.22 μmol/L	*Increase:* acute beryllium disease: (a chemical pneumonitis) occupational exposure; modern—aerospace industry; historical—beryllium

(continued)

Substance Tested (Specimen Needed, Reference Range [RR], and Critical Range [CR])	***Clinical Significance of Values***
RR: 2 ng/ml	mining, electronics, chemical plants, manufacture of fluorescent lights (inhalation, introduction into or under skin and/or conjunctiva) (berylliosis or granulomatosis) *NOTE:* Almost impossible to distinguish from sarcoidosis.
BISMUTH (BI)	
(urine, 24 hr) RR: <20 µg/L <95.7 nmol/L (plasma) RR: <1.0 µg/dl <47.9 mmol/L	*Increase:* bismuth used as a treatment for syphilis in the growing child when the mother has been treated during pregnancy; treatment of peptic ulcer with bismuth-containing preparations (Zolimidine, colloidal bismuth subcitrate); bismuth subcarbonate, subgallate, and subnitrate compounds (used as antiseptics, astringents, sedatives, and to treat diarrhea and inflamed skin) *Toxicity:* ulcerative stomatitis, anorexia, headache, rash, renal tubular damage, bluish line at gum margin, albuminuria; resembles lead poisoning, without the blood changes and paralysis
CYANIDE (CN RADICAL)	
(blood [5 ml]) RR: 0.004 mg/L or 0.15 µmol/L (nonsmokers) CR: >0.1 mg/L or >3.84 µmol/L	*Increase:* industrial exposure (pesticides, metallurgy); inhalation of hydrocyonic acid and fumes from burning nitrogen-containing products; ingestion of salts and latrile (derived from seeds of apricots, peaches, jetberry bush, toyon, bitter almonds, and some apple seeds) *Toxicity:* lethal dose <5 mg/kg body weight (small child) fatal dose = 5–25 seeds Death within 5 minutes of ingestion/inhalation
GOLD (AU)	
(colloidal gold in cerebrospinal fluid; CSF) RR: minute amount (serum) RR: 0–0.1 mg/L RR: Therapeutic 1.0–2.0 mg/L	*Increase:* rheumatoid arthritis if gold sodium thiomalate or gold thioglucose (aurothioglucose) is given parenterally; oral gold compound *Toxicity:* pruritus, dermatitis, stomatitis, albuminuria with or without nephrotic syndrome, agranulocytosis, thrombocytopenic purpura, and aplastic anemia
SILVER (AG)	
(serum—metal-free container) RR: 0.21 + 0.15 ng/dl 19.47 + 13.90 nmol/l	*Increase:* chemical conjunctivitis secondary to silver nitrate; gastroenteritis; (dose by mouth) grayish discoloration of mucous membranes;

Substance Tested (Specimen Needed, Reference Range [RR], and Critical Range [CR])	***Clinical Significance of Values***
	argyria (bluish gray skin discoloration from nose/eye drops over time or industrial exposure; Silvadene topically for burns; silver picrate (antiseptic) *Lethal dose:* 3.5–35 g total dose
THALLIUM (T1) (blood—metal-free container) RR: 0.5 μg/dl or 24.5 nmol/L CR: 10–800 μg/dl or 0.5–39.1 μmol/L (urine—metal-free container) RR: <2.0 μg/L or <9.78 nmol/L CR: 1.0–2.0 mg/L or 4.9–97.8 μmol/L	*Increase:* formerly used in ant, rat, roach poison *Toxicity:* thallitoxicosis or thallotoxicosis (ingestion of pesticides); hair loss, delerium, coma, paralysis, death *Lethal dose:* 5–50 mg

FEP = "free" erythrocyte protoporphyrin

APPENDIX VI

Vitamins in Human Nutrition

FAT-SOLUBLE

Vitamin A
Vitamin D
Vitamin E
Vitamin K

WATER-SOLUBLE

Ascorbic acid (vitamin C)
Biotin
Cobalamin (vitamin B_{12})
Folate (folic acid)
Niacin
Pyridoxine (vitamin B_6)
Riboflavin (vitamin B_2)
Thiamin (vitamin B_1)

Frances Fischbach: A MANUAL OF LABORATORY & DIAGNOSTIC TESTS, Fifth Edition.

APPENDIX VII

Table of Vitamins

Reference Range (RR) and Critical Range (CR)	*Clinical Significance of Values*	
	Increase	*Decrease*
FAT-SOLUBLE VITAMINS		
Vitamin A		
Retinol (serum) RR: 20–50 μg/dl 0.70–1.75 μmol/L CR: <10 μg/dl or <0.35 μmol/L indicates severe deficiency >100–2000 μg/dl (hypervitaminosis A) Carotene (serum) RR: 0.8–4.0 μg/ml or 1.5–7.4 μmol/L CR: >250 μg/dl indicates carotenemia	Activation of phagocytes and/or cytotoxic T cells Alopecia Amennorhea Arthralgia (gout) Birth defects Carotenodermia/aurantiasis Cheilosis Chronic nephritis Corticol hyperostoses Excessive dietary or supplement intake Hepatosplenomegaly Hypercholesterolemia Hyperlipemia Peeling of skin Permanent learning disabilities Pregnancy Premature epiphyseal closure Pseudotumor cerebri Spontaneous abortions	Acute infections Arthralgia (gout) Bile duct obstruction Bitot's spots Celiac disease Cirrhosis of the liver Congenital obstruction of the jejunum Cystic fibrosis Duodenal bypass Fat malabsorption syndrome Giardiasis Immunity compromised (cell-mediated responses and antibody response) Insufficient dietary intake Keratinization of lung, GI tract, and urinary epithelia Keratomalacia Measles Nyctalopia (night blindness) Oral contraceptives (carotene) Pancreatic surgery Protein–energy malnutrition, PEM (marasmus or kwashiorkor) Perifollicular hyperkeratosis (Darier's disease) Sprue Xerophthalmia Xerosis of the conjunctiva and cornea

(continued)

Reference Range (RR) and Critical Range (CR)	Clinical Significance of Values: Increase	Decrease
Vitamin D		
1,25 DHCC; calcitrol (serum) RR: 25–40 ng/ml for 25-(OH)D_3 20–45 pg/ml for 1,25-$(OH)_2D_3$ CR: Serum calcium levels of 12–16 mg/dl (vitamin D toxicity)	GI symptoms (anorexia, nausea, vomiting, constipation) Infants "Elfin facies," hypercalcemia with failure to thrive, mental retardation, stenosis of the aorta Metastatic extraosseous calcification Renal colic Supplements Williams' syndrome	Anticonvulsants Familial hypophosphatemic rickets, (diabetes mellitus, Falconi's syndrome, hypoparathyroidism, renal osteodystrophy, renal tubular acidosis) High phosphate or phytate intake Inadequate diet Inadequate exposure to sunlight (esp. elderly) Liver disease Malabsorption syndromes Osteomalacia (adults) Rachitic tetany Rickets (children)
Vitamin E*		
Tocopherol; TE (most active) RR: Plasma 0.8–1.2 mg/dl Deficiency: (plasma) <0.8 mg/dl (adults) <0.4 mg/dl (children) (serum) RR: 8.0–16.0 µg/ml (ratio of serum tocopherol/total lipid) Deficiency: ratio under 0.8 mg/g	LBW infants (sepsis, necrotizing enterocolitis) Vitamin E supplementation Increased bleeding tendency Impaired leukocyte formation Reduced cataract formation (with high beta-carotene and ascorbic acid levels)	Biliary atresia Ceroid deposits in muscle Cholestasis Dermatitis (flaky) Edema Malabsorption syndromes with steatorrhea Neurologic syndromes affecting the spinal cord, posterior columns and the retina (abeta- or hyperlipoproteinemia), blind loop syndrome, chronic pancreatitis, cystic fibrosis, inborn errors of metabolism, obstructive liver disease, short bowel syndrome) Premature infants (bronchopulmonary dysplasia, intraventricular hemorrhage, platelet dysfunction, retinopathy) Protein–energy malnourished children (PEM) Reperfusion injury

Reference Range (RR) and Critical Range	***Clinical Significance of Values***	
	Increase	***Decrease***
Vitamin K		
Phylloquinone (K^1)—plants; menaquinone (K_2 series) bacterial; menadione (K_3) synthetic RR: PIVKA 11 test (proteins induced in vitamin K absence). This test is superior. Plasma prothrombin concentration 80–120 μg/ml	G6PD deficiency Increased dietary intake or administered vitamin K preparation LBW infants (increased menadione) Anemia with Heinz bodies Hyperbilirubinemia Kernicterus (bilirubin encephalopathy) Loss of sucking reflex Postkernicterus syndrome	Breastfed infants (no vitamin K received) Conditions limiting absorption or synthesis of vitamin K Coumarin (warfarin) Excessive oral mineral oil Hypoprothrombinemia Lack of diet Lack of bile salts (external biliary fistulas, obstructive jaundice) Liver disease Nonabsorbable sulfonamides Salicylate therapy TPN
WATER-SOLUBLE VITAMINS		
Ascorbic Acid†		
(AA, vitamin C) RR: 28–84 μmol/L plasma 0.4–1.5 mg/dl plasma 114–301 nmol/108 cells (mixed leukocytes) 20–53 μg/108 cells (mixed leukocytes) CR: <11 μmol/L plasma ascorbate <0.2 mg/dl plasma ascorbate <57 nmol/108 cells (mixed leukoytes) <10 mg/108 cells (mixed leukocytes) Females consistently show higher vitamin	Decreased anticoagulant effect of heparin and warfarin (Coumarin) Diarrhea Overabsorption of iron Supplementation (alteration of tests for diabetes and occult blood)	Adult scurvy (acne, listlessness, deep muscle hemorrhages, swan neck hair deformity, gingivitis, perifollicular, hemorrhages and hyperkeratosis) Alcoholism Anemia (microcytic hypochromic) Burns Cold or heat stress Edema, lower extremities Gastric ulcers Impaired iron absorption Inadequate diet (esp. elderly men) Infantile scurvy (Barlow's disease, "pithed frog position") Inflammatory diseases, oxidative damage (proteins, DNA, human sperm DNA)

(continued)

Reference Range (RR) and Critical Range (CR)	Clinical Significance of Values: Increase	Clinical Significance of Values: Decrease
Ascorbic acid (continued) C levels in tissues and fluids than males. Plasma values are the best indicator of recent dietary intake. Leukocyte vitamin C levels are indicative of cellular stores and total body pool		Lactation Petechiae and ecchymoses Pregnancy Risk of cancer (esophagus, oral cavity, uterine, cervix) Smokers (decreased AA half-life) Thyrotoxicosis Toxicity from chemical carcinogens (anthracene, benzpyrene, organochloride pesticides, heavy metals, nitrosamines) Wound healing
Biotin (Plasma) RR: 0.82–2.87 nmol/L CR: <1.02 nmol/L deficiency Prenatal diagnosis of multiple carboxylase deficiency (MCD) by direct analysis of amniotic fluid for methylcitric acid or 3-hydroxyisovaleric acid		Alopecia Anorexia with nausea Antibiotics Biotin-responsive multiple carboxylase deficiency syndromes (MCD) Changes in mental status (depression) Glossitis (magenta hue) High fetal resorption rate Hyperesthesia (algesia) Immunodeficiency Increased serum, cholesterol and bile pigments Ingestion of large amounts (6/d) of *raw* egg white (avidin) Localized paresthesia Maculosquamous dermatitis of the extremities Myalgia Pallor TPN following gut resection

Reference Range (RR) and Critical Range (CR)	***Clinical Significance of Values*** *Increase*	*Decrease*
Cobalamin		
Vitamin B_{12} (Serum, overnight fast) RR: >200 pg/ml, 0.2–1.0 ng/ml CR: <160 pg/ml deficiency Fall in serum holo TCII (Assay of MMA levels, methylmalonyl-CoA-mutase in the liver: functional test, best indicator) (serum MMA) RR: 20–75 ng/ml (urinary MMA) RR: 0.8–3.0 µg/ml	Improved mental function in elderly receiving B_{12} supplements	Alcoholism Addisonian pernicious anemia Thalassemia Diet lacking microorganisms and animal foods (sole B_{12} sources) Distal sensory neuropathy ("glove and stockings") sensory loss Gastrectomy Gastric atrophy (superficial gastritis, hereditary–degenerative) Hypothyroidism Jaundice, mild (lemon yellow tint) Juvenile pernicious anemia (presents age 3–14) Lack of intrinsic factor (hereditary, congenital) Liver disease Pigmentation of skin creases and nailbeds (brownish) Polyendocrinopathy Pregnancy Renal disease Small intestine disorders (cancer, gluten-induced enteropathy–celiac disease, granulomatous lesions, intestinal resections, regional enteritis, "stagnant bowel" syndromes, tropical sprue) Subacute combined degeneration of the cord Tapeworms Tinnitus and noise-induced hearing loss (NIHL) Tongue—red, smooth, shining, painful

(continued)

Reference Range (RR) and Critical Rnge (CR)	***Clnical Significance of Values***	
	Increase	*Decrease*
Cobalamin (continued)		Vegans (and their breast-fed infants)
		Visual loss from optic atrophy
		Weakness
Folate		
(Folic acid)	Folacin; dominant form in serum and RBC	Alcohol, alcoholics
(pteroylglutamate, pteroylglutamic acid, 5-methyltetrahydrofolate)	Loss of seizure control	
	Acute renal failure	Breastfed infants of mothers on estrogen–progesterone contraceptives
(RBC folate: best indicator of status)	Active liver disease	Cervical dysplasia
RR: 200– 640 ng/ml whole blood, corrected to packed cell volume of 45%	RBC hemolysis	Cigarette smoking
	Supplemental folate (400 μg/4 mg/day—side effects	Drug therapy (phenytoin, primidone, barbiturates, cycloserine, azothioprine, oral contraceptives, antacids)
Tissue folate depletion (serum, dietary fluctuations) <160 ng/ml <360 nmol/L		Due to increased requirements
		Hematopoiesis (thalassemia major)
RR: 3–21 ng/ml 11.33–36.25 nmol/L		Increased metabolism
		Infancy
		Malignancy (lymphoproliferative)
CR: <1.5 ng/ml deficiency		Pregnancy
		HPV-16 infection
Negative folate balance: <7 nmol/L <3 ng/ml		Inadequate dietary intake
		Malabsorption syndromes (celiac disease, sprue, blind loop syndrome)
‡Other methods:		Megaloblastosis
Deoxyuridine suppression test (dU or dUST), a functional indicator of folate status; in vitro laboratory test that: (a) defines presence of megaloblastosis; (b) identifies which nutrient de-		Neural tube defects (NTD) (spina bifida, anencephaly)
		Pancytopenia
		Protection from malaria
		Psoriasis
		Renal dialysis
		Scurvy
		Tongue papillae atrophy (shiny, smooth)
		Vitamin B_{12} deficiency

Reference Range (RR) and Critical Range (CR)	***Clinical Significance of Values*** *Increase*	*Decrease*
Folate (continued) ficiency is responsible (folate or vitamin B_{12}) Formimino-glutamic acid (FIGLU)—after histidine loading		Increased mean corpuscular volume (MCV) Depression MTX-treated patients (methotrexate) Hyperhomocysteinemia TPN Rheumatoid arthritis
Niacin Nicotinic acid, niacinamide (urinary *N′*-methylnicatinamide, NMN) CR: <5.8 µmol/d (deficiency) <0.8 mg/d (deficiency)	Abnormal liver function As a hypolipidemic drug Atrial fibrillation Cystoid maculopathy Epigastric discomfort Glucose intolerance Gout, hyperuricemia Hyperglycemia Hypotension Pruritus Smooth, swollen tongue Upper body flushing	Alcoholics Carcinoid syndrome Casal's necklace Cirrhosis of the liver Diarrheal disease Diet lacking in niacin and tryptophan Dyssebacia Hartnup's disease Isoniazid therapy Pellegra dermatosa; glossitis (scarlet, raw beef) GI dysfunction CNS dysfunction Organic psychosis Encephalopathic syndrome
Pyridoxine (Vitamin B_6) RR: *Direct* Plasma pyridoxal 5′-phosphate (PLP) <30 nmol/L Plasma total vitamin B_6 <40 nmol/L Urinary 4-pyridoxic acid (4PA) <3.0 µmol/d (useful short-term index) Urinary total vitamin B_6 <0.5 µmol/d (invalid in persons receiving B_6 an-	Infants: neurologic symptoms and abdominal distress Peripheral neuropathy; progressive sensory ataxia; lower limb impairment	Alcoholism Anemias Asthma Breast cancer Cheilosis Coronary heart disease Depression and confusion Diabetes Drugs (iproniazid, cycloserine, penicillamine, ethinyl, estradiol, mestranol) Glossitis Hodgkin's disease Imparied interleukin-2 production Increased metabolic activity

(continued)

Reference Range (RR) and Critical Range (CR)	Clinical Significance of Values: Increase	Clinical Significance of Values: Decrease
Pyridoxine (continued) tagonists; ie, isoniazid, penicillamine, cycloserine) RR: *Indirect* [§]Erythrocyte alanine transaminase index (EALT/EGPT) >1.25 [‖]Erythrocyte aspartic transaminase index (EAST/EGOT) >1.80 [¶]2g L-tryptophan load; urinary xanthurenic acid >65 μmol/d [#]3g L-methionine load; urinary		Infants (abnormal electroencephalogram pattern, confusions) Irritability Lymphopenia Peripheral neuropathy Premenstrual syndrome (PMS) Seborrheic dermatosis Sickle cell anemia Smokers Stomatitis
Riboflavin (Vitamin B_2) RR: 80–269 μg/g (urine) 24–81 μmol/mol (urine) >40 nmol/dl (erythrocyte) >15 μg/dl (erythrocyte) CR: <30 μg riboflavin per gram creatinine indicates deficiency <27 nmol/dl (erythrocyte) deficient status <10 μg/dl (erythrocyte) deficient status		Alcoholism Angular stomatosis Ariboflavinosis Barbiturate use (long-term) Cheilosis Chronic diarrheas Dyssebacia (shark skin) Inadequate consumption of milk and other animal products Irritable bowel syndrome (IBS) Liver disease Normocytic anemia Nutritional amblyopia Oroaculogenital syndrome

Reference Range (RR) and Critical Range (CR)	***Clinical Significance of Values***	
	Increase	***Decrease***
Riboflavin (continued)		
Erythrocyte glutathion reductase assay (expressed in activity coefficients or AC). Test cannot be used in persons with glucose 6-phosphate deficiency AC <1.2 acceptable AC 1.2–1.4 low AC <1.4 deficient		Perleche (*Candida albicans* infection with cheilosis) Photophobia and lacrimation of eye Tongue (magenta hue) Use of phenothiazine derivative
Flavin adenine dinucleotide (FAD) stimulation test RR: stimulation <20%		
Thiamin		
(Vitamin B_1) RR: 10–64 ng/ml (serum or plasma) 79–178 nmol/L (whole blood) Late changes: <50 μg/d (urine) with elevated blood pyruvate RBC transketolase measurement (most reliable method) Enzyme assays—using TPP (thiamine pyrophosphate) RR: Stimulation of 0–15% Deficiency: Stimulation of >20%	Parenteral dosages	Alcoholism Beriberi Dry beriberi (peripheral neurologic changes; ie, symmetric footdrop) Infantile beriberi Wet beriberi Cardiovascular (high output/CHF, low output Shoshin disease) Wernicke-Korsakoff syndrome (acute hemorrhagic, polioencephalitis) Cerebral beriberi Dependency states (thiamine responsive: megaloblastic anemia, lactic acidosis, ketoaciduria, subacute necrotizing encephalopathy [SNE], Leigh's disease)

(continued)

Reference Range (RR) and Critical Range (CR)	Clinical Significance of Values: Increase	Clinical Significance of Values: Decrease
Thiamin (continued)		Dextrose infusions (frequent, long-continued or highly concentrated) Folate deficiency High-carbohydrate diet (mainly from milled [polished] rice) Hyperthyroidism Impaired absorption (ie, long-term diarrheas) Impaired utilization (ie, severe liver disease) Inadequate kilocalorie intake Increased requirements Fever Lactation Pregnancy Strenuous physical exertion Poor memory Renal dialysis TPN

*Concentration of vitamin E in newborns is less than half that of adults.
†Salivary vitamin C levels are not consistent; urinary vitamin C levels are not useful.
‡Infrequently used.
§EALT is bettern indicatior than EAST, standardized approach needed to compare results.
||Valid, but somewhat outdated indicator of hepatic vitamin B_6 status.
¶Limited data, figures based on three studies.
#24-hour urines, several collected over 1–3 weeks.

APPENDIX VIII

Minerals in Human Nutrition

I. Macronutrients (major minerals)
Essential at levels >100 mg/d
RDA established
Calcium, chloride,* magnesium, phosphorus, potassium,* sodium,* sulfur
Macronutrients are not listed in the table as they are explained in body of the text

II. Micronutrients (trace minerals)
Essential at levels of a few milligrams per day
RDA or ESADDI* established
Chromium,* cobalt,† copper,* fluorine,* iodine, iron, manganese,* molybdenum,* selenium, zinc

III. Micronutrients (ultratrace minerals)
Essential at levels <1 mg/d
No RDA or ESADDI established
Arsenic, boron, bromine, cadmium, lead, lithium, nickel, silicon, tin, vanadium

IV. Mineral elements found in the body without an assigned metabolic role. Aluminum, antimony, beryllium, bismuth, cyanide (an ion that forms salt with minerals), gold, mercury, silver, thallium, plus 20 others

*Estimated minimum requirements established.
†Cobalt is part of the vitamin B_{12} molecule.
RDA: Recommended Dietary Allowances, 1989.
ESADDI: Estimated Safe and Adequate Daily Dietary Intakes.

APPENDIX IX

Universal Precautions

Universal precautions are designed to protect healthcare workers and patients from exposure to blood-borne pathogens and other potentially infectious body substances. They are mandated by the Occupational Safety and Health Administration (OSHA) and include the following.

1. Wear personal protective equipment (aprons, gowns, gloves, goggles, face shields, masks, and CPR devices) when exposure to blood, blood droplets, and other body fluids is anticipated; these precautions are always mandated during invasive procedures.
2. Wear gloves when doing patient care if skin is cut, abraded, or chapped; when collecting or handling specimens or body fluids, cleaning specimen containers, or decontaminating. If contact with mucous membranes, nonintact skin, GI or GU tract, active bleeding wounds, venipuncture, vascular access procedures, or other invasive procedures is anticipated, then universal precautions must be observed.
3. Gowns, aprons, scrubs, or lab coats must cover exposed skin areas when there is a potential for splashing blood or body fluids on clothing; however, this protection is not required for routine care situations in which blood or body substances are not likely to be present. Perform all procedures in such a way such that splashing, spattering, or droplet formation is minimized.
4. Keep mouth-to-mouth emergency resuscitation equipment in strategic locations; make personal mouthpieces available for healthcare workers, since saliva is considered to be potentially infectious (even though it has not been implicated in HIV transmission).
5. Prevent injuries that can be caused by needles, scalpels, and other "sharps." Dispose of all these in puncture-resistant containers. Do not recap, bend, break by hand, or remove needles from disposable syringes. Tape "piggyback" needle devices in place to prevent accidental dislodging.
6. Remove torn or punctured gloves promptly. Thoroughly wash hands and other skin surfaces immediately if contaminated with blood or other body fluids.
7. Place and transport specimens in leak-proof receptacles properly sealed. Decontaminate or label as "biohazard" those fluids and tissues that present a potential problem. Warning labels and tags should contain a "signal work" or symbol (such as "biohazard," "biochemical material") and should be identified as such.

Frances Fischbach: A MANUAL OF LABORATORY & DIAGNOSTIC TESTS, Fifth Edition.

8. Eating, drinking, applying cosmetics or lip balm, and handling contact lenses are not permitted in work areas where there is a reasonable likelihood of exposure to blood or other body substances.
9. Healthcare workers should protect and always take care of themselves first—presume that **all** patients have hepatitis B or HIV. In cases of suspected HIV or hepatitis B (HBV) exposure, identify, obtain consent, and test for exposure if the patient consents to testing. If the patient refuses consent or outcome is positive, the healthcare worker **must** receive HIV antibody testing immediately. Advise HIV-negative person who has been exposed to seek medical evaluation of any acute febrile illness within 12 weeks of exposure to HIV and to retest in 6 to 12 weeks and 6 months after exposure. Some institutions offer prophylactic drug therapy or hepatitis B vaccinations to their employees. If exposed or injured, the healthcare worker must make the decision to accept drug therapy within a few hours of the incident.
10. Meanings of infection-control wordings are defined here.

    Blood-borne pathogens: organisms that can be transmitted from one person to another by exposure to the infected person's blood—the major pathogens include hepatitis B virus, hepatitis C virus, human immunodeficiency virus (HIV; the AIDS virus), and syphilis.

    Body substances: any fluids or solids that come out of or off of the human body—examples are saliva, sputum, urine, feces, wound drainage, and all the fluids referred to as "other potentially infectious materials" (see later).

    Exposure incident: the contact of blood or other body substances with an employee's mucous membranes (eyes, mouth), nonintact skin (skin with cuts, abrasions, dermatitis, or other); or contact by piercing or puncturing mucous membranes or skin with a contaminated item.

    Regulated (infectious) waste: items caked or saturated with blood or other potentially infectious materials; contaminated sharps; pathologic and microbiologic waste.

    Other potentially infectious materials (OPIM): body substances specifically designated by the CDC and OSHA that may transmit blood-borne pathogens include semen, vaginal secretions, cerebrospinal fluid, synovial fluid, pleural fluid, amniotic fluid, saliva in dental procedures, any body substance that is visibly contaminated with blood, and all body substances in situations for which it is difficult or impossible to determine whether blood is present.

INDEX

Page numbers followed by *f* indicate figures; those followed by *t* indicate tabular material.

A

C

D

E

F

G

J

K

L

M

N

O

P

Q

R

S

T

U

V

W

X

Y

Z